Be the Best
MyMAKit

D0568053

Use the registration code below to gain access to this online study companion. This a a single source for all your student resources that support the textbook. By following the registration instructions below you will link to a wealth of opportunities to further your understanding of your course material. Use this web-site in conjunction with your textbook for a multidimensional learning experience. Enjoy!

STEP 1: Register

All you need to get started is a valid email address and the access code below. To register, simply:

1. Go to **www.mymakit.com**.
2. Click "**Students**" under "**First-time users.**"
3. Find the appropriate book cover. Cover must match the textbook edition being used for your class.
4. Click "**Register**" beside your book cover.
5. Read the **License Agreement** and **Private Policy**. If you accept, click "**I Accept**."
6. Leave "**No**" selected under "**Do you have a Pearson account?**"
7. Using a coin scratch off the silver coating below to reveal your access code. Do not use a knife or other sharp object, which can damage the code.
8. Enter your access code in lowercase or uppercase, without the dashes.
9. Follow the on-screen instructions to complete registration.

During registration, you will establish a personal login name and password to use for logging into the Website. You will also be sent a registration confirmation email that contains your login name and password. Be sure to save this email.

Your Access Code is:

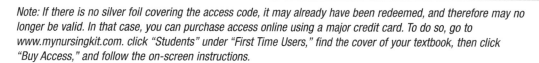

Note: If there is no silver foil covering the access code, it may already have been redeemed, and therefore may no longer be valid. In that case, you can purchase access online using a major credit card. To do so, go to www.mynursingkit.com. click "Students" under "First Time Users," find the cover of your textbook, then click "Buy Access," and follow the on-screen instructions.

STEP 2: Log in

1. Go to **www.mymakit.com** and click "**Students**" under "**Returning Users**."
2. Find the appropriate book cover. Click on "**Login**" next to your book cover.
3. Enter the login name and password that you created during registration. If unsure of this information, refer to your registration confirmation email.
4. Click "**Login**."

Instructors

For premium-level access that includes testing and lecture support materials, please go to **www.mymakit.com** and click Request Access under the Instructors bar. You may also click on the Instructor Registration and Student Handout documents for additional information. For further assistance contact your local Pearson representative or call 800-852-4508

Got technical questions?

Customer Technical Support: To obtain support, please visit us online anytime at http://247pearsoned.custhelp.com where you can search our knowledgebase for common solutions, view product alerts, and review all options for additional assistance.

SITE REQUIREMENTS

For the latest updates on Site Requirements, go to www.mymakit.com. Click "**Students**" under "**Returning Users**". Pick your book and click "**Login**". Click on "**Need help**" at bottom of page for site requirements and other frequently asked questions.

Important: Please read the Subscription and End-User License agreement, accessible from the book website's login page, before using the *mymakit* website. By using the website, you indicate that you have read, understood, and accepted the terms of this agreement.

BRIEF CONTENTS

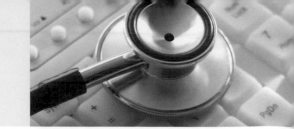

ADMINISTRATIVE
MEDICAL ASSISTING
Foundations and Practices

Christine Malone, MHA

Contributor:
Lorraine M. Papazian-Boyce,
M.S, C.P.C.

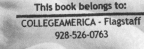
PEARSON

Upper Saddle River, New Jersey 07458

Library of Congress Cataloging-in-Publication Data

Malone, Christine.
  Administrative medical assisting : foundations and practice /
Christine Malone.
    p. ; cm.
  Includes bibliographical references and index.
  ISBN-13: 978-0-13-199932-9
  ISBN-10: 0-13-199932-X
  1. Medical assistants.   I. Title.
  [DNLM: 1. Practice Management, Medical.   2. Allied
Health Personnel.   W 80 M257a 2009]
  R728.8.M278 2009
  610.73´7—dc22
                                                    2008006040

Notice: The authors and the publisher of this volume have taken care that the information and technical recommendations contained herein are based on research and expert consultation, and are accurate and compatible with the standards generally accepted at the time of publication. Nevertheless, as new information becomes available, changes in clinical and technical practices become necessary. The reader is advised to carefully consult manufacturers' instructions and information material for all supplies and equipment before use, and to consult with a healthcare professional as necessary. This advice is especially important when using new supplies or equipment for clinical purposes. The authors and publisher disclaim all responsibility for any liability, loss, injury, or damage incurred as a consequence, directly or indirectly, of the use and application of any of the contents of this volume.

Publisher: Julie Levin Alexander
Publisher's Assistant: Regina Bruno
Executive Editor: Joan Gill
Associate Editor: Bronwen Glowacki
Editorial Assistant: Mary Ellen Ruitenberg
Director of Marketing: Karen Allman
Senior Marketing Manager: Harper Coles
Marketing Specialist: Michael Sirinides
Marketing Assistant: Judy Noh
Development: Triple SSS Press Media Development
Developmental Editor: Alexis Ferraro
Managing Production Editor: Patrick Walsh
Production Liaison: Julie Li
Production Editor: Karen Berry
Senior Media Editor: Amy Peltier

Media Project Manager: Rachel Collett
Manufacturing Manager: Ilene Sanford
Manufacturing Buyer: Pat Brown
Senior Design Coordinator: Maria Guglielmo
Interior Designer: Janice Bielawa
Cover Designer: Anthony Gemmellaro
Manager, Rights and Permissions: Zina Arabia
Manager, Visual Research: Beth Brenzel
Manager, Cover Visual Research and Permissions: Karen Sanatar
Image Permission Coordinator: Ang'john Ferreri
Composition: Laserwords
Printing and Binding: Quebecor World
Cover Printer: Phoenix Color Corporation

Credits and acknowledgments borrowed from other sources and reproduced, with permission, in this textbook appear on the appropriate pages in text.

Pearson® is a registered trademark of Pearson plc

Pearson Education Ltd., London
Pearson Education Singapore, Pte. Ltd
Pearson Education Canada, Inc.
Pearson Education-Japan
Pearson Education Australia PTY, Limited

Pearson Education North Asia, Ltd., Hong Kong
Pearson Educación de Mexico, S.A. de C.V.
Pearson Education Malaysia, Pte. Ltd.
Pearson Education Upper Saddle River, New Jersey

Prentice Hall
is an imprint of

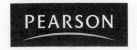

www.pearsonhighered.com

10 9 8 7 6 5 4 3 2 1
ISBN-13: 978-0-13-199932-9
ISBN-10:   0-13-199932-X

Dedication

To my Ian, whose life was a constant battle to improve the healthcare system for those who would come after him.

CONTENTS

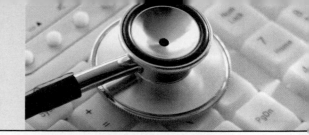

LIST OF PROCEDURES

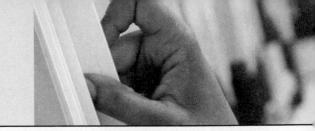

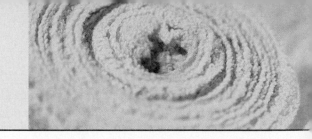

PREFACE

The Development of This Text

I was first inspired to write this textbook after reviewing countless administrative medical assisting textbooks and finding numerous inaccuracies and dated material in those texts. I found myself adopting texts currently available on the market, yet having to supplement the material with numerous handouts and case studies in order to ensure my students were fully competent in the administrative areas. As an instructor who has spent over 20 years in medical office management, I felt a textbook needed to be written by someone with extensive experience in the field of administrative medical office work.

In developing this text, it was my desire to complete a textbook that would fully address the administrative competencies of both the Accrediting Bureau of Health Education Schools (ABHES) and the Commission on Accreditation of Allied Health Education Programs (CAAHEP) for medical assisting programs.

How to Use This Text

The information in this textbook can be used by both ABHES and CAAHEP accredited schools or those schools applying for accreditation. This textbook meets both content and competency requirements in the administrative area.

The material in this text is divided into five sections. Section I is an introduction to the administrative medical assistant profession; Section II delves into the administrative responsibilities of the medical assistant; Section III focuses on responding to emergencies in the medical office; Section IV highlights the area of medical practice finances and the management of the medical office; and Section V outlines career strategies for the medical assistant.

Section I: Introduction to the Administrative Medical Assisting Profession

Section I begins with Chapter 1 and the history of medicine and healthcare, providing the medical assisting student with knowledge of how healthcare began, along with the milestones we've seen along the way. Chapter 2 gives the medical assisting student an overview of the history of medical assisting and a description of the roles and responsibilities of the many allied health professionals who work with medical assistants. Chapter 3 provides detailed coverage of the medical assisting field today, including the varied job duties and career opportunities for the professional medical office assistant. Chapter 3 also details many of the members of the healthcare team, such as physicians, nurses, and pharmacists, and outlines their duties and educational requirements. Chapter 4

provides the student with an understanding of medical law and ethics from the medical assistant's point of view. This chapter begins with an overview of the American legal system and works through medical malpractice, HIPAA legislation, and mandatory reporting requirements. Chapter 5 focuses on interpersonal communication skills for the medical assistant. This chapter highlights areas such as nonverbal communication, and communicating with patients who may present special challenges, such as the hearing impaired, or communicating with patients via interpreters. Section I ends with Chapter 6 on written communications. This chapter relays information on writing professional correspondence, how to chart in the patient's medical chart, how to correct errors in charting, and using email in a professional manner to communicate with patients.

Section II: Administrative Responsibilities of the Medical Assistant

Section II begins with Chapter 7 on telephone procedures. This chapter covers this topic in depth, including how to call in prescriptions and refill requests, taking emergency telephone calls, and documenting calls from patients. Chapter 8 focuses on the front desk and reception duties. This chapter covers how to prepare patient files, escorting patients, and maintaining the reception room in the medical office. Chapter 9 outlines patient appointment scheduling and includes information on both manual and computerized scheduling, scheduling patients for in- and outpatient procedures, and managing the physician's professional schedule. Chapter 10 works through medical records management from the various forms of charting (SOAP, POMR, etc.) to using flow charts, abbreviations, and charting patient communication. This chapter focuses on managing paper medical records, including filing systems. Chapter 10 also includes information on correcting errors in the medical chart and the legalities of retaining patient medical records. Chapter 11 presents information on electronic medical records and conducting research with medical records. This chapter includes information on converting paper medical records to electronic format, as well as how HIPAA legislation pertains to electronic medical records. Chapter 12 focuses on computers in the medical office. This chapter begins with the basics of computer anatomy and discusses the use of Internet search engines and personal digital assistants. Chapter 13 highlights the area of equipment, maintenance, and supply inventory in the medical office. This chapter presents an in-depth look at working with medical equipment, documenting maintenance of equipment, and all aspects of inventorying, ordering, and stocking supplies. Chapter 14 outlines the need for office policies and procedures, including instructions on writing office policies, how to write a mission statement, as well as creating a personnel manual. This chapter gives information regarding documentation of infection control procedures as well as creating a quality improvement and risk management procedure manual.

Section III: Responding to Emergencies in the Medical Office

Section III includes Chapter 15: Handling Medical Office Emergencies. This chapter presents the student with information on how to prevent accidents and injuries in the medical office. It presents the competencies medical assistants must have when performing life-saving procedures such as adult rescue breathing, cardiopulmonary resuscitation, and aiding patients in shock. It also presents information on the medical assistant's role in emergency preparedness and developing an environmental exposure plan.

Section IV: Medical Practice Finances and Management of the Medical Office

Section IV begins with Chapter 16: Insurance Billing and Authorizations. This chapter is an up-to-date and accurate view of how insurance billing and authorizations are handled in the medical office. The chapter covers topics from health insurance plans to all aspects of Medicare and Medicaid coverage, to filling out insurance billing forms. Chapter 16 also includes information on the use of COBRA coverage, flexible spending accounts, and health savings accounts. Chapter 17 provides the specifics of ICD-9-CM diagnostic coding. This chapter presents instructions for using the ICD-9-CM coding book and its various volumes, and educates students on how to avoid fraud in medical coding. Chapter 18: Procedural Coding describes the layout of the CPT coding book; provides steps for accurate CPT coding, including determining correct codes; and explains the relationship between accurate documentation and reimbursement. This chapter includes in-depth coverage of the use of modifiers in proper coding as well as the steps to follow to determine the proper evaluation and management (E&M) code. Chapter 19 focuses on billing, collections and credit. This chapter discusses the use of manual billing systems (pegboard) as well as computerized systems, and includes coverage of how to discuss fees with patients and collecting on patient accounts. Chapter 19 ends with a discussion of the use of collection agencies and small claims court. Chapter 20 focuses on payroll, accounts payable, and banking procedures. In this chapter, students are introduced to handling payroll in the medical office, reconciling bank statements, paying office invoices, and working with petty cash. Chapter 21 discusses the role of the medical office manager, including how to conduct an effective staff meeting, how to conduct interviews, and how to perform employee evaluations. Chapter 21 also discusses the topic of risk management in the medical office, including filing an incident report and ensuring employee safety.

Section V: Career Strategies for the Medical Assistant

Section V consists of Chapter 22: Competing in the Job Market. This chapter presents invaluable information on writing an effective resume and cover letter, preparing for an interview, and followup after an interview.

Pedagogical Features in This Textbook

The following special features appear throughout the text:

Learning Objectives: Specific learning objectives appear at the beginning of each chapter, stating what is to be achieved upon successful completion of the chapter.

Medical Assisting Competencies: Each chapter includes a list of CAAHEP entry-level competencies for CMAs and ABHES entry-level competencies for RMAs.

Competency Skills Performance: This feature lists all of the procedures presented in the chapter.

Key Terminology and Abbreviations: Terms and their definitions appear at the beginning of each chapter as well as in the narrative and the comprehensive glossary.

Case Study: A thought-provoking case study is presented at the beginning of each chapter, with critical thinking questions interspersed throughout the chapter. Students must rely on the content in the text and their own critical thinking skills to answer the questions.

Keys to Success: Each chapter contains brief, helpful tips containing practice advice for succeeding in the healthcare setting.

Informational Charts and Tables: Informative charts and tables appear throughout the text and summarize pertinent information for the reader. They provide students with visuals and comparisons to reinforce the lesson.

Color Photos: Color photos help to illustrate and reinforce the concepts presented in the text.

HIPAA Compliance Boxes: This feature contains helpful advice on how to apply the concepts presented in the text to create a HIPAA-compliant atmosphere in the healthcare setting.

In-Practice Boxes: These real-world scenarios with critical thinking questions present opportunities for readers to think about and apply the concepts presented in the text.

Procedures: For each competency, theory and rationale are discussed, required materials are listed, and the procedure is presented in the proper format with the task, conditions, and standards (time limits, required accuracy, or necessary achievement).

Concept Link: This visual aid provides a link to concepts presented in earlier or later chapters.

Chapter Summary: The chapter summary is an excellent review of the chapter content, often used for certification exams.

Chapter Review Questions: End-of-chapter questions are provided in multiple-choice, true/false, short answer, and research format, and help reinforce learning. The review questions measure the students' understanding of the material presented in the chapter. These tools are available for use by the student or by the instructor as an outcomes assessment.

Externship Application: This feature places the student in an externship site with a simulated situation the student may encounter.

Chapter Resources: This listing provides additional resources for the reader to consult for further information on the topics contained within the chapter.

Med Media: This link to the supplementary material available on the student CD describes the CD content as it relates to each chapter of the core student textbook.

ABOUT THE AUTHOR

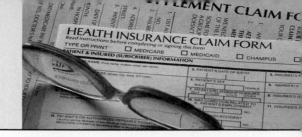

Christine Malone, B.S., M.H.A., studied management practice and theory at Henry Cogswell College, receiving her B.S. in Professional Management. She continued her education at the University of Washington, obtaining her Master's Degree in Health Administration. Christine is currently working toward her Ph.D. in Business Administration with a healthcare focus.

Christine has over 20 years' experience in the healthcare field, having spent time working as a dental assistant, a medical receptionist, an X-ray technician, medical clinic director, and as a consultant to healthcare providers, focusing on strategic management, efficient office flow, and human resource management. Since 2004, Christine has been teaching within the Health Professions Department at Everett Community College in Washington State. There she teaches Medical Office Management, Computer Applications in the Medical Office, Medical Practice Finances, Intercultural Communications in Healthcare, and Medical Law and Ethics. In 2006 Christine researched and developed a certificate program in Healthcare Risk Management. This series of three courses is offered via distance learning and provides the student who successfully completes the three courses a Certificate in Healthcare Risk Management.

Christine was elected to the Snohomish County Charter Review Commission, a one-year position from 2005–2006.

She is the cochair of the Young Careerists Group within the Business and Professional Women's Association of Greater Everett, a member of the American College of Healthcare Executives (ACHE), a member of the Washington State Healthcare Executive Forum (WSHEF), a member of the American Society for Healthcare Risk Management (ASHRM), a member of the American College of Medical Practice Executives (ACMPE), and is active in healthcare politics on both a local and national level. Christine has been the guest speaker at various events on healthcare issues and in continuing education meetings across Washington State and has received her certification in vocational teaching as well as in pediatric palliative care training.

Christine and her husband have five children and live in a 100-year-old home in Everett, Washington. In 1999, their third child, Ian, was injured due to medical negligence during his birth. Ian lived four and a half years before succumbing to his injuries in 2004. This was the genesis of Christine's work toward improving patient safety in healthcare. Her input has been sought by legislative committees, editorial boards, and many policymakers. A nationally recognized healthcare reform advocate, Christine has appeared on the *Today Show, NBC Nightly News, ABC Nightly News*, the CBC's *The National*, in *The New York Times, The Los Angeles Times*, and on *Salon.com*.

ACKNOWLEDGMENTS

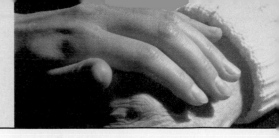

The author would like to extend a thank-you to Editor Joan Gill and to Alexis Breen Ferraro, Developmental Editor, for her experienced management and oversight of this project.

I would also like to extend a warm thank-you to the staff of the Kaanapali Beach Hotel in Maui, where much of the original draft was written. In addition, I'd like to thank my husband Dylan and children Corey, Mallory, Molly and Riley—thank you for your patience while this project was completed.

Last, but far from least, thank you to my colleagues at Everett Community College—Beth Adolphsen, CMA (AAMA); Karla Pouillon, RN, MEd; Julie Reiman, CMA (AAMA); and Francie Mooney, CMA (AAMA). You have not only welcomed me into your midst, you have been immensely helpful in showing me the wonderful world of educating such a valuable member of the healthcare team—the medical assistant.

Reviewers

The author and publisher wish to thank the following reviewers, all of whom provided valuable feedback and helped to shape the final text:

Michaelann M. Allen, M.A. Ed., C.M.A. (AAMA)
Medical Assisting Program Coordinator/Instructor
North Seattle Community College
Seattle, WA

Kristen Anderson, R.N./B.S.N.
MA Instructor
Southwest Wisconsin Technical College
Fennimore, WI

Vanessa Armor
Instructor, Medical Assisting
Ivy Tech Community College of Indiana
Gary, IN

Jennifer L. Barr, M.T., M.Ed., C.M.A. (AAMA)
Chairperson, Medical Assistant Technology
Sinclair Community College
Dayton, OH

Kay E. Biggs, B.S., C.M.A. (AAMA)
Coordinator, Advisor Medical Assisting Technology
Columbus State Community College
Gahanna, OH

Jeannie Bower, B.S.
Instructor, Allied Health Department
Central Pennsylvania College
Camp Hill, PA

Minda Brown, R.M.A.
Pima Medical Institute
Colorado Springs, CO

Janette Gallegos
Medical Assisting Instructor
Keiser University
Boca Raton, FL

Lisa M. Graese, C.M.T.
Instructor
Spokane Community College
Spokane, WA

Carol Hinricher
Program Director, Medical Information Technology
University of Montana College of Technology

Dolly R. Horton, C.M.A. (AAMA), B.S., M.Ed.
Medical Assisting Coordinator
Mayland Community College
Spruce Pine, NC

Rebecca Gibson-Lee, M.S.T.E., C.M.A. (AAMA), A.S.P.T.
Professor/Program Director Medical Assisting Technology
The University of Akron
Akron, OH

Robyn Gohsman, A.A.S., R.M.A. (AMT), C.M.A.S. (AMT)
Medical Assisting Program Director
Medical Careers Institute
Newport News, VA

Aimee Michaelis, V.A., Med.
Lead Instructor
Pima Medical Institute

Kinasha Myrick, C.M.A. (AAMA), C.A.H.I., B.B.A., M.A.
Medical Assistant/Coding Specialist Program Director
South Suburban College
South Holland, IL

Lisa Nagle, B.S.Ed., C.M.A. (AAMA)
Program Director, Medical Assisting
Augusta Technical College
Augusta, GA

Brigitte Niedzwiecki
Medical Assistant Program Director
Chippewa Valley Technical College

Tiffany Rosta, C.M.A. (AAMA)
Medical Instructor
Kaplan Career Institute
Pittsburgh, PA

Sulea Rucker, C.M.A. (AAMA)
Division Manager
San Joaquin Valley College
Modesto, CA

Judith D. Symons
McCann School of Business
Minersville, PA

Cynthia J. Watkins, R.N., M.S.N.
Medical Assisting Program Director
Lorain County Community College
Lorain, OH

THE LEARNING PACKAGE

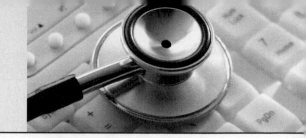

The Student Package

- Textbook

- Interactive CD ROM with exercises, learning games, skills review, medical office simulation for real-life application, skills videos, simulations, animations, resources, and audio glossary.

- Student Workbook that contains Chapter Outlines; Chapter Reviews; Learning Activities; Terminology Review; Critical Thinking Questions; Chapter Review Test, with Multiple Choice questions and additional True/False and Short Answer Questions; and Competency Check-Off Skill Sheets.

- MyMAKit is your key to student success. Use the code printed on the inside cover of this book to gain access to www.MyMAKit.com—the single source for all the resources that support this textbook!

The Instructional Package

- Instructor's Resource Guide with lesson plans, teaching tips, concepts for lecture, PowerPoint lecture slides, suggestions for classroom activities, answers to all textbook and workbook questions; and sample syllabus.

- CD ROM with Test Gen and over 2,000 test questions, and Classroom Management software.

- Transition Guides to help make text implementation easy.

- MyMAKit is your key to instructor success. Ask your sales representative how you can gain access to this single source for all the instructor resources that support this textbook!

Chapter Opener Features

Objectives

Each chapter opens with a list of learning objectives, which can be used to identify the material and skills the student show know upon successful completion of the chapter.

Case Study

Thought-provoking case studies provide scenarios that help students understand how the material presented in the chapter relates to the medical assisting profession.

MedMedia

This link to the accompanying CD ROM and Companion Website provides a description of the many interactive resources available to supplement the content in each chapter.

Critical Thinking Questions

Critical thinking questions are interspersed within the body of the chapter, and students must rely on the content in the text and their own critical thinking skills to answer the questions.

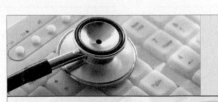

CHAPTER 2

Objectives

After completing this chapter, you should be able to:

- Define and spell the key terminology in this chapter.
- Describe the history of medical assisting.
- List the educational requirements of medical assisting.
- State the benefits of certifying or registering as a medical assistant.
- List the professional organizations that certify or register medical assistants.
- Name the benefits of membership in professional organizations.
- Define the scope of medical assisting.
- List the professional associations that certify other allied health professionals.

Medical Assisting Today

Case Study

Karla Wilkins and Carrie Smith, a medical assistant, were friends in high school. By the time the two unexpectedly meet at the local grocery store, they have not been in touch for several months. Carrie tells Karla about becoming certified as a medical assistant and includes such details as course load and topics. Looking confused, Karla responds, "If medical assistants don't *have* to be certified, why waste the time going to school? Why not just find a job and learn on the job?"

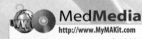

MedMedia
http://www.MyMAKit.com

Additional interactive resources and activities for this chapter can be found on http://www.MyMAKit.com. For a video, tips, audio glossary, legal and ethical scenarios, on-the-job scenarios, quizzes, and games related to the content of this chapter, please access the accompanying CD-ROM in this book.

Video
Legal and Ethical Scenario: *Medical Assisting Today*
On the Job Scenario: *Medical Assisting Today*
Tips
Multiple Choice Quiz
Audio Glossary
HIPAA Quiz
Games: Spelling Bee, Crossword, and Strikeout

—Critical Thinking Question 2-1—
Referring to the case study at the beginning of the chapter, what evidence supports the argument that medical assistants should have a standardized base of knowledge?

Medical Assisting Standards

This boxed feature identifies the CAAHEP and ABHES Entry-Level Standards for the medical assistant that are discussed in each chapter. The CAAHEP standards are identified according to learning domain (cognitive, psychomotor, or affective).

✚ MEDICAL ASSISTING STANDARDS

CAAHEP ENTRY-LEVEL STANDARDS	ABHES ENTRY-LEVEL COMPETENCIES
■ Recognize elements of fundamental writing skills (cognitive) ■ Organize technical information and summaries (cognitive) ■ Describe the process to follow if an error is made in patient care (cognitive) ■ Explain general office policies (psychomotor) ■ Use office hardware and software to maintain office systems (psychomotor) ■ Use Internet to access information related to the medical office (psychomotor) ■ Maintain organization by filing (psychomotor) ■ Incorporate the Patients' Bill of Rights into personal practice and medical office policies and procedures (psychomotor) ■ Apply ethical behaviors, including honesty/integrity in performance of medical assisting practice (affective)	■ Maintain confidentiality at all times ■ Be cognizant of ethical boundaries ■ Conduct work within scope of education, training, and ability ■ Orient patients to office policies and procedures ■ Adapt what is said to the recipient's level of comprehension ■ Adaptation for individualized needs ■ Apply computer concepts for office procedures ■ Exercise efficient time management ■ Fundamental writing skills

Medical Terminology and Abbreviations

Key Terminology

annotation—process of reading a document and highlighting pertinent information

body—main portion of a business letter

closing—ending portion of a business letter

electronic mail—message sent electronically from one person to another; also called e-mail

font—style of type

letterhead—professional-quality stationery with a business' contact information (e.g., name, address

Abbreviations

EKG—electrocardiogram

JCAHO—Joint Commission on the Accreditation of Healthcare Organizations

MLOCR—multiline optical character reader

OCR—optical character recognition

PDR—Physician's Desk Reference

UPS—United Parcel Service

USPS—United States Postal Service

The Medical Terminology and Abbreviations sections appear at the beginning of each chapter. The terms are listed in alphabetical order, a definition is provided, and the terminology appears in boldface on first introduction in the text. All terms are defined in the comprehensive glossary that appears at the back of the book, and phonetic pronunciations for difficult medical terminology are also provided.

Analyzing a Medical Term

You can often decipher the meaning of a medical term by breaking it down into its separate parts. Consider the following examples:

HEMAT/O/LOGY

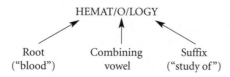

| Root ("blood") | Combining vowel | Suffix ("study of") |

The text also features a separate appendix of Medical Terminology Word Parts, designed to help students analyze medical terms; understand word parts and word part guidelines; and define basic medical terms and terms used to describe major body systems, body direction, and diseases and disease conditions.

Additional Features

Competency Skills Performance/Procedures

This unique text meets the highest standards outlined by CAAHEP and ABHES, and provides all of the tools needed for student success. This comprehensive text can be used by both ABHES-and CAAHEP-accredited schools or those applying for accreditation to meet both content and competency requirements in the administrative and clinical areas.

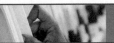 **PROCEDURE 9-8** **Schedule an Inpatient Admission**

Theory and Rationale
When patients require inpatient procedures or observations, physicians will ask medical assistants to schedule those patients for inpatient hospitalizations. Medical assistants who know the proper procedure help ensure that the scheduling process goes smoothly.

Materials
- Patient's chart
- Inpatient scheduling guidelines
- Calendar
- Telephone
- Notepad
- Pen

Competency
(Conditions) With the necessary materials, you will be able to **(Task)** schedule an inpatient admission **(Standards)** correctly within the time limit set by the instructor.

1. Call the patient's insurance carrier to obtain preauthorization for the procedure, the needed followup, and the allowable number of hospital days.
2. Document the preauthorization number in the patient's chart along with the name of the insurance company customer service representative spoken to.
3. Call the hospital admissions office with the patient's name, physician's name, and reason for admission.
4. Let the admissions office know when the physician would like the patient to be admitted.
5. Give the admissions office the patient's contact information, birth date, insurance information, and preauthorization number.
6. Instruct the patient when to arrive at the hospital and where to go once there.
7. Give the patient any specifics on what to bring (or not) to the hospital.
8. Chart all information in the patient's medical record, and give the chart to the physician for review.

A list of competencies appears at the beginning of each chapter in which procedures are presented. For each competency, Theory and Rationale are discussed, Required Materials are listed, and the procedure is presented in the proper format with the Conditions, Task, and Standards noted.

 COMPETENCY SKILLS PERFORMANCE

1. Schedule a new patient.
2. Establish an appointment matrix.
3. Schedule a patient appointment.
4. Use patient reminder cards.
5. Reschedule a missed patient appointment.
6. Manage the physician's professional schedule and travel.
7. Schedule a hospital procedure.
8. Schedule an inpatient admission.

Keys to Success

Helpful tips for career success are interspersed throughout the text to highlight the importance of professionalism

Keys to Success
ACCIDENTAL INJURY FILES

Keep patients' accidental injury files separate from those patients' general medical files. Then, when insurance companies request copies of patients' medical records due to the accidental injury, the copying task is far easier.

Using Abbreviations in Charting

Given that abbreviations can lead to confusion in health care, or even errors in patient care, medical assistants must be extremely careful when using abbreviations in patients' charts and ensure that the abbreviations are accepted by their facilities. Because different facilities may use different abbreviations for medical terms, when in doubt assistants should write out rather than abbreviate words. For example, one office may use the abbreviation "cx" to mean appointment cancellation. Another office may use the same abbreviation to indicate a cancer diagnosis.

Confusion among abbreviations can be avoided with a standard list of abbreviations between facilities. Chapter 6 lists abbreviations that are common in health care, as well as abbreviations that should never be used.

Concept Link

This visual link is a tool for providing concepts presented in earlier or later chapters.

In Practice

These real-life scenarios require students to pause and apply the knowledge presented in the chapter to answer critical thinking questions.

In Practice

The small physician's office where Jenny works as a front-desk medical assistant is on the first floor of a building where cars are parked outside the door. When Marion Wilson arrives for her appointment, she approaches the front desk and tells Jenny that she is going to leave her 2-year-old son sleeping in his car seat because Jenny can see the car from her desk. How should Jenny respond to Marion? What are some appropriate suggestions?

HIPAA Compliance

Patient confidentiality is an important part of Health Insurance Portability and Accountability Act (**HIPAA**) compliancy. The speaker-phone feature must only be used to discuss confidential patient information when parties unauthorized to have the patient's information are unable to overhear the conversation.

HIPAA Compliance

These feature boxes highlight the need-to-know law.

Electronic Medical Records

An entire chapter of this text is devoted to the important topic of electronic health records.

computer and have the added benefit of being small enough for physicians to carry with them from patient to patient. Most electronic medical records systems can be configured to work according to an office's specific needs. Figure 11-7 ◆ lists the functions many of these systems provide. One of the many benefits of such systems is the ability to access medical record information from many locations in the health care facility and to quickly search for and retrieve information in the patient's medical record (Figure 11-8 ◆).

In Practice

Dr. Jonas runs a private practice and makes rounds in two local hospitals. He uses one type of electronic medical records software in his private office and two other packages in the two hospitals. Not only must Dr. Jonas learn three software systems, he may at times be unable to move patient information between those systems due to incompatibility. What might Dr. Jonas do to address these issues?

Other Benefits of Electronic Medical Records

There are additional benefits to using electronic medical records, which are discussed in the following sections.

Electronic Signatures

An office that uses **electronic medical records** may use an **electronic signature.** In offices where medical notes are dictated and printed for patient files, an electronic signature or

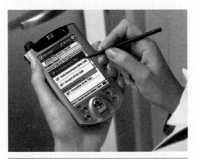

Figure 11-8 ◆ A handheld PDA.
Courtesy of Allscripts LLC.

rubber-stamp signature may replace handwritten signatures. In these offices, there must be a permanent record of the signer, as well as an original version of the signature on file.

Avoiding Medical Mistakes

Electronic medical records can be used to alert health care providers to possible medication reactions. This is especially helpful when treating patients who are cotreating with several specialists. The EMR software will typically have a safeguard mechanism built in that alerts the prescribing physician to any contraindicated medications a particular patient may have (Figure 11-9 ◆).

One of the most convincing arguments for converting paper medical records to an electronic format is based on patient safety. In 1999, the Institute of Medicine published a report called "To Err Is Human: Building a Safer Health System." This report stated, "At least 44,000 people, and perhaps as many

- ❑ Time-stamp recordings in the EMR/EHR
- ❑ Prescriptions printed or faxed to the pharmacy
- ❑ Printed patient education information that directly relates to the patient's care
- ❑ Search for a certain type of condition or certain age or geographic location of a group of patients
- ❑ Digital photos or X-rays attached in the patient's EMR/EHR
- ❑ Electronically ordered lab results, imaging items, or medical tests
- ❑ Electronic graphs of lab results of height, weight, or blood pressure data
- ❑ Letters to or about patients
- ❑ Electronic data transmission to other health care providers

Figure 11-7 ◆ Functions of an EMR/EHR.

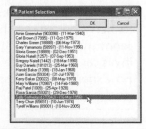

Figure 11-9 ◆ Selecting the right patient is easy with electronic medical records.
Courtesy of Medcin.

TABLE 15-3 TREATMENT FOR SHOCK
IN THE MEDICAL OFFICE

Cause	Treatment
Anaphylactic shock	Epinephrine
Cardiogenic shock	IV dopamine, immediate transport to the emergency room
Hemorrhagic shock	Stop bleeding, replace volume, immediate transport to the emergency room
Hypovolemic shock	Replace volume
Insulin shock	Sugar given to the patient by any means tolerated
Neurogenic shock	IV dopamine, immediate transport to the emergency room
Poisoning	Consult the poison center for treatment specific to the poison
Respiratory shock	Intubation and immediate transport to the emergency room
Sepsis	Fluids, IV dopamine, and immediate transport to the emergency room

Source: Beaman, N. and Fleming, L. Pearson's Comprehensive Medical Assisting, © 2007. Reprinted by permission of Pearson Education, Upper Saddle River, NJ.

Assisting Patients with Burns

Medical assistants may be required to assist with emergency burn victims. First, the assistants should try to determine the cause of the burn (e.g., chemical, fire, scalding). Medical staff who know the cause of a burn can provide better care. Some burns can be treated in the ambulatory care setting; others require hospital care. If possible, the medical assistant should immerse the burn in cool water, or soak sterile gauze in cool saline solution and apply the gauze to the burned area. In the event the burn was caused by a chemical, the medical assistant should attempt to flush the area with water. No matter what the cause of the burn, the medical assistant should seek the order of the physician in how to administer treatment to the patient.

Eye Treatment

Dust, dirt, chemicals, or other substances may get onto the surface of the eye and can be difficult for patients to safely remove on their own. Eye irrigations are an easy and comfortable way to remove these substances in the medical office. The procedure involves flowing a fluid across the eye and flushing the irritating substances from the surface Eyewash stations may also be used in the removal of dust, dirt and debris.

Emergency Preparedness

The medical assistant should be knowledgeable in the area of emergency preparedness. This includes knowing how to respond in the event of a man-made disaster, such as a terrorist event, and to a natural disaster, such as a hurricane.

Emergency Preparedness

This text includes the latest information on emergency preparedness and the medical assistant's role in protective practices.

Law and Ethics

Medical assistants face many situations that involve ethics and the law; therefore, a comprehensive chapter is provided to highlight the need-to-know law and present scenarios that may have a legal and ethical impact on patients. Informational tables and charts summarize key concepts.

Introduction

Medical assistants face many situations that involve ethics and law. Ethics deals with issues of right and wrong, whereas the law serves to uphold what society feels is right and wrong. Ethical issues often take more thought than legal ones, because people have differing ideas about what is right. The law, in contrast, tends to allow little room for opinion. Each state has unique laws governing health care and the medical-assisting profession. It is crucial for medical assistants to know the laws of their states and to uphold those laws at all times. That adherence to law, paired with a clear understanding of what society and the medical-assisting profession spell out with regard to ethics, can help the medical assistant build a solid career.

The Sources of Law

American law arises from varying sources. Court decisions establish **traditional law. Common law** comes from the English legal system. All states in America follow common law except Louisiana, which uses a system based on French law.

Key Terminology

common law—legislation that stems from the English legal system; also called traditional law (see following entry)

TABLE 2-5 COMPARING LICENSED, CERTIFIED, AND REGISTERED STATUSES		
Licensed	**Certified**	**Registered**
Usually pertains to a profession or occupation with a licensing requirement (e.g., licensed practical nurse [**LPN**]).	Usually pertains to a profession or occupation with a voluntary certification option (e.g., CMA (AAMA)).	May pertain to a profession or occupation with a registration requirement (e.g., RN); may also pertain to a profession or occupation with a voluntary registration option (e.g., RMA (AMT)).

Informational Charts and Tables

These appear throughout the text and summarize pertinent information for the reader. They provide students with visuals and comparisons to reinforce the lesson. In the specialty chapters they provide a quick reference for the disorders described in the chapter. Most tables include signs and symptoms, causes, diagnosis, and treatment.

Color Photos and Illustrations

Color photos and illustrations appear throughout the book to support the textual material presented and reinforce key concepts.

Bar-code scanner.

MEMORANDUM

Date: _____

To: _____

From: _____

Figure 6-12 ◆ Sample opening of an interoffice memo.

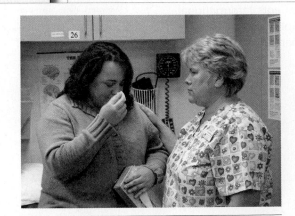

Figure 5-9 ◆ With an emotional patient, the medical assistant must remain calm.

Chapter Summary

Each chapter summary is an excellent review of the chapter content.

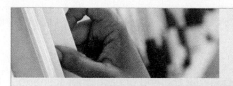

REVIEW

Chapter Summary

- Electronic medical records are the portions of a patient's medical record that are kept on a computer's hard drive or a medical office's computer network rather than on paper.
- Electronic medical records are gaining popularity over conventional paper files because they offer enhanced ease, efficiency, and accessibility.
- With paper charting, the patient's chart is only available to one staff member at a time. Electronic medical records make the patient's chart available to many healthcare team members at the same time.
- The conversion from paper to electronic medical record format is typically done over time. Once paper medical records are converted to electronic versions, those paper records must be appropriately destroyed.
- Medical offices should correct errors in a patient chart according to accepted protocol.
- By using electronic medical records, a medical office is able to perform tasks such as sending reminder post cards more easily than performing these same tasks with paper medical records.
- Other benefits of electronic medical records include using electronic signatures, avoiding medical mistakes, saving time, and communicating between staff members.

Chapter Review Questions

End-of-chapter questions are provided in multiple-choice, true/false, short answer, and research format, and help reinforce learning. The review questions measure the students' understanding of the material presented in the chapter. These tools are available for use by the student or by the instructor as an outcome assessment.

Chapter Review

Multiple Choice

1. At _____ minutes after a patient has missed an appointment, the medical assistant should call to reschedule.
   a. 5
   b. 10
   c. 15
   d. 60

2. A new patient is defined as someone who has:
   a. not been seen in the medical office for more than 1 year
   b. not been seen by any physician in the office for more than 3 years
   c. been seen by another physician in the office within the last year but is now seeing a new provider in the office
   d. all of the above

3. A new patient checklist is worthwhile when scheduling new patient appointments to ensure the medical assistant:
   a. gathers all necessary information from the new patient
   b. provides directions to the office, if needed
   c. gives information on parking arrangements
   d. all of the above

4. The medical office should ask new patients to arrive _____ minutes before their scheduled appointments to complete new patient paperwork.
   a. 5
   b. 15
   c. 25
   d. 35

5. Which of the following scheduling methods books several patients around the same time?
   a. Cluster booking
   b. Stream scheduling
   c. Set appointment time scheduling
   d. None of the above

True/False

T F 1. The time allowed for patient appointments remains constant from practitioner to practitioner.
T F 2. The appointment book is a legal document.
T F 3. Double booking is the process of allowing patients to arrive for appointments at their leisure.
T F 4. It is appropriate to tell chronically late patients that their appointments are 15 minutes before the times scheduled in the appointment book.
T F 5. It is unnecessary to chart a no-show appointment in a patient's chart.
T F 6. Medical offices that chart patients' missed appointments can help avoid losing malpractice lawsuits.
T F 7. When scheduling patients for procedures, it is important to disclose everything to expect.
T F 8. Administrative medical assistants do not arrange transportation services.
T F 9. A medical office's appointment scheduling system should be reviewed periodically to determine its efficiency.

Short Answer

1. What is one way to prepare the appointment schedule to allow appointments for patients who call and want same-day appointments?
2. Describe a triage notebook and its role in the medical office.
3. How can administrative medical assistants help patients remember to keep their appointments?
4. What is meant by a "no-show" appointment?
5. What can medical assistants do when they find that patients are waiting long periods for their appointments?
6. Describe how an appointment matrix is used in the medical office.

Research

1. Research online for companies that sell medical office appointment scheduling software. How do these companies compare to one another?
2. Interview someone who works in a medical office. Do the physicians in this office travel for out-of-town events related to their practice? If so, who in the office handles the scheduling arrangements?
3. What local resources are available in your area for arranging for medical language interpreters?

Externship Application Experience

This feature places the student in an externship site with a simulated situation the student may encounter. Critical thinking questions appear at the end of each brief scenario, and students must rely on the knowledge acquired in the chapter and their own critical thinking skills to answer each question.

Externship Application Experience

Sylvia Bissey, a patient of Dr. Borshack's for over 20 years, tells the medical assistant that she would like to get a copy of her husband's current lab results. The medical assistant explains that she will need a signed authorization from Mr. Bissey in order to release the information to his wife. Sylvia becomes upset and says, "I have *always* been given copies of his lab results in the past." How should the medical assistant respond to Sylvia?

Resource Guide

This listing provides additional information (organization contact information, websites, etc.) related to chapter content.

Resource Guide

American Heart Association
7272 Greenville Avenue
Dallas, TX 75231
Phone: (800) 242-8721
http://www.americanheart.org/

American Red Cross
www.redcross.org

Federal Emergency Management Agency (FEMA)
500 C Street SW
Washington, DC 20472
Disaster Assistance: (800) 621-FEMA
www.fema.gov

National Highway Traffic Safety Administration
1-888-327-4236

U.S. Department of Transportation (USDOT)
400 7th St., SW
Washington, DC 20590
www.dot.gov

U.S. National Library of Medicine
8600 Rockville Pike
Bethesda, MD 20894
http://www.nlm.nih.gov/medlineplus

MedMedia

Reminds students to visit and explore the Student CD to supplement chapter content.

 MedMedia

http://www.MyMAKit.com

More on this chapter, including interactive resources, can be found on the Student CD-ROM accompanying this textbook and on http://www.MyMAKit.com.

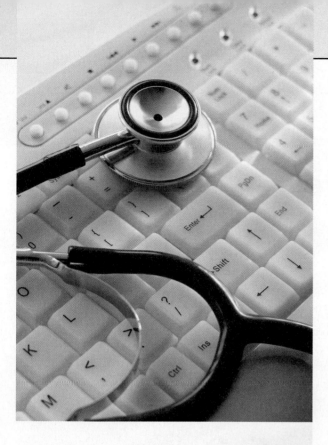

SECTION I

Introduction to the Administrative Medical Assisting Profession

My name is Sharon Martincak. I am a recent graduate of the medical assisting program at Everett Community College. I learned a lot about the importance of maintaining patient privacy in my training, and during my externship I realized how important that training was to my career as a medical assistant. Without this knowledge, I would be lost. It is important to know what information may be disclosed and what information cannot be disclosed about a patient. I am responsible for a lot of information about each patient and I am responsible for everything that is included in the patient's medical chart. I have had to deal with patients' friends, relatives, and insurance companies and I have to be aware of what I can disclose about the patient and what I cannot.

Every day I work with telephone messages, fax messages, and information that the patient entrusts to me. This information must be kept from anyone who is not supposed to have it. Medical assistants must be very careful in the way this information is used in order to protect both the patient and the physician. As a medical assistant, I am held liable for patient information and how it is used. I cannot stress enough the importance of knowing HIPAA privacy laws: this knowledge has made my job safer and easier.

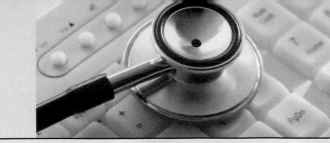

The History of Medicine and Health Care

Case Study

Dr. Kenyon will be giving a presentation on the history of medicine to a local community group. She has asked her medical assistant to prepare some background materials for this event. Because Dr. Kenyon is a surgeon, she wants her medical assistant to find information about early medical practices, including how patients were anesthetized and operated on in early days.

Objectives

After completing this chapter, you should be able to:

- Define and spell the key terminology in this chapter.
- Describe the history of medicine and health care.
- Identify early medical practices.
- Discuss the significant medical advances of previous centuries.
- Outline the roles played by health care pioneers.

MedMedia

http://www.MyMAKit.com

Additional interactive resources and activities for this chapter can be found on http://www.MyMAKit.com. For a video, tips, audio glossary, legal and ethical scenarios, on-the-job scenarios, quizzes, and games related to the content of this chapter, please access the accompanying CD-ROM in this book.

Video
Legal and Ethical Scenario: *History of Medicine and Health Care*
On the Job Scenario: *History of Medicine and Health Care*
Tips
Multiple Choice Quiz
Audio Glossary
HIPAA Quiz
Games: Spelling Bee, Crossword, and Strikeout

➕ MEDICAL ASSISTING STANDARDS

CAAHEP ENTRY-LEVEL STANDARDS	ABHES ENTRY-LEVEL COMPETENCIES
■ Differentiate between legal, ethical, and moral issues affecting healthcare (cognitive).	■ Be cognizant of ethical boundaries.

Introduction

Medicine has been practiced for a long time, but many of its advancements, including X-rays, medications, and anesthesia, are relatively new. Until the mid- to late 1800s, surgery was performed without anesthesia, and penicillin was not commonly used until the 1940s. Today, it would be hard to imagine health care without the advancements of the past century alone. Many of today's vaccinations were discovered in the 20th century, as were nearly all currently prescribed medications.

The Earliest Medical Practices

The history of medical treatment is rooted in ancient times. Cave paintings discovered in the Lascaux caves in France depict people using plants and herbs to treat illness. Using **radiocarbon dating**, these paintings have been estimated to date from 13,000 to 25,000 B.C. Even the emblem of the medical profession, the **caduceus**, derives from ancient times. This emblem, which depicts two snakes wrapped around a healing staff (Figure 1-1 ◆), reflects the early Greeks' use of nonpoisonous snakes to treat patients' wounds.

Ancient practitioners used nonpoisonous snakes and the roots, leaves, and flowers of plants to treat patients, but early medical treatments were often painful and sometimes fatal. In fact, the earliest medical treatments are thought to have killed patients nearly as often as diseases. Back then, most cultures believed demons or gods caused diseases and illnesses. As a result, most early medical practitioners were **faith healers** or **shamans** who were well versed in the superstitions of the day (Figure 1-2 ◆).

Critical Thinking Question 1-1
What are the historical roots of modern medicine?

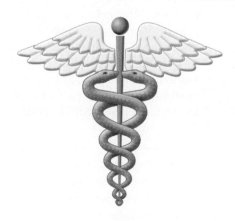

Figure 1-1 ◆ The caduceus is the emblem of the medical profession.

Key Terminology

American Red Cross—humanitarian organization that provides emergency assistance

anatomy—study of the structure and organization of living organisms

anesthesia—method of numbing a body area or rendering an individual unconscious

antisepsis—practice of preventing the growth and reproduction of bacteria and viruses

antiseptic—substance that prevents the growth and reproduction of bacteria and viruses

astrology—study of the planets and stars to try to understand how things work on Earth

autopsy—examination of a corpse to determine the cause of death

caduceus—emblem of the medical profession

chiropractic—system of therapy that corrects spine misalignments

chloroform—early method of general anesthesia used to render a patient unconscious

ether—early method of general anesthesia thought to be safer than chloroform

evidence-based medicine—theory that states health care methods should be scientifically proven

faith healer—practitioner who uses prayer rather than medicine to heal patients

Hippocrates—known as the "Father of Medicine"

Human Genome Project—project designed to map the human genes

pharmaceuticals—drugs, medicines, and chemical compounds

physiology—study of the mechanical, physical, and biochemical functions of living organisms

public health—overall health of a community

radiocarbon dating—procedure that measures a substance's carbon to determine its age

shaman—religious or spiritual figure

ultrasound—method of using sound waves to create three-dimensional images

Abbreviations

AHA—American Hospital Association
AMA—American Medical Association
CT—computed tomography
DNA—deoxyribonucleic acid

EKG—electrocardiograph
FAA—Federal Aviation Administration
JAMA—Journal of the American Medical Association

MRI—magnetic resonance imaging
TB—tuberculosis
WHO—World Health Organization

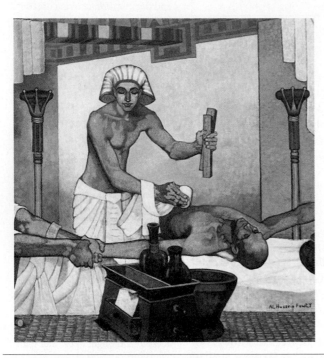

Figure 1-2 ◆ Most early medical practitioners were faith healers or shamans.

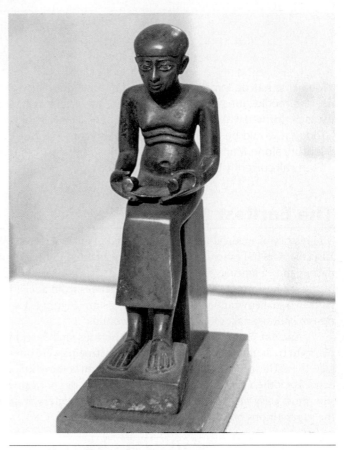

Figure 1-3 ◆ Imhotep (332–30 B.C.)

Early Egyptian Medicine

As far back as 3000 B.C., there is evidence that the Egyptians provided medical care for such conditions as tuberculosis and pneumonia. Other records suggest that they were performing surgery, as well. Fossils from this era indicate that an Egyptian patient underwent brain surgery and survived. The patient's skull bones had healed long before the patient died.

A practitioner named Imhotep, who lived from 2667 to 2648 B.C., is credited as founding Egyptian medicine in the Third Dynasty (Figure 1-3 ◆). He authored some of the original material on which the world's earliest known medical document, the *Edwin Smith Papyrus,* is based. Written around 1600 B.C., the *Papyrus* details the known cures, examination findings, and prognoses of the time and is thought to be a compilation of multiple authors.

Early Chinese Medicine

Classical Chinese medicine has been traced as far back as 2700 B.C. Much of it reflects the culture's beliefs that everything, including humans, is interconnected and that optimal health comes from living harmoniously in the world. Classical Chi-

nese practitioners believed the five methods in Figure 1-4 ◆ helped patients achieve good health. The Chinese also developed a list of the medical uses for many plants and herbs.

In the 1960s, the Chinese government commissioned 10 Western physicians to add scientific theory to classical Chinese medicine. The result, called traditional Chinese medicine, is taught in Chinese medical schools today.

1. Cure the patient's spirit.
2. Nourish the patient's body.
3. Give medications as needed.
4. Treat the entire body, not just the illness.
5. Use acupuncture.

Figure 1-4 ◆ Early Chinese Methods of Patient Treatment

Early Native American Medicine

Native Americans are among the earliest and most effective medical practitioners. Native American healers, whose practices date as far back as 40,000 years in the United States, believed they must always honor the patient's wishes and never force treatment. Though medical treatments varied among the Native American tribes, suicide was considered one of the highest forms of bravery. The elderly and sick of many tribes traditionally committed suicide during periods of famine.

When treatment was an option, both the Navaho and the Cherokee used herbs and such comfort measures as natural pain relievers. Patients who recovered were often thought to have supernatural powers. Because tribes lacked written language at the time, early Native American healers used oral means to pass their medical knowledge to younger tribe members.

The Father of Medicine

Hippocrates, known as the "Father of Medicine," helped shift medical care from a religious and superstitious practice to a scientific one by basing his practice of medicine on the belief that illness was the result of a physical condition. He believed that the body, rather than just one ailment, should be treated, and he was the first physician to note that some individuals recovered faster from their illnesses than others. Hippocrates, who lived from 460 B.C. to 377 B.C., founded a medical school on the island of Cos, Greece, where he taught his ideas. Around the fourth century B.C. he wrote *Ancient Medicine,* a book that described his medical theories, as well as the Hippocratic Oath, which is physicians' promise to treat their patients to the best of their abilities (Figure 1-5 ◆). Contemporary medical schools still recite the Hippocratic Oath at graduation.

—Critical Thinking Question 1-2—
Why was Hippocrates called "The Father of Medicine"?

Early European Medicine

Early European medicine used **astrology** to train physicians. The Greek physician Galen, who lived from 129 to 200 A.D. (Figure 1-6 ◆), is credited with advancing Hippocrates's work. As was common practice at the time, Galen advocated blood letting as a form of treatment. This treatment consisted of cutting into the patient's veins and allowing the patient to bleed. It was believed that patients may be ill because they had too much blood in their systems. Galen was the first physician to record a patient's pulse, although he failed to realize the pulse was related to the heart's action. He was also the first to document many parts of the human body. Since human **autopsies** were illegal during Galen's time, many of his findings were inaccurate because he studied dead animals.

The Hippocratic Oath

I swear by Apollo Physician, by Asclepias, by Health, by Heal All, and by all the gods and goddesses, that according to my ability and judgment, I will keep this oath and stipulation; to reckon him who taught me this art equally dear to me as my parents, and share my substance with him and relieve his necessities if required. To regard his offspring as on the same footing with my own brothers and to teach them this art if they should wish to learn it, without fee or stipulation; and that by precept, lecture, and every other mode of instruction I will impart a knowledge of my art to my own sons and to those of my teachers and to disciples bound by a stipulation and oath according to the law of medicine, but to none others.

I will follow that method of treatment which according to my ability and judgment, I consider for the benefit of my patients, and abstain from whatever is deleterious and mischievous. I will give not deadly medicine to anyone if asked, nor suggest any counsel.

Furthermore, I will not give to a woman an instrument to produce an abortion.

With Purity and with Holiness, I will pass my life and practice my art. I will not cut a person who is suffering with a stone, but will leave this to the practitioners of this work. Into whatever houses I enter I will go into them for the benefit of the sick and will abstain from every voluntary act of mischief and corruption; and further from the seduction of females or males, bond or free.

Whatever, in connection with my professional practice, or not in connection with it, I may see or hear in the lives of men which ought not to be spoken abroad, I will not divulge, as reckoning that all such should be kept secret.

While I continue to keep this oath inviolated, may it be granted to me to enjoy life and practice the art respected by all men, at all times, but should I trespass and violate this oath, may the reverse be my lot.

Figure 1-5 ◆ The Hippocratic Oath.

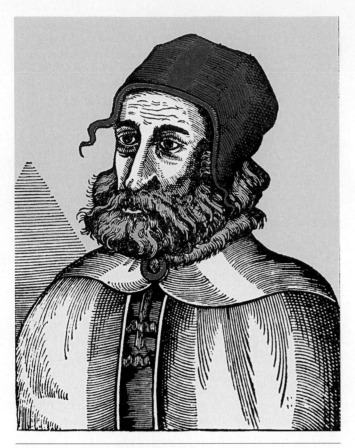

Figure 1-6 ◆ Galen (129–200 A.D.).

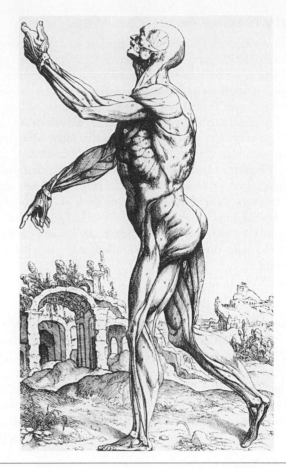

Figure 1-7 ◆ Andreas Vesalius (1514–1564), "Plate 25 from 'De Humani Corporis Fabrica,' Book II."

In addition to studying deceased animals, Galen experimented with live ones. He once publicly dissected a living pig to show that severing the laryngeal nerve stopped the pig from squealing. This nerve today is still known as "Galen's nerve." In other public experiments, Galen tied the ureters of living animals to show that urine comes from the kidneys and severed spinal cords to cause paralysis. Galen also performed many operations on living human patients, including cataract surgeries. To remove a cataract, he inserted a needle into the eye behind the lens and pulled back slightly.

Although Galen died in 200 A.D., his work was considered the authority on **anatomy** and **physiology** until the 16th century, when Andreas Vesalius corrected many of Galen's anatomy errors and wrote the first roughly correct anatomy textbook. Vesalius fared better than Galen, because Vesalius was able to perform autopsies on human bodies. The ban was lifted during Vesalius's time. He autopsied the bodies of executed criminals and commissioned artists to create drawings for his textbook (Figure 1-7 ◆).

The Turning Points of Modern Medicine

Medical practice changed dramatically in the 18th century. Chemistry knowledge advanced, and people began to believe that sickness and bacteria, rather than superstitions and reli-

gious beliefs, caused disease. A number of tools and discoveries helped advance medical study.

Medical Discoveries

A Dutch lens maker named Anton von Leeuwenhoek helped advance medical understanding by introducing the microscope in 1674 (Figure 1-8 ◆). German physicist Daniel Fahrenheit invented the mercury thermometer in 1714.

Surgeon John Hunter, who lived from 1728 to 1793, developed many of the surgical techniques that are still used today. In 1796, English physician Edward Jenner discovered the smallpox vaccine. He found that injecting patients with small amounts of material from smallpox blisters gave those patients immunity from the disease (Figure 1-9 ◆).

Jenner's smallpox discovery shifted medicine's focus from cures to prevention. **Public-health** and nutrition improvements, as well as pivotal medical discoveries that continued into the 19th century, would cause many diseases of the time to decline. In 1816, French physician Rene Laennec invented the stethoscope (Figure 1-10 ◆). At the time, Laennec was well known for extensively researching tuberculosis (**TB**) and for being the first physician to recognize cirrhosis of the liver as a disease.

CHAPTER 1   *The History of Medicine and Health Care*   ■   7

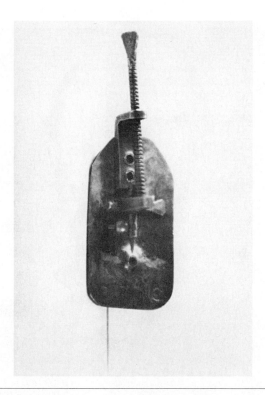

Figure 1-8 ◆ Anton Van Leeuwenhoek's prototype microscope.

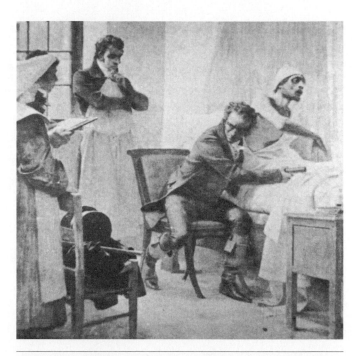

Figure 1-10 ◆ Rene Laennec using a stethoscope.

American physician and pharmacist Crawford W. Long was the first to employ modern **anesthesia** in 1842 when he used an **ether**-based anesthesia to remove a tumor from a patient's neck (Figure 1-11 ◆). Long went on to use his anesthesia technique in amputations and childbirth events. In 1846, American physician and pharmacist William Morton also used an ether-based anesthesia on a patient before removing a neck tumor. Morton tried to keep his compound secret, however, and later had it patented. Despite Morton's efforts, the compound's ingredients were quickly identified, and anesthesia use spread throughout Europe by the end of 1846.

Because ether had many side effects, **chloroform** replaced it as an anesthetic agent in 1853. Chloroform also had drawbacks, however. Many patients died when untrained

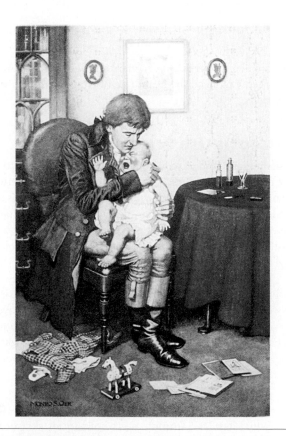

Figure 1-9 ◆ Dr. Edward Jenner administering vaccination against smallpox (to his son), 1789.

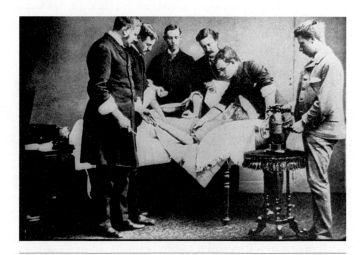

Figure 1-11 ◆ A patient receives anesthesia during surgery.

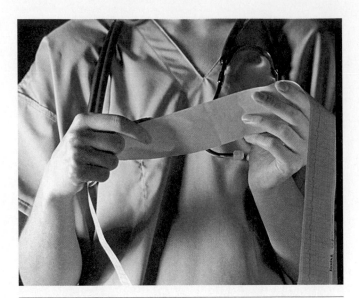

Figure 1-12 ◆ A physician reads an EKG strip.

practitioners used it improperly. Therefore, physicians reverted to the use of ether to anesthetize patients. The first effective topical anesthetic was used in 1859 for an opthalmic surgery. The substance, a form of cocaine, replaced salt and ice for numbing a small area.

In 1853, Scottish physician Alexander Wood invented the hypodermic needle, which allowed physicians to inject and extract liquids to and from patients' bodies. In 1903, Willem Einthoven, a physician in the Netherlands, invented the electrocardiograph (**EKG**) (Figure 1-12 ◆). This invention enabled physicians to record the electrical activity of a patient's heart.

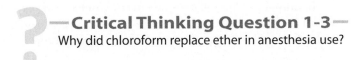

—Critical Thinking Question 1-3—
Why did chloroform replace ether in anesthesia use?

The Beginning of Hand Washing in Health Care

In 1847, Hungarian physician Ignaz Semmelweiss (Figure 1-13 ◆) noticed a dramatic difference in the death rate of new mothers from childbed fever when the women delivered their babies at home with the help of midwives rather than in hospitals with surgeons. Childbed fever was a condition caused by a severe vaginal or uterine infection. Women who delivered at home were far more likely to survive. Because he suspected poor hospital hygiene as the cause, Dr. Semmelweiss began an experiment that required physicians to wash their hands before treating women in childbirth. At the time, physicians failed to wash their hands between patients, often attending to women in childbirth after working with recently deceased patients. The

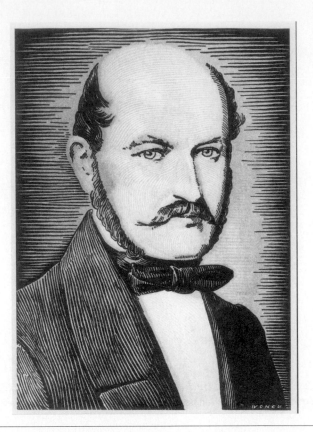

Figure 1-13 ◆ Ignaz Semmelweiss (1818–1865).

data from Semmelweiss's experiment showed that hand washing markedly reduced the death rate of women who delivered in hospitals.

Antisepsis Use in Health Care

Despite his landmark discovery, Semmelweiss received little respect from his colleagues. As a result, hand washing between patients only began to enjoy widespread use in hospitals after British surgeon Joseph Lister discovered in 1867 that an **antiseptic** on wounds helped prevent infection. Lister based his study of **antisepsis** on the discoveries of French biologist Louis Pasteur (Figure 1-14 ◆).

While Pasteur is best known for inventing pasteurization in 1862, a process that uses heat to destroy bacteria, he also worked to prevent anthrax transmission, and discovered the vaccine for rabies in 1885. Pasteur's pasteurization findings led to the use of heat in surgical-instrument sterilization. For all his work, Pasteur earned the title "Father of Preventive Medicine."

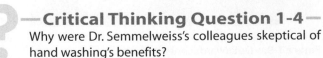

—Critical Thinking Question 1-4—
Why were Dr. Semmelweiss's colleagues skeptical of hand washing's benefits?

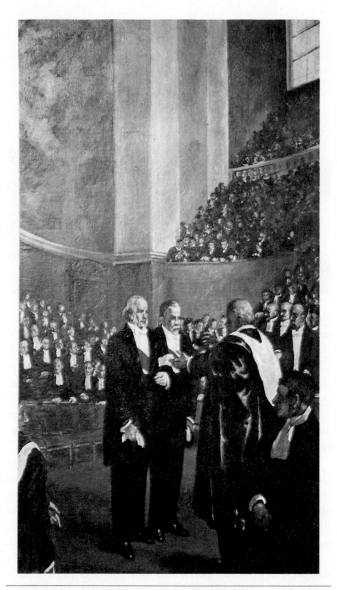

Figure 1-14 ◆ Joseph Lister and Louis Pasteur.

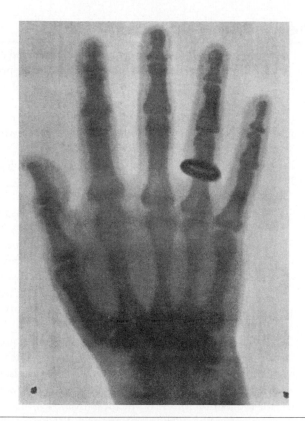

Figure 1-15 ◆ X-ray image of Roentgen's wife's hand, January 1896.

The Medical Value of X-Rays

Wilhem Roentgen revolutionized medical diagnosis in 1895 when he discovered X-rays while experimenting with vacuum tubes. His first X-ray image was of his wife's hand (Figure 1-15 ◆). Roentgen called the radiation rays he used "X" to indicate that they were unknown, but many of his colleagues called them Roentgen rays, a name that is still used in many languages today. In 1901, Roentgen received a Nobel Prize in physics for his discovery.

Chiropractic Practices in Medicine

In 1895, a man named D. D. Palmer started **chiropractic** practices when he found he could restore a man's hearing by correcting the man's spinal misalignment (Figure 1-16 ◆). (For more on chiropractic practices, see Chapter 3.)

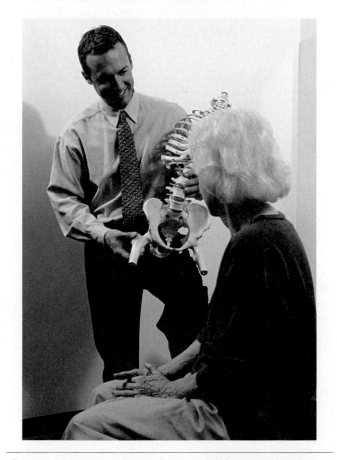

Figure 1-16 ◆ A chiropractor shows a model spine to a patient.

Medicine in the 20th Century

For many reasons, the 20th century is a notable era in medical treatment. Immunizations, a powerful weapon in disease prevention, are just one important 20th century advancement. Table 1-1 reviews the history of vaccines.

In 1901, biologist and physician Karl Landsteiner contributed to the development of modern medicine by creating the contemporary system of blood-group classification. For his discovery, Landsteiner won the Nobel Prize in physiology in 1930.

In 1928, Scottish scientist Alexander Fleming noticed circles of nongrowth around certain areas of mold in petri dishes. He believed the mold was releasing a substance that was inhibiting bacterial growth, and he named that substance penicillin. Penicillin was first used successfully in patient treatment in 1930 and came into popular use during World War II, when it was used to save the lives and limbs of wounded soldiers. Fleming won the Nobel Prize in 1945 for his discovery (Figure 1-17 ◆).

Scientists James Dewey Watson and Frances Harry Compton Crick also won a Nobel Prize. In 1953, the pair became the first to identify the genetic instructions for all living organisms: deoxyribonucleic acid (**DNA**). The men's groundbreaking work became the foundation for today's medical research.

Other critical medical inventions and discoveries followed. For example, John Hopps invented the first heart pacemaker in 1950, though this early device was large and painful, and mounted externally. While smaller external pacemakers were invented throughout the 1950s, they relied on external

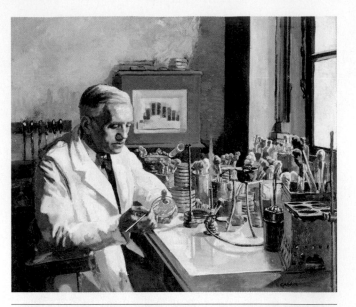

Figure 1-17 ◆ Sir Alexander Fleming (1881–1955). Scottish bacteriologist, discoverer of penicillin.

electrodes and had to be plugged into outlets. The first pacemaker was implanted in 1958 in Sweden, but it lasted only 3 hours. A second one was implanted into the same patient, and it lasted 2 days. That patient lived until 2001, having received 22 pacemakers in his lifetime.

The 1950s continued to be a decade of medical advances. During that time, the first open-heart surgery was performed successfully, the first heart-lung machine was used in surgery, and the first kidney was transplanted in a patient. A heart was first transplanted in a human by Dr. Christiaan Barnard in South Africa in 1967.

The 1970s ushered in the computed tomography (CT) scan and the advent of **ultrasound** technology. In 1982, the first artificial heart was implanted in patient Barney Clark. Clark survived for 112 days.

In 1990, the U.S. Department of Energy's Health and Environmental Research Program launched the **Human Genome Project,** an initiative aimed at identifying all the genes in human DNA. As the project progressed, several companies began using its research to determine if people had predispositions to such conditions as cancer, blood-clotting disorders, cystic fibrosis, and liver disease. Companies also began researching medicines that could be linked to a person's genetic makeup.

The Human Genome Project reached its goal in 2003 and its findings were made available to scientists worldwide. Scientists hope to use this information to learn how diseases work from the molecular level and thereby find cures for many diseases (Figure 1-18 ◆).

?—**Critical Thinking Question 1-5**—
How can research from the Human Genome Project improve the delivery of contemporary health care?

TABLE 1-1 VACCINE HISTORY

Vaccine	Year
Diphtheria	1923
Pertussis	1926
Tuberculosis	1927
Tetanus	1927
Yellow Fever	1935
Typhus	1937
Influenza	1945
Polio (Salk)	1952
Anthrax	1954
Polio (oral)	1962
Measles	1964
Mumps	1967
Rubella	1970
Chicken pox	1974
Pneumonia	1977
Meningitis	1978
Hepatitis B	1981
Haemonphilus influenzae type B (HiB)	1985
Hepatitis A	1992
Lyme disease	1998
Rotavirus	1998
Human papillomavirus	2006

Source: Centers for Disease Control: www.cdc.gov.

3. **Specialty**—Offer care to a certain patient type (e.g., children, burn victims, psychiatric patients, or patients undergoing drug or alcohol rehabilitation).
4. **Research**—Treat patients while researching certain disease types. Examples of these hospitals include cancer research facilities and Shriner's hospitals that care for children with spinal cord injuries, cleft palate, burns, or orthopedic conditions.

The History of the American Medical Association

The American Medical Association (**AMA**) was founded in 1847 at the University of Pennsylvania with the goals of "scientific advancement, standards for medical education, launching a program of medical ethics, and improved public health." It began organizing state and local associations in 1901, and its first meeting included 250 delegates from 28 states. Physician membership in the group went from 8,000 in 1900 to over 70,000 by 1910. At that point, the AMA counted fully half of licensed U.S. physicians among its membership.

The growth of AMA marked the beginning of "organized medicine." Table 1-2 lists AMA milestones.

TABLE 1-2 AMA MILESTONES

Year	Event
1847	The organization is founded.
1848	Makes dangers of "secretive remedies" the focus.
1858	Establishes Committee of Ethics.
1873	Sets up AMA Judicial Council.
1883	Launches *Journal of the American Medical Association* (**JAMA**).
1884	Supports experimentation on animals.
1897	Incorporates the organization.
1898	Starts Committee on Scientific Research to provide medical-research grants.
1899	Sets up Committee on National Legislation to represent group's interests in U.S. government.
1905	Launches Council on Pharmacy and Chemistry to set drug-manufacturing and advertising standards.
1912	Establishes Federation of State Medical Boards to deem group's rating of medical schools authoritative.
1948	Hires public relations firm to defeat government-run universal health care coverage.
1960	States that a blood alcohol level of 0.1% should be evidence of alcohol intoxication.
1970	Encourages the Federal Aviation Administration (**FAA**) to require all airlines to separate nonsmokers and smokers.
1974	Gives recommendations to ensure adequate protection of individuals used in human medical experimentation.
1982	Urges each state medical society to support laws to raise the legal drinking age to 21.
1988	Creates the Office of HIV/AIDS.
1995	Starts a campaign for liability reform.
2000	Supports Patients' Bill of Rights legislation in Congress.

Source: American Medical Association: www.ama-assn.org.

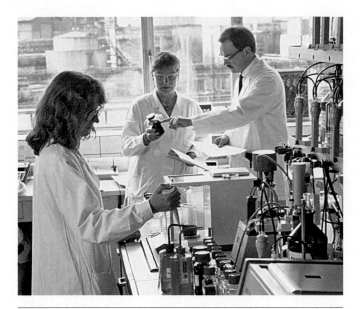

Figure 1-18 ◆ Scientists working in a laboratory.

Important Organizations in Medical History

Throughout the years, a number of entities have formed to advance varying facets of the medical profession.

The History of American Hospitals

Early American hospitals bore little resemblance to the hospitals of today, in large part because people preferred to receive medical care in their own homes in the country's early days.

Benjamin Franklin built the first American hospital in Philadelphia in 1751. By 1910, that hospital and others like it had begun to run like today's scientific institutions. They used antiseptics, focused on cleanliness, and relieved pain with medications. In 1921, National Hospital Day was first celebrated on May 12, the birthday of famous nurse Florence Nightingale (see the following section on important female figures in medicine). The holiday continues to be recognized during the week of Nightingale's birth every year.

According to the American Hospital Association (**AHA**), by 2005 the United States had 5,756 hospitals with staffed beds totaling near 1 million. Hospitals today fall into the four following categories:

1. **General or community**—Range from 10 beds to several hundred. Hospitals in this category, found in nearly every U.S. community, account for nearly 5,000 of the hospitals documented by the AHA in 2005.
2. **Teaching**—Found near university medical schools and have medical students, interns, and residents treating patients under the supervision of licensed physicians. In general, these facilities offer the same services as general hospitals (see preceding).

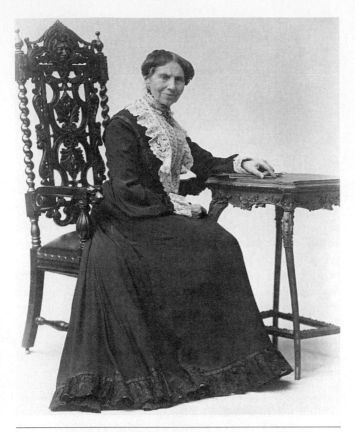

Figure 1-19 ◆ Clara Barton, founder of the American Red Cross.

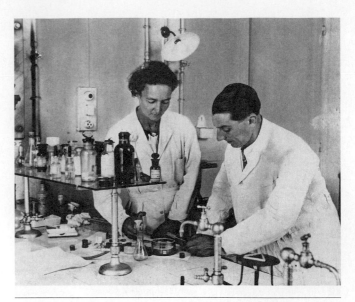

Figure 1-20 ◆ Marie Curie (1867–1934). Polish-born French physicist and her husband at work in the laboratory.

The Start of the American Red Cross

In 1881, a nurse named Clara Barton formed the **American Red Cross,** now one of the largest humanitarian organizations in the world (Figure 1-19 ◆). During her life, Barton was the most decorated American woman. She received the Iron Cross, the Cross of Imperial Russia, and the International Red Cross Medal. In 1904, at age 83, Barton founded the National First Aid Society.

Important Women in Health Care

Women like Clara Barton have featured prominently in medical history throughout the years.

The Work of Marie Curie

One of the first notable women in health care was Marie Curie (Figure 1-20 ◆). This Polish woman became the first female instructor at the Sorbonne in France, and, in 1903, she became the first woman in France to complete her doctorate. Curie was the first person to win two Nobel Prizes in two different fields, and to this day she remains the only woman to have done so. Curie's work with radium eventually caused her death from radiation poisoning in 1934.

The Role of Florence Nightingale

Florence Nightingale is known as the founder of nursing. She was born in Florence, Italy, in 1820. At the time, nursing had a poor reputation. Nurses followed armies around, providing care and cooking meals. Nightingale helped advance the care of the poor, advocating improved medical care and commitment to the nursing profession. In 1860, she opened a nursing school in England. That school, the Nightingale School of Nursing, is still training nurses today.

The Contributions of the Blackwell Sisters

In 1869, Nightingale opened the first women's medical school with Elizabeth Blackwell, the first woman to practice medicine in the United States with a degree (Figure 1-21 ◆). Given prejudices against women at the time, Blackwell herself had to apply to several medical schools before she was finally accepted by Geneva College in New York. She graduated at the top of her class. Although she was originally barred from practice in most hospitals because of her gender, Blackwell founded her own hospital in 1857, the New York Infirmary for Indigent Women and Children.

Blackwell's sister, Emily, was the third woman to earn a medical degree in the United States. The sisters worked together at the New York Infirmary for Indigent Women and Children for over 40 years. In 1868, they founded the Women's Medical College in New York. By 1899, the college had graduated nearly 400 women doctors.

In 1970, 8 percent of all U.S. physicians were women. By 1980, that number had exceeded 12 percent. As of 2004, the number of female physicians in the United States was nearly 27 percent.

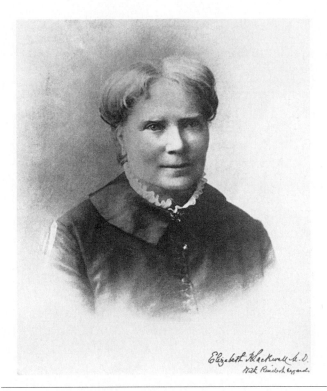

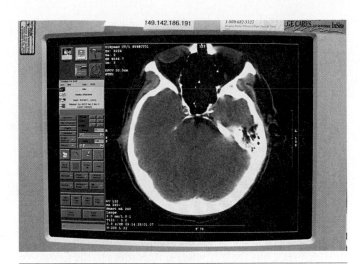

Figure 1-22 ◆ CT scan of a human brain.

Figure 1-21 ◆ First female physician in the United States, Elizabeth Blackwell.

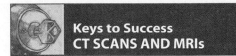

Keys to Success
CT SCANS AND MRIs

CT scans use X-rays to take three-dimensional images of the insides of objects (Figure 1-22 ◆).

MRI uses a large magnet to visualize the inside of an object (Figure 1-23 ◆).

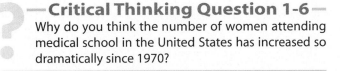

?—**Critical Thinking Question 1-6**—
Why do you think the number of women attending medical school in the United States has increased so dramatically since 1970?

The World Health Organization

In 1945, when diplomats met to form the United Nations, one of the items discussed was the setting up of a global health organization. The World Health Organization (**WHO**) was launched on April 17, 1948, a date celebrated today as World Health Day. The WHO is responsible for providing leadership on many global health issues. Some of the stated goals of the WHO are to shape the health research agenda, set the norms and standards for health issues worldwide, articulate evidence-based policy options, provide technical support to countries and to monitor and assess health trends around the globe.

Medical Care Today

From the 1950s to the 1980s, medical care advanced rapidly, with the discovery of numerous **pharmaceuticals**, **CT** scans, and magnetic resonance imaging (**MRI**).

Health care will likely continue to yield critical discoveries. Among the promising areas are stem-cell research, transplants, and chemistry in the area of pharmacology. There are, however, ongoing challenges. From 1950 to 1960, the cost of a

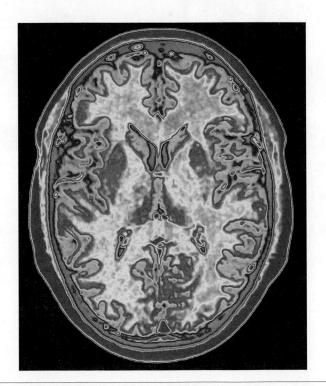

Figure 1-23 ◆ *MRI scan of a human brain.*

hospital stay doubled, causing many Americans, especially the elderly, to have difficulty affording care. Since 1990, health care costs in the United States have risen at double the rate of inflation. By 2000, 16 percent of all Americans, or 44 million people, were uninsured (PBS, 2006).

Evidence-Based Medicine

With health care costs in the United States rising far faster than inflation, eliminating costly and ineffective treatments is one way for the medical community to bring those costs under control. Evidence-based medicine has arisen as one solution to the problem.

Evidence-based medicine uses scientific findings, randomized controlled trials, and medical literature to find the most effective ways to treat disease. According to the Centre for Evidence-Based Medicine, "Evidence-based medicine is the conscientious, explicit, and judicious use of current best evidence in making decisions and the care of individual patients." In essence, this form of medicine is based on the idea that medical practice has a scientific method and that many traditional practices have no scientific basis and therefore can be costly and ineffective.

Physicians who practice evidence-based medicine are dedicated to treating patients with the most current, scientifically valid treatments (Figure 1-24 ◆). To keep abreast of drug trials and scientific studies, those providers must keep current with constant review of the medical literature.

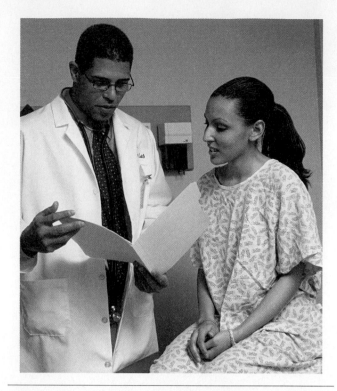

Figure 1-24 ◆ A physician reviews medical information with his patient.

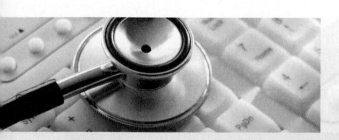

REVIEW

Chapter Summary

- The world's earliest medical practices have left a significant imprint on contemporary medical practices.
- Each of the world's centuries, dating back to ancient times, has contributed notable medical inventions and discoveries.
- Modern medical practices have built on the achievements of the past.
- A number of longstanding, pivotal organizations have formed throughout the years to further the advances of medical knowledge and achievement.

- Women have played a significant role in medicine throughout history.
- The future of health care continues to look promising, with recent advances including such practices as evidence-based medicine.

Chapter Review

Multiple Choice

1. Penicillin became commonly used during which of the following decades?
    a. 1920s
    b. 1930s
    c. 1940s
    d. 1950s

2. Who was known as "The Father of Medicine"?
    a. Hippocrates
    b. Galen
    c. Vesalius
    d. None of the above

3. Which early physician performed public displays of anatomy by cutting open live animals?
    a. Hippocrates
    b. Galen
    c. Vesalius
    d. None of the above

4. Which health care professional was the first to advocate that physicians wash their hands between patients?
    a. Fleming
    b. Pasteur
    c. Jenner
    d. Semmelweiss

5. Who discovered penicillin?
    a. Fleming
    b. Pasteur
    c. Jenner
    d. Semmelweiss

6. Who founded modern nursing?
    a. Clara Barton
    b. Florence Nightingale
    c. Marie Curie
    d. Elizabeth Blackwell

7. Who was the first woman to graduate from medical school in the United States?
    a. Clara Barton
    b. Florence Nightingale
    c. Marie Curie
    d. Elizabeth Blackwell

True/False

T F 1. Emily Blackwell founded the American Red Cross.
T F 2. One of the first physicians to use an ether-based compound as an anesthetic was given a U.S. patent for his concoction.
T F 3. The Human Genome Project has not yet been completed.
T F 4. The cost of health care in the United States is rising faster than the rate of inflation.
T F 5. Penicillin use became widespread during World War I.
T F 6. By the end of 2000, more than half of all medical school students were women.
T F 7. Marie Curie is the only woman to have won two Nobel prizes.

Short Answer

1. What is evidence-based medicine?

2. Why were Galen's anatomy findings only partially accurate?

3. Why was the letter *X* used in the name X-ray?

4. Who discovered the rabies vaccine?

5. How many pacemakers did the first internal-pacemaker patient receive, and how long did the patient live?

Research

1. Using the Internet as a resource, research the history of a commonly used medical instrument.

2. What is the history of the medical association in the state where you live?

3. Take one of the topics covered in this chapter on the history of medicine. Research this topic further to provide more details about how this innovation or invention has changed the way medicine is practiced.

Externship Application Experience

A patient asks the medical assistant to help identify resources for researching a physician-recommended vaccine. What should the medical assistant tell the patient? Which types of resources would help?

Resource Guide

American Hospital Association
One North Franklin
Chicago, IL 60606-3421
Phone: (312) 422-3000
http://www.aha.org/aha_app/index.jsp

Centers for Disease Control and Prevention
1600 Clifton Road
Atlanta, GA 30333
Phone: (404) 639-3311 / (404) 639-3534 / (800) 311-3435
http://www.cdc.gov/

Centre for Evidence-Based Medicine
Department of Primary Care
Old Road Campus
Headington, Oxford, OX3 7LF, United Kingdom
Phone: +44 (0)1865 226991
Fax: +44 (0)1865 226845
http://www.cebm.net/

Fisher, Leonard Everett. *The Hospitals.* New York: Holiday House, 1980.
Holland, Alex. *Voices of Qi: An Introductory Guide to Traditional Chinese Medicine.* Berkeley, CA: North Atlantic Books, Northwest Institute of Acupuncture and Oriental Medicine, 2000.

Human Genome Project
U.S. Department of Energy
1000 Independence Ave., SW
Washington, D.C. 20585
Phone: (800) 342-5363
Fax: (202) 586-4403
http://www.ornl.gov/sci/techresources/Human_Genome/home
.shtml

Maciocia, Giovanni. *The Foundations of Chinese Medicine: A Comprehensive Text for Acupuncturists and Herbalists.* New York: Churchill Livingstone, 2005.

PBS's Health Care Crisis: Health Care Timeline
Issues TV
18 Twin Ponds Drive
Bedford Hills, NY 10507-1208
Phone: (800) 752-9727
e-mail: issuestv@aol.com
http://www.pbs.org/healthcarecrisis/history.htm

Porter, R. *The Greatest Benefit to Mankind: A Medical History of Humanity from Antiquity to the Present.* New York: W.W. Norton and Company, 1999.

Shriner's Hospital for Children
2900 Rocky Point Drive
Tampa, FL 33607
Phone: (800) 237-5055
http://www.shrinershq.org/Hospitals/_Hospitals_for_Children/

Vallejo-Manzur, F., et al. (2003). "The resuscitation greats. Andreas Vesalius: The concept of an artificial airway." *Resuscitation* 56:3–7.
Wells, Susan. *Out of the Dead House: Nineteenth-Century Women Physicians and the Writing of Medicine.* Madison, WI: University of Wisconsin Press, 2001.

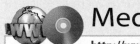 Med**Media**

http://www.MyMAKit.com

More on this chapter, including interactive resources, can be found on the Student CD-ROM accompanying this textbook and on http://www.MyMAKit.com.

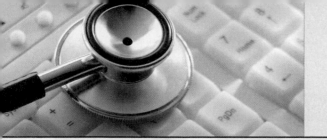

Objectives

After completing this chapter, you should be able to:

- Define and spell the key terminology in this chapter.
- Describe the history of medical assisting.
- List the educational requirements of medical assisting.
- State the benefits of certifying or registering as a medical assistant.
- List the professional organizations that certify or register medical assistants.
- Name the benefits of membership in professional organizations.
- Define the scope of medical assisting.
- List the professional associations that certify other allied health professionals.

Medical Assisting Today

Case Study

Karla Wilkins and Carrie Smith, a medical assistant, were friends in high school. By the time the two unexpectedly meet at the local grocery store, they have not been in touch for several months. Carrie tells Karla about becoming certified as a medical assistant and includes such details as course load and topics. Looking confused, Karla responds, "If medical assistants don't *have* to be certified, why waste the time going to school? Why not just find a job and learn on the job?"

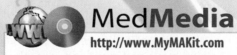

MedMedia
http://www.MyMAKit.com

Additional interactive resources and activities for this chapter can be found on http://www.MyMAKit.com. For a video, tips, audio glossary, legal and ethical scenarios, on-the-job scenarios, quizzes, and games related to the content of this chapter, please access the accompanying CD-ROM in this book.

Video
Legal and Ethical Scenario: *Medical Assisting Today*
On the Job Scenario: *Medical Assisting Today*
Tips
Multiple Choice Quiz
Audio Glossary
HIPAA Quiz
Games: Spelling Bee, Crossword, and Strikeout

Key Terminology

accredited—endorsed by a reputable overseeing agency

Accrediting Bureau of Health Education School (ABHES)—agency that helps support the certification of medical assistants through program endorsement

administrative—pertaining to office functions (e.g., computer operation, medical records management, coding and billing)

American Association of Medical Assistants (AAMA)—national, professional association for medical assistants

American Medical Technologists (AMT)—national, professional association for medical technologists

associate degree—degree awarded by community colleges after a roughly 2-year course of study

certified medical assistant (CMA)—graduate of an accredited medical assisting program who has passed the certification examination of the American Association of Medical Assistants (AAMA) (see preceding entry)

clinical—pertaining to direct patient care (e.g., drawing blood samples, taking vital signs, assisting with surgery)

Commission of Accreditation of Allied Health Education Programs (CAAHEP)—agency supporting the process of medical-assisting certification through program endorsement

community college—educational institution that provides 2-year undergraduate education

competency—skill in a defined area

externship—final phase of an accredited medical-assisting program

recertification—process of certificate renewal

registered medical assistant (RMA)—credential awarded a medical assistant who has passed the RMA certification examination

role delineation chart—list created by the AAMA (see preceding entry) that identifies all clinical, administrative, and general procedures of medical assisting

scope of practice—range of skills a health care professional is expected to have and operate within

technical educational program—program designed to give students skills without higher

✚ MEDICAL ASSISTING STANDARDS

CAAHEP ENTRY-LEVEL STANDARDS	ABHES ENTRY-LEVEL COMPETENCIES
■ Differentiate between legal, ethical, and moral issues affecting healthcare (cognitive) ■ Discuss legal scope of practice for medical assistants (cognitive) ■ Explore the issue of confidentiality as it applies to the medical assistant (cognitive) ■ Respond to issues of confidentiality (psychomotor) ■ Perform within scope of practice (psychomotor) ■ Practice within the standard of care for a medical assistant (psychomotor) ■ Apply local, state and federal health care legislation and regulation appropriate to the medical assisting practice setting (psychomotor) ■ Apply ethical behaviors, including honesty/integrity in performance of medical assisting practice (affective) ■ Demonstrate awareness of the consequences of not working within the legal scope of practice (affective) ■ Recognize the importance of local, state, and federal legislation and regulations in the practice setting (affective)	■ Adapt to change. ■ Evidence a responsible attitude. ■ Allied health professions and credentialing. ■ Maintain licenses and accreditation.

✓ COMPETENCY SKILLS PERFORMANCE

1. Adapt to change.

Introduction

With dramatic changes in health care over the past decade, including shorter hospital stays and managed care, physicians must rely on allied health personnel like medical assistants to help care for patients. With technology advancing and patient safety increasingly a focal point, many physicians today insist on hiring medical assistants who have been formally trained in accredited medical assisting programs. Part of this training includes complete knowledge of the medical assistant's role in patient care.

The History of the Medical Assisting Profession

Traditionally, physicians hired nurses to work in their offices. With a shortage of nurses, physicians began to seek other qualified staff who could fulfill administrative and clinical duties. As a result, the demand for formally trained medical assistants began to rise.

When medical assisting began in the early 1950s, the Kansas Medical Assistants Society formed a professional organization for those in the field. A year later, the organization voted to

Key Terminology *(continued)*

education; also called vocational program
(see following)

vocational program—program designed
to give students skills without higher education; also called technical educational
program (see preceding)

Abbreviations

AAMA—American Association for Medical Assistants

AAMT—American Association of Medical
Transcriptionists

AAPC—American Academy of Professional Coders

ABHES—Accrediting Bureau of Health Education Schools

AHIMA—American Health Information
Management Association

AMA—American Medical Association

AMT—American Medical Technologists

CAAHEP—Commission on Accreditation
of Allied Health Education Programs

CEU—continuing education unit

CLC—certified laboratory consultant

CMA—certified medical assistant

CMAS—certified medical administrative
specialist

CMT—certified medical transcriptionist

COLT—certified office laboratory technician

CPC—certified professional coder

CPR—cardiopulmonary resuscitation

HIPAA—Health Insurance Portability and
Accountability Act

LPN—licensed practical nurse

MLT—medical laboratory technician

MT—medical technologist

NP—nurse practitioner

PA—physician assistant

RMA—registered medical assistant

RPT—registered phlebotomy technician

rename itself the **American Association of Medical Assistants**
(AAMA). At the time, medical assistants lacked formal education; physicians trained most of their assistants on the job, and
the AAMA held educational sessions designed to increase the
professionalism of medical assisting. Since 1957, the AAMA has
kept its national headquarters in Chicago, IL.

The first AAMA president was Maxine Williams. Williams
was a strong advocate for medical assisting. In 1959, she donated $200 of her own money to begin a fund to help needy
students pursue their goal of becoming medical assistants. This
fund, which still exists today, is called the Maxine Williams
Scholarship Fund.

In 1978, the U.S. Department of Education followed suit
of the **AMA** and recognized medical assisting as a profession.
In 1991, the AAMA approved the current definition of medical assisting as, "... an allied health profession whose practitioners function as members of the health care delivery team
and perform administrative and clinical procedures" (AAMA,
2007). Table 2-1 lists other AAMA milestones.

Today, medical assistants of both sexes are well trained,
valuable members of the health care team (Figure 2-1 ◆).

TABLE 2-1 HISTORY OF THE AAMA

Year	Event
1961	Establishes certifying board.
1962	Offers sample exam.
1963	Holds first exams.
1977	Engages National Board of Medical Examiners as a test consultant.
1978	Gives exam in January and June at nationwide centers.
1980	Allows medical assistants to recertify via continuing education or exam.
1998	Requires exam candidates to complete medical assisting programs accredited by the Commission on Accreditation of Allied Health Education Programs (CAAHEP).
1999	Makes graduates of medical assisting programs accredited by the Accrediting Bureau of Health Education Schools eligible for the exam.
2002	Places certified medical assistant pin in space aboard a NASA shuttle.
2003	Renders recertification mandatory for certified medical assisting credential; adds October exam.
2005	Makes health care provider–level cardiopulmonary resuscitation mandatory to maintaining medical assisting certification.

Source: American Association for Medical Assistants: www.aama-ntl.org.

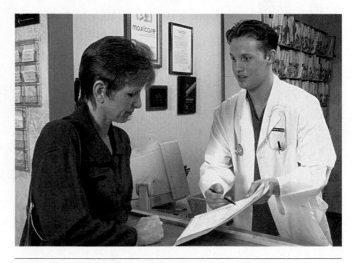

Figure 2-1 ◆ A medical assistant goes over paperwork with a
patient.

General, Clinical, and Administrative Skills* of the CMA (AAMA)

General Skills

◆ Communication
- Recognize and respect cultural diversity
- Adapt communications to individual's understanding
- Employ professional telephone and interpersonal techniques
- Recognize and respond effectively to verbal, nonverbal, and written communications
- Utilize and apply medical terminology appropriately
- Receive, organize, prioritize, store, and maintain transmittable information utilizing electronic technology
- Serve as "communication liaison" between the physician and patient
- Serve as patient advocate professional and health coach in a team approach in health care
- Identify basics of office emergency preparedness

◆ Legal Concepts
- Perform within legal (including federal and state statutes, regulations, opinions, and rulings) and ethical boundaries
- Document patient communication and clinical treatments accurately and appropriately
- Maintain medical records
- Follow employer's established policies dealing with the health care contract
- Comply with established risk management and safety procedures
- Recognize professional credentialing criteria
- Identify and respond to issues of confidentiality

◆ Instruction
- Function as a health care advocate to meet individual's needs
- Educate individuals in office policies and procedures
- Educate the patient within the scope of practice and as directed by supervising physician in health maintenance, disease prevention, and compliance with patient's treatment plan
- Identify community resources for health maintenance and disease prevention to meet individual patient needs
- Maintain current list of community resources, including those for emergency preparedness and other patient care needs
- Collaborate with local community resources for emergency preparedness
- Educate patients in their responsibilities relating to third-party reimbursements

◆ Operational Functions
- Perform inventory of supplies and equipment
- Perform routine maintenance of administrative and clinical equipment
- Apply computer and other electronic equipment techniques to support office operations
- Perform methods of quality control

Clinical Skills

◆ Fundamental Principles
- Identify the roles and responsibilities of the medical assistant in the clinical setting
- Identify the roles and responsibilities of other team members in the medical office
- Apply principles of aseptic technique and infection control
- Practice Standard Precautions, including handwashing and disposal of biohazardous materials
- Perform sterilization techniques
- Comply with quality assurance practices

◆ Diagnostic Procedures
- Collect and process specimens
- Perform CLIA-waived tests
- Perform electrocardiography and respiratory testing
- Perform phlebotomy, including venipuncture and capillary puncture
- Utilize knowledge of principles of radiology

◆ Patient Care
- Perform initial-response screening following protocols approved by supervising physician
- Obtain, evaluate, and record patient history employing critical thinking skills
- Obtain vital signs
- Prepare and maintain examination and treatment areas
- Prepare patient for examinations, procedures and treatments
- Assist with examinations, procedures, and treatments
- Maintain examination/treatment rooms, including inventory of supplies and equipment
- Prepare and administer oral and parenteral (excluding IV) medications and immunizations (as directed by supervising physician and as permitted by state law)
- Utilize knowledge of principles of IV therapy
- Maintain medication and immunization records
- Screen and follow up test results
- Recognize and respond to emergencies

Administrative Skills

◆ Administrative Procedures
- Schedule, coordinate, and monitor appointments
- Schedule inpatient/outpatient admissions and procedures
- Apply third-party and managed care policies, procedures, and guidelines
- Establish, organize, and maintain patient medical record
- File medical records appropriately

◆ Practice Finances
- Perform procedural and diagnostic coding for reimbursement
- Perform billing and collection procedures
- Perform administrative functions, including book-keeping and financial procedures
- Prepare submittable ("clean") insurance forms

Figure 2-2 ◆ General, clinical, and administrative skills of the CMA (AAMA).

*All skills require decision making based on critical thinking concepts.
Reprinted by permission of The American Association of Medical Assistants.

20

—Critical Thinking Question 2-1—

Referring to the case study at the beginning of the chapter, what evidence supports the argument that medical assistants should have a standardized base of knowledge?

In Practice

In coming years, the scope of medical assisting will expand to meet the needs of an aging population and to fill a continued nursing shortage. As it does, new graduates will acquire new skills. How will current medical assistants keep their skills up to date? What resources can assistants use to further their training?

Education Requirements of the Medical Assistant

Vocational programs, **technical educational programs**, and **community colleges** all offer medical-assisting education. Programs take from 6 months to 2 years to complete. Many 2-year programs award **associate degrees** as well as medical assisting certificates.

Medical Assisting Accreditation

Medical assisting programs are **accredited** by one of two associations: (1) **Commission of Accreditation of Allied Health Education Programs (CAAHEP)** or (2) **Accrediting Bureau of Health Education Schools (ABHES)**. The AAMA curriculum review board approves the work of both agencies. As of 2002, the CAAHEP had accredited roughly 500 medical assisting programs in the United States, while the ABHES had accredited another 170.

—Critical Thinking Question 2-2 —

Why do medical assistants who have completed accredited programs have more health care knowledge than those lacking formal training?

Accredited medical-assisting programs must teach in all areas of the AAMA Occupational Analysis Grid, which lists medical-assisting competencies for graduation, including those in the administrative, clinical, and general areas (Figure 2-2 ◆). The AAMA composes the Occupational Analysis Grid by randomly and periodically surveying medical assistants nationwide to determine their job duties.

Achieving Certified or Registered Medical Assistant Status

Medical assisting certification or registration is voluntary, but the AAMA strongly encourages it as a means of guaranteeing competency. Many physicians require medical assistants to have

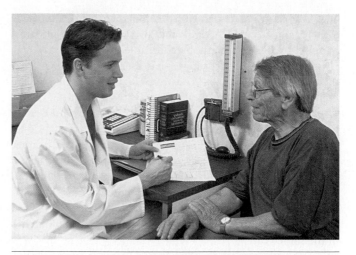

Figure 2-3 ◆ Certification or registration means medical assistants have educations that render them able to behave legally and ethically.

certification or registration as a condition of employment, in part because many malpractice insurance carriers offer discounts to physicians who employ only certified or registered medical assistants. Certification or registration means medical assistants have trained to a standard required by the AAMA, which implies they have educations that render them able to behave legally and ethically and help avoid patient injuries as well as breaches of patient confidentiality (Figure 2-3 ◆). Figure 2-4 ◆ outlines the Medical Assistant's Creed.

—Critical Thinking Question 2-3—

How do certification or registration discounts on physicians' medical malpractice insurance policies impact job opportunities for medical assistants?

As of January 5, 2009, the CMA (AAMA) Certification Examination began to be offered via computer-based testing. Candidates are able to select locations and flexible testing times at conveniently located computer-based testing centers throughout the United States.

The exam fee for the computer-based test is $125 for CAAHEP and ABHES graduating students, recent CAAHEP

I believe in the principles and purposes of the profession of medical assisting.

I endeavor to be more effective.

I aspire to render greater service.

I protect the confidence entrusted to me.

I am dedicated to the care and well-being of all patients.

I am loyal to my physician-employer.

I am true to the ethics of my profession.

I am strengthened by compassion, courage, and faith.

Figure 2-4 ◆ Medical Assistant's Creed

and ABHES graduates, and AAMA members. The exam fee is $250 for non-recent CAAHEP and ABHES graduates and non-members. Exam fees are non-refundable.

After taking the computer-based exam, preliminary immediate pass/fail results will be provided. Official scores will be mailed within five to six weeks directly to candidates.

The CMA (AAMA) Certification/Recertification Examination is currently offered three times a year in January, June, and October through 2008. Eligible candidates can take it either on the last Friday in January, the last Saturday in June, or the fourth Friday in October. This is a pencil and paper examination.

The application deadline for the January exam is October 1 of the preceding year.

The application deadline for the June exam is March 1 of the same year.

The application deadline for the October exam is July 1 of the same year. *The October 24, 2008 examination will be the last pencil and paper examination to be administered.*

Beginning in January 2009, the CMA (AAMA) Certification/Recertification Examination will be computer-based. A pencil and paper examination will no longer be offered. The deadline to apply for the January 2009 examination is August 1, 2008.

The AAMA will inform the applicant of application status within 75 days after the application postmark deadline. Applicants also can inquire about enrollment status via e-mail <mailto:info@aama-ntl.org>. It is important to include the following information in the e-mail:

- Your name
- Your graduation date
- Your accreditation code
- OR
- Your school name, school city and school state.

In addition to applying for the exam, applicants must pay a fee and provide appropriate documentation. AAMA members and CAAHEP program graduates both enjoy significant enrollment fee discounts. Documentation requirements depend on the applicant's enrollment category. Applicants fall into one of the two following categories:

- 1—Graduating student or recent graduate of a CAAHEP or an ABHES accredited medical assisting program.
- 2—Nonrecent graduate of a CAAHEP or an ABHES accredited medical assisting program.

Since 1998, applicants for the Certification Examination for Medical Assistants have been required to complete accredited medical assisting programs that include classes in clinical

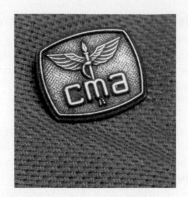

Figure 2-5 ◆ CMA (AAMA) pin.
Reprinted by permission of American Association of Medical Assistants (AAMA).

and administrative competencies (Table 2-3) and end with a required **externship** of a minimum number of hours.

Externships involve working as a medical assistant under a physician's supervision. Externships can run anywhere from 60 to 240 hours, but many medical-assisting programs require externships of more than 240 hours. While externships are unpaid, students earn credits toward their medical assisting certificates.

After taking the certification examination, applicants can wait up to 12 weeks to receive their scores. Students who complete accredited programs and pass the Certification Examination for Medical Assistants earn the title of **certified medical assistant (CMA)** (AAMA) (Figure 2-5 ◆). Those who fail the exam may take it the next time it is offered.

?—Critical Thinking Question 2-4—

How could Carrie explain to Karla how an externship supports the educational goals of an accredited medical-assisting program?

HIPAA Compliance

All accredited medical-assisting programs include training on Health Insurance Portability and Accountability Act (**HIPAA**) regulations. HIPAA is critical for all health care professionals, because it provides a roadmap to avoiding patient-safety errors and malpractice lawsuits through vigilance to patient privacy. ∞ Chapter 4 details HIPAA and its implications for the medical assistant.

TABLE 2-3 SAMPLE ACCREDITED MEDICAL ASSISTING CLASSES

Medical terminology	Medical law and ethics	Clinical surgical skills
Phlebotomy skills	Introduction to pharmacology	Clinical ambulatory skills
Intercultural communications	Administrative and office management skills	Medical billing and coding
Medical practice finances	Computer applications in the medical office	Anatomy and physiology
Medication administration	Disease and pathology	Cardiopulmonary resuscitation (**CPR**) and first
Clinical laboratory skills	Patient relations	aid skills
		Externship

TABLE 2-4 RMA EXAMINATION CONTENT OUTLINE		
General Medical Assisting Knowledge *(41 percent of exam)*	**Administrative Medical Assisting** *(24 percent of exam)*	**Clinical Medical Assisting** *(35 percent of exam)*
Anatomy and physiology Medical terminology Medical law Medical ethics Human relations Patient education	Insurance knowledge Financial aptitude and bookkeeping Medical receptionist/secretarial/clerical skills	Asepsis Sterilization Instruments Vital signs and mensurations Physical examinations Clinical pharmacology Minor surgery Therapeutic modalities Laboratory procedures Electrocardiography First aid

Recertifying in Medical Assisting

To maintain CMA (AAMA) status, medical assistants must complete **recertification** every 5 years. They can retake the Certification Examination for Medical Assistants or acquire 60 continuing education units (**CEUs**) in administrative, clinical, or general categories by attending informational seminars or lectures. Recertification via CEU is discounted for AAMA members.

Becoming a Registered Medical Assistant

Another medical-assisting credential, this one received through the **American Medical Technologists (AMT)** agency, is **registered medical assistant (RMA)** (AMT). Since 1972, assistants can earn RMA (AMT) status by taking a voluntary certification exam that today is given on paper or electronically. Table 2-4 outlines the exam's content.

To sit for the RMA (AMT) certification exam, a medical assistant must meet one of the following requirements:

1. Graduation from a:
   - Medical assistant program accredited by the ABHES or CAAHEP
   or
   - Medical assistant program with institutional accreditation by a regional or national accrediting commission that is approved by the U.S. Department of Education and that includes at least 720 hours of training in medical assisting skills and a clinical externship
   or
   - Formal medical services training program of the U.S. Armed Forces

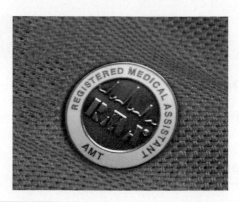

Figure 2-6 ◆ RMA (AMT) pin.
Reprinted by permission of American Medical Technologists (AMT).

2. At least 5 years of medical-assisting employment experience, no more than two of which may have been as an instructor in a medical-assistant program

In addition to one of the preceding requirements, applicants must also be:

- Of good moral character
- At least 18 years old
- A graduate of an accredited high school or acceptable equivalent

In paper format, the RMA (AMT) exam is available at least four times a year, depending on exam location. The electronic version is available every day of the year, except Sundays and holidays, at over 200 locations in the United States and Canada. In the electronic version, scores appear on the screen moments after students complete the exam. With the paper version, notification can be expected within 4 weeks.

Applicants who pass the exam earn the RMA (AMT) distinction (Figure 2-6 ◆). Those who fail can retake the exam 90 days after their initial attempts. The AMT has no formal recertification requirement.

Gaining Multiple Medical-Assisting Statuses

Medical assistants who are certified by both the AAMA and the AMT can use both CMA (AAMA) and RMA (AMT) credentials. Both CMAs (AAMA) and RMAs (AMT) are encouraged to join their local, state, and federal professional organizations. Although these organizations require fees to join, they help medical assistants maintain the skills needed in today's competitive job market through such benefits as:

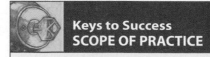

Keys to Success
SCOPE OF PRACTICE

Each state's Health Department outlines the exact scope of practice for medical assisting in that state.

PROCEDURE 2-1 Adapt to Change

Theory and Rationale

Because physicians, supervisors, or office managers will often ask medical assistants to start a new task, it is crucial for medical assistants to adapt efficiently and effectively to changing priorities.

Materials

- Notepad
- Pen

Competency

(**Conditions**) With the necessary materials, you will be able to (**Task**) adapt to change when given a new task (**Standards**) within the time limit set by the instructor.

1. Listen closely as a new task is requested.
2. Ask questions to clarify the request, if needed.
3. Take notes about the task, if needed.
4. Begin working on the new task while maintaining a positive and professional attitude.

- Educational presentations that offer CEUs
- Access to information on upcoming legislation related to the profession
- Subscription to professional journals
- Group insurance plans
- Professional malpractice insurance policies
- Networking opportunities

The Medical Assistant's Scope of Practice

Each state dictates the **scope of practice** for medical assisting. To practice according to local laws, medical assistants must know, and stay on top of, the legal parameters in their state.

Currently, medical assistants must work under the direction and supervision of physicians, nurse practitioners (**NP**s), or physician assistants (**PA**s). In coming years, the scope of practice in medical assisting is expected to grow. While medical assisting is not currently a licensed profession, that may change. Table 2-5 compares licensed, certified, and registered statuses.

Patient Education

It is important for patients to understand the knowledge, skills, and scope of practice of all health care professionals, including the medical assistant. When patients incorrectly identify the medical assistant as a nurse, they should be politely corrected so they understand the medical assistant's role. For example, the medical assistant might say, "I am Dr. Smith's medical assistant. I have different skills from a nurse, and we perform different duties in the physician's office."

The Requirements of Other Allied Health Associations

Health care is a very diverse community of professionals who work together as a team to care for patients. Allied health professionals have industry-specific associations; some have certification or registration exams. Postname initials indicate a professional's certification or registration status.

The American Medical Technologists (AMT)

In addition to the RMA (AMT) certification discussed previously, the AMT (Figure 2-7 ◆) offers certification or registration as medical technologist (**MT**), medical laboratory

TABLE 2-5 COMPARING LICENSED, CERTIFIED, AND REGISTERED STATUSES

Licensed	Certified	Registered
Usually pertains to a profession or occupation with a licensing requirement (e.g., licensed practical nurse [**LPN**]).	Usually pertains to a profession or occupation with a voluntary certification option (e.g., CMA (AAMA)).	May pertain to a profession or occupation with a registration requirement (e.g., RN); may also pertain to a profession or occupation with a voluntary registration option (e.g., RMA (AMT)).

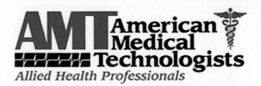

Figure 2-7 ◆ Logo for the American Medical Technologists Association (AMT).
Reprinted by permission.

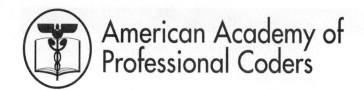

Figure 2-8 ◆ Logo for the American Academy of Professional Coders (AAPC).
Reprinted by permission.

technician (**MLT**), certified office laboratory technician (**COLT**), certified laboratory consultant (**CLC**), certified medical administrative specialist (**CMAS**), and registered phlebotomy technician (**RPT**).

The American Academy of Professional Coders (AAPC)

The American Academy of Professional Coders (**AAPC**) (Figure 2-8 ◆) is an organization for professionals focusing on medical billing and coding. The AAPC offers a voluntary credentialing program with examinations that confer certified professional coder (**CPC**) status.

The American Health Information Management Association (AHIMA)

The American Health Information Management Association (**AHIMA**) is a national organization of professionals who work in the field of medical records, coding, and health information

management. This group was founded in 1928 to improve the quality of medical records. Currently, it is working to educate its membership on the changes required as health care records move toward becoming electronic.

The Association for Healthcare Documentation Integrity

In 1978, The Association for Healthcare Documentation Integrity (AHDI) was established as part of an effort to achieve recognition for the medical transcription profession. AHDI sets standards of education and practice for the medical transcription profession, and offers a voluntary certification exam to individuals who wish to become Certified Medical Transcriptionists (CMTs). The **CMT** credential is awarded upon successfully passing the AHDI certification examination for medical transcriptionists (Figure 2-9 ◆)

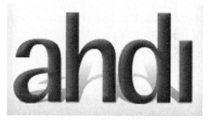

Figure 2-9 ◆ Logo for the Association for Healthcare Documentation Integrity.
Reprinted by permission.

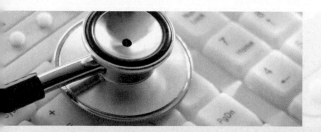

REVIEW

Chapter Summary

- The medical assisting profession has a long history of advocating for the patient in the medical office.
- Types of certifications and registrations in the field dictate the educational requirements of medical assisting.
- Medical-assisting certification or registration can help the medical assistant stay abreast of industry developments and maintain the skills needed to remain competitive in the workplace.

- Like certification and registration, professional organizations offer a number of benefits aimed at keeping the medical assistant optimally efficient and effective.
- The scope of medical-assisting practice is expected to continue to grow and change.
- Medical assisting is just one allied health profession that has created organizations to keep its members aligned and active.

Chapter Review

Multiple Choice

1. The certification examination is offered through the AAMA _____ time(s) each year.
   a. 1
   b. 2
   c. 3
   d. 4

2. To recertify as CMAs (AAMA), medical assistants must:
   a. obtain 60 hours of CEUs within 5 years
   b. retake the Certification Examination for Medical Assistants
   c. obtain permission from their employers
   d. A or B

3. The first president of the AAMA was:
   a. Elizabeth Blackwell
   b. Maxine Williams
   c. Clara Barton
   d. none of the above

4. In what year did the U.S. Department of Education recognize medical assisting as a profession?
   a. 1958
   b. 1968
   c. 1978
   d. 1988

5. Medical assistants must work under the direction of:
   a. physicians
   b. nurse practitioners
   c. physician assistants
   d. all of the above

6. The AMT offers certification or registration to which of the following groups of professionals?
   a. CMAs (AAMA)
   b. CMAS
   c. CPCs
   d. All of the above

7. The term *certified* usually refers to professions that offer which type of certification?
   a. Voluntary
   b. Required
   c. Licensed
   d. None of the above

True/False

T F 1. Accredited medical-assisting programs must include externships.

T F 2. Malpractice insurance carriers may offer discounts to physicians who hire only certified or registered medical assistants.

T F 3. The scope of medical-assisting practice varies from state to state.

T F 4. One requirement of the AMT RMA examination is to be at least 21 years of age.

T F 5. Certification or registration signals that the medical assistant has been trained to a certain standard.

T F 6. AHIMA focuses mainly on the area of medical records, billing, and coding.

T F 7. The term *licensed* usually refers to a profession that is *required* to be licensed.

Short Answer

1. Name the types of education facilities that may offer accredited medical-assisting programs.

2. What are the benefits of professional medical-assisting organizations?

Chapter Review (continued)

3. What is the purpose of the role delineation chart?

4. Which two agencies accredit medical-assisting programs?

5. Why is the scope of medical-assisting practice soon expected to grow?

6. Why is it important to correct patients who misidentify medical assistants?

Research

1. Where does your local medical assisting association meet?

2. How would you go about becoming a member of your local medical assisting group?

3. What is the scope of practice of a medical assistant in your state?

Externship Application Experience

A patient at the externship site asks the medical assistant to differentiate between a nurse and a medical assistant. How should the medical assistant respond?

Resource Guide

American Academy of Professional Coders
2480 South 3850 West, Suite B
Salt Lake City, UT 84120
Phone: 800-626-2633
Fax: 801-236-2258
e-mail: info@aapc.com, www.aapc.com

American Association of Medical Assistants
20 N. Wacker Dr., Ste. 1575
Chicago, IL 60606
Phone: (312) 899-1500
Fax: (312) 899-1259
www.aama-ntl.org

American Association of Medical Transcription
4230 Kiernan Avenue, Suite 130
Modesto, CA 95356
Phone: (800) 982-2182
Fax: (209) 527-9633
e-mail: www.aamt.org

American Health Information Management Association
233 N. Michigan Avenue, 21st Floor
Chicago, IL 60601-5800
Phone: (312) 233-1100
Fax: (312) 233-1090
e-mail: info@ahima.org, www.ahima.org

American Medical Technologists
10700 West Higgins Road, Suite 150
Rosemont, IL 60018
Phone: (800) 275-1268
Fax: (847) 823-0458
www.amt1.com

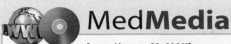

MedMedia

http://www.MyMAKit.com

More on this chapter, including interactive resources, can be found on the Student CD-ROM accompanying this textbook and on http://www.MyMAKit.com.

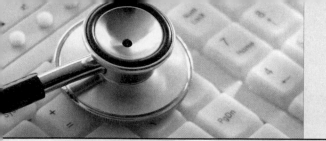

Objectives

After completing this chapter, you should be able to:

- Define and spell the key terminology in this chapter.
- List the qualities of a good medical assistant.
- Describe the proper attire of a medical assistant.
- List techniques for improving time-management skills.
- List career opportunities for the medical assistant.
- Define the jobs of other members of the health care team and their education requirements.
- Define various medical practice specializations.
- Outline the scope of complementary alternative medicine.

The Medical Assisting Career: Roles and Responsibilities

Case Study

William Johanson is a patient of Dr. Chan's. Because the medical assistant is responsible for arranging specialist referrals for patients, Dr. Chan has asked the medical assistant to arrange for Mr. Johanson to see a podiatrist and an ophthalmologist as part of his diabetes care plan. Mr. Johanson is unsure what those specialists do.

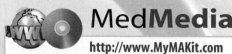

MedMedia

http://www.MyMAKit.com

Additional interactive resources and activities for this chapter can be found on http://www.MyMAKit.com. For a video, tips, audio glossary, legal and ethical scenarios, on-the-job scenarios, quizzes, and games related to the content of this chapter, please access the accompanying CD-ROM in this book.

Video: *Patient Care*
Legal and Ethical Scenario: *Your Career as a Medical Assistant: Roles and Responsibilities*
On the Job Scenario: *Your Career as a Medical Assistant: Roles and Responsibilities Tips*
Multiple Choice Quiz
Audio Glossary
HIPAA Quiz
Games: Spelling Bee, Crossword, and Strikeout

Key Terminology

accredited—endorsed by a reputable organization

administrative skills—clerical-type jobs (e.g., typing, filing)

advocate—one who defends or acts on behalf of another

ambulatory care centers—health care clinics where patients are seen for short visits

attitude—state of mind; way of carrying one's self

body language—nonverbal means of communication (e.g., gestures, expressions)

clinical skills—abilities gained through hands-on patient care

confidentiality—state of privacy or secrecy

courtesy—polite behavior

credibility—quality of inspiring belief

dependability—capable of being relied on

empathy—ability to identify with and understand another person's feelings

flexibility—willingness to change when needed or requested

initiative—energy or aptitude displayed in starting a task without prompting

loyalty—devotion to another

multidisciplinary—combining many fields of study

rapport—trust and affection between parties

respect—to hold in high esteem

Abbreviations

ACPE—Accreditation Council for Pharmacy Education

ADN—associate degree in nursing

AMA—American Medical Association

BSN—bachelor of science degree in nursing

CAM—complementary alternative medicine

DEA—Drug Enforcement Agency

DME—durable medical equipment

FDA—Federal Drug Administration

HIPAA—Health Insurance Portability and Accountability Act

LPN—licensed practical nurse

LVN—licensed vocational nurse

✛ MEDICAL ASSISTING STANDARDS

CAAHEP ENTRY-LEVEL STANDARDS	ABHES ENTRY-LEVEL COMPETENCIES
■ Differentiate between legal, ethical, and moral issues affecting healthcare (cognitive) ■ Identify the role of self boundaries in the health care environment (cognitive) ■ Recognize the role of patient advocacy in the practice of medical assisting (cognitive) ■ Identify time management principles (cognitive) ■ Discuss legal scope of practice for medical assistants (cognitive) ■ Explore issue of confidentiality as it applies to the medical assistant (cognitive) ■ Discuss licensure and certification as it applies to healthcare providers (cognitive) ■ Report relevant information to others succinctly and accurately (psychomotor) ■ Explain general office policies (psychomotor) ■ Document patient care (psychomotor) ■ Document patient education (psychomotor) ■ Advocate on behalf of patients (psychomotor) ■ Respond to issues of confidentiality (psychomotor) ■ Perform within scope of practice (psychomotor) ■ Apply ethical behaviors, including honesty/integrity in performance of medical assisting practice (affective) ■ Examine the impact personal ethics and morals may have on the individual's practice (affective) ■ Demonstrate awareness of diversity in providing patient care (affective) ■ Demonstrate empathy in communicating with patients, family, and staff (affective)	■ Adapt to change. ■ Project a positive attitude. ■ Be cognizant of ethical boundaries. ■ Evidence a responsible attitude. ■ Conduct work within scope of education, training, and ability. ■ Professional components. ■ Exercise efficient time management. ■ Allied health professions and credentialing. ■ Be a team player. ■ Exhibit initiative.

Introduction

Medical assistants, along with physicians, pharmacists, nurses, and other staff, work as part of a health care team that cares for patients. Some patients receive care from multiple specialists, while others see only single primary care physicians. To be most effective, medical assistants must practice the art of listening to patients and relay information effectively between patients and all other members of the health care team.

Abbreviations *(continued)*

MPJE—Multistate Pharmacy
Jurisprudence Exam
NAPLEX—North American Pharmacist
Licensure Exam

NP—nurse practitioner
OTC—over the counter

PA—physician assistant
RN—registered nurse

Choosing Medical Assisting as a Career

Because medical assisting today is a career with multiple responsibilities, it requires a set of unique qualities.

Understanding Medical Assisting Responsibilities

As mentioned earlier, the medical assistant helps the physician on the health care team provide patient care. To help keep patients safe, the medical assistant must practice good **clinical skills,** which include taking vital signs, collecting specimens, and administering medications and immunizations. Specific clinical duties for the medical assistant depend on the scope of practice in the state where the medical assistant is employed.

While patient care is part of medical assisting, the medical assistant's main responsibility is to be the patient's **advocate.** Because medical assistants will likely spend more time with patients than the physicians, medical assistants must develop a **rapport** with patients. Patients must be able to trust medical assistants, because those patients are more likely to share their personal information with assistants they trust. Patients may feel uncomfortable sharing their personal information with physicians, especially physicians they do not trust (Figure 3-1 ◆).

?— Critical Thinking Question 3-1—

Referring to the case study at the beginning of the chapter, why is the process of building trust with Mr. Johanson an important part of patient advocacy? In what way can the medical assistant in the case study gain Mr. Johanson's trust?

In addition to clinical skills, medical assistants are responsible for performing **administrative skills,** such as appointment scheduling for physicians and insurance processing. The types of administrative duties medical assistants perform depend on the type and size of practice, as well as the assistants' preferences. Assistants may choose to apply for positions that have responsibilities weighted in the clerical or clinical arenas. In small clinics, medical assistants often perform both administrative and clinical functions. In large offices, job duties are often more specialized. Medical assistants in these offices may work in the clinical or administrative areas exclusively (Figure 3-2 ◆).

Identifying Positive Medical Assisting Qualities

To be highly valued in today's competitive job market, medical assistants should have good clinical and administrative skills. The most sought-after assistants can perform varied duties in

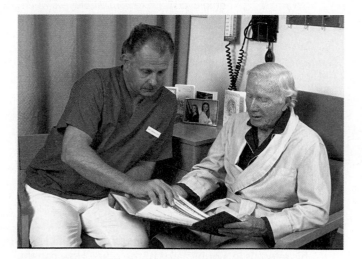

Figure 3-1 ◆ Medical assistants must develop a rapport with patients.

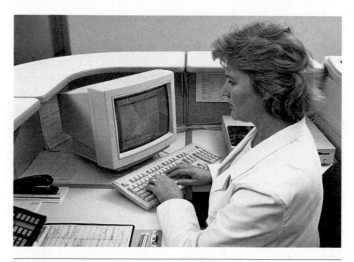

Figure 3-2 ◆ This medical assistant's responsibilities are weighted in the clerical arena.

the medical office, applying their skills where those skills are needed most. To ensure they gain the proper skills, medical assistants should complete **accredited** programs. They should have a good understanding of medical terminology, and they should be well versed in the scope of their professional duties.

In addition to the proper background and training, good medical assistants have sound interpersonal skills. For a list of some desired qualities, see Table 3-1. Because many patients will stop seeing physicians when they feel uncomfortable with the office staff, patients should always feel welcome and cared for in the medical office. Good medical assistants remember patients' names. It helps make patients feel important and builds patient rapport.

In Practice

A new patient in town, Isaiah Rodriguez, arrives at the office needing a physician. According to Isaiah, his last physician had an unpleasant receptionist. Isaiah tells the medical assistant, "If I didn't like my doctor so much, I would have found another one." He adds that the person who answered his call for this appointment seemed like she was in a hurry. How should the medical assistant handle this situation? What can the medical assistant say to Isaiah? Should the medical assistant bring the situation to the doctor's attention? Why or why not?

Effective medical assistants communicate well with patients as well as with other members of the health care team. Medical assistants should have **empathy** for others, and they should be comfortable in their role as patient advocates. In a country as diverse as the United States, good medical assistants know the prevailing cultural customs in their areas and can keep their personal beliefs separate from patient care. Good medical assistants also maintain patient confidentiality, disclosing personal patient information only when directed to do so by a patient or a court order.

Living and working in the same community can pose special challenges for health care staff who work with private patient information. Medical assistants know confidential patient information and are obligated by the Health Insurance Portability and Accountability Act (**HIPAA**), as well as ethical considerations, to keep that information private. In small communities, patients may ask about other patients outside the office. Medical assistants should never breach patient privacy, whatever the setting.

HIPAA Compliance

The Health Insurance Portability and Accountability Act (HIPAA) requires that medical assistants carefully guard patient confidentiality. Medical assistants should never release patient information without a patient's written authorization or a court order.

TABLE 3-1 DESIRABLE MEDICAL ASSISTING QUALITIES

Quality	Explanation
Loyalty	■ Being faithful to one's employer, performing to the best of one's abilities, and arriving to work on time and ready to perform the job. Loyalty is staying with an employer through good days and bad.
Respect	■ Treating coworkers and patients with honor. Staff should demonstrate respect for physicians by using the title "Doctor" in front of patients, and doctors should show respect for their staff in return. Any corrective comments or disciplinary action should occur in private.
Dependability	■ Completing tasks on time and to the best of one's abilities. Dependability is arriving to work on time and staying to the end of the assigned shift. Late arrivals and frequent cancellations disrupt the whole office. Emergencies do happen, but dependable employees can generally be counted on to arrive and work when scheduled.
Courtesy	■ Extending kind words and compassion to patients and coworkers. Professional words and actions demonstrate courtesy.
Initiative	■ Taking action without being asked. A person with initiative knows what needs to be done and does it.
Flexibility	■ Willingness to exceed the job description whenever needed by changing one's schedule, if needed, or replacing someone who cannot work. Flexibility is the willingness to work late when the physician is running late and patients are still in the office. This is the ultimate sign of teamwork.
Credibility	■ Trustworthiness. Credibility is the feeling employers have toward employees when those employees have demonstrated that they are open and honest in their communications and actions.
Confidentiality	■ Ability to keep patient information private, to avoid sharing that information with inappropriate parties, like coworkers or neighbors.
Attitude	■ Overall approach. Positive attitudes foster positive work environments, while poor attitudes cultivate poor ones.

?— Critical Thinking Question 3-2—

Imagine Mr. Johanson asks the medical assistant about his referrals in a public area of the office. How can the medical assistant best answer Mr. Johanson's questions while maintaining the patient's privacy?

**Keys to Success
PATIENT CONFIDENTIALITY**

The job of protecting patient confidentiality extends beyond the work day. Never discuss patients by name outside the office, even when with coworkers. Always imagine that the patients, or people who know them, can hear the conversation. Imagine how breaching patient confidentiality would affect you and the physician.

TABLE 3-2 BODY LANGUAGE IN DIFFERENT CULTURES	
Culture	**Examples**
Asian-Pacific	■ An open mouth, as when yawning, is considered rude. ■ Smiling can mean happiness, anger, confusion, or sadness. ■ Pointing with fingers is considered rude.
Chinese	■ Being physically intimidating, especially with an older person, is considered very rude. ■ Pointing is appropriate with an open hand, not just one finger.
Japanese	■ Bowing is a traditional greeting. ■ Staring is considered rude. ■ Standing with the hands in pockets is considered rude. ■ The "OK" symbol, the thumb and forefinger joined in a circle, may be interpreted as the signal for money.
Korean	■ Prolonged direct eye contact is considered rude. ■ Entering a room without knocking is considered rude. ■ Spitting and burping in public is acceptable.
Filipino	■ Hugging upon first meeting is acceptable. ■ Greetings include raised eyebrows. ■ Staring is considered rude.
Arabic	■ Failing to face a person while speaking is considered rude. ■ Men stand when women enter a room. ■ Men may shake hands with women only when the women offer their hands. ■ Only the right hand is used for eating.
Hispanic	■ Pointing with the index finger has a sexual meaning. ■ Standing closely together is appropriate.

Like ethical behavior, a professional image is a critical part of medical assisting. Medical assistants are often patients' first contact with the office, and their behavior and appearance directly reflect the office and the physicians. Demonstrating professionalism means avoiding eating, drinking, and chewing gum while working or in patient view and maintaining a professional attitude. Part of maintaining a professional attitude includes remaining calm and polite and preventing patients from sensing any stress or irritation. Good medical assistants keep their personal feelings to themselves, never indicating disagreement with patients' health care or lifestyle choices. **Body language**, like facial expressions, may indicate disapproval. (Table 3-2) provides examples of body language in different cultures.

— Critical Thinking Question 3-3—
Imagine Dr. Chan is referring Mr. Johanson to a podiatrist the medical assistant dislikes. How might the medical assistant disguise his feelings in front of Mr. Johanson?

Good medical assistants give the same level of professional care to all patients, even those who are rude and unpleasant. Good assistants also use proper grammar when communicating with patients, and that means avoiding slang terms or phrases. Patients who speak English as a second language may be unfamiliar with these terms and misinterpret their meanings.

Good personal hygiene, like professional behavior, is part of a professional image. Medical assistants should practice good personal hygiene for their body and their clothing. For example, American Medical Association (**AMA**) studies have shown that artificial nails may harbor bacteria, which is difficult to remove with hand washing. As a result, artificial nails should not be worn on the job. Medical assistants should also avoid wearing excessive or obtrusive jewelry, because hands will be washed and gloves donned several times a day. Body piercings, except for posts in the ear lobes, should not be visible, and tattoos and other body art should be covered during office hours. Hair should be clean and pulled back, and scented lotions and perfumes should be minimized out of respect for patients with allergies.

Uniforms, including shoes, should be clean and in good repair (Figure 3-3 ◆). The medical assistant's nametag should be in plain view and clearly identify the name and role of the medical assistant. Policies for dress, jewelry, hairstyles, piercings, and tattoos will vary from office to office, so medical assistants should review these policies when they are hired.

Understanding the Medical Assistant's Role Outside of the Office

In some ways, health care workers are held to a higher standard than those in many other fields. The medical assistant's professional image is expected to extend beyond the medical office, and the rules of patient confidentiality apply in all environments. When medical assistants work in the communities where they live, they are likely to see patients outside the clinical setting. Medical assistants must remember that they represent the medical office at all times, not just during business hours.

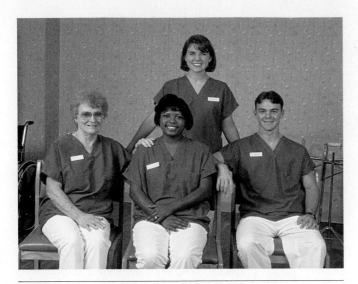

Figure 3-3 ◆ The medical assistant must maintain a professional image.

Keys to Success
MAINTAINING A PROFESSIONAL IMAGE

- **Leave personal problems at home.** As much as possible, avoid bringing personal problems to work. When personal problems become overwhelming, consider taking a day or two off to address them.
- **Avoid office gossip.** Refuse to gossip and spread rumors, because doing so is unproductive and can be harmful. Even when true, office information should be kept confidential. Consider how you would feel if you were the subject of the material.
- **Conduct no personal business during work hours.** Personal business takes time from the employer. Respect your employer's time, and conduct personal business, like telephone calls, during breaks or before or after work. Remember that patients may overhear your conversations, so always act professionally and courteously. When you must make a personal call during business hours, do so from a private room or outside the building.
- **Stay out of office politics.** Avoid office politics, because they are particularly destructive. Do not take credit for coworkers' accomplishments or blame others for your mistakes.
- **Do not procrastinate.** Practice prioritization rather than procrastination. Rank activities so you can complete them in an acceptable time frame. When a project seems too big to handle, try breaking it into smaller pieces or seek help.

Critical Thinking Question 3-4
Referring to the case study at the beginning of the chapter, imagine the medical assistant is leaving the office at the end of his shift when Dr. Chan asks him to schedule the referral for Mr. Johanson. How should the medical assistant handle this situation?

Managing Time Effectively in the Medical Office

In a busy health care setting, demands on the medical assistant's time can seem overwhelming. Depending on the office, one medical assistant may support several physicians. Especially in these situations, it is important for medical assistants to track their job duties and to know who to consult when their priorities conflict.

Good organization is key to medical-office time management. A time-management outline, which prioritizes projects, is one way for medical assistants to manage their time effectively. Writing down tasks is a good habit to develop. On paper, it is easier to divide big projects into smaller tasks or to organize tasks into a workable schedule. List items according to their due dates, and then categorize those items depending on how long they will take to complete. To stay on top of tasks, at the end of each day make a "to-do" list for the following day (Figure 3-4 ◆). Crossing items off the list as they are completed gives a sense of accomplishment and helps to ensure all items are completed.

If these techniques fail to help the medical assistant manage time effectively, try keeping a journal of each activity and the time it takes. Figure 3-5 ◆ lists the steps involved in creating and using such a time-management journal.

It is important for medical assistants to collaborate with their supervisors on time-management initiatives. Office man-

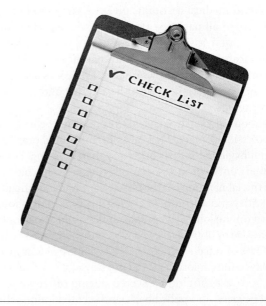

Figure 3-4 ◆ Using a checklist is a good way to stay organized.

1. At the beginning of the work day, place a notepad and pen in the clinic jacket.

2. Each time you perform a task, list the task and the exact time it took from beginning to end.

3. Note any conflicts, such as overlapping requests from supervisors.

4. At the end of the day, analyze the data. Determine if any tasks were unneeded or could be combined. For example, you might be making multiple trips to the file room for patients' charts instead of pulling all charts at the beginning of each shift. You might need data from more than one day to obtain an accurate picture of an average work day.

5. When you find no tasks to omit or combine, schedule a meeting with your supervisor to try to achieve a more efficient workflow.

Figure 3-5 ◆ Steps to Creating and Using a Time-Management Journal

Working in Health Care Today

Health care is constantly changing and growing. As the population ages and the demand for health care continues to rise, more and more patients will seek physicians' care and medical-assisting careers will grow more promising. The U.S. Department of Labor Bureau of Labor Statistics projects medical assisting to be the fastest-growing occupation from 2004 to 2014. According to the U.S. Department of Labor Web site (2006–2007), job prospects ". . . should be best for medical assistants with formal training or experience, particularly those with certification."

The Medical Assistant's Career Opportunities

Medical assistants today can work in a variety of health care specialties or in more administrative capacities, such as in insurance companies. According to the U.S. Department of Labor, 6 out of 10 medical assistants today work in **ambulatory care centers** under the direction of physicians; 14 percent work in public and private hospitals, including inpatient and outpatient facilities; and 11 percent work in the offices of other health practitioners, such as chiropractors, optometrists, and podiatrists. The remaining medical assistants work in public and private educational services, state and local government agencies, employment services, medical and diagnostic laboratories, and nursing care facilities.

Medical assistants earn varying amounts depending on their experience and skill levels and locations. In the United States in 2004, the median annual earnings of medical assistants was $24,610. Table 3-3 lists average medical assistant wages by place of employment.

TABLE 3-3 AVERAGE MEDICAL ASSISTANT EARNINGS (2004)

Place of Employment	Average Earnings
Colleges, universities, and professional schools	$27,490
Outpatient care centers	$25,360
General medical and surgical hospitals	$25,160
Physician offices	$24,930
Offices of other health practitioners	$21,930

Source: U.S. Department of Labor: www.dol.gov (2006–2007).

Members of the Health Care Team

Today's health care team is **multidisciplinary.** Many different types of providers and medical specialists help provide a patient's care. Medical assistants should have a good working knowledge of the types of care these professionals provide so they can accurately relay information to patients when doctors make referrals, as well as direct patients to the appropriate members of the health care team.

Working with Physicians

The term *physician* refers to a medical doctor or doctor of osteopathy. Many people use these terms interchangeably, but generally the term refers to one who practices medicine. Physicians typically head the health care team, directing other medical-office staff. Physicians diagnose and treat patients, as well as refer patients to other members of the health care team (Figure 3-6 ◆).

The Physician's Education Requirements
Medical training for physicians varies around the world, but all physicians must pass a licensure examination to practice medicine in the United States, as well as in whichever states they wish to practice.

In the United States, physicians must first obtain at least a 4-year undergraduate or bachelor's degree, which usually consists of varied premedical courses. After that, they must then attend 4 years of medical school, followed by a residency program. Residency programs usually concentrate on the fields the physicians wish to practice in, such as dermatology or emergency medicine. Residency programs vary from 2 to 6 years.

The Pharmacist's Role

Pharmacists play an important role in patient care. They distribute the drugs prescribed by health care providers and educate patients about the medications they are taking (Figure 3-7 ◆). Some pharmacists work for pharmacies, while others own them. Many large health care facilities including hospitals have pharmacies on their premises, which can be

agers and physicians should strive to keep their employees happy and efficient, and medical assistants who raise concerns about their use of time show that they are responsible members of the health care team.

Binker Physical Therapy LLC

72192 76ᵗʰ Ave. W., Suite 101
Wynnwood, WA 98088

Molly K. Malone PT
Espen Ford OT

Phone: 425-555-9991
Fax: 425-555-9995

Date _____

Patient's Name _____

Diagnosis_____

_____

ICD-9 Codes _____

Requested Treatment _____

☐ Evaluate & Treat

☐ Specific Treatment _____

_____

_____

Frequency: _____ times per week for _____ weeks.

Precautions _____

_____

_____

Physician Re-check Date _____

Physician's signature below constitutes letter of medical necessity.

_____
Physician's Signature

Figure 3-6 ◆ Sample referral form for sending a patient out for physical therapy.

Beth Williams, MD
Windy City Clinic
123 Michigan Avenue
Chicago, IL 60000
Telephone (200) 555-9876

Name _Jane Doe_ Age _56_

Address _____

Date _2/14/xx_

Rx _Estrace 1 mg_

Sig. _i q̄ AM_
Disp. # 100

Substitution Permissible _____ M.D.

"Prescriber must hand-write "Brand Necessary" or "Brand Medically Necessary" in the space below in order for a brand name product to be dispensed." _Brand Necessary_

B Williams M.D.

Refill 0 1 2 ③ 4 5 6

Figure 3-7 ◆ Sample prescription.

American Pharmacist Licensure Exam (**NAPLEX**), which tests pharmacy skills and knowledge. The District of Columbia and 43 of the United States also require pharmacists to pass the Multistate Pharmacy Jurisprudence Exam (**MPJE**), which tests knowledge of pharmacy law.

As of 2004, 89 colleges of pharmacy were accredited in the United States. Pharmacy programs grant the degree of Doctor of Pharmacy (Pharm D), which requires at least 6 years of college, including extensive courses in all aspects of drug therapy.

The Role of the Physician's Assistant

Physician assistants (**PAs**) are clinicians who are licensed to practice medicine under the supervision of a physician or a surgeon. PAs can treat patients, including taking medical histories, performing examinations, interpreting laboratory tests and x-rays, and making diagnoses. PAs will often perform such tasks as suturing, splinting, and casting. In 48 states, PAs can also prescribe medications.

The Physician Assistant's Education Requirements

As of 2006, there were 135 accredited PA programs in the United States. All states require PAs to complete an accredited, formal education program and pass a national exam to obtain a license.

convenient for patients. Some pharmacists work for drug manufacturers researching new medications.

Pharmacists who work in community or retail pharmacies often counsel patients and answer questions about medications, both prescriptions and over-the-counter (**OTC**) medications, including possible side effects or drug interactions. Pharmacists may also advise patients about the use of durable medical equipment (**DME**), diet, exercise, or stress management.

The Pharmacist's Education Requirements

A license to practice pharmacy is required in all 50 of the United States, the District of Columbia, and all U.S. territories. To obtain a license to practice, pharmacists must graduate from a college of pharmacy that is accredited by the Accreditation Council for Pharmacy Education (**ACPE**) and pass an examination. All states require pharmacists to pass the North

PA programs are generally 2 or more years long, and admission requirements vary. Many programs require at least 2 years of college and some health care experience before admission.

The Role of the Nurse Practitioner

Nurse practitioners (**NPs**) provide services similar to those of the PA. The main differences between these two professions are that the NP is also a trained nurse, and NPs require more training than PAs. Most NPs have advanced nursing degrees and many are able to open their own clinical practices, depending on the laws in their states. NPs are also allowed to prescribe medications and have Drug Enforcement Administration (**DEA**) registration numbers in most states. NPs can serve as patients' primary care providers and can see patients of all ages.

The Nurse Practitioner's Education Requirements

To be licensed as NPs, applicants must first complete the education and training needed to be a registered nurse (**RN**). In most states, NPs are also required to have a master's degree in nursing. Once applicants have secured their RN degree, they must complete an advanced nursing education program. Many of these programs specialize in a field like family practice, adult health, acute care, or women's health. NPs must be licensed by the states where they practice.

The Role of the Nurse

Nurses are employed in varied health care settings. Nurses may work in hospitals, with insurance companies, or in home health care settings. In most medical practices today, nurses perform triage roles or help physicians with complex cases (Figure 3-8 ◆). Medical assistants assist the physician in other cases.

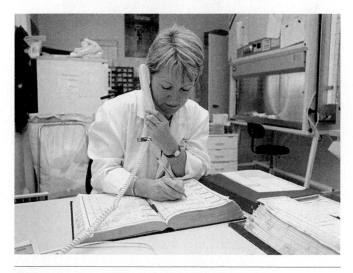

Figure 3-8 ◆ A nurse performing telephone triage.

Education Requirements for Nurses

Unlike the education requirements of many other health care professions, nursing education has many levels. A bachelor degree in nursing (BSN) requires 4 years of education, while an associate degree in nursing (ADN) takes 2 years. RNs may attend programs from 2 to 3 years long. Licensed practical nurses (**LPNs**) normally attend 1-year nursing programs, as do licensed vocational nurses (**LVNs**). The scope of practice for nurses varies from state to state. Typically, nurses with more advanced degrees (e.g., RN or **BSN**) have higher level duties than LPNs or LVNs.

Medical Practice Specializations

Medical and surgical specialties today are varied. Table 3-4 lists several common medical specialties and the services they provide. Table 3-5 outlines several common surgical specialties.

?— Critical Thinking Question 3-5—

Medical assistants are often asked to complete the referral for the physician to such specialists as podiatrists and ophthalmologists. What type of information could the medical assistant keep on hand to help answer patient questions?

Complementary and Alternative Medicine

Complementary and alternative medicine (**CAM**) is another term for holistic or natural medicine. CAM providers treat patients with such alternative practices as chiropractic treatments (Figure 3-9 ◆), acupuncture, naturopathy, massage, biofeedback, hypnosis, and dietary supplements. For examples of these treatments, see Table 3-6.

In the United States, CAM is a $10 billion per year industry. Most of those revenues come directly from patients, not their insurance carriers, because traditional health insurance does not cover many CAM therapies. Medical assistants must alert patients that CAM therapies may not be reimbursed. With any treatment, it is always good to verify a patient's coverage with the insurance carrier.

Because alternate therapies may not be covered by traditional insurance, the CAM industry, especially the dietary supplements industry, is highly competitive for the consumer's dollar. A 2002 survey by the American Medical Association (AMA) found that 36 percent of adults in the United States said they use some form of CAM. Most of those surveyed (54.9 percent) said they use CAM with conventional medicine.

Applying CAM Approaches

Many traditional health care providers recommend or use some CAM techniques with their patients, but CAM health care providers may advise their patients to avoid traditional

TABLE 3-4 COMMON MEDICAL SPECIALTIES

Specialty Type	Service(s) Provided
Allergist	Diagnoses and treats allergic conditions
Cardiologist	Diagnoses and treats heart and cardiovascular system conditions
Dermatologist	Diagnoses and treats skin disorders
Emergency physician	Treats patients with emergent needs, such as in emergency rooms
Endocrinologist	Diagnoses and treats hormone-related disorders
Family practitioner	Acts as a primary care physician for patients of all ages, treating varied illnesses and performing routine screenings (e.g., physical examinations)
Gastroenterologist	Diagnoses and treats disorders related to the stomach and intestines
General practitioner	Same as the family practice physician (see preceding), except may not accept child patients
Gerontologist	Diagnoses and treats conditions of the elderly population
Gynecologist	Diagnoses and treats conditions related to the female reproductive system
Hematologist	Diagnoses and treats conditions associated with blood disorders
Infertility practitioner	Diagnoses and treats disorders related to infertility problems and helps achieve pregnancy via medical means
Intensive care physician	Treats patients in the hospital intensive care unit
Internist	Focuses on the prevention and treatment of adult diseases
Neonatologist	Diagnoses and treats newborns
Nephrologist	Diagnoses and treats conditions associated with the kidneys
Obstetrician	Treats pregnant women through the postpartum period
Oncologist	Diagnoses and treats patients with cancerous conditions
Ophthalmologist	Diagnoses and treats eye conditions
Orthopedist	Diagnoses and treats conditions associated with the musculoskeletal system
Otolaryngologist	Diagnoses and treats conditions associated with the ears, nose, and throat
Pediatrician	Treats children
Podiatrist	Diagnoses and treats feet conditions
Proctologist	Diagnoses and treats conditions associated with the colon, rectum, and anus
Psychiatrist	Diagnoses and treats mental disorders
Pulmonologist	Diagnoses and treats conditions associated with the respiratory system
Radiologist	Interprets radiographs (x-rays) and other imaging studies (e.g., ultrasounds or mammograms)
Rheumatologist	Diagnoses and treats conditions associated with arthritis or other joint disorders
Urologist	Diagnoses and treats conditions associated with the urinary system

TABLE 3-5 COMMON SURGICAL SPECIALTIES

Surgical Specialty Type	Description
Cardiothoracic	Treats chest diseases and heart and lung conditions
Cosmetic	Repairs or reconstructs body parts, either due to accidents or disease or as elective surgery
General	Treats varied surgical cases
Maxillofacial	Repairs face and mouth disorders
Neurological	Repairs disorders of the neurologic system
Orthopedic	Repairs conditions of the musculoskeletal system
Vascular	Repairs conditions of the blood vessels

medicine. Most patients who use CAM do so because they want more natural, drug-free types of treatment. Some patients may wish to pursue some form of CAM while undergoing traditional medical treatment. For example, a patient receiving chemotherapy for cancer may use massage for relaxation and comfort.

Even when an office does not endorse or practice CAM, patients will often ask for advice on treatments or supplements

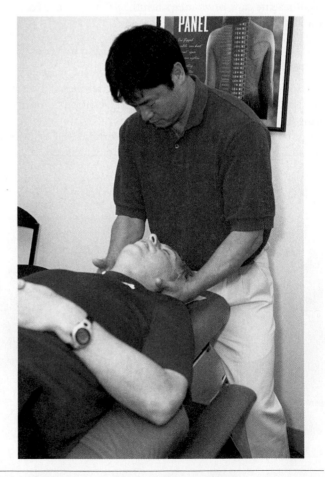

Figure 3-9 ◆ A chiropractor adjusting his patient.

TABLE 3-6 COMPLEMENTARY AND ALTERNATIVE MEDICINE EXAMPLES

Treatment Type	Treatment Objective
Acupressure	Use hand pressure on various body areas to restore balance.
Acupuncture	Insert needles into various body areas to restore balance.
Biofeedback	Teach patients to control their involuntary body responses to treat pain and disease.
Chiropractic	Manipulate the spine and extremities to rectify misalignments, relieve pain, and treat disease.
Dietary supplements	Administer such substances as vitamins, herbs, or minerals, usually by mouth, to promote health and treat certain diseases.
Hypnosis	Induce a trance-like state to access the subconscious mind.
Magnetic therapy	Apply magnets to various body areas to correct the body's energy fields.
Massage	Use touch to relieve pain and encourage muscle relaxation.
Naturopathy	Use nutrition and exercise to promote healing and well-being.
Yoga	Use breathing exercises and poses to encourage relaxation and flexibility.

Keys to Success
DIETARY SUPPLEMENTS

Many patients take dietary supplements in addition to prescribed medications. Because physicians do not prescribe those supplements, patients may fail to mention them when listing their medications. Because some supplements can conflict with medications, be sure to ask patients about any supplements they may be taking when helping those patients complete their medical history forms.

supplements. Products may contain vastly different ingredients, even when they are marketed as the same items.

Given that dietary supplements need not meet standard requirements, the FDA requires that all manufacturers of dietary supplements refrain from stating that their products treat or cure disease. The agency also requires that disclaimers accompany any benefits on product labels. A sample disclaimer might read, "This statement has not been evaluated by the Food and Drug Administration. This product is not intended to diagnose, treat, cure, or prevent disease" (Figure 3-10 ◆).

Because vitamins and minerals are needed in the diet to achieve optimal health, the FDA has established recommended

they have heard about from friends, family, neighbors, or advertisements. As a result, all members of the health care team, including the medical assistant, should have a working knowledge of each of the common CAM therapies.

With Food and Drug Administration (**FDA**) regulations absent from many CAM therapies, patients should always be advised to investigate thoroughly any alternative therapy and discuss that therapy with their physician before starting it. Patients have the right to seek CAM, either with or instead of traditional medicine, so health care workers should respect that right even when it conflicts with their personal beliefs.

The Role of Dietary Supplements

In 1994, Congress passed the Dietary Supplement and Education Act, which defines dietary supplements as products that are:

- Intended to supplement a diet
- Made of one or more dietary ingredient (e.g., vitamins, minerals, or herbs)
- Intended for oral administration
- Labeled as dietary supplements

Although all medications must meet FDA approval, dietary supplements do not have to be proven effective or safe. Products found to be ineffective or unsafe will likely be removed from the market, but they do not require approval to appear on the market. In addition, there is no standard within dietary

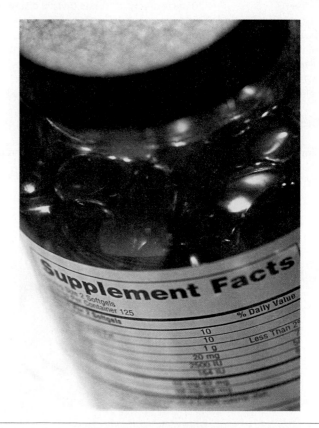

Figure 3-10 ◆ A dietary supplement label.

daily amounts for them. Many people take vitamins and minerals supplements even when eating well balanced diets. Medical assistants should therefore have a good working knowledge of dietary supplements and should regularly ask patients which supplements they are taking. Medical assistants should know the uses of supplements and any possible adverse reactions. Table 3-7 lists common dietary supplements with their recommended daily amounts, benefits, and possible adverse reactions.

TABLE 3-7 COMMON DIETARY SUPPLEMENTS

Supplement	Recommended Daily Amount	Intended Benefits	Possible Adverse Reactions
Vitamin A	5000 IU	Protects cells from free radicals that can cause disease	Birth defects, bone abnormalities, liver disease
Vitamin B6	2 mg	Treats asthma and heart disease	Balance problems, decreased sense of touch
Vitamin B12	6 micrograms	Aids in metabolism, formation of red blood cells, and maintenance of the central nervous system	Skin rash
Vitamin C	60 mg	Increases the body's reactions to free radicals	Gastrointestinal distress
Vitamin D	400 IU	Treats tuberculosis, rheumatoid arthritis, and skin disorders	Bone demineralization, tendonitis
Vitamin E	30 IU	Increases the body's reactions to free radicals	Increased blood coagulation, stroke
Vitamin K	80 micrograms	Aids in blood clotting	Temporary redness of the face and neck
Biotin	300 micrograms	Treats brittle fingernails and thinning hair	None noted
Calcium	1000 mg	Prevents osteoarthritis and strengthens teeth and bones	Constipation, bloating, gas, and flatulence
Chromium	120 micrograms	Helps regulate glucose levels	At high levels, anemia and liver dysfunction
Copper	2 mg	Treats arthritis and serves as an antioxidant and anticancer agent	Nausea, vomiting, and diarrhea
Folate	400 micrograms	Reduces risk of neural tube defects in the fetus	Sleep changes
Iodine	150 micrograms	Treats thyroid disorders	Acne, skin rash
Iron	18 mg	Treats anemia	Nausea, vomiting, bloating
Magnesium	400 mg	Treats various heart disorders	Diarrhea
Manganese	2 mg	Treats osteoarthritis and premenstrual syndrome	Increase liver dysfunction
Niacin	20 mg	Decreases cholesterol	Stomach pain, vomiting, nausea, diarrhea
Potassium chloride	3400 mg	Treats hypertension	Nausea, vomiting, diarrhea
Selenium	70 micrograms	Decreases cancer risk	Tissue damage of the hair, nails, nervous system, and teeth
Thiamin	1.5 mg	Helps protect against metabolic changes in alcoholics	None noted
Zinc	15 mg	Prevents and lessens the severity of the common cold	Nausea and vomiting

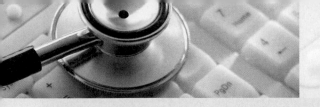

REVIEW

Chapter Summary

- Medical assistants perform varied tasks, both clinical and administrative, and keep the medical office running smoothly. The scope of medical assisting is expected to expand and to continue offering varied challenges and responsibilities.
- Effective medical assistants today have sound clinical and administrative skills, good interpersonal skills, and a professional image that extends outside the office.
- Organization and the proper tools are key to efficient time management in the medical office.
- Many medical assistants work in ambulatory care settings, insurance companies, and other care settings, but the growing nature of the industry will continue to offer assistants new and varied career opportunities with other members of the health care profession.
- Because the medical assistant is just one member of the health care team, that person should know the roles and responsibilities of other staff and learn to interface with those staff properly.
- Contemporary medical and surgical specialities offer patients a wide variety of services and treatments.
- Complementary alternative medicine (CAM) is a growing alternative to traditional medical techniques.

Chapter Review

Multiple Choice

1. _____ is being faithful to the employer, performing to the best of one's abilities, and arriving to work on time.
   a. Loyalty
   b. Respect
   c. Courtesy
   d. Initiative

2. _____ is treating others in a manner that honors them.
   a. Loyalty
   b. Respect
   c. Courtesy
   d. Dependability

3. _____ is completing tasks on time and to the best of one's abilities, arriving to work on time, and staying to the end of the shift.
   a. Loyalty
   b. Respect
   c. Courtesy
   d. Dependability

4. _____ is extending kind words and compassion to others and keeping words and actions professional.
   a. Respect
   b. Courtesy
   c. Initiative
   d. Dependability

5. _____ is completing tasks without waiting to be asked.
   a. Respect
   b. Courtesy
   c. Initiative
   d. Dependability

6. Which of the following professional degrees has many associated levels of education?
   a. Physician
   b. Nurse
   c. Physician assistant
   d. Pharmacist

7. The American Medical Association (AMA) has shown that _____ may harbor bacteria that are not removed with normal washing.
   a. artificial nails
   b. tattoos
   c. nylon stockings
   d. all of the above

True/False

T F 1. According to the U.S. Department of Labor Bureau of Labor Statistics, medical assisting is projected to be the fastest growing occupation from 2004 to 2012.

T F 2. Massage uses touch to relieve pain and encourage muscle relaxation.

T F 3. Acupuncture is the practice of inducing a trance-like state.

Chapter Review (continued)

T F 4. Natural medicine is sometimes called holistic medicine.

T F 5. CAM services are nearly always covered in full by health insurance.

T F 6. Chiropractic is only for the treatment of back pain.

T F 7. The FDA has very strict regulations regarding the manufacture of dietary supplements.

T F 8. Medical assistants are not obligated to maintain professional images when outside the office.

Short Answer

1. What is the pharmacist's role on the patient's health care team?

2. Explain how a PA differs from an NP.

3. Why would a patient seek CAM services?

4. Explain why medical assistants should not wear scented perfumes, lotions, or colognes while working.

5. Explain why it is important for medical assistants to know their coworkers' job duties.

Research

1. Think back to your last visit as a patient with a health care provider. Did the staff you encountered act in a professional manner? Describe the visit and what you felt was professional, or unprofessional, about the actions.

2. Speak with some of your friends about how they would describe professionalism in the health care setting. What is the same or different about their ideas?

3. Using the Internet as a resource, look up definitions for professionalism. What do you find?

Externship Application Experience

Markus is helping his patient, Sun Chien, complete her paperwork on her first office visit when she mentions that she is taking a number of herbal supplements. When Markus asks Sun to name those supplements so he can list them on her history form, she tells him she does not believe the doctor will care about them. How should Markus respond to Sun?

Resource Guide

American Association of Medical Assistants
20 N. Wacker Dr., Suite 1575
Chicago, IL 60606
Phone: (312) 899-1500
Fax: (312) 899-1259
www.aama-ntl.org

Harris, Philip R., and Robert T. Moran. *Managing Cultural Differences.* Houston: Gulf Publishing Co., 1977.

National Center for Complementary and Alternative Medicine
9000 Rockville Pike
Bethesda, MD 20892
http://nccam.nih.gov/

U.S. Department of Labor Bureau of Labor Statistics
Postal Square Building
2 Massachusetts Ave., NE
Washington, DC 20212-0001
Phone: (202) 691-5200
Fax: (202) 691-6325
www.bls.gov/

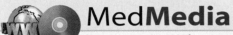

Med**Media**
http://www.MyMAKit.com

More on this chapter, including interactive resources, can be found on the Student CD-ROM accompanying this textbook and on http://www.MyMAKit.com.

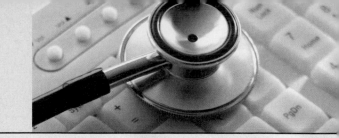

CHAPTER 4

Medical Law and Ethics

Case Study

Victoria Mason is a medical assistant in Dr. Kozlowski's office. Victoria takes a telephone call from a man named Bart. He tells Victoria that one of his employees is a patient of Dr. Kozlowski's and asks her to tell him when his employee was last in the office and what treatment she received.

Objectives

After completing this chapter, you should be able to:

- Define and spell the key terminology in this chapter.
- Classify varied laws as they apply to health care.
- Describe malpractice, defenses to malpractice, and the different types of malpractice insurance policies.
- Outline the physician's public duties.
- Compare the duties of the physician and the patient in the physician-patient relationship.
- List ways in which administrative medical assistants can help maintain patient confidentiality.
- Describe the history of the Health Insurance Portability and Accountability Act (HIPAA) and how it affects health care clinics.
- Describe varied federal and local organizations and the qualities health care professionals need to comply with those organizations.
- Define the conscience clause and how it applies to health care professionals.
- Explain why each health care profession has a code of ethics.
- Discuss the patients' bill of rights.
- Identify the monitoring agencies that address ambulatory health care.

 MedMedia

http://www.MyMAKit.com

Additional interactive resources and activities for this chapter can be found on http://www.MyMAKit.com. For a video, tips, audio glossary, legal and ethical scenarios, on-the-job scenarios, quizzes, and games related to the content of this chapter, please access the accompanying CD-ROM in this book.

Video: *Protecting Patient Privacy*
Legal and Ethical Scenario: *Medical Law and Ethics*
On the Job Scenario: *Medical Law and Ethics*
Tips
Multiple Choice Quiz
Audio Glossary
HIPAA Quiz
Games: Spelling Bee, Crossword, and Strikeout

⊕ MEDICAL ASSISTING STANDARDS

CAAHEP ENTRY-LEVEL STANDARDS	ABHES ENTRY-LEVEL COMPETENCIES
■ Identify the role of self boundaries in the health care environment (cognitive) ■ Recognize the role of patient advocacy in the practice of medical assisting (cognitive) ■ Discuss licensure and certification as it applies to healthcare providers (cognitive) ■ Compare and contrast physician and medical assistant roles in terms of standard of care (cognitive) ■ Compare criminal and civil laws as it applies to the practicing medical assistant (cognitive) ■ Provide an example of tort law as it would apply to a medical assistant (cognitive) ■ Explain how the following impact the medical assistant's practice and give examples: a. Negligence; b. Malpractice; c. Statute of Limitations; d. Good Samaritan Act; e. Uniform Anatomical Gift Act; f. Living will/Advanced directive; g. Medical durable power of attorney (cognitive) ■ Identify how the Americans with Disabilities Act (ADA) applies to the medical assisting profession (cognitive) ■ Discuss all levels of governmental legislation and regulation as they apply to medical facilities (cognitive) ■ Compare personal, professional, and organizational ethics (cognitive) ■ Discuss the role of cultural, social, and ethnic diversity in ethical performance of medical assisting practice (cognitive) ■ Identify where to report illegal and/or unsafe activities and behaviors that affect, health, safety, and welfare of others (cognitive) ■ Identify the effect personal ethics may have on professional performance (cognitive) ■ Report relevant information to others succinctly and accurately (psychomotor) ■ Explain general office policies (psychomotor) ■ Document patient care (psychomotor) ■ Document patient education (psychomotor) ■ Advocate on behalf of patients (psychomotor)	■ Adapt to change. ■ Project a positive attitude. ■ Be cognizant of ethical boundaries. ■ Evidence a responsible attitude. ■ Conduct work within scope of education, training, and ability. ■ Professional components. ■ Maintain licenses and accreditation. ■ Maintain liability coverage. ■ Monitor legislation related to current healthcare issues and practices. ■ Follow established policy in initiating or terminating medical treatment.

Key Terminology

administrative law—legislation passed by governmental agencies

advance directives—directions for medical staff to follow in the event the patient cannot speak for themselves

appeal—request for review of a denied service or claim, in an attempt to see the insurance company's denial reversed or overturned

assault—threat of touching or doing harm to another without their consent

assumption of risk—defense to medical malpractice in which the physician must prove the patient was fully informed of a procedure's risks

battery—act of touching or abusing another person without the person's consent

bioethics—issues surrounding life-and-death situations in health care (e.g., cloning, artificial insemination, abortion)

civil law—legislation that governs actions between two or more citizens

commercial law—legislation that relates to businesses

common law—legislation that stems from the English legal system; also called traditional law (see following entry)

comparative negligence—defense to medical malpractice in which the physician proves the patient was partly responsible for the patient's injury

conscience clauses—statements that allow health care workers to refuse to perform job tasks based on religious or personal objections

constitutional law—legislation that is based on the U.S. Constitution

contract law—legislation that relates to contracts

contributory negligence—defense to medical malpractice in which the physician proves an injury would not have occurred if not for the patient's actions

criminal law—legislation that relates to crimes

damages—money a patient is awarded for damages or injuries the patient sustained

defamation of character—act of saying negative things about a person that harm the person in some way

Key Terminology *(continued)*

discovery rule—legislation that states the statute of limitations begins when an injury was discovered or should have been discovered

duress—act of coercing someone into an act

expert witness—person in a lawsuit who is considered an expert in a given field

expressed consent—agreement, either verbally or in writing, from the patient before a procedure is performed

expressed contract—agreement to a contract, either verbally or in writing

Four Ds of Negligence—elements patients must prove in malpractice (i.e., duty, dereliction of duty, direct cause, and damages)

fraud—deceitful act done to conceal the truth

Good Samaritan Act—law that protects a person performing life-saving care to a stranger outside the medical setting

Health Insurance Portability and Accountability Act (HIPAA)—legislation that addresses patient privacy

immunity—state of being held unaccountable for one's actions

implied consent—agreement through actions only

implied contract—agreement to a contract through actions only

informed consent—process in which a physician reviews with a patient the risks

associated with a procedure, the risks of nontreatment, and accepted treatment alternatives

intentional tort—act of purposefully harming another

international law—legislation that relates to two or more countries

invasion of privacy—act of providing another person's information without that person's permission

malfeasance—state of performing an incorrect treatment

malpractice insurance policy—insurance to cover actions that have hurt a patient

misfeasance—state of performing a procedure incorrectly

negligence—action or inaction that injures another

nonfeasance—state of delaying or failing to perform a treatment

Patient Care Partnership—A list from the American Hospital Association (AHA) of patients' expectations, rights, and responsibilities while under care in the hospital setting

portability—state of being able to move an insurance policy from one employer to another

precedence—legal decision that sets the standard for subsequent, like cases

public law—legislation that relates to citizens

regulatory law—legislation that relates to government regulations

res judicata—Latin phrase for "the thing has been decided"

respondeat superior—Latin phrase for "let the master answer"

segregation—act of keeping two parties apart due to such differences as race or gender

settled—state in which when an offer of money is extended and accepted to drop a lawsuit

standard of care—care a reasonable provider with the same skills would provide in the same circumstances

statute of limitations—period after an injury happens within which a patient may file a malpractice lawsuit

tort of outrage—to intentionally inflict emotional upset on another

tort law—legislation that relates to one party injuring another

traditional law—also known as common law (see preceding entry)

undue influence—to persuade someone to do something they do not want to do

unintentional tort—to harm another person accidentally

Abbreviations

AAMA—American Association of Medical Assistants

ADA—Americans with Disabilities Act

AHA—American Hospital Association

AHIMA—American Health Information Management Association

AIDS—acquired immune deficiency syndrome

AMA—American Medical Association

CDC—Centers for Disease Control

CLIA—Clinical Laboratory Improvement Amendments Act

CMA—certified medical assistant

CMS—Centers for Medical and Medicaid Services

CPR—cardiopulmonary resuscitation

CPT—Current Procedural Terminology

DEA—Drug Enforcement Agency

DNR—do not resuscitate

EIN—employer identification number

FDA—Food and Drug Administration

HIPAA—Health Insurance Portability and Accountability Act

HIV—human immunodeficiency virus

IRS—Internal Revenue Service

JCAHO—Joint Commission on the Accreditation of Healthcare Organizations

MSA—medical savings account

OSHA—Occupational Safety and Health Act

STD—sexually transmitted disease

MEDICAL ASSISTING STANDARDS (CONTINUED)

CAAHEP ENTRY-LEVEL STANDARDS	ABHES ENTRY-LEVEL COMPETENCIES
■ Respond to issues of confidentiality (psychomotor) ■ Perform within scope of practice (psychomotor) ■ Apply HIPAA rules in regard to privacy/release of information (psychomotor) ■ Practice within the standard of care for a medical assistant (psychomotor) ■ Incorporate the Patients' Bill of Rights into personal practice and medical office policies and procedures (psychomotor) ■ Develop a plan for separation of personal and professional ethics (psychomotor) ■ Apply ethical behaviors, including honesty/integrity in performance of medical assisting practice (affective) ■ Examine the impact personal ethics and morals may have on the individual's practice (affective) ■ Demonstrate awareness of diversity in providing patient care (affective) ■ Demonstrate empathy in communicating with patients, family, and staff (affective)	

✓ **COMPETENCY SKILLS PERFORMANCE**

1. Prepare an informed consent for treatment form.
2. Obtain authorization for the release of patient medical records.
3. Respond to a request for copies of a patient's medical record.

Introduction

Medical assistants face many situations that involve ethics and law. Ethics deals with issues of right and wrong, whereas the law serves to uphold what society feels is right and wrong. Ethical issues often take more thought than legal ones, because people have differing ideas about what is right. The law, in contrast, tends to allow little room for opinion. Each state has unique laws governing health care and the medical-assisting profession. It is crucial for medical assistants to know the laws of their states and to uphold those laws at all times. That adherence to law, paired with a clear understanding of what society and the medical-assisting profession spell out with regard to ethics, can help the medical assistant build a solid career.

The Sources of Law

American law arises from varying sources. Court decisions establish **traditional law. Common law** comes from the English legal system. All states in America follow common law except Louisiana, which uses a system based on French law.

Courts set **precedence** when they decide cases. *Roe v. Wade,* for example, caused all states to revamp their legal approaches to abortion. Similarly, *Brown* v. *Board of Education* forced states to address the issue of segregation. **Segregation** is an example of how courts can overrule decisions and set new precedence. Years ago, court decisions deemed segregation a legal practice. Subsequent court decisions ruled segregation illegal, however, and thereby reversed the legal precedence.

Statutes are laws created by federal, state, or local legislators. Statutes are upheld by law enforcement, and cases may end up in local, state, or federal court systems. Medicare, Medicaid, and the Food and Drug Administration (**FDA**) are all agencies that create health-care-related statutes.

Administrative Law

Administrative law, also called **regulatory law,** is passed by governmental agencies such as the Internal Revenue Service (**IRS**). Administrative law addresses issues of taxation, public transportation, manufacturing, the environment, and public broadcasting.

Comparing Public and Private Law

The United States' judicial system has two main branches of law: (1) public and (2) private. **Public law** focuses on issues between the government and citizens, such as criminal law, **constitutional law**, administrative law, and **international law**. Private or **civil law** focuses on issues between two or more citizens.

Criminal Law

Criminal law, also called penal law, focuses on the public's safety and welfare, addressing people who commit crimes or other illegal offenses. Classified by severity as felonies or misdemeanors, criminal law varies from one state to another. While all states have laws against such serious crimes as rape or murder, the laws for less serious crimes like theft or drug use may vary from one jurisdiction to another.

Felonies

Felonies are considered serious crimes, whereas misdemeanors are considered less serious offenses. States have varying definitions for each. Table 4-1 lists general felony categories. Some states, like New Jersey, classify felonies in four degrees. Other

TABLE 4-1 FELONY CATEGORIES	
Felony Degree	**Action of Person Being Charged**
First	Committed the crime
Second	Was at the scene of the crime and assisted in the crime
Third	Assisted in the crime before the crime occurred
Fourth	Assisted the person who committed the crime after the fact

states place felonies in "classes," like Class A or Class 1. In cases like these, Class 1 is the most serious while Class 6 is the least.

Misdemeanors

Like felony classifications, misdemeanor classifications vary from state to state. Misdemeanors include such crimes as petty theft, prostitution, simple **assault,** and disorderly conduct. Because they are considered lesser crimes than felonies, misdemeanors are generally punished with lesser sentences.

Civil Law

The medical profession is primarily concerned with civil law, because it deals with issues relating to **contract law, commercial law**, and tort law. Contract and commercial laws address the rights and obligations one has to another, such as the doctor-patient relationship. Tort law deals with the injuries one has suffered at the hands of another, such as cases of medical malpractice.

Tort Law

Tort law deals with situations in which someone has been injured by another's actions or inactions. Torts are one of two types: unintentional or intentional. An **unintentional tort** occurs when a mistake is made. The vast majority of medical malpractice cases fall into this category, because unintentional torts usually involve negligence. **Negligence** is defined as an act that a reasonable health care provider would not have done or the omission of an act that a reasonable health care provider would have done. In contrast, an **intentional tort** occurs when someone purposefully does something that injures someone else. Table 4-2 defines intentional torts and gives health care examples.

—Critical Thinking Question 4-1—
How does the case study outlined at the beginning of this chapter illustrate one of the torts in Table 4-2? Please specify the tort.

Understanding and Classifying Consent

Before patients are accepted for care in a medical office, they must give their consent to be examined and/or treated by the physician or health care provider and sign a consent form. Figure 4-1 ◆ lists the information that must be included on a consent form.

Only certain parties are legally able to sign consent forms (Figure 4-2 ◆). Consent forms must be written in the languages patients speak. Most facilities that treat patients from other cultures have consent forms in multiple languages.

Health care has two types of consent: (1) implied and (2) expressed. **Implied consent** is given when patients indicate through action only that they agree to submit. When patients are told they need to give blood samples and roll up their sleeves while saying nothing, they give implied consent (Figure 4-3 ◆).

TABLE 4-2 INTENTIONAL TORTS

Assault	Unauthorized attempt or threat to touch another person. *Example:* Telling a patient their temperature will be taken whether they want it or not after they refuse to allow it.
Battery	Actual physical touching of another person without the person's consent; includes physical abuse. *Example:* Taking a patient's temperature against the patient's will.
Defamation of character	Making or publishing false or malicious statements about another person's character or reputation. *Example:* Telling patients they should not see the cardiologist across the street because that cardiologist has a drinking problem.
Duress	Act of coercing someone into an act. *Example:* Telling patients they must have a tetanus vaccine or they will develop a life-threatening infection. The patients feel they have no choice but to comply, even though they do not want the vaccine.
Fraud	Deceitful act made to conceal the truth. *Example:* Falsifying a patient's medical record to conceal a medical mistake.
Invasion of privacy	Releasing private information about another person without the person's consent. *Example:* Releasing a patient's medical records without the patient's consent or a court order.
Tort of outrage	Intentionally inflicting emotional distress on another person. *Example:* The physician yells at a patient for failing to follow instructions.
Undue influence	Intentionally persuading people to do things they do not want to do. *Example:* Convincing single mothers that they should give their children up for adoption when they clearly do not want to.

- Name of the procedure to be performed
- Name of the physician who will perform the procedure
- Name of the person administering the anesthesia (if applicable)
- Any potential risks to the patient from the procedure
- Any risks to the patient if the procedure is *not* elected
- Any accepted alternative treatments and their risks
- Any exclusions the patient has requested
- A statement indicating that all the patient's questions have been answered
- The patient's and witnesses' signatures and the date signed

Figure 4-1 ◆ Necessary Consent Form Information

- Any mentally competent adult over age 18
- The parent or legal guardian of a child, mentally incompetent adult, or temporarily incapacitated adult
- Emancipated minors, defined as under age 18 but:
  - Are married or self-supporting and responsible for their debts
  - Have received a court order declaring them emancipated
- A minor who is:
  - In the armed services
  - Being seen for treatment for sexually transmitted diseases
  - Pregnant
  - Being seen for information regarding birth control or abortion
  - Being seen for treatment regarding drug or alcohol abuse

Figure 4-2 ◆ Parties Who Can Sign a Consent Form

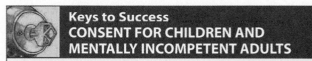

Keys to Success
CONSENT FOR CHILDREN AND MENTALLY INCOMPETENT ADULTS

Children or people who are mentally incompetent or temporarily incapacitated cannot legally give consent, just as they cannot legally enter into contracts. The parents or guardians of these patients must give consent for these patients.

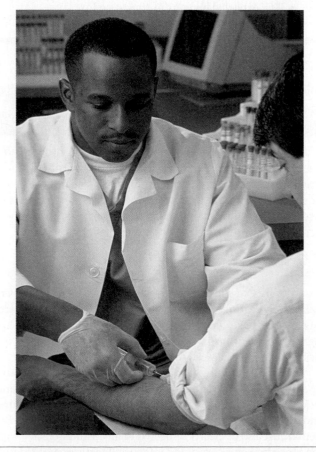

Figure 4-3 ◆ This patient has given implied consent to have his blood drawn.

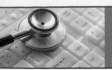

PROCEDURE 4-1 Prepare an Informed Consent for Treatment Form

Theory and Rationale

While the task of explaining the procedures, risks, and alternatives falls to the physician, the medical assistant is often the person who discusses the paperwork with the patient and obtains the patient's signature.

Materials

- Informed consent for treatment form
- Blue or black ink pen
- Copy machine

Competency

(**Conditions**) With the necessary materials, you will be able to (**Task**) prepare an informed consent for treatment form (**Standards**) correctly within the time limit set by the instructor.

1. As the physician goes over the details of the upcoming procedure with the patient, fill in the informed consent form. The form must include:
   - The name of the procedure or treatment to be performed
   - The expected benefits of the procedure
   - Any possible risks of the procedure
   - Any accepted alternatives to the procedure and the risks or benefits associated with each
   - The fact that the patient may choose to forego the procedure and the possible risks or benefits associated with that choice
2. Be certain the form lists the patient's name, birth date, and the place the procedure is to be performed (in office, hospital, etc.).
3. Show the consent form to the physician for him/her to verify that all information is correct.
4. After the physician has left the room, go over the form with the patient. If the patient has further questions about the procedure, have the patient wait in the treatment room while you ask the physician to return to answer the questions. If the patient has no further questions about the procedure, have the patient sign the consent form.
5. Sign the consent form as a witness to the patient's signature.
6. Go over any specifics with the patient about the procedure day, such as any restrictions to eating or drinking on the day of the surgery, or where the patient should park the car.
7. Make a copy of the consent form for the patient. Place the original form in the patient's file.

Keys to Success
SIGNING CONSENT FORMS

Patients must never be coerced or threatened into signing consent forms. Consent must be gained voluntarily and only after the patient has been fully informed of the procedure. Patients who fail to completely understand procedures, have any unanswered questions, or cannot read consent forms should never sign those forms.

Keys to Success
OBTAINING INFORMED CONSENT

The physician is responsible for obtaining informed consent. For the consent to be truly "informed," however, patients must have the opportunity to ask the physician any and all questions. This task should never be delegated to the medical assistant. Instead, it is appropriate for the medical assistant to witness the patient's signature on the consent form.

Keys to Success
WHEN PATIENTS REFUSE TREATMENT

Physicians have the right to refuse to perform elective surgery on patients who refuse to receive blood if needed.

Expressed consent occurs when patients agree either verbally or in writing to consent to a procedure. In health care, any invasive procedure should be done only after a patient has signed a consent form. This helps prove the patient knew the risks involved and agreed to them before the service.

Whether consent is implied or expressed, it must always be informed, meaning patients must be told the benefits and risks of any procedure, the risks of not having the procedure, and any accepted alternative treatments to the procedure. Patients must also be clearly informed of any pain associated with the procedure or recovery and if they will require any assistance after the procedure.

Patients may refuse treatment for any reason, including religious and personal beliefs. For example, a patient with end-stage cancer may refuse chemotherapy because the side effects may decrease the quality of life. A Jehovah's Witness may refuse blood products on religious grounds. When patients refuse treatment, they or their parents or guardians must sign a refusal-of-consent form. This form must indicate that the patient was given information on the risks and benefits of having the procedure or not.

Medical Malpractice

Doctors are sued for varied reasons. Some are sued for making serious errors, such as giving the wrong medications, performing the wrong surgeries, or failing to properly diagnose or treat patients. Other doctors, though few, commit Medicare or insurance fraud, or falsify patient records to conceal errors.

Malpractice is one of three types:

- **Malfeasance** is performing an incorrect treatment, such as operating on the wrong patient.
- **Misfeasance** is performing a treatment incorrectly, such as operating on a patient's arm and accidentally severing a nerve, leaving the patient without the use of the arm.
- **Nonfeasance** is delaying or failing to perform treatment, such as telling a patient a tumor does not need to be removed and the patient later has a bad outcome due to the non-removal of the tumor.

The Doctrine of Respondeat Superior

Staff in the medical office can cause the office to be sued. If the medical assistant makes an error, for example, the lawsuit will usually be filed against the doctor who employs the medical assistant. This is called the doctrine of **respondeat superior**, which is Latin for, "Let the master answer." Under this doctrine, physicians are responsible for the actions of their health care employees (Figure 4-4 ◆). Medical assistants can still be named in malpractice lawsuits, however, so each should seriously consider carrying a **malpractice insurance policy**. Because medical assistants have a low risk of injuring patients, insur-

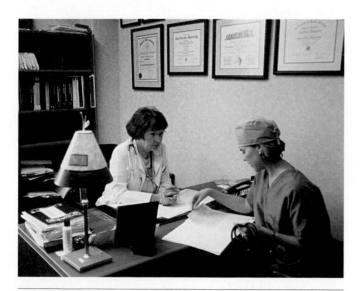

Figure 4-4 ◆ The physician and medical assistant work closely together to maintain safe care for their patients.

Keys to Success
THE DOCTRINE OF RESPONDEAT SUPERIOR

The doctrine of respondeat superior only covers employees performing within their scope of practice at the time of injury. In other words, a health care worker performing a duty outside the scope of practice in the worker's state is not covered by the physician's malpractice insurance policy.

ance rates are generally low. Policies are available through local or state medical-assisting associations.

Types of Malpractice Insurance Policies

Malpractice insurance policies are one of two types: (1) claims-made and (2) occurrence policies. Claims-made policies protect policyholders from malpractice claims only when the insurance company insuring the policyholders at the time of the alleged malpractice is the same company at the time the claim is filed in court. Assume, for example, that on June 1, 2007, Dr. Rasheem is covered under a claims-made policy provided by Allied Insurance when she performs an alleged malpractice event. If Dr. Rasheem is still covered by Allied Insurance when the claim is filed on December 10, 2007, she will be covered. If, however, she switches to a different insurance company before the filing date, Allied Insurance will not cover her. With her new plan, Dr. Rasheem could purchase a "tail" to cover her for the alleged malpractice incidence. A tail is a rider on the new policy that states the new company will cover any events for a certain period before the policy's purchase.

The second type of malpractice insurance policy, occurrence policies, cover policyholders regardless of when claims are filed provided the policies were in effect at the time of the alleged malpractice events. If Dr. Rasheem is covered by Unified Insurance under an occurrence-made policy on June 1, 2007, when an alleged malpractice event occurs, and then switches to a different company before the claim filing date of December 10, 2007, she would still be covered for the claim under her Unified Insurance policy.

Keys to Success
INDIVIDUAL MALPRACTICE INSURANCE POLICIES FOR MEDICAL ASSISTANTS

Individual malpractice insurance policies for medical assistants are fairly inexpensive. For medical assistants working full time, rates are usually less than $100 per year for policies that cover up to $1 million per malpractice occurrence. For a quick online quote on malpractice insurance premiums, visit www.hpso.com.

Proving Medical Malpractice

The vast majority of medical malpractice lawsuits fail to make it to court. They are either **settled,** meaning the two sides agree on a financial award to the injured patient, or they are dismissed due to lack of proof. To prove medical malpractice, the patient must prove all of the following **Four Ds of Negligence:**

- **Duty**—Physicians have a duty to care for patients once they have taken those patients on. The patients must prove the physician breached this duty.
- **Dereliction of duty**—Physicians must meet **standard of care** guidelines for a health care provider with the same training, in the same location, under the same circumstances. The patients must prove the physician failed to perform to this standard.
- **Direct cause**—Patients must prove that the physicians' actions, or lack of action, directly caused the patients' injuries.
- **Damages**—Patients must prove they sustained **damages** due to the negligence.

Medical Malpractice Awards

Personal injury attorneys accept about 1 out of every 20 cases they review, but most cases are found in the physician's favor. Only 1 in 10 cases accepted by an attorney result in an award or a settlement for the patient. When injured patients win cases, judges or juries may make one of the three following types of awards:

- **Nominal**—These are small awards or payments that are made when the negligence is proven but the damages are minimal.
- **Compensatory**—This is money that is awarded to the patient or the patient's family to compensate for the cost of medical care, the disability, mental suffering, any loss of income, and the loss of future income due to the injury.
- **Punitive**—Awards like these are made when judges or juries feel the health care providers should be punished for their actions. Courts may feel the providers were reckless or purposefully ignored signals that should have alerted them to the injuries. Punitive damages are typically high dollar amounts. Several states do not allow for punitive damages.

Preventing Medical Malpractice Claims

Patients file malpractice lawsuits for many reasons; lack of understanding is chief among them. Scientific advances in health care have allowed doctors to perform procedures that were considered too risky until recently. As procedures have become more complicated, patient risk has increased, and this has increased the likelihood of both poor outcomes and malpractice lawsuits, especially when the physician has failed to thoroughly explain the risks to patients. Physicians can help avoid lawsuits by completely explaining the risks of the procedures and ob-

taining the patients' **informed consent.** Informed consent should be written in detail and signed by both the patient and the health care provider (Figure 4-5 ◆).

Another means of lawsuit reduction has been gaining popularity recently, and that is if health care providers apologize to patients those patients will be less likely to file malpractice claims. Many believe that patients sue because they are angry and only pursue legal recourse because they failed to receive acknowledgments of the errors, and apologies. In research activities at the University of Michigan, health care providers were instructed to apologize to their patients when errors occurred. After one year, malpractice defense costs decreased from $3 million to $1 million. Today, 29 states have laws that allow health care providers to apologize to patients after injuries without those apologies used as proof of negligence in lawsuits.

Defending Against Medical Malpractice Claims

Once a medical malpractice suit has been filed, the best defense is the medical record. Especially in the area of medical malpractice, an accurate and complete medical record is paramount. This record is the authoritative description of all care given a patient. It has all consent forms signed by the patient, as well as descriptions of the questions the patient asked and the answers the physician gave about needed care or treatment. ∞ For more on the medical record, see Chapter 10.

The Statute of Limitations

Each state has a **statute of limitations** that sets the time within which an injured patient can file a malpractice lawsuit. Normally, this statute begins from the date of the injury. According to something called the **discovery rule,** some states allow the statute to begin when the injury was discovered or should have been discovered. This rule helps in cases in which the patient fails to discover the injury for several years after the injury has

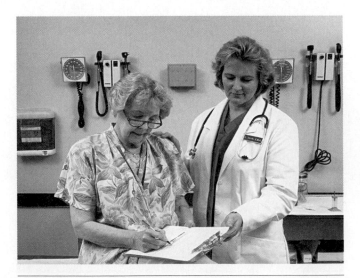

Figure 4-5 ◆ The medical assistant will frequently witness a patient's signature on a consent form.

**Keys to Success
PATIENT SAFETY**

Every member of the health care team is responsible for patient safety. Any team member who witnesses something that seems wrong is compelled to speak with the physician about it out of the patient's hearing range. Team members who remain silent may be considered partly responsible for patients' injuries.

occurred. Other states allow the statute to begin when a minor child turns 18, allowing injured children to bring suits on their own behalf once they reach adulthood. Table 4-3 outlines the statute of limitations for each state.

Using Assumption of Risk as a Defense

Assumption of risk is a defense to medical malpractice physicians can use to prove they made the patients aware of the risks of their procedures. Under this defense, patients cannot sue the physicians when one of those risks occurs. This defense relies, however, on a detailed consent form signed by the patient.

Contributory and Comparative Negligence

The **contributory negligence** defense is one in which physicians may have been at fault for patients' injuries but can prove that the patient aggravated their injuries or in some way worsened them. For example, assume a physician sends a patient home with a sling instead of a cast and tells the patient to limit the motion of the arm to avoid aggravating the injury. If the patient then lifts groceries, worsening the fracture, that patient could be proven to have contributed to negligence.

Most states give patients no awards in contributory negligence cases. When awards are allowed, the court will normally assign a percentage of the award based on how responsible the patient was for the injury. For example, if the court finds the physician is 50 percent responsible for an injury and the patient is also 50 percent responsible, the physician will be ordered to pay 50 percent of the damages. These types of cases are typically called **comparative negligence**.

Immunity from Negligence Suits

The Feres doctrine was passed in response to a 1950 U.S. Supreme Court ruling regarding the Federal Tort Claims Act of 1946. The doctrine prevents members of the armed services from suing the U.S. federal government, its officials, or its facilities, unless an intentional tort was committed. Lawsuits derived from a person acting within their scope of practice and discharged military personnel are examined on an individual basis with regard to the Federal Tort Claims Act, as exemplified in *Brown v. United States* and *Sherer v. United States*.

Res Judicata and Res Ipsa Locuitur

Res judicata is Latin for the phrase, "The thing has been decided." If patients lose their malpractice lawsuits, they cannot bring other suits against the physician for the same injuries. Once a case has been decided in a physician's favor, the case must be dropped. Conversely, when the court awards a patient damages, the physician can appeal the decision in the hope that the patient will settle for less than the awarded amount or the case will be found in the physician's favor.

Under the doctrine of res ipsa locuitur, the Latin phrase for, "The thing speaks for itself," physicians must prove what they did was correct. In all other malpractice cases, the patient must prove the physician's negligence. Cases of res ipsa locuitur are ones in which the malpractice is obvious. A wrong limb may have been amputated or an instrument left inside a patient.

The Standard of Care

The standard of care is a crucial tool for deciding most medical malpractice cases. The standard of care is the care a reasonably prudent person, in the same circumstances, with the same level of training, would perform. To determine if a health care provider has performed within the standard of care, one or both sides in the lawsuit will call on **expert witnesses**. An expert witness is a health care professional who is licensed or certified in the same specialty as the physician involved in the lawsuit. While expert witnesses must be licensed or certified, they need not be licensed or certified in the state where they are testifying.

Tort Reform

Some sources claim that the number of malpractice cases has risen over the past few years, causing an increase in medical malpractice insurance premiums, but those sources are mistaken. The medical malpractice insurance industry is cyclical, exhibiting the ups and downs of any other insurance industry. In fact, the number of malpractice cases that have awarded money to patients has decreased over the past decade and, once inflation is factored in, the amount of money awarded to patients has remained flat. Medical malpractice insurance carriers make most of their profits by investing premiums in the stock market. As the stock market ebbs and flows, so do the profits of insurance carriers.

Capping the Money Awarded to Injured Patients

About half the states in America have capped the awards that can be given to injured patients. These caps typically range from $250,000 to $1 million and fail to factor in the severity of injuries, the number of physicians' prior malpractice cases, or if patients were injured due to physicians' reckless behavior.

Studies have shown that capping the money awarded to injured patients has not lowered medical malpractice

TABLE 4-3 STATUTE OF LIMITATIONS IN EACH STATE

State	Statute of Limitations for Medical Malpractice
Alabama	2 years from the date of injury or 6 months from the date the injury was discovered to a maximum of 4 years from the date of injury.
Alaska	2 years from the date of injury.
Arizona	2 years from the date of injury.
Arkansas	2 years from the date of injury.
California	3 years from the date of injury or 1 year from the date the injury was discovered or should have been discovered. In the event a foreign object is found inside the plaintiff, the statute begins at the date the object was discovered or should have been discovered.
Colorado	2 years from the date of injury or date the injury was discovered or should have been discovered to a maximum of 3 years from the date of injury.
Connecticut	2 years from the date of injury or date the injury was discovered or should have been discovered to a maximum of 3 years from the date of injury.
Delaware	2 years from the date of injury or within 3 years if the injury was unknown and could not reasonably have been discovered.
Florida	2 years from the date of injury or date the injury was discovered or should have been discovered to a maximum of 4 years from the date of injury.
Georgia	2 years from the date of injury.
Hawaii	2 years from the date of injury or reasonable date of discovery. In the event an object is left inside a patient, a claim may be filed up to 1 year from the date of discovery. All claims must be filed within 6 years of the injury.
Idaho	2 years from the date of injury.
Illinois	2 years from the date of injury or up to 4 years if the injury could not reasonably have been discovered within 2 years.
Indiana	2 years from the date of injury.
Iowa	2 years from the date of injury or discovery of the injury. All claims must be filed within 6 years of the injury.
Kansas	2 years from the date of injury or up to 4 years if the injury could not reasonably have been discovered within 2 years.
Kentucky	1 year from the date of injury or up to 5 years if the injury could not reasonably have been discovered within 1 year.
Louisiana	3 years from the date of injury.
Maine	3 years from the date of injury.
Maryland	5 years from the date of injury or 3 years from the date the injury was discovered, whichever is greater.
Massachusetts	3 years from the date of injury or 3 years from the date of discovery. All claims must be filed within 7 years of the date of injury.
Michigan	2 years from the date of injury or 6 months from the date of discovery. All claims must be filed within 6 years of the date of injury.
Minnesota	4 years from the date of injury.
Mississippi	2 years from the date of injury or 2 years from the date of discovery. All claims must be filed within 7 years of the date of injury.
Missouri	2 years from the date of injury or date of discovery up to 10 years from the date of injury.
Montana	3 years from the date of injury or discovery up to 5 years from the date of injury.
Nebraska	2 years from the date of the injury or 1 year from the date the injury was discovered. All claims must be filed within 10 years of the date of injury.
Nevada	4 years from the date of injury.
New Hampshire	2 years from the date of the injury. In the event a foreign object is left inside a patient, the claim must be filed within 2 years of the discovery.
New Jersey	2 years from the date of the injury or 2 years from the date the injury was discovered or should have been discovered.
New Mexico	3 years from the date of injury.
New York	30 months from the date of injury. In the event a foreign object is left inside a patient, the claim must be filed within 1 year of the discovery.
North Carolina	3 years from the date of injury or the date the injury was discovered or should have been discovered. All claims must be filed within 10 years of the injury.
North Dakota	2 years from the date of injury or the date the injury was discovered or should have been discovered. All claims must be filed within 6 years of the injury.
Ohio	1 year from the date of injury. In the event a foreign object is left inside a patient, the claim must be filed within 1 year of the discovery.
Oklahoma	2 years from the date of injury.
Oregon	2 years from the date of injury or the date the injury was discovered or should have been discovered. All claims must be filed within 5 years of the injury.
Pennsylvania	2 years from the date of injury.
Rhode Island	3 years from the date of injury.

TABLE 4-3 STATUE OF LIMITATIONS IN EACH STATE (CONTINUED)

State	Statue of Limitations for Medical Malpractice
South Carolina	3 years from the date of injury or the date the injury was discovered or should have been discovered. In the event a foreign object is left inside a patient, the claim must be filed within 2 years of the discovery. All claims must be filed within 6 years of the date of injury.
South Dakota	2 years from the date of injury.
Tennessee	1 year from the date of injury.
Texas	2 years from the date of injury.
Utah	2 years from the date of injury or the date the injury was discovered or should have been discovered. In the event a foreign object is left inside a patient, the claim must be filed within 1 year of the discovery. All claims must be filed within 4 years of the date of injury.
Vermont	3 years from the date of injury or 2 years from the date injury was discovered or should have been discovered. All claims must be filed within 7 years of the injury.
Virginia	2 years from the date of injury or the date the injury was discovered or should have been discovered. In the event a foreign object is left inside a patient, the claim must be filed within 1 year of the discovery. All claims must be filed within 10 years of the date of injury.
Washington, D.C.	3 years from the date of injury.
Washington State	3 years from the date of injury or 1 year from the date the injury was discovered or should have been discovered. All claims must be filed within 8 years of the injury.
West Virginia	2 years from the date of injury or the date the injury was discovered or should have been discovered.
Wisconsin	3 years from the date of injury or 1 year from the date the injury was discovered or should have been discovered. All claims must be filed within 5 years of the injury.
Wyoming	2 years from the date of injury or the date the injury was discovered or should have been discovered.

Source: Expert Law.

premiums. Instead, premiums have continued to rise, even in states with caps. For example, a study performed by the Rand Corporation in 2004 found that caps on awards in the state of California resulted in payment of up to 30 percent less to injured patients than in states where no cap exists. In addition, this study found that patients who suffer the most severe injuries are typically compensated far less than patients with similar injuries in states without caps. Figure 4-6 ◆ outlines each state's record for providing safe care to patients.

There is a social cost of capping awards to injured patients, as well, and it is high. With too little money to cover their medical costs and expenses after an injury, patients often rely on their states' public health care systems (Medicaid), which means the taxpayers in those states pay for the injuries instead of the providers who are responsible for them.

Repeat Offender Providers

Studies in many states have shown that the vast majority of patient injuries arise from the same small handful of health care providers. Public Citizen, a nonprofit consumer rights group, performed a study in 1998 comparing the malpractice payouts in the United States to the number of doctors making payments. Their findings concluded that 5.9 percent of U.S. physicians were responsible for 57.8 percent of all medical malpractice payouts. In some states, like Kentucky, these providers are carefully disciplined to avoid injuring other patients. Other states, like Washington, have far worse records. In states like Washington, multiple offenders are likely to continue practicing and injuring patients. Figure 4-7 ◆ compares the number of health care providers in the United States who paid for a malpractice suit or settlement.

The Physician's Public Duties and Consequences

Physicians have certain responsibilities surrounding the reporting of certain events. Physicians who deliver babies must report birth certificates, for example. Physicians who are the last to care for patients who have died are typically responsible for completing death certificates. All states list reporting requirements in the event of certain infectious or communicable diseases. Such lists can be obtained from state or local health departments and should be updated yearly.

Reporting Vaccine Injuries

According to the 1986 National Childhood Vaccine Injury Act, vaccine injuries must be reported by physicians' offices to alert other physicians to possibly contaminated batches of vaccine. To report a vaccine injury, the medical assistant should obtain the patient's name and age, as well as the name and lot number of the vaccine. The call must be documented in the patient's file.

Reporting Cases of Abuse

Any incapacitated person, elderly person, or child who shows signs of suspected abuse or neglect must be protected. To that end, physicians are required to report all cases of suspected

State	Overall Grade	Access to Care	Quality and Patient Safety	Public Health and Injury Prevention	Medical Liability Environment
Alabama	D+	D+	C-	D+	D-
Alaska	C+	B+	D+	D	C-
Arizona	D+	D+	C	C-	D-
Arkansas	D	D+	D	D	F
California	B	C	C+	A+	A+
Colorado	C	C+	D-	D+	B-
Conneticut	B	A-	A+	B	F
Delaware	C+	B-	A-	C+	D-
Dist. of Columbia	B	A+	A-	D+	F
Florida	C-	C-	B-	D-	D
Georgia	C+	D+	A	C	B-
Hawaii	C-	C+	D+	C+	D-
Idaho	D	D	D	D-	D
Illinois	C	B+	C	D+	D
Indiana	D+	C-	D	C	D-
Iowa	C+	B-	A-	C	D-
Kansas	C-	B-	F	D	D
Kentucky	C-	C	C	C	D-
Louisiana	C-	C-	B	D	D
Maine	B-	A	C+	C-	D
Maryland	B-	B+	B+	A+	F
Massachusetts	B	A	B	A-	D-
Michigan	B-	B+	B+	A	D-
Minnesota	C+	B+	C+	C	D-
Mississippi	C-	C	C+	D-	D-
Missouri	C+	B+	C-	D+	C-
Montana	C	C+	D-	F	A-
Nebraska	C-	C+	C-	D+	D+
Nevada	C-	D+	F	D-	A-
New Hampshire	C	B+	D-	C-	D-
New Jersey	C+	C+	A+	B+	F
New Mexico	D+	D+	C-	D+	D-
New York	C+	B-	B-	A+	D-
North Carolina	C-	C-	C	B+	F
North Dakota	C-	B-	D	D	D
Ohio	C+	A-	B-	D	D
Oklahoma	D+	C-	D-	C-	D-
Oregon	C-	C+	D	B+	D-
Pennsylvania	B-	A	A-	C-	F
Rhode Island	B-	A	B+	C-	F
South Carolina	B-	C	B+	D	B+
South Dakota	D+	C+	F	F	D
Tennessee	C-	C	C	D+	F
Texas	C	D+	D+	D	A+
Utah	D	D+	D-	D	D
Vermont	C	B+	C	C	F
Virginia	D+	C-	D+	C	F
Washington	D+	C	D	B-	D-
West Virginia	C+	C+	A	D	D
Wisconsin	C-	B-	D+	D+	D
Wyoming	D+	C+	D-	D-	F

Figure 4-6 ◆ Chart of information from the American College of Emergency Physicians regarding access to quality care in states with and without caps on malpractice awards.
Reprinted by permission of American College of Emergency Physicians®.

child abuse to the proper authorities. After accidents, abuse is thought to be the second leading cause of death in children under age 5. When patients of any age sustain violent injuries, including injuries from gunshots or knives or criminal acts (like assault), attempted suicide, or rape, those injuries must be reported. The law protects health care workers from being sued for reporting suspected abuse.

Revoking Medical Licenses

Each state has its own medical practice acts. These acts list the duties and responsibilities of the physician and outline the actions that may be cause for disciplinary action, including suspension or revocation of the physician's license. In general, the more serious the action, the more serious the disciplinary ac-

Number of Payments Reported	Number of Doctors	Percent/Total Doctors in United States	Total Number of Payments	Total Amount of Payments	Percent of Total Number of Payments
All	147,378	17.6	219,272	$38,993,664,850	100
1	107,260	12.8	107,260	$18,131,973,750	48.9
2 or more	40,118	4.8	112,012	$20,861,691,100	51.1
3 or more	14,293	1.7	60,362	$11,084,300,850	27.5
4 or more	6,193	0.7	36,063	$6,481,629,350	16.5
5 or more	3,071	0.4	23,576	$4,073,749,100	10.8

Figure 4-7 ◆ Public Citizen study outlines the small number of physicians responsible for the vast number of malpractice payouts. *Reprinted with permission.*

tion. For example, physicians who are convicted of felonies or proven to have abused patients may face license revocation.

The Physician-Patient Relationship

Both physicians and patients have responsibilities in their relationships.

The Role of the Patient

Patients are free to choose their physicians within the guidelines of their managed care plans. They can also choose whether they want to begin care or limit their care. Patients have the right to understand their treatment components, as well as side effects or benefits. All this information must be detailed for the patient before the procedure.

The Role of the Physician

Physicians have the right to refuse treatment to new patients, or even existing ones, unless those patients have life-threatening, emergent conditions. With proper notification, physicians can change their policies or their availabilities. When physicians are away from their practice for a period, like vacation, they must arrange for other physicians to cover their practice in the event of emergency. To simply close an office, with no emergency referral, may be seen as abandonment of the patient and may result in a malpractice lawsuit.

Contracts in Health Care

A contract is an agreement between two or more parties. All contracts must have the three following components:

1. An offer (the initiation of the contract)
2. Acceptance of the offer (both parties agree to the terms of the contract)
3. Some form of consideration (the exchange of fees for service)

Contracts can be verbal or written. In health care, a contract may be initiated when a patient calls the office to sched-

ule an appointment. The offer is accepted when the medical assistant schedules the appointment. The patient is obligated to pay a fee for the service of seeing the physician, and the physician is obligated to treat the patient.

Physicians and patients operate using two types of contracts: (1) implied and (2) expressed.

Implied Contracts

Much like in implied consent discussed earlier, in an **implied contract**, nothing is written or spoken. Instead, patients imply through their actions alone that they agree to the contracts. For example, simply by arriving for care at the medical office patients imply that they will abide by the patient's portion of the doctor-patient contract and will pay for the services (Figure 4-8 ◆).

Expressed Contracts

Unlike implied contracts, **expressed contracts** have elements that are spoken or written. Expressed contracts occur when patients either verbally or in writing state that they will be responsible for their portion of contracts. For example, patients

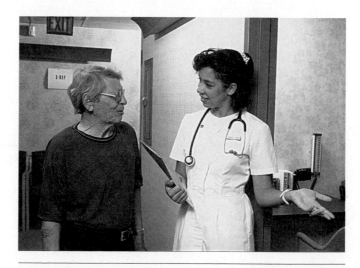

Figure 4-8 ◆ By arriving for care at the medical office, the patient implies that they will abide by the patient's portion of the doctor-patient contract and pay for services.

who sign payment agreements stating they will make payments of $100 per month for the next 6 months enter into an expressed contract. Figure 4-9 ◆ shows a sample expressed contract.

Terminating Contracts

The doctor-patient contract is typically resolved once the patient has completed the prescribed course of treatment outlined by the physician. While the patient may choose to end the doctor-patient relationship at any time, the physician must follow legal protocol to end the relationship.

Patients may choose to end their physician relationship for varied reasons, and they may or may not share those reasons with their provider. When patients do state reasons for ending their medical relationship, those reasons must be charted in the

---

September 4, 2009

I, *Walter Backous*, agree to make payments of $100 per month to Morton Family Practice. My payment will be made by the *15th* of each month and will begin on the *15th of September, 2009*.

Walter Backous	*9/11/09*
Parent or Guardian's Signature	Date
John Smith	*9/11/09*
Witness's Signature	Date

Figure 4-9 ◆ Sample Expressed Contract Agreement.

patients' charts. Physicians should send the patients letters acknowledging the termination and offer to refer the patients to other health care providers, if desired.

For their part, physicians may choose to terminate the doctor-patient relationship due to patients' noncompliance with treatment programs. They may also end patient relationships for personal reasons. Whatever the reason, physicians must follow legal protocol to avoid accusations of patient abandonment. This protocol includes sending a letter to a patient indicating the intent to terminate the relationship. This letter must include:

- A statement clearly indicating the intent to terminate the relationship
- The reason for the desire to terminate the relationship
- A statement that the patient's medical records will be available for transfer to another physician
- An offer to refer the patient to another physician
- A statement strongly encouraging the patient to seek care with another physician as needed

Figure 4-10 ◆ is a sample termination letter.

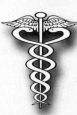

Wilma Steinman, MD
Woodway Family Practice
2413 NW Greenlake Ave.
Milford, CA 12345

August 25, 2009

Gloria Sanchez
891 NW Wallingford Ave.
Milford, CA 12345

Dear Ms. Sanchez:

Because you have missed your last four follow-up appointments to monitor your condition, I will no longer be able to provide you medical services. I believe your condition requires attention and strongly encourage you to seek care with a physician. When you have chosen a new physician, please advise this office by requesting, in writing, the transfer of your medical records.

If you wish, I would be happy to give you a referral. I will be available to treat you for no longer than 30 days from the receipt of this letter.

Sincerely,

Wilma Steinman, M.D.

Wilma Steinman, M.D.

Figure 4-10 ◆ Sample Termination-of-Care Letter

A termination-of-care letter must give the patient at least 30 days to find another physician. During that time, the present physician must continue to see the patient if the patient desires. Termination letters should be sent via certified mail with a signed return receipt requested. Copies of termination letters and signed receipts must be placed in patients' medical records.

The Good Samaritan Act

The **Good Samaritan Act** protects health care workers from being sued when they render first aid in emergency situations outside the medical setting. If, for example, health care workers rendered cardiopulmonary resuscitation (**CPR**) at their local grocery store and the patient died or survived with poor outcomes, those health care workers would be protected. All states have Good Samaritan Acts, although only Vermont requires those with CPR knowledge to stop and render first aid to victims.

Maintaining Patient Confidentiality Through Proper Records Handling

Because medical assistants are patient advocates, they must keep patients' best interests, notably patient confidentiality, at the forefront of their work. Medical assistants must never reveal patient information without a patient's signed consent or a court order. As a result, when patients' family members call the office, medical assistants can tell them nothing about the patients. Similarly, medical assistants are forbidden from releasing information to insurance companies, even bills for services, without patients' consent.

? — Critical Thinking Question 4-2—
Referring back to the case study at the beginning of this chapter, assume that Victoria revealed information about Dr. Kozlowski's patient to the patient's employer. What is the potential impact on Victoria?

Releasing Medical Records

Requests for patients' medical records are common. Patients may need to see specialists, obtain second opinions, or seek care at different facilities. Any request for copies of patients' medical records must be accompanied by the patients' signed authorization. The medical assistant must be certain the authorization is directed to the correct facility and that it contains a date for when the signature was made. In addition to verifying the authorization, the medical assistant must also be completely clear about the nature of the request. Patients may authorize the release of their entire records, or they may authorize the release of information for one date of service only. Some physicians require their staff to alert them of any requests for records. In these offices, the medical assistant pulls the patient's file, attaches the request for copies, and gives the file to the physician for review.

Before sending any copies of medical records, however, the medical assistant must review the file to ensure that it is complete and that it contains only information about that patient. Some facilities provide counseling services that include patients and their family members. For these records, the medical assistant must obliterate any non–patient specific information before sending copies.

In rare cases, medical offices may release original patient records. These requests are most often received via subpoena for court cases in which the judge or attorneys wish to see original material. When original medical records are required, the medical assistant should make a complete copy of every item in the chart, and keep the copies in the office, recorded in a log, as proof of the contents at the time of release.

Occasionally patients will ask to rescind the authorization to release information previously given. When this occurs, the patient will need to sign a separate form that states their previously given authorization is now rescinded. Many legal documents used for obtaining medical records have a disclosure included that states the amount of time the authorization is to be valid. For example, a form may say, "This authorization is valid for 90 days from the date of the signature." In the event one of these forms is used, the patient will not need to sign a separate form in order to rescind the authorization, unless the patient wishes to withdraw their authorization before the 90 day time period.

Accommodating Subpoenas of Medical Records

Occasionally, medical offices may receive a subpoena for patients' medical records. Subpoenas may arise from lawsuits due to injury, such as from a car accident. A judge must sign a subpoena, which authorizes the physician to release the information without the patient's signature. Medical facilities are not required to notify the patient of the subpoena, but many will as a courtesy. HIPAA requires medical facilities to keep records of all patient-record disclosures, however, and to make those records available to patients upon request.

? — Critical Thinking Question 4-3—
In the case study at the beginning of the chapter, imagine the patient's employer obtained a subpoena for her medical information. How would the medical assistant determine which information to release? What is the proper procedure?

Disclosing Minors' Medical Information

In most states, children under 18 may receive certain types of medical treatment without their parents' consent. Such treatments are limited to those for family planning (i.e., birth control or abortion), sexually transmitted diseases (**STDs**), mental health, human immunodeficiency virus (HIV), acquired immune deficiency syndrome (AIDS), or alcohol or drug rehabilitation. Because laws for releasing minors' information vary from state to state, medical assistants must be very clear about the laws in the states where they practice.

PROCEDURE 4-2 Obtain Authorization for the Release of Patient Medical Records

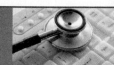

Theory and Rationale

The release of patient medical records requires strict attention to detail and relevant laws. **The Health Insurance Portability and Accountability Act (HIPAA)** requires health care providers to obtain patients' consent to release those patients' health information. The ability to properly obtain authorization for the release of patient medical records is vital to the medical assistant.

Materials

- Release-of-records authorization form
- Blue or black ink pen
- Copy machine
- Patient medical record

Competency

(**Conditions**) With the necessary materials, you will be able to (**Task**) obtain an authorization to release information from a patient (**Standards**) correctly within the time limit set by the instructor.

1. When the patient states all or a portion of the patient's records is to be released to a third party, ask the patient to sign and date a release-of-records form.
2. Verify the address where the patient would like the copies of the record sent.
3. Verify the records the patient would like released. If the patient requests specific release dates, ask the patient to write those dates on the release-of-records form.
4. Verify if the patient would like super-protected information (**HIV/AIDS**, mental health, drug or alcohol rehabilitation information, sexually transmitted disease information, or information about family planning), and ask the patient to check the appropriate box on the authorization form to allow the release of that information.
5. Identify which information in the medical record must be copied.
6. Copy the appropriate documents from the medical record.
7. Send the copies to the requested location.
8. Make a notation of the release of information in the patient's medical record.

PROCEDURE 4-3 Respond to a Request for Copies of a Patient's Medical Record

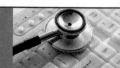

Theory and Rationale

Releasing personal patient information without the patient's consent or a court order violates HIPAA. In fact, improperly copying documents in a patient's medical record could subject the physician to a lawsuit. Therefore, knowing how to properly respond to a request for copies of the patient's medical record is imperative for the medical assistant.

Materials

- Release-of-records authorization form
- Blue or black ink pen
- Copy machine
- Patient's medical record

Competency

(**Conditions**) With the necessary materials, you will be able to (**Task**) respond to a request for copies of a patient's medical record (**Standards**) correctly within the time limit set by the instructor.

1. Verify that the release-of-records form has been signed and dated by the patient or the patient's legal representative.
2. Carefully review the release form for any specific date or information requests.
3. Check if the patient has authorized release of super-protected information (HIV/AIDS, mental health, drug or alcohol rehabilitation information, sexually transmitted disease information, or information about family planning).
4. Verify that you have the correct patient file.
5. Locate the documents to be copied.
6. Review the documents to be copied to verify that they carry the correct patient name and contain the information requested in the authorization to release information and only that information.
7. Copy the appropriate documents.
8. Send the copies to the requesting agency.
9. File the release-of-records request in the patient's medical record with a notation of the documents that were copied and sent.

Minors may receive copies of only those documents their parents cannot see. For example, minors could request and receive copies of their STD treatments, but they could not receive copies of the vaccines they received. Parents, in contrast, could receive copies of their children's vaccination record, not their STD treatments.

Guarding Super-Protected Medical Information

A few areas of medical information are considered "super-protected." While the definition varies from state to state, super-protected information is usually any material pertaining to family planning; STDs; mental illness; HIV or AIDS treatment, diagnosis, or testing; and alcohol or drug rehabilitation. Super-protected information normally requires a separate authorization before it can be released to a third party. In other words, if the medical assistant were to receive a request for copies of a patient's file, she would be unable to release super-protected information without a specific request from the patient.

Faxing Medical Records

Medical records should be faxed only when no other method of data transfer is available, because the risk of unintended recipients is too high. The American Health Information Management Association (**AHIMA**) recommends fax use for confidential patient information only when sending copies via postal service or messenger does not suffice. Medical offices should use a HIPAA-compliant fax cover sheet such as the one in Figure 4-11 ◆ any time they fax patient information.

Disclosing Medical Records Improperly

Disclosing confidential patient information without proper authorization or subpoena is cause for a lawsuit. Patients who feel they have been harmed by improper disclosure may sue a medical office for defamation of character, invasion of privacy, or breach of confidentiality. When information is disclosed improperly, the office is responsible for reporting the event to the HIPAA authorities.

The Health Insurance Portability and Accountability Act (HIPAA)

The Health Insurance Portability and Accountability Act (HIPAA) of 1996 was enacted to reform health care mainly by:

1. Improving **portability** and continuity in group and individual insurance
2. Combatting waste, fraud, and abuse in health insurance and health care delivery
3. Promoting the use of medical savings accounts (**MSAs**)
4. Improving access to long-term care services and coverage
5. Simplifying health insurance administration
6. Providing a means of paying for reforms and related initiatives

HIPAA is divided into the seven following titles:

Title I	Health Care Access, Portability, and Renewability
Title II	Preventing Health Care Fraud and Abuse; Administrative Simplification; Medical Liability Reform
Title III	Tax-Related Health Provisions
Title IV	Application and Enforcement of Group Health Plan Requirements
Title V	Revenue Offsets
Title XI	General Provisions, Peer Review, Administrative Simplification
Title XXVII	Assuring Portability, Availability, and Renewability of Health Insurance Coverage

HIPAA titles are nonsequential because some portions of the original legislation failed to pass.

Title II of HIPAA

Title II of HIPAA, which relates to health care providers, has three main goals, which are to:

- Prevent fraud and abuse in health care delivery and payment
- Improve Medicare and other programs through an efficient and effective standard
- Establish standards and requirements for all electronic transmission of certain health information

Title II dictated that, by July 2002, all health care providers begin using employer identification numbers (**EINs**) whenever they transmitted patient data electronically. The second portion of Title II imposed a privacy rule that addressed the:

- Rights individuals should have for their private health information
- Procedures that should be established for patients to exercise their rights to private health information
- Uses and disclosures of private patient health information that should be authorized or required

This rule required all providers of health care or health care products to notify patients in writing how the patients' private health information would be handled and under what circumstances it would be released. The deadline for compliance was April 2003.

The third portion of Title II addresses the issue of electronically transmitting private health information. HIPAA mandated security measures to standardize electronic claim formats and eliminate outdated forms. The Security Ruling in Title II outlines the security measures that must be in place for health care providers to submit patient health information electronically.

HIPAA and Computer Privacy

HIPAA requires password protection for all computers used in health care. All employees who access the computers must have their own passwords and log off when leaving their desks. In ad-

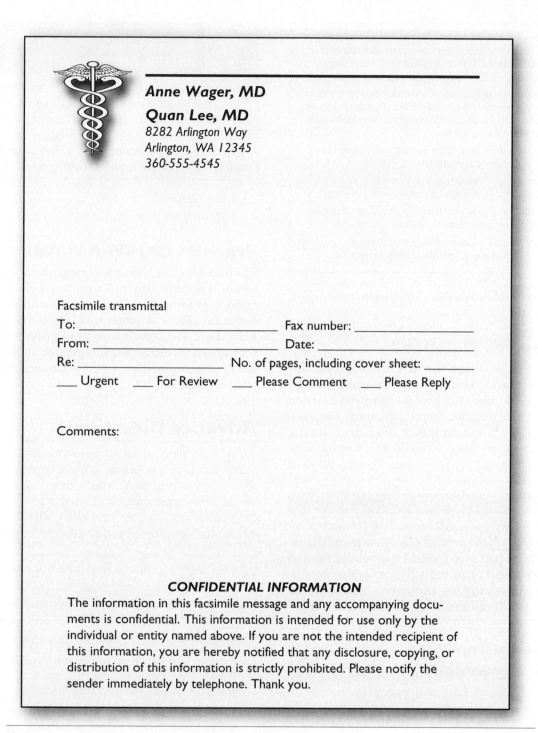

Anne Wager, MD

Quan Lee, MD
8282 Arlington Way
Arlington, WA 12345
360-555-4545

Facsimile transmittal

To: _____   Fax number: _____

From: _____   Date: _____

Re: _____   No. of pages, including cover sheet: _____

___ Urgent   ___ For Review   ___ Please Comment   ___ Please Reply

Comments:

CONFIDENTIAL INFORMATION
The information in this facsimile message and any accompanying documents is confidential. This information is intended for use only by the individual or entity named above. If you are not the intended recipient of this information, you are hereby notified that any disclosure, copying, or distribution of this information is strictly prohibited. Please notify the sender immediately by telephone. Thank you.

Figure 4-11 ◆ Sample HIPAA-Compliant Fax Cover Sheet

dition, computers must face away from patient areas of the clinic. Figure 4-12 ◆ outlines other computer-related requirements in the ambulatory setting.

The HIPAA Privacy Officer

While every member of the medical office should be well versed in HIPAA, every office must designate one person as the HIPAA privacy officer. The privacy officer is responsible for overseeing all aspects of the office's HIPAA compliance and helping patients who may question or file complaints about suspected violations.

 — Critical Thinking Question 4-4 —
Assume that the patient was fired after the medical office gave her employer her private health information without her permission. How should she go about filing a complaint with HIPAA authorities?

To be HIPAA compliant, the medical office must keep its computer systems secure. Knowing the proper procedure for keeping private patient information from being inappropriately viewed is an important function of the administrative medical assistant.

1. Before stepping away from an office computer for a moment or for the evening, be certain the computer is logged out so no one can obtain private patient information without logging in with a password.
2. Look around the desk area to be certain nothing in sight has private information viewable.
3. Cover or remove any files or papers that may contain patient information and may be be viewable to patients.
4. When returning to the workstation, log back into the computer system using a personal password.
5. Ensure that your password is changed periodically and that it is not written anywhere near the computer station.

Figure 4-12 ◆ HIPAA Compliancy for Computers in the Ambulatory Setting

HIPAA Records Violations

Patients who believe medical offices have inappropriately disclosed medical information may contact HIPAA authorities directly. Every medical office must have the complaint forms on file and help patients filing the proper paperwork. Normally, HIPAA authorities will only issue fines or written warnings when violations were intentional or offices have logged a number of violations.

HIPAA Compliance

Patients can give anyone verbal access to their medical information by notifying the medical office in writing. Such information becomes part of the patients' permanent medical records. For example, if Julius Reiman gives written permission for his wife, Ruth, to have knowledge of his care, the physician can talk to Ruth about Julius's care or condition.

The HIPAA Business Associate Agreement

HIPAA legislation stipulates that only those persons in the office who must have access to private patient information should have access. The office cleaners may work for the physician, but they do not need access to any private patient information.

Employees of medical offices are covered under HIPAA and are required to keep confidential information from leaving the office. Anyone who is not an employee of the medical office but may come into contact with private patient information must sign a HIPAA Business Associate Agreement. Such people include:

- Copy-machine repairperson
- Computer software support technician
- Medical assistant externing in the clinic
- Medical assistant performing a shadow project
- Consultants
- Professional staff (e.g., accountants or lawyers)

Keys to Success
WHAT IS AN EMPLOYEE?

Employees are people who work for wages and have payroll taxes taken out of their checks. People who work for the office but have no payroll taxes taken from their checks are not employees. These people must sign a HIPAA Business Associate Agreement if they might come into contact with patient private health information.

- Cleaning staff
- Transcriptionists

Penalties for HIPAA Violations

The fines for HIPAA violations range from $100 to $25,000. Criminal penalties may also apply if it is determined that an individual knowingly obtained or disclosed personal health information without the proper authority. The most severe penalties under HIPAA legislation apply to anyone who commits an offense with the intent to sell, transfer, or use another person's health information. Figure 4-13 ◆ outlines the penalties for HIPAA violations.

Advance Directives

Today, many patients use **advance directives** to outline their wishes should they be unable to speak for themselves. Advance directives consist of living wills, orders outlining patients' desire to not be resuscitated, and durable power of attorney for health care. Any "Do Not Resuscitate" (**DNR**) order must be written and signed by the patient's doctor. A copy should rest in

General penalty for the failure to comply with requirements and standards:

- Not more than $100 for each violation up to a $25,000 for all violations of an identical requirement during a calendar year.

Wrongful disclosure of protected health information:

- A person who knowingly and in violation of HIPAA regulations:
  - Uses or causes to be used a unique health identifier
  - Obtains private health information relating to an individual
  - Discloses individually identifiable health information to another person

  Shall be punished by:
  - A fine of not more than $50,000, imprisoned for not more than 1 year, or both
  - If the offense is committed under false pretenses, be fined not more that $100,000, imprisoned for not more than 5 years, or both
  - If the offense is done with the intent to sell, transfer, or use private health information for commercial purposes or to cause harm, be fined not more than $250,000, imprisoned not more than 10 years, or both

Figure 4-13 ◆ Penalties for HIPAA Violations

the patient's file. Concealing or altering an advance directive is a misdemeanor. Creating an advanced directive falsely is a felony.

Living wills, which are legal in every state, state patients' desires should those patients become incapacitated (Figure 4-14 ◆). Instructions address patients' desire for life-support procedures.

Patients may sometimes give durable power of attorney to other people. The power of attorney names people who can speak or act for the patients in the event the patients cannot speak for themselves. Power-of-attorney documents normally address patients' desires for life support, but authorized parties may do such things as sign contracts or access bank accounts (Figure 4-15 ◆).

Employment Law and Health Care

Title VII of the Civil Rights Act of 1964 was passed to protect employees from discrimination in the workplace. Under this act, employers cannot refuse to hire, refuse to equally compensate, or fire an employee based on race, color, sex, religion, or national origin.

During an interview, candidates cannot be asked questions that would reveal their age, marital status, religion, height, weight, or arrest record unless the information somehow relates to the job for which they are interviewing. For example, candidates who must reach objects on a shelf during the day can be polled about height to ensure they have the proper reach. Arrests are a forbidden topic, because mistakes can be made in the criminal justice system. Employers can, however, ask about convictions, as well as drug use. Drug screening before employment is also legal.

Sexual Harassment

Title VII of the Civil Rights Act protects employees against sexual harassment. Sexual harassment is defined as any unwelcome sexual advance or request for sexual favors in the workplace. This can include verbal or physical conduct of a sexual nature if it is used as a condition of employment, is a basis for promotion, or creates a hostile workplace. In plain terms, sexual harassment occurs when one employee feels uncomfortable with another employee on a sexual level.

To keep from being sued for allowing a hostile work environment, employers must act on any employee complaints. Employees who are being sexually harassed but fail to complain to the employer cannot sue the employer for allowing a hostile work environment. The employer must be given a chance to remedy the situation.

The Americans with Disabilities Act and Healthcare Employment

The Americans with Disabilities Act (**ADA**) prohibits employers from refusing to hire people with disabilities unless those disabilities prevent the people from performing the job. Employers would be justified in turning down wheelchair candidates for ditch-digging jobs, for example. A written, complete job description that includes any physical duties that are required helps candidates know if they can meet the requirements (Figure 4-16 ◆).

The ADA applies only to employers with 15 or more employees, and a disability is defined as any condition that causes a person's major life activities to be limited. The act covers those who are HIV infected or have AIDS, cancer, a history of mental illness, and alcoholism.

The ADA's Requirements

The ADA requires employers to provide their employees basic accommodations, such as extra-wide parking spaces close to the door, accessible bathrooms, break rooms, and work-area accommodations. If an employer has 15 or more employees and one of those employees suddenly becomes disabled, the employer must provide accommodations so the employee can continue to work. However, the employer has 2 years to provide the accommodations, and the accommodations must be reasonable.

The Conscience Clause

A **conscience clause**, adopted in many states, outlines a health care worker's ability to refuse to participate in actions or care for reasons of religion or conscience. Usually, this clause is used when health care workers do not wish to be involved in abortion procedures, although it has recently been used when pharmacists do not wish to dispense certain pregnancy-preventing medications. When medical assistants have religious or conscientious objections to any actions or procedures in the office, they should familiarize themselves with the laws in their state and should fully inform their employer.

The Patients' Bill of Rights

The American Hospital Association (AHA) first adopted a Patients' Bill of Rights in 1972 and modified it in 1992. The AHA revamped this document in 2003, renaming the new version The Patient Care Partnership. This agreement is provided to all patients upon entering the inpatient hospital setting. The Patient Care Partnership outlines patients' expectations, rights and responsibilities while in the hospital setting. Expectations are listed in areas such as the quality of care the patient can expect to receive, and a clean and safe environment should be provided to all patients.

Patients should expect to be involved in their care while in the hospital and should be involved in discussing their condition with the medical providers. These discussions should include the patient's treatment plan. Patients are directed to provide their health care team with all information relating to their treatment, including past illnesses and allergic reactions. Within the **Patient Care Partnership**, patients are told they should expect protection of their privacy while in the hospital setting, to be properly prepared for discharge when the time comes, and to be provided with help in filing insurance claims, if needed. The Patient Care Partnership can be viewed on the American Hospital Association website: http://www.aha.org.

LIVING WILL OF _____

I, _____, a resident of the City of _____,
_____ County, State of _____, being of sound and dispos-
ing mind, memory and understanding, do hereby willfully and voluntarily make, publish, and declare this to
be my LIVING WILL, making known my desire that my life shall not be artificially prolonged under the
circumstances set forth below, and do hereby declare:

1. This instrument is directed to my family, my physician(s), my attorney, my clergyman, any medical facility in
   whose care I happen to be, and to any individual who may become responsible for my health, welfare, or
   affairs.

2. Death is as much a reality as birth, growth, maturity, and old age. It is the one certainty of life. Let this
   statement stand as an expression of my wishes now that I am still of sound mind, for the time when I may
   no longer take part in decisions for my own future.

3. If at any time I should have a terminal condition and my attending physician has determined that there can
   be no recovery from such condition and my death is imminent, where the application of life-prolonging
   procedures and "heroic measures" would serve only to artificially prolong the dying process, I direct that
   such procedures be withheld or withdrawn, and that I be permitted to die naturally. I do not fear death
   itself as much as the indignities of deterioration, dependence, and hopeless pain. I therefore ask that
   medication be mercifully administered to me and that any medical procedures be performed on me which
   are deemed necessary to provide me with comfort or care or to alleviate pain.

4. In the absence of my ability to give directions regarding the use of such life-prolonging procedures, it is my
   intention that this declaration shall be honored by my family and physician as the final expression of my
   legal right to refuse medical or surgical treatment and accept the consequences for such refusal.

5. In the event that I am diagnosed as comatose, incompetent, or otherwise mentally or physically incapable of
   communication, I appoint _____ to
   make binding decisions concerning my medical treatment.

6. If I have been diagnosed as pregnant and my physician knows that diagnosis, this declaration shall have no
   force or effect during the course of my pregnancy.

7. I understand the full import of this declaration and I am emotionally and mentally competent to make this
   declaration. I hope you, who care for me, will feel morally bound to follow its mandate. I recognize that this
   appears to place a heavy responsibility on you, but it is with the intention of relieving you of such responsibility and of placing it on myself, in accordance with my strong convictions, that this statement is made.

IN WITNESS WHEREOF, I have hereunto subscribed my name and affixed my seal at _____,
_____, this _____ day of _____, 20 _____, in the presence of the
subscribing witnesses whom I have requested to become attesting witnesses hereto. _____

                                                                              Declarant

The declarant is known to me and I believe him/her to be of sound mind.

_____Witness   Address

_____Witness   Address

Subscribed and acknowledged, before me by _____, and subscribed and sworn
   to before the witnesses, on the _____ day of _____, 20_____.

_____

(SEAL)
NOTARY PUBLIC State of _____ My Commission
   Expires:_____

Copies of this instrument have been given to:

Receipt and acknowledged & date:

Figure 4-14 ◆ Sample living will.

DURABLE POWER OF ATTORNEY FOR HEALTH CARE

I, _____,

(Printed or typed full name)

am of sound mind, and I voluntarily make this designation. I designate _____, (insert name of patient advocate) my _____, (Spouse, child, friend . . .) living at _____

(Address of patient advocate) as my patient advocate to make care, custody and medical treatment decisions for me in the event I become unable to participate in medical treatment decisions. If my first choice cannot serve, I designate

_____ (Name of successor) living at _____

_____ (Address of successor) to serve as patient advocate.

The determination of when I am unable to participate in medical treatment decisions shall be made by my attending physician and another physician or licensed psychologist.

In making decisions for me, my patient advocate shall follow my wishes of which he or she is aware, whether expressed orally, in a living will, or in this designation.

My patient advocate has authority to consent to or refuse treatment on my behalf, to arrange medical services for me, including admission to a hospital or nursing care facility, and to pay for such services with my funds. My patient advocate shall have access to any of my medical records to which I have a right.

My specific wishes concerning health care are the following: (if none, write "none")

_____

_____

_____

_____

_____

_____

I may change my mind at any time by communicating in any manner that this designation does not reflect my wishes.

It is my intent that my family, the medical facility, and any doctors, nurses and other medical personnel involved in my care shall have no civil or criminal liability for honoring my wishes as expressed in this designation or for implementing the decisions of my patient advocate.

Photostatic copies of this document, after it is signed and witnessed, shall have the same legal force as the original document.

I sign this document after careful consideration. I understand its meaning and I accept its consequences.

Signed: _____ Date: _____

Address: _____

NOTICE REGARDING WITNESSES

You must have two adult witnesses who will not receive your assets when you die (whether you die with or without a will), and who are not your spouse, child, grandchild, brother or sister, an employee of a company through which you have life or health insurance, or an employee at the health care facility where you are a patient.

STATEMENT OF WITNESSES

We sign below as witnesses. This declaration was signed in our presence.

The declarant appears to be of sound mind, and to be making this designation voluntarily, without duress, fraud or undue influence.

Signed by witness: _____

(Print or type full name)

Address: _____

Signed by witness: _____

(Print or type full name)

Address: _____

Figure 4-15 ◆ Sample Durable Power of Attorney for Healthcare

Job Title: Certified Medical Assistant
Department: Pediatrics
Reports To: Clinical Manager

SUMMARY:

Under general supervision, is responsible for the physical care of patients through tasks of routine difficulty; responsible for maintaining the clinical area of the clinic.

ESSENTIAL DUTIES AND RESPONSIBILITIES:

Includes the following. Other duties may be assigned. Assists physicians with surgical procedures. Takes and records patients' blood pressure, temperature, pulse, respiration and weight. Makes routine entries into patients' charts. Shares responsibilities for use of equipment and supplies. Administers specified medication, by injection, orally or topically, and notes time and amount on patients' charts. Sterilizes equipment and supplies. Makes suggestions to improve work methods, trains new employees; makes routine entries into logs, records supplies and materials used. Completes requisitions for supplies and forwards to supervisor for approval.

QUALIFICATIONS:

To perform this job successfully, an individual must be able to perform each essential duty satisfactorily. The requirements listed below are representative of the knowledge, skill, and/or ability required. Reasonable accommodations may be made to enable individuals with disabilities to perform the essential functions.

EDUCATION:

Successful completion of an accredited medical assisting program.

LANGUAGE SKILLS:

Ability to read and comprehend simple instructions, short correspondence, and memos. Ability to write simple correspondence. Ability to effectively present information in one-on-one and small group situations to patients and other employees of the organization.

MATHEMATICAL SKILLS:

Ability to add and subtract two digit numbers and to multiply and divide with 10's and 100's. Ability to perform these operations using units of American money and weight measurement, volume and distance.

REASONING ABILITY:

Ability to apply common sense understanding to carry out instructions furnished in written, oral, or diagram form.

CERTIFICATES, LICENSES, REGISTRATIONS:

Must have certification of completion of CMA (AAMA) or RMA (AMT) certification examination.

PHYSICAL DEMANDS:

The physical demands described here are representative of those that must be met by an employee to successfully perform the essential functions of this job. Reasonable accommodations may be made to enable individuals with disabilities to perform the essential functions. While performing the duties of this job, the employee is regularly required to stand; walk; use hands to finger, handle, or feel; reach with hands and arms; and talk or hear. The employee is occasionally required to sit; climb or balance; and stoop, kneel, crouch, or crawl. The employee must regularly lift and/or move up to 50 pounds. Specific vision abilities required by this job include close vision, distance vision, color vision, peripheral vision, depth perception, and ability to adjust focus.

The employee must have the ability to work overtime hours.

WORK ENVIRONMENT:

The work environment characteristics described here are representative of those an employee encounters while performing the essential functions of this job. Reasonable accommodations may be made to enable individuals with disabilities to perform the essential functions. While performing the duties of this job, the employee is occasionally exposed to outside weather conditions. The noise level in the work environment is usually moderate.

Figure 4-16 ◆ Sample Detailed Job Description.

I. Information Disclosure You have the right to receive accurate and easily understood information about your health plan, health care professionals, and health care facilities. If you speak another language, have a physical or mental disability, or just do not understand something, assistance will be provided so you can make informed health care decisions.

II. Choice of Providers and Plans You have the right to a choice of health care providers that is sufficient to provide you with access to appropriate high-quality health care.

III. Access to Emergency Services If you have severe pain, an injury, or a sudden illness that convinces you that your health is in serious jeopardy, you have the right to receive screening and stabilization emergency services whenever and wherever needed, without prior authorization or financial penalty.

IV. Participation in Treatment Decisions You have the right to know all your treatment options and to participate in decisions about your care. Parents, guardians, family members, or other individuals that you designate can represent you if you cannot make your own decisions.

V. Respect and Nondiscrimination You have a right to considerate, respectful, and nondiscriminatory care from your doctors, health plan representatives, and other health care providers.

VI. Confidentiality of Health Information You have the right to talk in confidence with health care providers and to have your health care information protected. You also have the right to review and copy your own medical record and request that your physician amend your record if it is not accurate, relevant, or complete.

VII. Complaints and Appeals You have the right to a fair, fast, and objective review of any complaint you have against your health plan, doctors, hospitals, or other health care personnel. This includes complaints about waiting times, operating hours, the conduct of health care personnel, and the adequacy of health care facilities.

Figure 4-17 ◆ Patients' Bill of Rights

In March 1997, President Bill Clinton appointed a committee to study the quality of health care in the United States. As part of its work, the committee issued a list of Consumer Bill of Rights and Responsibilities, which contained the Patients' Bill of Rights in Figure 4-17 ◆.

Many states have enacted their own patients' bills of rights. Contents vary, but most include patients' rights for obtaining care, completing the **appeal** process, and handing abuses by insurance carriers.

OSHA and Ambulatory Care

Under the Occupational Safety and Health Act (**OSHA**), employers are required to provide a safe working environment for their employees. OSHA controls and monitors employers for compliance, and employees can make complaints directly to OSHA if they feel their workplace is unsafe.

With regard to health care, OSHA has rules that protect workers from exposure to blood-borne pathogens. OSHA requires health care workers use standard precautions when likely to come into direct contact with patients, and that protective equipment is used to protect from blood and bodily fluids. Figure 4-18 ◆ list the standard precautions recommended by the Centers for Disease Control (**CDC**).

Under OSHA rules, all health care facilities must keep a list of all employees who might be exposed to blood-borne pathogens. All facilities must have a written exposure control plan that outlines the steps to follow in the event of an accidental needle stick or other blood-borne exposure (Figure 4-19 ◆). In many states, OSHA also dictates that any employee who is exposed to bodily fluids in the workplace must be given a Hepatitis B vaccine free of charge.

The Clinical Laboratory Improvement Amendments Act (CLIA) and Ambulatory Care

The Centers for Medicare and Medicaid Services (**CMS**) regulates all laboratory testing performed on humans in the United States, with the exception of testing done for medical research. CMS achieves this regulation via the Clinical Laboratory

Hand Washing

☒ Wash hands after touching blood, body fluids, secretions, excretions, and contaminated items, whether or not gloves are worn.

☒ Wash hands immediately after gloves are removed, between patient contacts, and when otherwise indicated to avoid transfer of microorganisms to other patients or environments. It may be necessary to wash hands between tasks and procedures on the same patient to prevent cross-contamination of different body sites.

☒ Use a plain soap for routine hand washing.

☒ Use an antimicrobial agent for specific circumstances, as defined by the infection-control program.

Gloves

☒ Wear gloves when touching blood, body fluids, secretions, excretions, and contaminated items.

☒ Put on clean gloves just before touching mucous membranes and nonintact skin.

☒ Change gloves between tasks and procedures on the same patient after contact with material that may contain a high concentration of microorganisms.

☒ Remove gloves promptly after use, before touching noncontaminated items and environmental surfaces, and before treating another patient.

Mask, Eye Protection, Face Shield

☒ Wear a mask and eye protection or a face shield to protect mucous membranes of the eyes, nose, and mouth during procedures and patient-care activities that are likely to generate splashes or sprays of blood, body fluids, secretions, and excretions.

Gown

☒ Wear a gown to protect skin and to prevent soiling of clothing during procedures and patient care activities that are likely to generate splashes or sprays of blood, body fluids, secretions, or excretions.

☒ Remove a soiled gown as promptly as possible.

Patient-Care Equipment

☒ Handle used patient care equipment soiled with blood, body fluids, secretions, and excretions in a manner that prevents skin and mucous membrane exposures, contamination of clothing, and transfer of microorganisms to other patients and environments.

☒ Ensure that reusable equipment is not used for the care of another patient until it has been cleaned and reprocessed appropriately.

☒ Ensure that single-use items are discarded properly.

Environmental Control

☒ Ensure that the facility has adequate procedures for the routine care, cleaning, and disinfection of environmental surfaces, beds, bedrails, bedside equipment, and other frequently touched surfaces.

Linen

☒ Handle, transport, and process used linen soiled with blood, body fluids, secretions, and excretions in a manner that prevents skin and mucous membrane exposures and contamination of clothing.

Occupational Health and Bloodborne Pathogens

☒ Take care to prevent injuries when using needles, scalpels, and other sharp instruments or devices; when handling sharp instruments after procedures; when cleaning used instruments; and when disposing of used needles.

☒ Never recap used needles, or otherwise manipulate them using both hands or use any other technique that involves directly the point of a needle toward any part of the body.

☒ Do not remove used needles from disposable syringes by hand, and do not bend, break, or otherwise manipulate used needles by hand.

☒ Place used disposable syringes and needles, scalpel blades, and other sharp items in appropriate puncture-resistant containers.

☒ Use mouthpieces, resuscitation bags, or other ventilation devices as alternatives to mouth-to-mouth resuscitation methods in areas where the need for resuscitation is predictable.

Patient Placement

☒ Place a patient who contaminates the environment or who does not or cannot be expected to assist in maintaining appropriate hygiene or environmental control in a private room.

Figure 4-18 ◆ CDC Recommended Standard Precautions

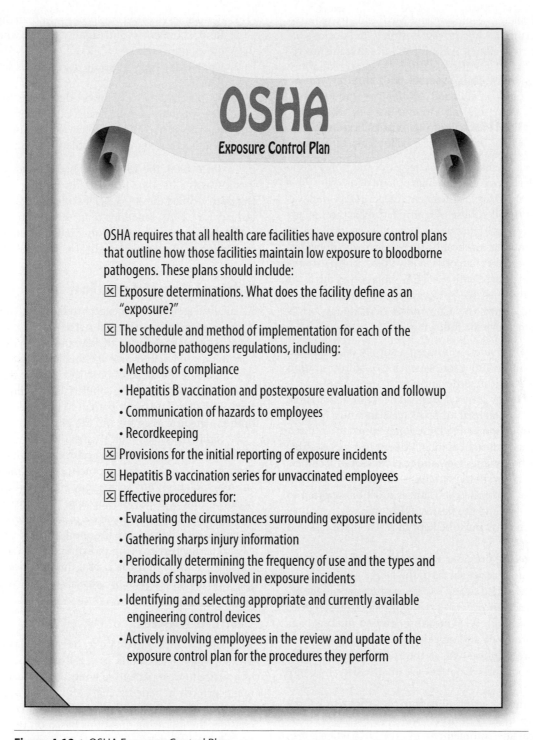

Figure 4-19 ◆ OSHA Exposure Control Plan

Improvement Amendments Act (**CLIA**) of 1988. These rules apply to any lab that is performing any work with specimens, including ambulatory care settings, and are in place to ensure safe, accurate laboratory testing. CLIA regulations are based on the complexity of the test method. The more complicated the test, the more stringent the requirements. Every facility that performs laboratory testing must establish a quality assurance program that includes quality control, personnel policies, patient test management, and proficiency testing. Facilities are inspected every 2 years to ensure compliance with federal CLIA regulations.

The Joint Commission on the Accreditation of Healthcare Organizations (JCAHO) and Ambulatory Care

The Joint Commission on the Accreditation of Healthcare Organizations (**JCAHO**), often simply called the Joint Commission, is a private organization that sets standards for health care administration and patient safety. Hospitals that receive federal funding, such as Medicare and Medicaid, are required to be JCAHO certified, while private hospitals and doctor's offices are not. Many facilities, including clinics that are not required to be JCAHO certified still seek this accreditation, because it is a sign of excellence in patient safety.

The Controlled Substances Act

The Controlled Substances Act of 1970 regulates the manufacture, distribution, and dispensing of narcotics and nonnarcotic drugs that are considered to have a high potential for abuse. This act is enforced by the Drug Enforcement Agency (**DEA**) and was designed to limit the illegal use of controlled substances in addition to preventing substance abuse by health care professionals. This law requires that any health care provider who dispenses, administers, or prescribes narcotics or any other controlled substances must be registered with the DEA. Violation of this act is a criminal offense punishable by fines and/or imprisonment.

Compliance with the Controlled Substances Act is mandatory and includes the following:

■ Health care providers who keep a supply of controlled substances in the office for dispensing or administration must use a triplicate order form from the DEA.

■ A record of every controlled substance transaction must be kept and maintained for 2 to 3 years and must be available for inspection by the DEA at any time.

■ All controlled substances must be kept in a locked cabinet out of the patient's view and only those staff members who need access should have it.

■ Any theft of controlled substances must be reported to the local police and the nearest DEA office.

■ Prescription pads must be kept in a safe place to avoid theft.

■ Any health care provider who ceases practice must return all unused order forms to the DEA.

■ Keep only a limited supply of prescription pads in the office. Rather than ordering enough pads to last a year, order just enough for a month or two so missing pads will be more easily and quickly noticed.

■ Keep no prescription pads in the examination rooms or any other location where they are unattended and could be stolen.

■ Inventory the prescription pads in the office regularly so theft will be quickly noticed.

■ Notify local law enforcement and the DEA when a prescription pad is stolen.

Medical Ethics

Medical ethics are what govern the behavior of health care professionals. Each professional association has its own code of ethics that details the actions that are considered ethical by that profession. The American Association of Medical Assistants (**AAMA**) has a code of ethics that addresses five areas the medical assistant must strive for. Those areas are to:

1. Render services with respect for human dignity
2. Respect patient confidentiality, except when the law requires information
3. Uphold the honor and high principles set forth by the AAMA
4. Continually improve knowledge and skills for the benefit of patients and the health care team
5. Participate in community services that promote the good health and welfare of the general public

Since 1999, the AAMA has had a policy of sanctioning medical assistants who violate its disciplinary standards. Under this policy, called the AAMA's Disciplinary Standards and Procedures for CMAs, sanctions range from being denied eligibility to sit for the certification examination to permanent revocation of the certified medical assistant (**CMA**) credential.

Ethical Considerations

All medical assistants can expect to face legal and ethical situations that may require them to act to protect the patient yet remain within the bounds of law and the scope of practice. Sometimes, physicians may ask medical assistants to perform duties outside the scope of practice. Because this is illegal, the medical assistant should be comfortable declining to accept the task. To do so could cause patient injury and a lawsuit against both the medical assistant and the physician.

Similarly, most medical assistants will witness the physician or other members of the health care team perform procedures outside of the scope of practice for the medical assistant. In some practices, physicians may train medical assistants to perform some of these tasks. Because there are variations, medical assistants must be fully versed in their states' scopes of practice. Some procedures, like the application of a cast, may seem easy to perform after being shown by the physician, but if it is outside the scope of medical-assisting practice, it may be illegal to perform even with the physician's supervision.

Ethical Model

An unethical physician may ask the medical assistant to break the law. Medical assistants are legally bound by law and scope of practice to treat patients lawfully and ethically and to document correctly in patients' charts. If medical assistants wonder whether actions cross ethical or legal boundaries, they should consider the following questions based on the Blanchard and Peale Ethical Model:

1. Is the action legal?
2. Is the action ethical?
3. How will the action make me feel?
4. How would I feel if the action, and my involvement, was published in the local newspaper? If I had to explain my actions to my child/spouse/parent?

If the medical assistant is uncomfortable with any of the answers to these four questions, the action likely crosses an ethical or legal boundary and the medical assistant should decline to participate. Any local Association of Medical Assistants chapter is a good place to call when in doubt about an action. Bad actions can hinder future employment. Prospective employers must believe new staff are ethical and will practice within their legal scopes of practice. Medical assistants who are associated with a medical practice or a physician who is practicing unethically or illegally will unfortunately gain that same reputation.

In Practice

Jan has been working as an administrative medical assistant for Dr. Borse for 7 years. Dr. Borse frequently asks Jan to add charges to a patient account for services he did not perform.

Jan is paid well and feels she is harming no patients by complying with the doctor's requests. Dr. Borse says he only submits the false claims to make up for the money he loses by treating Medicare and Medicaid patients. One day, Dr. Borse is arrested for insurance fraud; he eventually serves 2 years in prison and loses his license to practice medicine. Jan has a very hard time getting a new job. Dr. Borse's story has been in all the local papers, and employers do not want to work with unethical staff.

How could Jan have changed the course of events? What advice would have helped Jan while she was working with Dr. Borse?

Raising Ethical Issues in Health Care

The American Medical Association (AMA) has outlined several areas surrounding ethics in the management of patient care. A few appear in Figure 4-20 ◆.

- With regard to organ transplantation, physicians must not consider age in the decision of who gets the organ. Priority must be given to the patient who has the strongest chance of obtaining long-term benefit; a person's individual worth to society must not be considered.
- With regard to clinical research, physicians must fully inform any patient involved in research and must give those patients the highest level of respect and care. The goal of any research program must be to obtain some type of scientific data.
- With regard to obstetrics, physicians must perform abortions within the boundaries of state and federal laws. If physicians do not wish to perform abortions, they must refer patients to physicians who will perform the procedure. If a patient undergoes genetic testing, the physician must give the results to both parents.

Figure 4-20 ◆ AMA Ethical Viewpoints

Other ethical standpoints by the AMA include areas surrounding finances in the healthcare setting. These include:

- Patient care should not be dictated by the patient's ability to pay. In other words, a physician should not order expensive tests for a patient who can pay and skip tests for one who cannot.
- Physicians can charge for missed appointments only when they notify the patients ahead of time.
- Patients must be able to receive copies of their medical record, regardless of any amounts owed the office. The physician cannot hold the medical record hostage for payment of the bill.
- Physicians can charge interest on medical bills in accordance with state law if they notify patients ahead of time.
- Fees for service must be reasonable and fair and must be based on Current Procedural Terminology (**CPT**) code guidelines regarding the nature of the care involved.

Bioethics

As medical technology advances, the issue of **bioethics** will continue to expand current thought, as well as some individuals' comfort zones. Bioethics addresses areas that affect human life. Examples are cloning, the use of embryonic stem cells, in-vitro fertilization, and abortion. Within bioethics, what is right for one person may not be right for another. The goal is to make decisions on a case-by-case basis, taking into consideration the individuals who are involved.

The Uniform Anatomical Gift Act

Several human organs can be transplanted, including the corneas, liver, kidney, heart, lung, and skin, but every year approximately 6000 Americans die waiting for organ transplants. To address the donation of human organs, the National Conference of Commissioners for Uniform State Laws passed the Uniform Anatomical Gift Act. Most states allow people to indicate their wish to become organ donors by making a notation on their driver's license. All states abide by the following rules:

- Donors must be mentally competent and over age 18 to donate their own bodies.
- A physician who is also on the transplant team must not determine the death of the donor.
- No financial compensation may be made for organ donation.

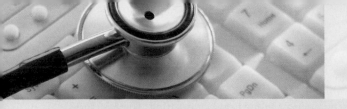

REVIEW

Chapter Summary

- U.S. laws arise from varying sources to achieve varying legal purposes.
- Malpractice is a serious, wide-ranging issue in health care that the medical assistant can address both individually and as a member of the health care team.
- Physicians have a number of public duties to perform to ensure patient safety and confidentiality are upheld.
- Medical assistants play a crucial role in patient confidentiality procedures.
- The Health Insurance Portability and Accountability Act (HIPAA) is in place to help steer the proper direction of contemporary health care.

- The various federal and state organizations driving current health care practices demand compliance from all members of the medical staff.
- Health care professionals must be vigilant about all relevant legislation, including the conscience clause, patients' bill of rights, and codes of ethics.
- Medical ethics govern the behavior of health care professionals. Each professional association has its own code of ethics that details the actions that are considered ethical by that profession

Chapter Review

Multiple Choice

1. *Res judicata* is Latin for:
   a. The physician is responsible
   b. The thing speaks for itself
   c. Let the master answer
   d. None of the above

2. _____ is the unauthorized attempt or threat to touch another person.
   a. Assault
   b. Battery
   c. Duress
   d. Invasion of privacy

3. _____ is releasing private information about another person without the person's consent.
   a. Assault
   b. Battery
   c. Duress
   d. Invasion of privacy

4. _____ is the actual physical touching of another person without the person's consent; it includes physical abuse.
   a. Assault
   b. Battery
   c. Duress
   d. Invasion of privacy

5. _____ is the act of coercing someone into an act.
   a. Assault
   b. Battery
   c. Duress
   d. Invasion of privacy

True/False

T F 1. In most states, children under age 18 may receive medical attention for a sexually transmitted disease without parental consent.

T F 2. Patients win most medical malpractice cases.
T F 3. Patients may refuse treatment for any reason.
T F 4. Hospitals that receive federal funding, such as Medicare and Medicaid, are required to be JCAHO certified.
T F 5. The statute of limitations for medical malpractice cases is the same in every state.
T F 6. Classes of felony crimes are the same in every state.
T F 7. The physician must report any vaccine injuries.

Short Answer

1. What are the four steps in an ethical model, and how do they apply to an everyday situation, such as talking about a patient with coworkers outside the medical office?
2. What is the Good Samaritan Act?
3. What are the Four Ds of Negligence?
4. Differentiate implied consent from expressed consent.
5. Explain what is meant by "informed consent."
6. Define the conscience clause, and explain how it pertains to health care professionals.
7. Describe the steps the physician must take to legally terminate the physician-patient relationship.
8. Explain the function of the HIPAA Privacy Officer in the medical office.

Research

1. Are there caps on the medical malpractice awards allowed in your state? If so, what are they?
2. Search the Internet for a medical malpractice case. What were the specifics of the case?
3. Search the Internet for a medical ethical case. What were the specifics of the case?

Externship Application Experience

Joe Rutigliano is a patient of Dr. Mallory's. As Joe is leaving the office after his appointment, he overhears Dr. Mallory and her medical assistant discussing his treatment plan in the hallway. He believes other patients also overhear their conversation, and he is upset. What should the medical assistant do?

Resource Guide

American Association of Medical Assistants
20 N. Wacker Dr., Suite 1575
Chicago, IL 60606
Phone: (312) 899-1500
Fax: (312) 899-1259
http://www.aama-ntl.org/

Bioethics.com
http://bioethicsnews.com

Health Care Providers Service Organization
159 E. County Line Road
Hatboro, PA 19040-1218
Phone: (800) 982-9491
Fax: (800) 739-8818
www.hpso.com

Public Citizen
1600 20th St. NW
Washington, DC. 20009
Phone: (202) 588-1000
www.citizen.org

Sorry Works
P.O. Box 531
Glen Carbon, IL 62034
Phone: (618) 559-8168
http://www.sorryworks.net/

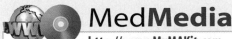

MedMedia
http://www.MyMAKit.com

More on this chapter, including interactive resources, can be found on the Student CD-ROM accompanying this textbook and on http://www.MyMAKit.com.

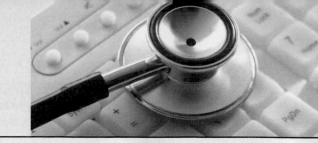

CHAPTER 5

Interpersonal Communication Skills

Case Study

Katerina Bolshoy is a Russian patient who speaks broken English. The medical assistant, who does not speak Katerina's language, must schedule several appointments for Katerina, as well as explain insurance coverage to her.

Objectives

After completing this chapter, you should be able to:

- Define and spell the key terminology in this chapter.
- Describe both verbal and nonverbal communication and how each can be used most effectively.
- List various listening skills.
- Identify communication barriers and how to overcome them.
- List techniques for communicating effectively with distressed patients.
- Describe techniques for communicating effectively with difficult patients.
- List ways to adapt communication skills to patients from different cultures.
- Name community resources for patient referrals.
- Explain how to communicate effectively with members of the health care team.
- Outline a plan for creating patient-education materials.

 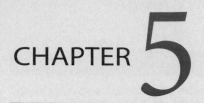

MedMedia

http://www.MyMAKit.com

Additional interactive resources and activities for this chapter can be found on http://www.MyMAKit.com. For videos, tips, audio glossary, legal and ethical scenarios, on-the-job scenarios, quizzes, and games related to the content of this chapter, please access the accompanying CD-ROM in this book.

Videos: *Getting Along with Coworkers; Housekeeping 101; The Angry Patient; When English Is Not the Language*
Legal and Ethical Scenario: *Interpersonal Communication Skills*
On the Job Scenario: *Interpersonal Communication Skills*
Tips
Multiple Choice Quiz
Audio Glossary
HIPAA Quiz
Games: Spelling Bee, Crossword, and Strikeout

MEDICAL ASSISTING STANDARDS

CAAHEP ENTRY-LEVEL STANDARDS	ABHES ENTRY-LEVEL COMPETENCIES
■ Identify styles and types of verbal communication (cognitive)	■ Adapt to change
■ Identify nonverbal communication (cognitive)	■ Maintain confidentiality at all times
■ Recognize communication barriers (cognitive)	■ Project a positive attitude
■ Identify techniques for overcoming communication barriers (cognitive)	■ Be cognizant of ethical boundaries
■ Recognize the elements of oral communication using a sender-receiver process (cognitive)	■ Evidence a responsible attitude
■ Differentiate between subjective and objective information (cognitive)	■ Conduct work within scope of education, training, and ability
■ Identify resources and adaptations that are required based on individual needs, i.e., culture and environment, developmental life stage, language, and physical threats to communication (cognitive)	■ Adaptation for individualized needs
■ Discuss the role of assertiveness in effective professional communication (cognitive)	■ Instruct patients with special needs
■ Report relevant information to others succinctly and accurately (psychomotor)	■ Teach patients methods of health promotion and disease prevention
■ Instruct patients according to their needs to promote health maintenance and disease prevention (psychomotor)	■ Locate resources and information for patients and employers
■ Demonstrate empathy in communicating with patients, family, and staff (affective)	■ Instruct patients with special needs
■ Apply active listening skills (affective)	■ Professional components
■ Use appropriate body language and other nonverbal skills in communicating with patients, family, and staff (affective)	■ Monitor legislation related to current healthcare issues and practices
■ Demonstrate awareness of the territorial boundaries of the person with whom communicating (affective)	■ Orient patients to office policies and procedures
■ Demonstrate sensitivity appropriate to the message being delivered (affective)	■ Adapt what is said to the recipient's level of comprehension
■ Demonstrate awareness of how an individual's personal appearance affects anticipated responses (affective)	■ Use proper telephone techniques
■ Demonstrate recognition of the patient's level of understanding in communications (affective)	■ Follow established policy in initiating or terminating medical treatment
■ Analyze communications in providing appropriate responses/feedback (affective)	■ Be courteous and diplomatic
■ Recognize and protect personal boundaries in communicating with others (affective)	■ Serve as a liaison between the physician and others
■ Demonstrate respect for individual diversity, incorporating awareness of one's own biases in areas including gender, race, religion, age, and economic status (affective)	■ Exercise efficient time management
■ Apply ethical behaviors, including honesty/integrity in performance of medical assisting practice (affective)	■ Receive, organize, prioritize, and transmit information expediently

Key Terminology

assess—determine patients' learning needs and how to meet them

body language—set of nonverbal means of communication (e.g., facial expressions)

close-ended question—question that can be answered with "yes" or "no"

discriminating—acting against a person's interest due to a perceived difference in race, gender, economic, or other status

documenting—process of capturing information in the patient's chart

empathy—identification with another person's feelings

evaluation—process of verifying a patient's progress

examples—illustrations of concepts or ideas

feedback—information that is reflected in an interpersonal exchange

implementing—process of taking action; putting a plan in place

open-ended question—question that requires more than a "yes" or "no" answer

personal space—area around a person deemed the "comfort zone"

planning—process of researching the actions or steps needed to implement a plan or project

professional distance—professional relationship

reflecting—process of repeating information that is communicated

stereotyping—process of shaping an opinion based solely on something like race, gender, or economic status

sympathy—pity

✓ **COMPETENCY SKILLS PERFORMANCE**

1. Use effective listening skills in patient interviews.
2. Communicate with a hearing-impaired patient.
3. Communicate with a sight-impaired patient.
4. Communicate with patients via interpreters.
5. Prepare a patient's specialist referral.
6. Identify community resources.
7. Use the Internet to find patient education materials.

Introduction

Communication is the process of sharing ideas between two or more people; it is sending and receiving messages verbally and nonverbally. Communication skills are vital for anyone working in health care, including the medical assistant. The medical assistant must share information accurately with patients, physicians, and coworkers and respond appropriately. The medical assistant must have a positive attitude and present information pleasantly.

Verbal Communication

Communication takes different forms. Verbal communication uses spoken words. Professional medical assistants adopt polite tones of voice, avoid slang, and use proper grammar. Figure 5-1 ◆ outlines the "Five Cs" of better communication.

Communication must be geared to patients' ability to understand, which often means using basic terms rather than medical terminology. This applies even when patients are also health care professionals. Such patients may work in different fields and lack knowledge in the procedures they are undergoing.

Some patients may be embarrassed to admit a lack of understanding, and that can be dangerous. Patients who fail to understand may fail to follow medical directions. **Feedback,** which involves questioning patients to ensure comprehension, is the best way to avoid this situation. Medical assistants must ensure that patients understand what is being said. When communication barriers like language or disabilities limit patient comprehension, medical assistants must arrange for interpreters or family members to help facilitate the patient exchange.

Part of medical assisting is communicating carefully to ensure patients never feel demeaned. Sometimes, communication can be unintentionally offensive. Tone of voice, facial expression, and projection are all critical. Medical assistants who project the image that something is important inspire patients to do the same.

? **— Critical Thinking Question 5-1—**
How can the medical assistant enhance communication with non-native English speakers like Katerina?

Using Nonverbal Communication

Some communication is verbal, while other communication is nonverbal. Nonverbal communication includes writing, using body language, and therapeutic touch.

 Keys to Success
ENGLISH AS A SECOND LANGUAGE

Remember that patients may not use English as their primary language. As a result, they may fail to understand phrases or slang common in English.

☒ **Content**—Address all areas of interest and fully answer all questions.

☒ **Conciseness**—Get to the point; say what needs to be said in as few words as possible.

☒ **Clarity**—Choose words that accurately and precisely convey meaning.

☒ **Coherence**—Create a logical, easy-to-follow train of thought.

☒ **Check**—Ask for feedback or clarification to ensure comprehension.

Figure 5-1 ◆ The five Cs of better communication.

Writing as a Means of Communication

Written communication is one form of nonverbal communication that is crucial to both medical documentation and patient education. Medical assistants should use patients' charts both to capture patient information and to document that patients have understood the information given them.

In health care, patients typically receive written instructions after verbal instructions. Figure 5-2 ♦ provides a sample

of written instructions. ∞ Chapter 6 goes into written communication in detail.

Critical Thinking Question 5-2

What is the value of written communication for patients like Katerina, who speak English as a second language? What characteristics would make that written communication most effective?

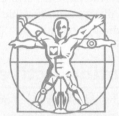

Wilma Steinman, MD
Woodway Family Practice
2413 NW Greenlake Ave.
Milford, CA 12345

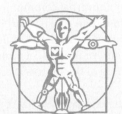

Your child has eczema, which can be a long-term condition. It is important to use the cream medication at the first sign of a breakout and to continue using the medication until the rash has cleared up.

Following are some facts and tips about eczema:

❑ Eczema is a condition of extremely dry skin. Your child should drink plenty of liquids throughout the day and avoid any perfumed lotions or soaps.

❑ Eczema is not contagious. Your child can continue to go to school and to participate in all other activities.

❑ To avoid skin breakdowns, have your child keep short fingernails and avoid scratching.

❑ If the rashes seem to worsen, call the office.

_____
Parent or Guardian's Signature

Figure 5-2 ♦ Sample written instructions.

Keys to Success
BODY LANGUAGE AND CULTURE

Different cultures have different body-language norms. Some cultures consider direct eye contact a sign of disrespect, for example. As patient advocates, medical assistants must know the norms of their patients' cultures and observe those norms as signs of respect for patients' needs.

Reading and Using Body Language

Research has shown that nonverbal communication sends primary messages more often than spoken words, and **body language** is an important part of nonverbal communication. Facial expressions, gestures, and eye movements can say more than words. For example, a shrug of the shoulders can be interpreted as a lack of interest.

Body language can help clarify verbal communication. A patient may, for example, claim to feel no pain but grimace when touched. The real message, then, is that the patient needs attention. Medical assistants should use nonverbal communication to ensure patient exchanges are effective and accurate. When patients say one thing but do another, medical assistants should ask appropriate questions to ensure that patients provide accurate information.

Patients will read medical assistants' body language as well, so it is important for medical assistants to use neutral stances, even when patients are difficult. Medical assistants should always be professional and nonjudgmental, whatever the patient communication. Patients need to trust their medical assistants and should feel comfortable sharing personal information (Figure 5-3 ◆).

Therapeutic Touch

Nonverbal communication includes the use of touch. Touch can be very helpful to some patients. For example, touching a patient's arm during a time of sadness can relay a sense of kindness that most patients will appreciate. A patient in a good deal of emotional pain may appreciate a hand on the arm or shoulder (Figure 5-4 ◆).

Some patients prefer no touch. All people have a comfort zone called **personal space.** In general, personal space varies by culture. People from some cultures desire closeness, while others do not. Medical assistants can determine patients' personal spaces by observing how those patients react to differing levels of interaction. If, for example, the medical assistant reaches out to touch the patient's arm and the patient pulls away, the patient is likely uncomfortable and the medical assistant should withdraw the hand.

Demonstrating Active Listening

Medical assistants should always focus on patients' body language and spoken words. Active listening is the process of giving full attention during an exchange and minimizing interruptions. In the medical office, interruptions like telephone calls tell patients that they are less important than the callers.

Active listening is more listening than talking. This means the medical assistant should listen without interruption while the patient speaks, and then give the patient feedback so they feel understood. This is especially important when the patient is angry or upset. When medical assistants try to hurry conversations or fail to show **empathy** for patients, situations may worsen. Empathy, which is identification for patients' feelings, differs from **sympathy,** which is pity.

Because patients spend more time with the medical assistant than with the doctor, they often feel more comfortable sharing information with the medical assistant. Studies have shown that patients grow less likely to share information as a

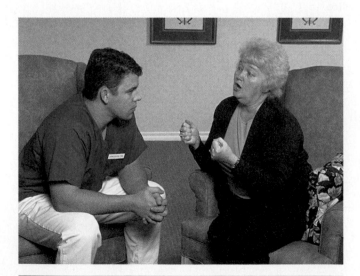

Figure 5-3 ◆ This patient's body language reflects her anger. The medical assistant must remain calm and show the patient with his body language that he is listening and he cares.

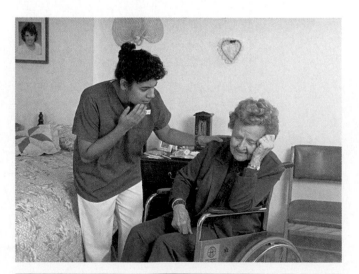

Figure 5-4 ◆ A medical assistant comforts a patient in distress.

**Keys to Success
EMPATHETIC LISTENING**

Part of empathetic listening is making direct eye contact with the patient, nodding, and keeping an interested facial expression.

person's authority rises. Therefore, the medical assistant should share any patient concerns with the physician, chart all medically relevant information, and notify the doctor when appropriate.

Interviewing the Patient

Administrative medical assistants are often asked to obtain information from patients in the office. Medical assistants should always remain professional and organized and begin any patient conversation with introductions. With a working pen to document information in patient charts, the assistant should then conduct the interview in a private room. When the interview concludes, the medical assistant should let the patient know who will be entering the room next and when. When the medical assistant expects the physician or other provider to be delayed, the patient should be informed.

Employing Interviewing Techniques

Medical assistants may use different communication styles when interviewing patients. Some are more appropriate than others depending on the patient and the situation. **Open-ended questions** are appropriate when more than a "yes" or "no" response is needed. An example is, "Mrs. Dow, would you please

describe your symptoms?" **Close-ended questions,** in contrast, can be answered with "yes" or "no." An example of this type of question is, "Mrs. Dow, have you had anything to eat or drink since midnight last night?"

Reflecting is another interviewing technique. This is the practice of repeating the patient's statement so the patient knows they have been understood. This technique allows the medical assistant to clarify parts of conversations. For example, a medical assistant might say, "Mrs. Dow, you said that for 2 weeks you have been having pain in your right shoulder and arm, and that the pain has been running down to your right hand. Is that right?"

Asking for **examples** is a technique that may help the medical assistant better understand the patient. In this case, a medical assistant may say, "With '1' being no pain, and '10' being extreme pain, can you tell me how you would rate the pain level you are having, Mrs. Dow?"

Allowing for periods of silence in conversations gives patients time to collect their thoughts or to think of answers. When patients fail to answer questions right away, the medical assistant should give them time before asking more questions.

Another communication tool to use when speaking with patients is the indirect question. An indirect question is considered polite, especially when speaking with strangers. A sample direct question is, "Where is your son?" An indirect question is, "I was wondering if you know where your son is?" Figure 5-5 ◆ lists some common indirect phrases.

─ Critical Thinking Question 5-3─
How does the reflecting conversation technique help ensure that medical assistants understand the concerns of patients like Katerina? What sort of questions would support this technique?

PROCEDURE 5-1 Use Effective Listening Skills in Patient Interviews

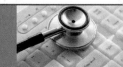

Theory and Rationale
Effective listening skills are vital for the medical assistant. By listening carefully to the patient and documenting appropriately, the medical assistant performs a valued function for the physician. Watching for the patient's nonverbal communication and paraphrasing the patient's statements verifies comprehension.

Materials
■ Patient history form
■ Pen

Competency
(**Conditions**) With the necessary materials, you will be able to
(**Task**) use effective listening skills in interviewing the patient
(**Standards**) correctly within the time limit set by the instructor.

1. Smile, and introduce yourself to the patient.
2. Identify the patient by verifying the patient's birth date.
3. Verify that you have the correct patient chart.
4. Maintain a professional persona.
5. Maintain eye contact with the patient.
6. Ask the patient open-ended questions.
7. Do not interrupt the patient.
8. Paraphrase the patient's statements to verify comprehension.
9. Watch for the patient's nonverbal communication.
10. Summarize the patient's statements, and conclude the interview.
11. Document appropriate information in the patient's file.

Do you know . . . ?

I was wondering . . . .

Can you tell me . . . ?

Do you happen to know . . . ?

I'd like to know. . . .

Have you any idea . . . ?

Figure 5-5 ◆ Common phrases used for asking indirect questions.

Identifying Factors That Hinder Communication

Various factors can impede communication. Culture is one, because messages can be perceived differently. Medical assistants will encounter patients who think differently than they do, but assistants must treat all patients with dignity and respect. **Stereotyping** is prejudging patients based solely on gender, ethnic background, or other identifying factor. **Discriminating** is taking some sort of action against a person based solely on a stereotype. Whatever the medical assistant's personal feelings about a patient, he or she must always remain professional.

Communicating in Special Circumstances

Patients who are young, hearing impaired, sight impaired, mentally unable to understand, or sedated present special communication challenges. In all cases, medical assistants must always include the patients and their interpreters or guardians in conversations. Patients should always feel part of the process.

Communicating with Hearing-Impaired Patients

Communicating with hearing-impaired patients presents some special challenges. Many hearing-impaired people can read lips. When this is the case, medical assistants must speak slowly, facing the patient in a well-lighted room. The medical assistant can touch patients' arms to get their attention, and then begin the conversation (Figure 5-6 ◆).

When hearing-impaired patients have an interpreter, the conversation is still with the patient, not the interpreter. Medical assistants should face their patients and speak with them directly.

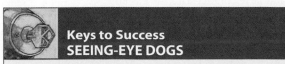

Keys to Success
SEEING-EYE DOGS

To ensure patient safety and honor the Americans with Disabilities Act (ADA), patients with service animals like seeing-eye dogs must be allowed to keep the animals with them at all times. These animals are working; however, so medical assistants should not pet or play with them unless invited to do so by the patient.

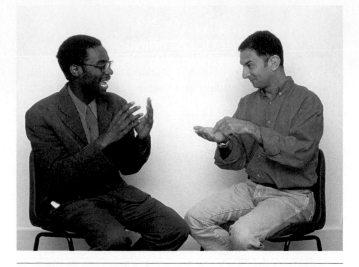

Figure 5-6 ◆ Hearing-impaired patients will often bring an interpreter.

Communicating with Sight-Impaired Patients

Patients with sight impairments present communication challenges as well as raise special considerations about medical facilities. Medical assistants must escort patients who cannot see well to treatment rooms or the rest room, being careful to alert the patients to any steps, ramps, or slopes. Once to the treatment room, the medical assistant should place the patient's hand on the chair or table where the patient should sit (Figure 5-7 ◆). The medical assistant should then familiarize the patient with the room's layout and important features, such as the sink and door.

Sight-impaired patients often bring service animals to the medical office. These animals must stay with the patients throughout the visit, including when the patients use the restroom or visit the lab or radiology facilities.

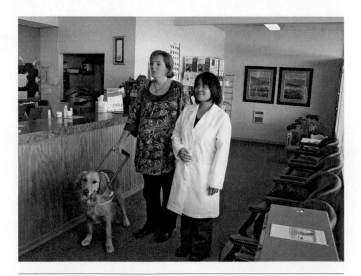

Figure 5-7 ◆ The medical assistant will need to assist the sight-impaired patient while in the office.

PROCEDURE 5-2 Communicate with a Hearing-Impaired Patient

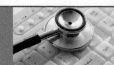

Theory and Rationale

Communicating with hearing-impaired patients is a skill needed in any medical facility. Knowing how to get the patient's attention and how to communicate professionally and accurately is an important skill to master.

Materials

■ Patient's file
■ Blue or black pen

Competency

(**Conditions**) With the necessary materials, you will be able to (**Task**) communicate with a hearing-impaired patient (**Standards**) correctly within the time limit set by the instructor.

1. Alert the patient that you are ready to take him to the examination room by entering the reception area, touching the patient's arm to get his attention, and motioning to follow.

2. If the patient has an interpreter, also have the interpreter enter the examination room.

3. When speaking, look directly at the patient and speak slowly.

4. When the patient can read lips, verify understanding through patient questioning. When comprehension is lacking, write instructions for the patient.

5. When asking a patient to change into a gown, ask the patient to flip a switch or crack the door open when ready. People with hearing impairments cannot hear a knock to announce the physician's arrival.

6. At the end of the patient's visit, chart all communications, including verification of the patient's understanding.

Communicating with Patients with Speech Impairments

For the medical assistant, patients with speech impairments may be difficult to understand. When communication is difficult, the medical assistant should ask patients to repeat themselves.

If medical assistants cannot understand patients upon repetition, those medical assistants should ask the patients to write down what they are saying. At no time should the medical assistant act frustrated or hurried. Part of patient advocacy is being certain to correctly relate patient information to the physician.

PROCEDURE 5-3 Communicate with Sight-Impaired Patients

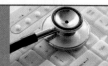

Theory and Rationale

Communicating with sight-impaired patients is a skill needed in any medical facility. The administrative medical assistant may be called on to gather information from sight-impaired patients to facilitate paperwork completion in the office.

Materials

■ Patient's file
■ Blue or black pen

Competency

(**Conditions**) With the necessary materials, you will be able to (**Task**) communicate with a sight-impaired patient (**Standards**) correctly within the time limit set by the instructor.

1. Alert the patient that you are ready to visit the examination room by entering the reception area, touching the patient's arm, and offering your arm for the patient to hold.

2. Ensure any service animal accompanies the patient to the examination room.

3. Alert the patient to any steps, doorways, ramps, or slopes along the way.

4. Take the patient to a private area, outside of other patients' views or hearing ranges.

5. Place the patient's hand on the chair or table where sitting is desired.

6. Arrange for any service animal to sit directly next to the patient.

7. Ask the patient the questions on the history form, and write down the answers. Ensure the patient's responses are clearly understood.

8. At the end of the patient's visit, chart all communications, including how the patient's understanding was verified.

9. Sign and date the patient history form and note that the history form was completed for the patient due to sight impairment.

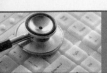

PROCEDURE 5-4 Communicate with Patients Via Interpreters

Theory and Rationale

Communicating with a patient via an interpreter is something the administrative medical assistant may need to do both over the telephone when scheduling an appointment, and when the patient arrives in the office for a visit. It is imperative that patients understand the information being communicated to them and that healthcare professionals understand what patients are communicating.

Materials

- Patient's file
- Pen

Competency

(**Conditions**) With the necessary materials, you will be able to (**Task**) communicate with a patient via an interpreter

(**Standards**) correctly within the time limit set by the instructor.

1. When the patient arrives in the office with an interpreter, obtain the name of the interpreter and verify the spelling.
2. Obtain the interpreter's contact information for the patient's medical record. If the interpreter has a business card, attach it to the patient's file.
3. Communicate with the patient directly; do not speak directly to the interpreter.
4. When any of the interpreter's comments are unclear, ask for clarification.
5. Document all essential parts of the interview in the patient's chart.

Communicating with Patients via Interpreters

Patients who cannot communicate due to language barriers should be accompanied to the medical office by interpreters (Figure 5-8 ◆). The office may arrange interpreters, or the patient may bring a friend or family member to serve the role. The most important issues are that patients can understand the information being communicated to them and that health care professionals clearly understand what the patients are communicating. In communities with a high proportion of patients who speak languages other than English, the medical office will likely seek medical professionals who speak the community's prevalent language, in which case interpreters may be unneeded. The names and contact information of interpreters who accompany patients should be clearly noted in the patients' files so the interpreters can be contacted for comment or clarification.

Communicating with Mentally Ill Patients

Most patients who are mentally incompetent visit the medical office with their legal guardians. The medical assistant should speak with such patients first and then their guardians. Some patients have a mental illness and are mentally incompetent to speak for themselves. In these situations, the medical assistant must be certain the patient understands any instructions. Some effective techniques are to repeat patients' statements, ask patients to repeat what they have been told, or demonstrate the skills the patients have been shown.

Communicating with Angry or Distressed Patients

To avoid angering or distressing patients, the medical assistant should try to avoid the emotions' triggers. For example, the medical assistant can help avoid anger over a bill by reviewing the bill with the patient. The medical assistant should always explain things up front and give the patient written information on any relevant office policies.

When patients become angry or distressed, the medical assistant must always remain calm and professional (Figure 5-9 ◆). Typically, the best response to an angry patient is, "I'm sorry you're upset. Let's see if we can work this out." Most patients calm when the medical assistant responds calmly and demonstrates a sincere desire to help.

Communicating with Young Patients

When communicating with young patients, it is important that the medical assistant use words and questions the patients will understand. When the patients cannot articulate their feelings,

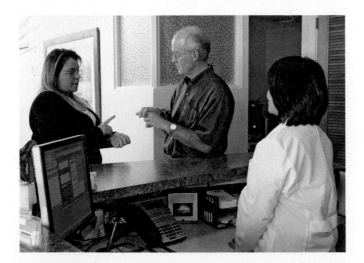

Figure 5-8 ◆ Interpreters should accompany those patients who cannot communicate due to language barriers.

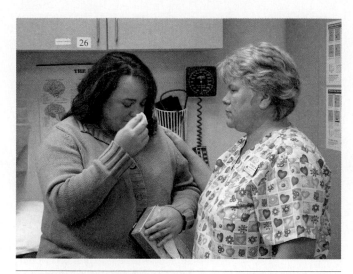

Figure 5-9 ◆ With an emotional patient, the medical assistant must remain calm.

**Keys to Success
WORKING WITH YOUNG PATIENTS**

Treat young patients with respect. Do not lie to them. Misinformation about pain, for example, can instill long-standing distrust in health care professionals. Be honest, and demonstrate on stuffed animals or dolls first so the patients can understand the plan and prepare.

the medical assistant can have them draw pictures. When talking to a young patient, the medical assistant should sit down in order to be at eye level with the patient. Before beginning any procedure on a young patient, even a simple one, the medical assistant should explain the procedure and show the equipment that will be used (Figure 5-10 ◆).

Young patients may at times be subjected to undesirable procedures. Vaccinations and blood draws, for example, may be uncomfortable and may require the patient to remain still for a few

moments. For these types of procedures, parents may be helpful in or out of the room. Medical assistants should use their best judgment about parent presence and reassure the patient as much as possible. When the procedure concludes, the medical assistant should always praise the patient for being brave or "grown up." To help the patients view the medical office in a positive light, the office may reward young patients with a small prize, like a sticker.

Communicating with Grieving Patients

Communicating with grieving patients can be uniquely challenging. First, medical assistants must remember that the patients may be grieving for unique reasons: the loss of a loved one, a job, or a relationship. Patients may also grieve the diagnoses of chronic or terminal illnesses. Second, medical assistants must remember that people feel grief in individual ways. Therefore, medical assistants should never belittle someone for feeling grief. Every person is entitled to grieve and for whatever reason. People feel what they feel. Medical assistants are not entitled to judge why.

Dr. Elizabeth Kübler-Ross was a pioneer in the field of working with dying or grieving patients. She advocated hospice care and wrote several books about the dying process. Kübler-Ross developed a list of the five stages of grief, noting that not every person experiences the stages in the same way or for the same period (Table 5-1).

It is important to remember that there is no "right" way to grieve. Medical assistants should listen to grieving patients and allow those patients time to express themselves. As appropriate, medical assistants should touch patients reassuringly on the arm or shoulder. Because there is no right thing to say, medical assistants should focus on offering support and empathy. Medical assistants can also offer information as needed. With physicians' permission, medical assistants can refer patients to a number of community and national resources that are available through hospice or other support groups (Table 5-2).

Defense Mechanisms

Defense mechanisms are people's characteristic, usually unconscious, ways of protecting themselves in stressful situations. Just as everyone has physical defenses that combat disease, everyone also has mental and emotional defenses to deal with stress and **anxiety**. These mechanisms may be engaged consciously or unconsciously, usually in combination with others. Table 5-3 lists some common defense mechanisms the MA may encounter in patients. The MA should also examine his or her own defense mechanisms as they arise in interactions with patients and coworkers.

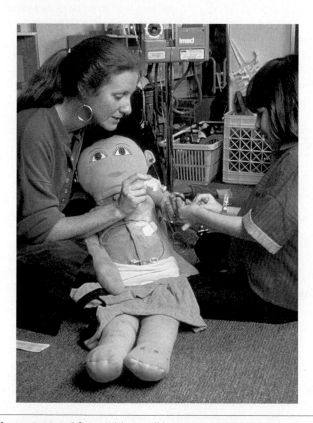

Figure 5-10 ◆ Often children will be more relaxed if the medical assistant demonstrates the procedure on a doll first.

TABLE 5-1 KÜBLER-ROSS' FIVE STAGES OF GRIEF

Stage	Description
Denial	Patients refuse to believe what is happening or has happened to them. This stage lasts until the patients accept the deaths or diagnoses.
Anger	Patients become angry, perhaps with the people who have died or the physicians who have given them the diagnoses. Patients may also become angry with God.
Bargaining	Patients try to make promises in return for the people who have died or new, nonterminal diagnoses (e.g., "I'll spend 20 hours a week doing volunteer work if God will bring back George").
Depression	Deep sadness over the loss sets in. Patients should seek help via counseling and/or medications, if needed.
Acceptance	Patients accept the deaths or diagnoses and begin to move on.

Reprinted with permission of Scribner, an imprint of Simon & Schuster Adult Publishing Group, from On Death and Dying by Dr. Elisabeth Kübler-Ross. Copyright © 1969 by Elisabeth Kübler Ross; copyright renewed © 1997 by Elisabeth Kübler Ross. All rights reserved.

TABLE 5-2 NATIONAL RESOURCES

Organization	Focus Area(s)
American Cancer Society www.cancer.org	Patients, families, friends and survivors of cancer
American Diabetes Association www.diabetes.org	Diabetes and related nutrition and recipes, prevention, and research
American Lung Association www.lungusa.org	Hayfever, asthma, lung cancer, and other respiratory illnesses
National Domestic Violence Hotline www.ndvh.org	Domestic violence, including a toll-free number to call 24 hours per day, 365 days per year
International Child Abuse Network www.yesican.org	Twenty-four-hour chat groups on child abuse, incest, and parenting; Web site is in English and Spanish
American Heart Association www.americanheart.org	Heart attack/stroke warning signs, high blood pressure, and healthy lifestyles; Web site is in English and Spanish
Centers for Disease Control HIV/AIDS www.cdc.gov/hiv/	Information on HIV/AIDS transmission, current research, and Internet links to testing centers or support groups

TABLE 5-3 COMMON DEFENSE MECHANISMS

Compensation	Trying to overcome some inability or inferiority. It helps to maintain one's self-respect and raise self-esteem.
Conversion	Changing an emotional problem into a physical symptom or other method of release that eases tension and anxiety related to conflict.
Denial	Avoiding or escaping the unpleasant or distasteful realities of living by ignoring or refusing to admit their existence.
Displacement	Transferring into another situation an emotion that was felt in a past situation where its expression would have been socially unacceptable.
Identification	Unconsciously imitating the mannerisms, behavior, and feelings of another person.
Overcompensation	Repressing unconscious attitudes and wishes and replacing them with conscious attitudes and behavior that are the opposite of the unconscious ones. Often referred to as *reaction formation*.
Projection	Blaming someone else for one's own failures or for specific events.
Rationalization	Explaining, excusing, or defending ideas, actions, and feelings. It helps to "save face" in embarrassing and anxiety-producing situations.
Regression	Escaping frustration and conflict anxiety by returning to methods used at an earlier stage of life.
Repression	Unconsciously storing unpleasant, unacceptable thoughts, desires, and impulses in the mind. The repressed information does not enter conscious awareness and may not be remembered unless there is an emotional trigger. Repression is sometimes termed *selective forgetting*.
Substitution	Accepting something in place of a desired object or need when the original cannot be obtained. The substitution helps to achieve at least some fulfillment.
Suppression	Storing away or forgetting unpleasant, emotionally painful experiences. This is a conscious forcing of unpleasant, anxiety-producing experiences into the unconscious mind.

Source: Frazier, Margie, Morgan, Connie. Clinical Medical Assisting: Foundations and Practice, First Edition. © 2008. Reprinted by permission of Pearson Education, Inc. Upper Saddle River, NJ.

**Keys to Success
THE INFLUENCE OF CULTURE AND AGE**

The following are examples of different approaches to the same situation—a patient has just been diagnosed with insulin-dependent diabetes.

- You are teaching a 7-year-old boy how to give himself insulin injections. It is natural for the child to be worried. He may not listen well or remember instructions. One way to handle the situation is to find out more about the child's home situation, then instruct one or both parents in giving the insulin injection along with the child. The child will feel more secure when his parents are involved. It also satisfies the child's emotional needs, paving the way for easier learning. A parent or responsible caretaker should be present in the room during the teaching experience.
- A woman with a hearing impairment who is on Medicare and social security thinks she is going to die because she has no money for insulin and syringes. Explain that you will help her contact the appropriate agencies to help pay for the medications. Stress that she should contact you if she needs any other help. By relieving her concerns about money, you now have a patient ready to learn.
- A Chicano man learns he will have to take insulin for the rest of his life. He tells you, "I might as well die!" After talking with the man, you learn he is afraid he will no longer be able to work. Assure him that working should not be a problem. Tell him that learning how to take care of himself will help him continue taking care of his family.

**Keys to Success
PROFESSIONAL COMMUNICATION
WITH PATIENTS**

Medical assistants should conceal all personal stress from patients; voice and body language should mask any negative feelings. When medical assistants cannot keep their patient interactions free of personal stresses, they should consider asking their employer to find a temporary replacement.

of hearing. In addition, medical assistants should always use proper forms of address when speaking with patients. Elderly patients, for example, may prefer to be called either "Mrs. Thompson" or "Margaret."

To ensure patient respect, medical assistants should not assume they can shorten anyone's name; it is rude to shorten a person's name without permission. It is acceptable with permission, however. Take a patient named Richard, for example. The medical assistant should ask the patient if he would like to be called Richard. If he indicates he prefers to be called Rick, then the medical assistant should make a note in his chart so that all members of the health care team can address him properly.

The medical assistant should never use pet names for patients, like "Honey" or "Sweetie." It could offend some patients. The medical assistant should also avoid referring to patients as their conditions, such as "Back pain is in Room 2." In the same vein, the medical assistant should maintain patient confidentiality by only calling out full patient names outside the hearing of other patients.

HIPAA Compliance

To be Health Insurance Portability and Accountability Act (HIPAA)–compliant, the medical assistant should not call patients by their full names in the reception area. Instead, the assistant should use first or last name only. When two patients have the same first name, the last name is appropriate. For example, instead of "Jim," the medical assistant should call out "Mr. Costas."

Keeping a Professional Distance

It is important, both for the patient and the medical assistant, to keep a **professional distance,** but doing so can be difficult. Most health care professionals chose the field because they care about people and find it hard to remain detached when patients are hurting, dying, or in need. Medical assistants could become very stressed if they became attached to every patient, and some patients may take advantage of medical assistants who are willing to go above and beyond the call of duty. Medical assistants need not abandon their concern for patients. They simply must keep a professional distance to maintain a professional image.

In addition to maintaining a professional distance, medical assistants must be very careful to avoid revealing personal details about themselves or the physician. It is acceptable for medical assistants to reveal an engagement when a patient notices an

Defense mechanisms protect a person's self-esteem but do not effectively deal with conflict. It is important to recognize the coping style of the patient, the patient's family, staff, and physicians. For example, one of the most common defense mechanisms is denial. A patient with a serious condition may refuse to believe what is happening. This refusal to accept reality is a factor in the patient's treatment and education.

An understanding of the psychological principles discussed in this chapter will improve your therapeutic communication skills and your interactions with patients.

Maintaining Professional Patient Communication

The most effective medical assistants form positive relationships with their patients through mutual respect and professionalism. Medical assistants must be role models and earn their patients' trust and admiration. In short, medical assistants are professionals and must always act like ones. Medical assistants' bad days should always be hidden from patients, and any personal problems or coworker difficulties should be continually concealed.

Medical assistants must speak respectfully and appropriately to patients, as well as to anyone within the patients' ranges

Keys to Success
COMMUNITY RESOURCES

Do not offer to drive patients to the store or to pay for prescriptions. Medical assistants serve patients best by finding them the appropriate community resources and making referrals with the doctor's permission.

engagement ring, but the assistants should not tell the patient where they live or discuss personal relationships. Such details have no place in the patient–health care professional relationship.

Communicating with Coworkers

The medical assistant must maintain professional communication with coworkers and the doctors at all times while in the office. The medical assistant should minimize any nonwork conversations, remembering that patients may overhear them.

Just as in any work setting, the medical assistant may dislike some coworkers. Personal feelings aside, all members of the health care team should treat each other professionally and respectfully. Should medical assistants ever need to speak to a supervisor about coworkers, they should do so in a private setting. They should be professional, stating only facts, not opinions.

When communicating with the doctor in front of patients, the medical assistant must always address the doctor as "Dr." Even when the doctor is relaxed and informal, patients must have a level of respect for the doctor as an authority, and that image starts with the behavior of the other members of the health care team. Similarly, patients should never suspect that medical assistants are irritated with the physician.

All members of the health care team should be careful to use correct medical terminology and no slang when speaking with physicians and coworkers. The medical assistant should speak slowly, confidently, and always honestly. Jokes and nonwork conversation have no place in the medical office when patients are present.

In Practice

Mark Minton, medical assistant, is completing paperwork in the reception area. Two of his coworkers, who are standing behind him at the front desk, begin a conversation about last night's episode of their favorite television show. Their conversation is loud enough to be heard in the reception area. What should Mark do?

Communicating with Other Facilities

Patient confidentiality is the most important factor when communicating with other facilities. When medical assistants schedule patients in another facility, they should give those facilities only the information they need to schedule the patients. This usually includes patient name and contact information, reason for referral, referring physician, and patient's insurance carrier. Any other information about the patient should come from the patient.

When making appointments for patients with other facilities, medical assistants must be out of hearing range of all other patients in the office. The assistants should have a telephone location for these types of calls, one that is not in the clinic hallway or at the front desk. Calling from the treatment room where the patient is waiting or from a private area is best.

Educating the Patient

Any patient education the medical assistant does in the office must be done under the direction of the physician. Part of patient education includes helping patients accept their condition and providing positive reinforcement. To educate patients properly, the medical assistant must first **assess** the best way to teach them. For this step, the medical assistant will want to know how much pain patients are experiencing or if they are distressed. Patients cannot fully comprehend information when distracted by pain or anxiety.

After assessment, the medical assistant must gather the patient's information. Normally, this is found in the patient's medical record, but the medical assistant might need to gather information from the doctor, the patient's family members, or other health care facilities.

Planning the patient's education includes taking the information gathered during the assessment and determining how to proceed in educating the patient. This step may include gathering pamphlets or printed information on the patient's condition or gathering equipment that will be used to demonstrate a new skill to the patient.

The **implementing** step is the actual teaching phase. During this step, it may help for the medical assistant to demonstrate what they want the patient to learn and then have the patient demonstrate the skill. For example, the medical assistant might show the patient how to use a pair of crutches and then ask the patient to demonstrate using the crutches (Figure 5-11 ◆).

The next step in patient education is **documenting** what has been taught to the patient, the tools used in the teaching process, how well the patient demonstrated the skill, and any concerns the medical assistant may have, such as a patient who states an unwillingness to follow the doctor's instructions.

The **evaluation** step of patient education involves checking to see how well patients are using the information given to them. Some evaluation may need to be done over the phone if the doctor asks patients to call in to let the medical assistant know how they are doing. If the medical assistant discovers a patient is failing to comply with the doctor's instructions, either because they are unable or unwilling, the medical assistant will need to determine if there is a misunderstanding. If the patient is refusing to follow through, the refusal must be charted and the doctor notified right away. Patients have the right to refuse treatment, but if they do so, their choices must be clearly documented.

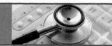

PROCEDURE 5-5   Prepare a Patient's Specialist Referral

Theory and Rationale

Administrative medical assistants are often required to schedule patients to see specialists. This procedure must always be done in a private place and preferably with the patient present. Knowing the steps in this procedure, and how to communicate the necessary information to the patient, is part of being a patient's advocate in the medical office.

Materials

■ Telephone
■ Blue or black ink pen
■ Patient's file
■ Referral form to a specialist

Competency

(**Conditions**) With the necessary materials, you will be able to (**Task**) prepare a referral for a patient to see a specialist (**Standards**) correctly within the time limit set by the instructor.

1. Verify the patient file is correct.
2. Verify the referral form for the specialist is correct.

3. Verify the doctor's instructions (e.g., What does the doctor want the patient to be seen for? How soon does the patient need to be seen?).
4. Choose a private location, out of the hearing range of other patients.
5. If the pending referral is not an emergency and the patient is in the clinic, ask the patient for a convenient time or day to see the specialist.
6. Call the specialist's office, and ask to speak to the person who handles the schedule.
7. Provide personal identification and the name of the referring doctor or clinic.
8. State the reason for the call.
9. Give patient information as requested by the specialist's office.
10. Set an appointment date and time. If the patient is in the clinic, verify the date and time.
11. Document the appointment's date and time on the referral form. If the patient is in the clinic, give the patient the referral form. Choose to mail the referral form when there is time before the appointment.
12. Document the call's results in the patient's chart.

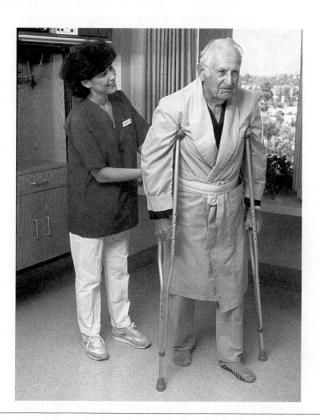

Figure 5-11 ◆ An MA assisting a man learning to use crutches.

Working Through Miscommunication

Miscommunication can be disastrous, so medical assistants must be careful to be completely clear and watch for signs that patients may not understand instructions fully. Communicating with the patient cannot be hurried, so assistants will need to ensure they are comfortable with patients' levels of understanding before moving on.

Taking Time for Patient Education

Depending on the disease or illness, patient education can take several visits. Serious illnesses can be difficult to comprehend, and patients may need multiple visits to comprehend all the

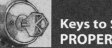

Keys to Success
PROPER CHARTING

The party who signs the patient's medical chart is assumed to have performed the tasks described. For example if, after entering information on patient instruction, the medical assistant signs the chart, the assistant indicates that he or she did the teaching. When that is not the case, notes must reflect the facts.

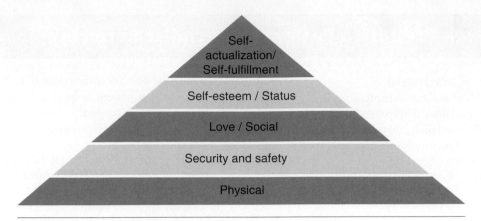

Figure 5-12 ◆ Maslow's hierarchy of needs.

relevant information. When patients are willing to bring family members, those family members can be very helpful in patient-education initiatives. Written instructions or information are also helpful, because they serve as reference materials outside the medical office.

Maslow's Hierarchy of Needs

Patients must be ready to learn for education to occur. They must be motivated and see a need to learn what the medical assistant is trying to teach. Abraham Maslow was an American psychiatrist who came up with a theory that said people will be motivated by their needs and that lower level needs must be met before higher ones. For example, it is impossible to teach people about proper nutrition when they cannot access food.

Maslow arranged human needs on a pyramid with basic needs at the bottom and higher needs at the top. The medical assistant's job is to determine where patients are on this chart before teaching those patients new skills (Figure 5-12 ◆).

Establishing a Proper Learning Environment

The teaching environment must be conducive to learning. It must be quiet and free from interruptions, and it should be well lighted. Hallways, the reception area, and any locations in view of other patients are inappropriate places for teaching. Patients must feel relaxed, comfortable, and able to ask questions (Figure 5-13 ◆).

Assume the medical assistant is teaching a patient how to use a piece of equipment. The equipment should be in the office, and the medical assistant should be very familiar with the equipment's use and repair. The medical assistant should always provide written instructions on how to use any machinery.

Medical assistants must have solid knowledge of the skills they are trying to teach. When assistants are uncomfortable or less knowledgeable, they should request help before teaching patients. If patients ask a question and medical assistants do not know the answer, the assistants should admit they do not know and let the patients know they will find the answer and get back to them.

Using Teaching Resources

Teaching resources may be available for purchase, or the medical office can create its own. The medical assistant may use such teaching tools as audiocassettes, compact disks (CDs), food labels, videos, or pamphlets in helping to demonstrate a new skill to a patient. Because people learn through seeing, hearing, and touching, and different patients may have different learning styles, the medical assistant may need to incorporate more than one teaching approach to educate the patient.

Appreciating the Patient's Skills and Abilities

Before teaching patients new skills, the medical assistant must be aware of any of the patients' physical impairments. For example, assistants must know if patients cannot open a bottle of pills due to severe arthritis, especially when educating about medication use throughout the day. In cases like these, the medical assistant may need to improvise and devise other ways to help patients accomplish the doctor's directives.

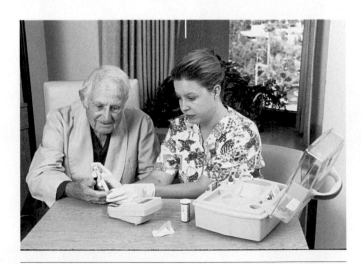

Figure 5-13 ◆ A quiet environment is the best place to teach a patient a new skill.

Keys to Success
PREVENTING CHILDHOOD INJURIES

Preventable injuries are the leading cause of childhood death in the United States. Medical assistants working in family practices or pediatric offices should have educational materials on how to keep children safe and distribute them to new parents. Simple tips for preventing choking, drowning accidents, and fire hazards can help prevent tragedies.

Factoring Culture into Patient Education

Patients' cultures may prevent the medical assistant from teaching those patients certain skills. It is important for the medical assistant to know this and to come up with alternatives that are acceptable to both the physician and the patient. An example would be a medical assistant teaching a patient about proper nutrition. If the patient's culture is one that does not consume meat, the medical assistant must consult the physician regarding alternatives.

Factoring Finances into Patient Education

Financial difficulties may prevent patients from achieving desired educational goals. For example, patients may be unable to pay for appropriate shoes to begin a walking or exercise program. The medical assistant must address any such restrictions before undertaking education.

In Practice

Dr. Lopez has asked the medical assistant to schedule Sara Hardy for three followup visits, but Sara is not covered by insurance and states that she can afford just one visit. How should the medical assistant proceed?

Teaching Patients about Preventive Medicine

Studies have shown that if people practiced preventive medicine, they would greatly reduce the cost of health care in the United States. Preventive medicine includes mammograms or prostate exams, yearly physical exams, and scheduled immunizations for children. Medical assistants should promote health screenings to patients. They should keep educational literature available and ask patients about their last physical examinations to encourage screening appointments.

Preventing Medication Errors

Medication errors are far too common and are mostly preventable. Medical assistants can help prevent such errors by properly teaching patients about their medications. Patients do not always read the information the pharmacist gives them, and they sometimes fail to take time to consult with the pharmacist. Figure 5-14 ◆ is a sample medication-teaching tool that can be implemented in any medical office.

```
Name of
medication:_____

Dosage:_____

You will be taking this medication _____ times each
day.

This medication is being prescribed for the following
health condition:_____

Possible side effects of this medication include:
_____

If you experience any of the following signs or symp-
toms, please call the office right away:_____
_____
```

Figure 5-14 ◆ Sample medication-teaching tool.

Keys to Success
PREVENTING INJURIES IN THE ELDERLY

Falls are common with the elderly, and they are preventable. Practices that treat elderly patients should distribute pamphlets detailing how to prevent falls. Such pamphlets should include details like removing throw rugs and ensuring steps are lined with slip-resistant material.

Keys to Success
IS THE INFORMATION PRACTICAL FOR THE PATIENT'S LIFESTYLE?

Be sure to think or ask about patients' lifestyles before teaching them about the medications they need to take. Do they work nights? If a prescription says to take a medication three times per day, does that mean patients must rise in the middle of the night? Ensure patients are clear on how to administer medications and know the proper administration routes.

Providing Dieting or Weight-Loss Information

Because patients will ask for information on dieting or weight loss, medical assistants should have information on hand to teach basic nutrition. This information should include copies of the new food guide (MyPyramid) and information on reading food labels (Figures 5-15 ◆ and 5-16 ◆). The

MyPyramid food guide outlines the types of foods and food groups that are necessary for a balanced diet. Many people are unaware of the proper foods to eat to maintain a healthy lifestyle and giving this information to the patient is one way to help them make healthy changes in their diet. However, the physician must authorize any information given to patients.

Anatomy of MyPyramid

One size doesn't fit all
USDA's new MyPyramid symbolizes a personalized approach to healthy eating and physical activity. The symbol has been designed to be simple. It has been developed to remind consumers to make healthy food choices and to be active every day. The different parts of the symbol are described below.

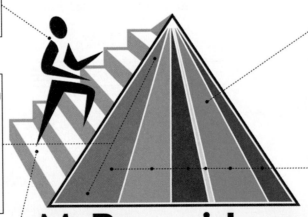

Activity
Activity is represented by the steps and the person climbing them, as a reminder of the importance of daily physical activity.

Moderation
Moderation is represented by the narrowing of each food group from bottom to top. The wider base stands for foods with little or no solid fats or added sugars. These should be selected more often. The narrower top area stands for foods containing more added sugars and solid fats. The more active you are, the more of these foods you can fit into your diet.

Personalization
Personalization is shown by the person on the steps, the slogan, and the URL. Find the kinds and amounts of food to eat each day at MyPyramid.gov.

Proportionality
Proportionality is shown by the different widths of the food group bands. The widths suggest how much food a person should choose from each group. The widths are just a general guide, not exact proportions. Check the website for how much is right for you.

Variety
Variety is symbolized by the 6 color bands representing the 5 food groups of the Pyramid and oils. This illustrates that foods from all groups are needed each day for good health.

Gradual Improvement
Gradual improvement is encouraged by the slogan. It suggests that individuals can benefit from taking small steps to improve their diet and lifestyle each day.

USDA U.S. Department of Agriculture Center for Nutrition Policy and Promotion April 2005 CNPP-16

USDA is an equal opportunity provider and employer.

| GRAINS | VEGETABLES | FRUITS | OILS | MILK | MEAT& BEANS |

Figure 5-15 ◆ MyPyramid food guide.

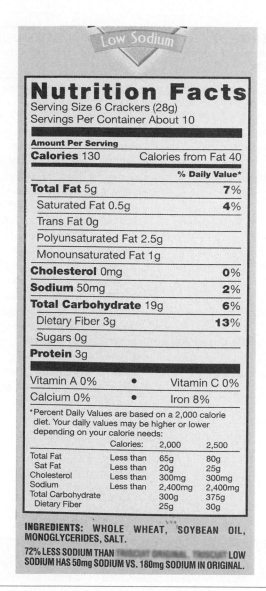

Nutrition Facts
Serving Size 6 Crackers (28g)
Servings Per Container About 10

Amount Per Serving	
Calories 130	Calories from Fat 40

	% Daily Value*
Total Fat 5g	7%
Saturated Fat 0.5g	4%
Trans Fat 0g	
Polyunsaturated Fat 2.5g	
Monounsaturated Fat 1g	
Cholesterol 0mg	0%
Sodium 50mg	2%
Total Carbohydrate 19g	6%
Dietary Fiber 3g	13%
Sugars 0g	
Protein 3g	

Vitamin A 0%	•	Vitamin C 0%
Calcium 0%	•	Iron 8%

*Percent Daily Values are based on a 2,000 calorie diet. Your daily values may be higher or lower depending on your calorie needs:

		Calories:	2,000	2,500
Total Fat	Less than		65g	80g
Sat Fat	Less than		20g	25g
Cholesterol	Less than		300mg	300mg
Sodium	Less than		2,400mg	2,400mg
Total Carbohydrate			300g	375g
Dietary Fiber			25g	30g

INGREDIENTS: WHOLE WHEAT, SOYBEAN OIL, MONOGLYCERIDES, SALT.

72% LESS SODIUM THAN ████████ ████████ ████████ LOW SODIUM HAS 50mg SODIUM VS. 180mg SODIUM IN ORIGINAL.

Figure 5-16 ◆ Food label listing nutritional information.

Delivering Information on Exercise

Teaching patients about exercise is a common task. Medical assistants should have pamphlets on the benefits of exercise. Patients must be taught the importance of easing into exercise programs, how to stretch and warm up properly, and how to keep from injuring themselves. Any patient over age 35 or with any underlying health conditions should seek the advice of their physician before beginning any new exercise program.

Educating Patients about Stress Reduction

Most people are under various levels of stress every day. Sometimes that stress gets to be too much to handle, and it impedes health. Having information on how to handle and reduce stress is one tool to help patients to maintain good health. Many physicians suggest their patients find a mechanism for reducing stress that works best for that patient's lifestyle. Some ideas for stress reduction are:

- **Breathing exercises.** Deep, slow breathing is believed to relax the muscles, oxygenate the blood, and calm the mind.
- **Meditation.** This technique goes a step further than deep breathing exercises. With meditation, the mind is literally focused on nothing—taking the stressful thoughts or situation out of mind for a period of time.
- **Guided imagery.** This technique is taught to women who take childbirth education classes. With this technique, the patient closes their eyes and thinks of a pleasant situation to focus upon.
- **Visualization.** Taking guided imagery one step further, visualization is the technique of thinking of a task that needs to be done and thinking of doing it well. During a stressful situation, this technique might be used to visualize a resolution that is less stressful.
- **Exercise.** Many people find that exercise has the benefit of reducing stress.
- **Sex.** Though in stressful situations many people tend to have less sex, physicians recommend sex as a stress reliever.
- **Music.** Listening to relaxing music is a well known mechanism for reducing stress levels.
- **Yoga.** This type of exercise incorporates breathing techniques and imagery, which can greatly reduce a person's stress level.

Teaching Patients about Smoking Cessation and Substance Abuse

Patients who smoke or abuse other substances will sometimes ask for help in stopping. Physicians may advise patients to stop smoking for health-related reasons. Therefore, medical assistants should have information that has been approved by the physician on hand to give to patients to let them know what resources are available, both locally and nationally or on the Internet. The American Cancer Society (ACS) Web site (www.cancer.org) contains valuable resources for persons who wish to quit smoking. The ACS points out that tobacco addiction is both psychological and physical. For this reason, most people who wish to quit smoking may need to try some combination of medicine, some method to change personal habits, and some level of emotional support. On the ACS Web site, patients or healthcare professionals can find links to information on:

- Using nicotine replacement therapy
- Various nicotine substitutes
- Choosing the right method to quit smoking
- Telephone support to help stop smoking
- Support groups
- Success rates

The National Institute on Drug Abuse (NIDA) maintains a Web site (www.nida.nih.gov), which provides a wealth of information on drug abuse and addiction. There the patient or healthcare professional will find information and resources for combating abuse of:

- Alcohol
- Club drugs
- Cocaine
- Heroin
- Inhalants
- LSD
- Marijuana
- Ecstasy
- Methamphetamine
- PCP
- Prescription medications
- Tobacco
- Anabolic steroids

Using the Internet for Education

The Internet has patient education materials, but the medical assistant should use only reputable Web sites to gather information on conditions, medications, or illnesses (Table 5-3). Reputable Web sites are typically those that are associated with a university or college, the government, reputable news sources, and nonprofit organizations. Web sites that are maintained as "personal sites"—sites that are created and maintained by one person containing that person's beliefs—are not typically considered a reputable source for patient education materials. The physician should approve any material before the assistant gives it to patients.

TABLE 5-3 REPUTABLE WEB SITES FOR PATIENT EDUCATION

Web Site	Information
American Lung Association	Smoking cessation, asthma, hay fever, lung cancer (www.lungusa.org)
American Diabetes Associations	Nutrition and recipes, weight loss and exercise, diabetes prevention (www.diabetes.org)
Hospice	Guides for caregivers of and patients with terminal illnesses, talking to children about death, pain control, advance directives, finding a local hospice, healing after a loss (www.americanhospice.org)
American Heart Association	High blood pressure, controlling cholesterol levels, diet, and nutrition (www.americanheart.org)
Alzheimer's Association	Living with Alzheimer's, guides for caregivers (www.alz.org)
American Parkinson Disease Association	Local support groups (www.apdaparkinson.org)
ALS Association	Local support groups, guides for caregivers (www.alsa.org)

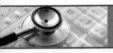

PROCEDURE 5-6 Identify Community Resources

Theory and Rationale

Medical assistants will frequently be asked to give patients referrals to community resources at the physician's request. Having this information in an easy and quick to locate format is one way to provide patients with excellent care.

Materials

- A computer with Internet access
- Written pamphlets and brochures
- Telephone directories

Competency

(**Conditions**) With the necessary materials, you will be able to (**Task**) identify community resources (**Standards**) correctly within the time limit set by the instructor.

1. Locate the name, address, telephone number, and website address for each of the following need categories in your community:
   a. Homeless services
   b. HIV/AIDS resources
   c. Disability services
   d. Domestic violence services
   e. Public assistance
   f. Housing authority/services
   g. Ombudsman services
   h. Foster care for children
   i. Foster care for adults
   j. Senior services
   k. Legal aid
   l. Rape victim services
   m. Crime victim services
   n. Culturally specific services (Native American, Military, etc.)
   o. Medical assistant services (Medicaid, etc.)
2. Identify at least 1–3 resources for each need category.
3. Create a written document to give to patients.

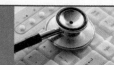

PROCEDURE 5-7 Use the Internet to Find Patient Education Materials

Theory and Rationale

Locating educational resources on the Internet is a fast way to find information. Often, the information can be printed and distributed to patients or incorporated into an educational piece created by the medical office.

Materials

- Computer and printer
- Patient chart
- Blue or black pen

Competency

(**Conditions**) With the necessary materials, you will be able to (**Task**) use the Internet to find patient education materials

(**Standards**) correctly within the time limit set by the instructor.

1. Using the computer, locate reputable Web sites for desired materials.
2. Print copies of materials.
3. Show materials to the physician for approval.
4. Give/mail the materials to the patient.
5. Explain the materials to the patient as needed.
6. Place a copy of the materials in the patient's file.
7. Document how the materials were given to the patient and any verbal education provided with the materials.

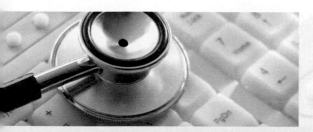

REVIEW

Chapter Summary

- Good communication skills are vital to anyone who works in health care, but especially for the medical assistant, who must demonstrate superior verbal and nonverbal communication.
- Listening is a crucial component of communication in health care.
- The medical assistant must identify barriers to communication and work to overcome them using the appropriate tools and techniques.
- Patient populations, including those with special needs and/or disabilities, dictate the ways in which the medical assistant should interact with them.
- A number of community resources are available when it comes time for patient referrals.

- Just as they do with patients, medical assistants must communicate properly, professionally, and respectfully with the other members of the health care team.
- Patient education is a vital part of the medical assistant's job duties
- Patient education consists of supplying information about the patient's condition and treatment options and on supplying the patient with resources where they might seek further information.

Chapter Review

Multiple Choice

1. What is the proper way to address an elderly patient?
   a. Mrs. _____
   b. By first name
   c. "Honey" or "Sweetie"
   d. None of the above

2. The opinion that all people living in homeless shelters are likely to have lice is an example of:
   a. Stereotyping
   b. Discriminating

3. Which of the following is *not* an example of keeping a professional distance?
   a. Giving a patient transportation options to the clinic
   b. Offering to pay a patient's copayment
   c. Reviewing a patient's billing charges with the patient
   d. None of the above

4. When calling another facility to schedule a patient, the most important factor to remember is:
   a. End the call quickly
   b. Get the earliest appointment
   c. Maintain patient confidentiality
   d. All of the above

True/False

T F 1. Body language is far less important than verbal communication.

T F 2. Empathy and sympathy are really the same thing.

T F 3. When working with a hearing-impaired patient, the medical assistant should speak directly to the interpreter.

T F 4. When working with child patients, it is best to communicate directly with the parent during the visit rather than the child.

T F 5. Addressing the physician as "Dr." in front of patients gives patients the impression that the doctor is an authority figure who should be respected.

T F 6. Part of developing a good patient relationship includes sharing personal problems with the patients.

T F 7. Sometimes, patient communication may take more than one visit.

T F 8. Patients will often share more information with the medical assistant that they will with the physician.

T F 9. It is best to use proper medical terminology when speaking with patients to demonstrate intelligence.

T F 10. A clinic's office policy dictates whether to allow service animals to accompany their owners to treatment rooms.

Short Answer

1. What is a good communication technique to use with angry patients?

2. Name the five stages of grief.

3. Why would writing down patient instructions help the patient?

4. What is the difference between an open-ended question and a close-ended question?

5. When might it be appropriate to use therapeutic touch with a patient?

6. Describe the method you would use to communicate effectively with a hearing-impaired patient.

Research

1. Search the Internet for books to read about communication skills. Which ones sound as if they might be helpful to the medical assistant?

2. What are the local resources for hearing-impaired people in your area?

3. What are the local resources for sight-impaired people in your area?

Externship Application Experience

Dr. Roberts wants Beth Parcher, a sight-impaired patient, to be scheduled for a series of physical therapy appointments and has asked the medical assistant to schedule the appointments.

How will the medical assistant ensure Beth completely understands what Dr. Roberts wants her to do? How will the assistant ensure Beth is clear about the appointments scheduled for her?

Resource Guide

American Lung Association
61 Broadway, 6th Floor
New York, NY 10006
1-800-LUNGUSA
www.lungusa.org

American Diabetes Association
ATTN: National Call Center
1701 North Beauregard Street
Alexandria, VA 22311
1-800-DIABETES
www.diabetes.org

American Hospice Foundation
2120 L Street NW, Suite 200
Washington, DC 20037
1-800-347-1413
www.americanhospice.org

American Heart Association National Center
7272 Greenville Avenue
Dallas, TX 75231
1-800-AHA-USA-1
www.americanheart.org

Alzheimer's Association
225 N. Michigan Ave, Floor 17
Chicago, IL 60601
(312) 335-5886
www.alz.org

American Parkinson Disease Association Inc.
135 Parkinson Avenue
Staten Island, NY 10305
1-800-223-2732
www.apdaparkinson.org

The ALS Association
27001 Agoura Road, Suite 150
Calabasas Hills, CA 91301
(818) 880-9007
www.alsa.org

Online Communication Skills Test
http://discoveryhealth.queendom.com/

Seven Challenges: A guide to cooperative communication skills
http://www.newconversations.net/

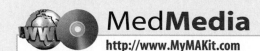

Med**Media**
http://www.MyMAKit.com

More on this chapter, including interactive resources, can be found on the Student CD-ROM accompanying this textbook and on http://www.MyMAKit.com.

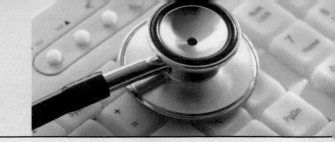

CHAPTER 6

Written Communication

Case Study

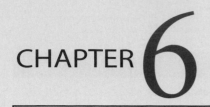

D r. Calvin Jones brings the medical assistant a business card from the medical equipment salesperson he just had lunch with and asks the assistant to type a letter to the salesperson. In the letter, the physician would like to thank the salesperson for showing him a new electrocardiogram (**EKG**) machine and indicate that while he is uninterested in purchasing the machine now, the salesperson should call after the first of the year to assess the physician's willingness to purchase one at that time.

Objectives

After completing this chapter, you should be able to:

- Define and spell the key terminology in this chapter.
- Use correct grammar, spelling, and punctuation in all professional written communication.
- Discuss how to compose a patient letter.
- Detail the process of proofreading a business letter.
- List accepted health care abbreviations.
- Describe appropriate memo use in the medical office.
- Classify mail, including its size and postage requirements.
- Develop a policy for incoming and outgoing e-mail to patients.
- Manage incoming mail and correspondence.

Med**Media**

http://www.MyMAKit.com

Additional interactive resources and activities for this chapter can be found on http://www.MyMAKit.com. For a video, tips, audio glossary, legal and ethical scenarios, on-the-job scenarios, quizzes, and games related to the content of this chapter, please access the accompanying CD-ROM in this book.

Video
Legal and Ethical Scenario: *Written Communication*
On the Job Scenario: *Written Communication*
Tips
Multiple Choice Quiz
Audio Glossary
HIPAA Quiz
Games: Spelling Bee, Crossword, and Strikeout

⊕ MEDICAL ASSISTING STANDARDS

CAAHEP ENTRY-LEVEL STANDARDS	ABHES ENTRY-LEVEL COMPETENCIES
■ Recognize elements of fundamental writing skills (cognitive) ■ Discuss applications of electronic technology in effective communication (cognitive) ■ Organize technical information and summaries (cognitive) ■ Report relevant information to others succinctly and accurately (psychomotor) ■ Explain general office policies (psychomotor) ■ Instruct patients according to their needs to promote health maintenance and disease prevention (psychomotor) ■ Compose professional/business letters (psychomotor) ■ Use office hardware and software to maintain office systems (psychomotor) ■ Analyze communications in providing appropriate responses/feedback (affective)	■ Adapt to change ■ Maintain confidentiality at all times ■ Project a positive attitude ■ Be cognizant of ethical boundaries ■ Evidence a responsible attitude ■ Conduct work within scope of education, training, and ability ■ Application of electronic technology ■ Apply computer concepts for office procedures ■ Be courteous and diplomatic ■ Serve as a liaison between the physician and others ■ Receive, organize, prioritize, and transmit information expediently ■ Fundamental writing skills

✓ COMPETENCY SKILLS PERFORMANCE

1. Compose a business letter.
2. Prepare a document for photocopying.
3. Send a letter to a patient about a missed appointment.
4. Proofread written documents.
5. Fold documents for window envelopes.
6. Open and sort mail.
7. Annotate written correspondence.

Introduction

The ability to compose written documents is key for the administrative medical assistant. Physicians regularly ask medical assistants to type the letters they send to patients and other health care providers. Often, physicians will provide just basic facts and ask their medical assistants to compose letters with more detail. To perform these tasks well, the medical assistant must understand medical terminology as well as proper grammar, sentence structure, and punctuation.

Key Terminology

annotation—process of reading a document and highlighting pertinent information

body—main portion of a business letter

closing—ending portion of a business letter

electronic mail—message sent electronically from one person to another; also called e-mail

font—style of type

letterhead—professional-quality stationery with a business' contact information (e.g., name, address, telephone and fax numbers)

logo—image that represents a business entity or brand

memo—interoffice note

postage meter—electronic scale used for weighing packages and printing postage labels

proofreading—process of reading and reviewing a document for errors

proofreader's marks—notations used when reading and reviewing a document for errors; see also *proofreading*

reference initials—in a professional letter, the all-capital initials of the author followed by the all-lowercase initials of the person who typed the letter (e.g., AJF/cmm)

salutation—greeting

spell check—software that verifies word spellings

subject line—in a professional letter, the subject of the letter

thesaurus—resource for locating alternate words with similar meanings

Abbreviations

EKG—electrocardiogram

JCAHO—Joint Commission on the Accreditation of Healthcare Organizations

MLOCR—multiline optical character reader

OCR—optical character recognition

PDR—Physician's Desk Reference

UPS—United Parcel Service

USPS—United States Postal Service

Writing to Patients and Other Health Care Professionals

Any written correspondence from the medical office reflects the physician and the office. Typographical, grammatical, and punctuation errors are not only confusing; they reflect poorly on the medical office and may endanger the patient. Therefore, as a general rule, letters to patients and other health care professionals should be accurate, professional, and to the point. Each paragraph should address one topic and have no more than three to six sentences (Figure 6-1 ◆).

To compose and correct documents properly, every medical office should have a comprehensive medical dictionary, a **thesaurus** for acceptable alternate words, a desk dictionary, current coding books for procedure and diagnostic coding, and a *Physician's Desk Reference* (**PDR**) (Figures 6-2 ◆ through 6-4 ◆).

The Role of Spell-Checking

To help ensure written correspondence is error free, most computer software programs have built-in **spell-check** abilities, but medical assistants should not rely on such programs alone.

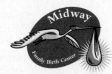

Jack Tsong, MD
Midway Family Birth Center
55 Long Island Way
Seattle, WA 12345

July 25, 2008

Suzanne Haufe
4728 California Ave E
Seattle, WA 12345

Dear Suzanne:

On behalf of my entire staff, I would like to welcome you to Midway Family Birth Center. Our goal is to provide our patients the highest quality service. If you ever feel we fall short, please bring it to my attention. I would consider it a personal favor.

It is an honor that you have placed your care in our hands. We look forward to working with you to meet your health goals.

Sincerely,

Jack Tsong, MD

Jack Tsong, MD
JKT/cmm

Figure 6-1 ◆ Sample patient letter.

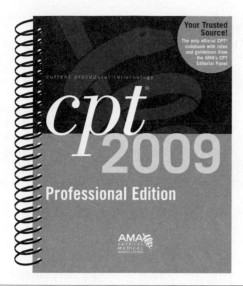

Figure 6-2 ✦ Current Procedural Terminology (CPT) 2007 Professional Edition coding book.
Reprinted by permission of the American Medical Association.

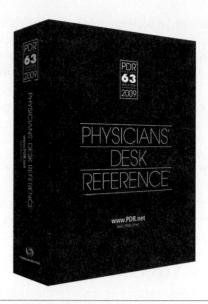

Figure 6-4 ✦ Physician's Desk Reference (PDR).
Reprinted by permission of Thomson Healthcare.

Some words may pass spell checking because they are spelled correctly, but they may be used incorrectly. For example, the words "two," "to," and "too" all pass computerized spell checking, but each has a distinct meaning that is sometimes confused. An understanding of meaning is therefore important. Also, many spelling-verification programs lack the ability to check medical terms. As a result, medical assistants should keep medical dictionaries on hand for supplementary reference. While spell-check programs can be valuable tools, the medical assistant should take the time to read all documents for errors before giving those documents to physicians for final review and signing.

?—**Critical Thinking Question 6-1**—
Referring to the case study at the beginning of this chapter, how can the medical assistant help ensure the typed letter contains no errors?

Proper Spelling, Grammar, and Punctuation Use

Many words in the English language, especially medical words, are commonly misspelled. Table 6-1 gives some examples. When medical assistants are unsure of correct spellings of medical terms, they should consult a comprehensive medical dictionary. Commonly used medical dictionaries include *Taber's Cyclopedic Medical Dictionary* and *Mosby's Medical Dictionary*.

Like accurate spelling, proper grammar is essential to a medical office's written correspondence. Poor grammar is

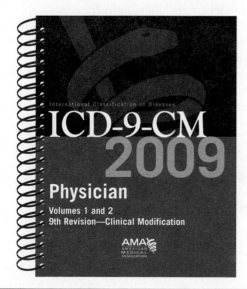

Figure 6-3 ✦ International Classification of Diseases, 9th Edition, Clinical Modification (ICD-9-CM) coding book.
Reprinted by permission of the American Medical Association.

TABLE 6-1 COMMONLY MISSPELLED WORDS

acceptable	accidentally	accommodate
acquire	a lot	apparent
believe	calendar	category
cemetery	changeable	collectible
column	conscience	conscientious
conscious	discipline	embarrass
foreign	gauge	guarantee
harass	height	immediate
inoculate	judgment	leisure
liaison	maintenance	maneuver
miniature	minuscule	noticeable
occurrence	personnel	possession
privilege	publicly	questionnaire
receive	recommend	referred
relevant	schedule	threshold

unprofessional and reflects poorly on the physician and the office. Part of the medical assistant's role is to correct any grammar issues in physicians' drafts but retain the original intent of the content. Table 6-2 identifies common grammatical errors.

?— Critical Thinking Question 6-2—

What are the possible ramifications for Dr. Jones if the medical assistant does not use accurate grammar, spelling, and punctuation?

Proper punctuation is another vital focus area in written documentation. Table 6-3 outlines the rules of use for common punctuation marks.

Sentence Structure

In order to compose a proper sentence, certain components must be present. Every sentence must have a subject and a predicate in order to be a proper sentence. The subject is whom or what the sentence is about. The predicate is the word that says something about the subject. As an example, consider the sentence: "The patient arrived at 2:00 P.M." The subject is the word that the verb describes. In the example sentence, the verb "arrived" is describing the subject "patient." The predicate is what the subject did. In the example sentence, the predicate is "arrived at 2:00 P.M."

Numbers in Correspondence

In general, medical assistants should use words for quantities from one to ten in office correspondence but numbers for quantities over ten, like 24 or 876. When writing any unit of measurement, however, such as a medication dosage or weight or height, numbers always apply. For example, the medical assistant should type, "The patient is taking 5 milligrams of the medication every hour." Numbers also always apply for the time of day, such as "1 P.M."

TABLE 6-2 COMMON GRAMMATICAL ERRORS

Error	Example
Noun/verb mismatch	"The office feels this is a bad idea." (The office cannot feel, but people can.)
Adjective used as a verb	"I did good on that exam." (The word *well* should replace *good*.)
Sentence that ends with a preposition	"This is something we need to work on." (A proper rewrite is, "This is something on which we need to work.")
Run-on sentence	"This lab is a dangerous place, patients should not be back here." (A semicolon should replace the comma.)
Misuse of words that sound alike but differ in spellings and meanings	"Their here, just two quiet." (The sentence should read, "They're here, just too quiet.")

TABLE 6-3 RULES OF USE FOR COMMON PUNCTUATION MARKS

Mark	Use(s)
Period (.)	Indicates the end of a sentence and separates the part of an abbreviation.
Comma (,)	Separates words, phrases, or two independent clauses and sets off elements that interrupt or add information in a sentence.
Semicolon (;)	Sets apart independent clauses and items in a list that contain commas.
Colon (:)	Follows a salutation in a business letter, precedes a list, separates independent clauses, helps express time.
Apostrophe (')	Indicates a missing letter from a contracted word and the possessive case of nouns.
Diagonal (/)	Separates the numbers in dates (e.g., 6/1/07) and fractions (e.g., 1/2) and sometimes indicates abbreviations (e.g., w/o).
Parentheses ( )	Sets off part of a sentence that is not part of the main thought.
Quotation marks (" ")	Indicates a direct quote.
Ellipsis (. . .)	Shows that a thought trails off or represents missing material (e.g., "I was going to, but . . .").

Rules for Medical-Term Plurals

The rules for creating plurals of medical terms can create confusion. Table 6-4 serves as a guide to the proper approaches.

Components of the Business Letter

All business letters, including those from medical offices, have the same basic components. First, each letter should appear on **letterhead**. Most medical offices have professionally printed letterhead that carries the offices' names and addresses, telephone and fax numbers, e-mail addresses, and physicians' names (Figure 6-5 ◆). Letterhead may also contain a **logo,** some form of artwork that indicates the type of practice or other item of significance. For example, a pediatric office might have a

TABLE 6-4 PLURALIZATION RULES FOR MEDICAL TERMS

Singular Form	Plural	Example
a	ae	bulla to bullae
ax	aces	thorax to thoraces
ex or ix	ices	appendix to appendices
on	a	ganglion to ganglia
um	a	ilium to illia
us	i	mellitus to melliti
y	ies	idiosyncrasy to idiosyncrasies
nx	ges	phalanx to phalanges

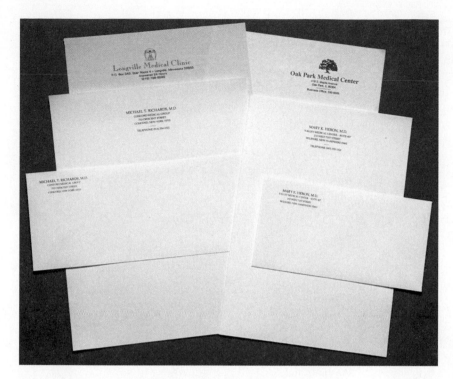

Figure 6-5 ◆ Sample physician letterhead stationery and envelopes.

logo that depicts children, while a chiropractic office might have a logo that includes a spine.

After letterhead, every piece of correspondence that is composed in the medical office must contain a nonabbreviated date, such as May 26, 2008, three lines down from the letterhead content at the top. Normally, a letter carries the date that the physician wrote or dictated it, not the date the medical assistant types it.

Three to six lines after the date comes the next component of the business letter: the inside address. The inside address appears against the left margin and includes the recipient's name, title, company name, and address (Figure 6-6 ◆). Except for state name, the inside address includes no abbreviations. Table 6-5 lists the two-letter abbreviation for each state.

The **salutation** component of the business letter serves as the greeting. It typically appears two lines down from the inside address and carries the same name as the inside address. The salutations of formal letters should include the recipients' proper names and courtesy titles, such as "Dear Dr. Hagen." Table 6-6 provides guidelines for courtesy titles. For more informal correspondence, such as between two physicians who know each other well, salutations may use first names only, as

in "Dear Shawn." When unsure of name spellings, medical assistants should ask for verification.

Critical Thinking Question 6-3

Which courtesy title is appropriate for a letter to a sales representative, and why?

The **subject line** is that part of the business letter that describes the letter's purpose. The subject line should appear two lines down from the salutation after the abbreviation "RE:" to indicate "regarding." A subject line might read, "RE: Sally Luder," for example. The subject line is the patient's name when the letter is about the patient (Figure 6-7 ◆).

The **body** is the main part of the business letter. It should start two lines down from the subject line, and each of its paragraphs should address only one issue, as mentioned earlier (see Figure 6-7).

The **closing** part of the letter typically appears two lines down from the ending portion of the body. The most common closing in a business letter is "Sincerely," but closing choice is at

Shawn D. Hagen, DC
19713 Scriber Lake Road
Lynnwood, WA 98036

Figure 6-6 ◆ Sample inside address.

TABLE 6-5 TWO-LETTER STATE ABBREVIATIONS

State	Abbreviation	State	Abbreviation
Alaska	AK	North Carolina	NC
Alabama	AL	North Dakota	ND
Arkansas	AR	Nebraska	NE
Arizona	AZ	New Hampshire	NH
California	CA	New Jersey	NJ
Colorado	CO	New Mexico	NM
Connecticut	CT	Nevada	NV
Delaware	DE	New York	NY
Florida	FL	Ohio	OH
Georgia	GA	Oklahoma	OK
Hawaii	HI	Oregon	OR
Iowa	IA	Pennsylvania	PA
Idaho	ID	Rhode Island	RI
Illinois	IL	South Carolina	SC
Indiana	IN	South Dakota	SD
Kansas	KS	Tennessee	TN
Kentucky	KY	Texas	TX
Louisiana	LA	Utah	UT
Massachusetts	MA	Virginia	VA
Maryland	MD	Vermont	VT
Maine	ME	Washington	WA
Michigan	MI	Wisconsin	WI
Missouri	MO	West Virginia	WV
Mississippi	MS	Wyoming	WY
Montana	MT		

the physician's discretion. Four or five lines should be left between the closing and the physician's typed name to accommodate the physician's handwritten signature (see Figure 6-7).

Reference initials typically appear four to five lines down from the closing. Reference initials include the all-capital initials of the physician who wrote the letter, followed by the all-lowercase initials of the medical assistant who typed the letter (Figure 6-8 ◆).

Any information that may be enclosed with the letter should be indicated in the form of an enclosure notification two lines down from the reference initials. Such information can be indicated as "Enclosures" or "ENC.," followed by the number of items that are enclosed in parentheses. For example, a letter with two enclosures would have an enclosure notification that reads "Enclosures (2)" or "ENC. (2)." When there are no enclosures, this notation is omitted.

When the letter is to be copied to another party, the notation "c:" followed by that party's name should appear two lines down from the enclosure indication. For example, when Sally Luder is to receive a copy of the letter, the copy notation would read, "c: Sally Luder."

Sometimes, business letters exceed one page. When they do, all subsequent pages must begin with the date of the letter, followed by the subject line. Pages after the first page require no letterhead, but they should appear on paper that matches the color and quality of the letterhead. Subsequent pages should be numbered.

TABLE 6-6 GUIDELINES FOR COURTESY TITLES

- ■ "Mr." is the appropriate title for males.
- ■ Professional titles like "MD" or "DO" replace the courtesy title. For example, "John Aye, MD," should replace "Mr. John Aye."
- ■ "Ms." is used when a woman's marital status is unknown, or when the woman prefers.
- ■ "Mrs." is used for a married woman.
- ■ "Miss" is used for a young girl or an unmarried woman who prefers it. When in doubt, use "Ms." rather than "Miss."
- ■ Two people at the same address should appear separately (e.g., "Mr. Joseph Paterniti and Ms. Beth Dorio").

Keys to Success
SIGNING LETTERS FOR THE PHYSICIAN

Occasionally, physicians will be out of the office when letters must be mailed, so they may ask their medical assistants to send those letters without their signatures. The review process, however, should remain the same. The physicians should still read or otherwise review the letters and give their approvals before the letters are sent. Approved letters can be stamped with lines like, "Read but not signed due to time constraints." When offices lack preprinted stamps like this, the medical assistant can print the physician's name where the signature belongs and follow the printing with a personal signature to indicate that the assistant signed for the physician.

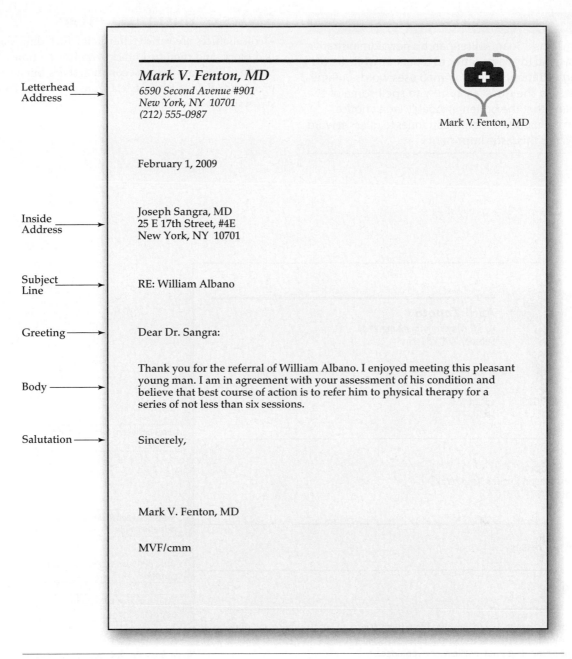

Letterhead Address →

Mark V. Fenton, MD
6590 Second Avenue #901
New York, NY 10701
(212) 555-0987

Mark V. Fenton, MD

February 1, 2009

Inside Address →

Joseph Sangra, MD
25 E 17th Street, #4E
New York, NY 10701

Subject Line →

RE: William Albano

Greeting →

Dear Dr. Sangra:

Body →

Thank you for the referral of William Albano. I enjoyed meeting this pleasant young man. I am in agreement with your assessment of his condition and believe that best course of action is to refer him to physical therapy for a series of not less than six sessions.

Salutation →

Sincerely,

Mark V. Fenton, MD

MVF/cmm

Figure 6-7 ◆ Sample business letter.

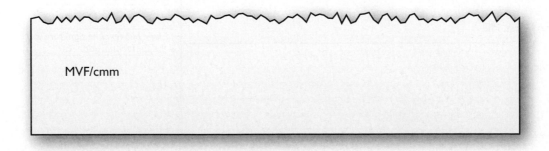

MVF/cmm

Figure 6-8 ◆ Sample reference initials.

In Practice

Dr. Mohammad asks Joanne Brennan, his new administrative medical assistant, to type a letter to a patient while he dictates. During dictation, Dr. Mohammad uses words unfamiliar to Joanne, so she guesses at how to spell some of the words, thinking that the patient probably won't notice.

What may happen if Joanne continues to guess at word spellings? Why is this issue important?

Styles of Business Letters

Medical offices use varied letter styles, including block, modified block, and modified block with indentations. Block and modified block are the most common styles, but the physician's preference dictates letter style. Figure 6-9 ◆ describes different styles and gives examples.

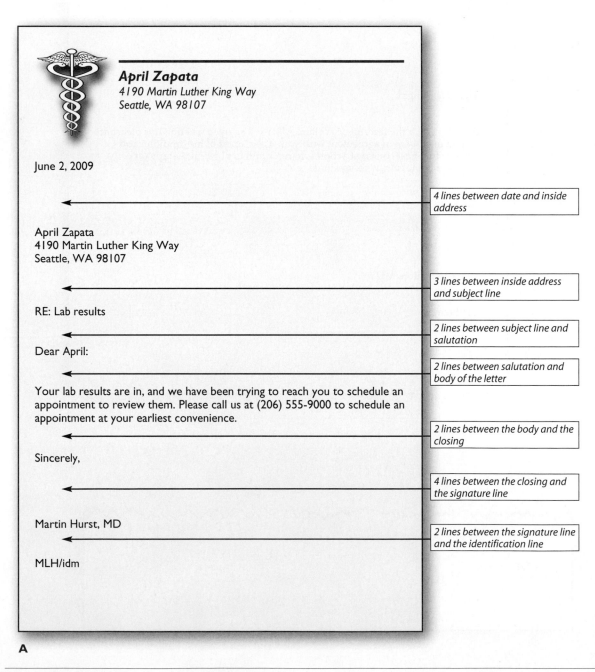

Figure 6-9 ◆ Styles of business letters. A. Block style.

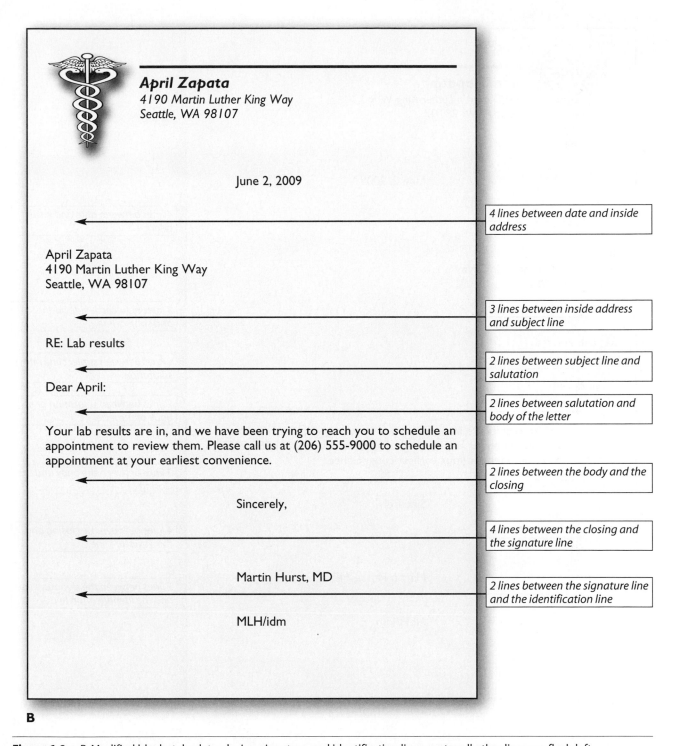

April Zapata
4190 Martin Luther King Way
Seattle, WA 98107

June 2, 2009

4 lines between date and inside address

April Zapata
4190 Martin Luther King Way
Seattle, WA 98107

3 lines between inside address and subject line

RE: Lab results

2 lines between subject line and salutation

Dear April:

2 lines between salutation and body of the letter

Your lab results are in, and we have been trying to reach you to schedule an appointment to review them. Please call us at (206) 555-9000 to schedule an appointment at your earliest convenience.

2 lines between the body and the closing

Sincerely,

4 lines between the closing and the signature line

Martin Hurst, MD

2 lines between the signature line and the identification line

MLH/idm

B

Figure 6-9 ◆ B. Modified block style: date, closing, signature, and identification lines center, all other lines are flush left.

Using Fonts in Typed Communication

All word-processing software comes with a set of **fonts**, which are different styles of type. Professional letters should appear in 10- to 12-point formal fonts, like Times New Roman, Garamond, or Arial (Figure 6-10 ◆). While informal fonts may function for things like interoffice informational sheets, they are considered inappropriate for professional business letters.

Sending Letters to Patients

Medical offices send letters to patients for a number of reasons, including to communicate changes in office policy or procedure. Personalized letters serve to notify patients they need or have missed appointments. Whatever the reasons they are sent, patient letters should be professional and accurate. Copies of all written patient correspondence should be filed in the patients' medical records.

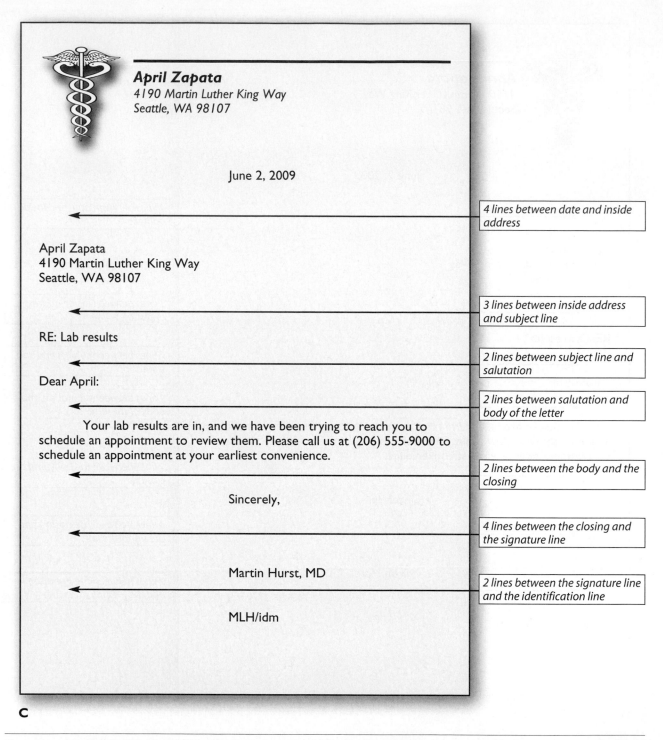

April Zapata
4190 Martin Luther King Way
Seattle, WA 98107

June 2, 2009

← *4 lines between date and inside address*

April Zapata
4190 Martin Luther King Way
Seattle, WA 98107

← *3 lines between inside address and subject line*

RE: Lab results

← *2 lines between subject line and salutation*

Dear April:

← *2 lines between salutation and body of the letter*

  Your lab results are in, and we have been trying to reach you to schedule an appointment to review them. Please call us at (206) 555-9000 to schedule an appointment at your earliest convenience.

← *2 lines between the body and the closing*

     Sincerely,

← *4 lines between the closing and the signature line*

     Martin Hurst, MD

← *2 lines between the signature line and the identification line*

     MLH/idm

C

Figure 6-9 ◆ C. Modified block with identations: resembles modified block style, except that each paragraph is indented five spaces.

Arial 10-point font	Arial 12-point font
Garamond 10-point font	Garamond 12-point font
Times New Roman 10-point font	Times New Roman 12-point font

Figure 6-10 ◆ Sample fonts.

Proofreading

As discussed earlier, while most word-processing software can check spelling and grammar, such programs are neither fail-safe nor complete substitutes for manual error-checking processes. Because most documents today are composed electronically, medical assistants can proofread and correct those documents before printing. **Proofreading** is the process of checking written information for spelling or other errors. Some-

PROCEDURE 6-1 Compose a Business Letter

Theory and Rationale

Administrative medical assistants often compose business letters from physicians. Because these letters directly reflect the physicians, they must be professional, grammatically correct, and free of typographical errors.

Materials

■ Computer with word-processing software
■ Information for the letter

Competency

(**Conditions**) With the necessary materials, you will be able to (**Task**) compose a business letter (**Standards**) correctly within the time limit set by the instructor.

1. Determine the recipient and content of the letter.
2. Using the word-processing software, type the date of the letter.
3. Type the recipient of the letter.
4. Type the subject line.
5. Type the greeting of the letter.
6. Type the body of the letter.
7. Type the salutation.
8. Indicate enclosures, if any.
9. Indicate if a copy of the letter will be sent to another party.
10. Enter the initials of the letter's author, followed by your initials as the typist.
11. Perform complete electronic spelling and grammar checks.
12. Print the letter.
13. On paper, perform manual spelling and grammar checks.
14. Give the letter to the physician for a signature.
15. Address an envelope.
16. Send the letter.

---

times, proofreading includes modifying a letter's style (e.g., line format) to make the letter more appealing on paper.

Proofreading requires medical assistants to read documents slowly and check that the documents are clear and logically organized. To indicate needed changes, medical assistants place **proofreader's marks** on printed documents (Figure 6-11 ◆).

To catch all errors, medical assistants should read all letters at least twice. Documents should be printed only after they have been proofread. Once documents are printed, medical assistants should proofread them one last time to determine if format changes, like more or less space between lines, would make the documents more attractive.

PROCEDURE 6-2 Prepare a Document for Photocopying

Theory and Rationale

Many documents in the medical office will need to be photocopied. Often, originals are sent to the patient and copies are kept in the patient's file. The medical assistant must be familiar with how the photocopier works and the steps to take to correctly copy needed documents.

Materials

■ Photocopier
■ Document to be copied
■ Envelope
■ Patient medical record

Competency

(**Conditions**) With the necessary materials, you will be able to (**Task**) prepare a document for photocopying (**Standards**) correctly within the time limit set by the instructor.

1. Turn the photocopy machine on and allow time for it to warm up.
2. Place the document to be copied face down on the glass surface of the photocopier, following the diagram on the photocopier.
3. Indicate the number of copies needed by entering the number in the appropriate place on the photocopier.
4. Press the "copy" button on the photocopier.
5. Once the copy has been made, remove the original.
6. Place the original document into an envelope to be mailed to the patient.
7. Place the photocopy of the document into the patient's file.

style of type

wf	Wrong font (size or style of type)
lc	lower Case letter
lc	Set in LOWER CASE
C	Capital letter
Caps	SET IN capitals
c + lc	Set in lower case with INITIAL CAPITALS
sc	SET IN small capitals
c + sc	SET IN SMALL CAPITALS with initial capitals
rom.	Set in roman type
ital.	Set in italic type
ital. caps	SET IN ITALIC capitals
lf	Set in lightface type
bf	Set in boldface type
bf ital.	Set in boldface italic
bf caps	Set in boldface CAPITALS
	Superior letter b
	Inferior figure 2

position

	Move to right
	Move to left
ctr	Center
	Lower (letters or words)
	Raise (letters or words)
	Straighten type (horizontally)
	Align type (vertically)
tr	Transpose
tr	Transpose (order letters of or words)

spacing

ld in	Insert lead (space) between lines
Or ld	Take out lead
	Close up; take out space
	Close up partly; leave some space
Eq #	Equalize space between words
#	Insert space (or more space)
Space out	More space between words

insertion and deletion

the/)	Caret (insert marginal addition
	Delete (take it out)
	Delete and close up
l	Correct letter or word marked
Stet	Let it stand (all matter above dots)

paragraphing

	Begin a paragraph
No ¶	No paragraph.
Run in	Run in or run on
flush	No indention

punctuation

(Use caret in text to show point of insertion)

⊙	Insert period
	Insert comma
⊙	Insert colon
;/	Insert semicolon
	Insert quotation marks
	Insert single quotes
	Insert apostrophe
(set)?	Insert question mark
!	Insert exclamation point
=/	Insert hyphen
	Insert one-em dash
(/)	Insert parentheses
[/]	Insert brackets

miscellaneous

⊗	Replace broken or imperfect type
	Reverse (upside down type)
(sp)	Spell out (twenty gr)
Au/(?)	Query to author
Ed/(?)	Query to editor
	Mark off or break start new line

Figure 6-11 ◆ Proofreader's marks.

Working with Accepted Abbreviations

Abbreviations are common in medical terminology. For all members of the health care team, however, it is essential to use only accepted abbreviations in office communication. The Joint Commission on the Accreditation of Healthcare Organizations (**JCAHO**) has identified the standard abbreviations its members are required to use, as well as avoid. Table 6-7 lists the latter. JCAHO prepared this list due to the growing concern that the use of more than one abbreviation for the same medical term created a situation where confusion, misdiagnosis, or even injury to the patient could occur. In the medical office, lists like these help staff maintain consistent terminology and avoid confusion and errors. Medical assistants who are unclear about abbreviations should

PROCEDURE 6-3 Send a Letter to a Patient about a Missed Appointment

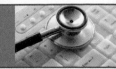

Theory and Rationale

Administrative medical assistants regularly write professional letters to patients. These letters may be sent for a variety of reasons when the physician wishes to communicate in writing with the patient, such as when the patient misses an appointment. Often, written communication is used when the physician desires written proof of what was said to the patient. Strict attention to detail helps avoid miscommunication between the patient and the medical office.

Materials

- Computer with word-processing software
- Patient medical record

Competency

(**Conditions**) With the necessary materials, you will be able to (**Task**) send a letter to a patient regarding a missed appoint-

ment (**Standards**) correctly within the time limit set by the instructor.

1. Using the word-processing software, type the date at the top of the letter.
2. Type the patient's name and mailing address.
3. For the subject line, type "RE: Missed Appointment."
4. In the body of the letter, describe the appointment that was missed, including its date.
5. Per the physician's instructions or office policy, list the reasons the patient should call to reschedule the missed appointment.
6. Copy the letter for the patient's file.
7. Obtain the signature of the letter's author (you or the physician).
8. Send the patient the original letter.

---

always err on the side of caution and spell out the corresponding words.

Creating Memos for the Office

A **memo** is a type of interoffice correspondence. Memos are a quick and efficient means of communication. They require no postage and are designed to have clear messages. Office man-

agers might compose memos to communicate with their entire staff, or staff members may write memos to communicate with other staff.

Most memos begin with the word "MEMO" or "MEMORANDUM" at their tops. Below that, typically the date, recipient, and author appear (Figure 6-12 ◆). Many medical offices preprint memo paper, but some print memo paper on an as-needed basis.

PROCEDURE 6-4 Proofread Written Documents

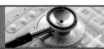

Theory and Rationale

Proofreading skills are imperative to the administrative medical assistant, because the composition of written documents is a large part of administrative medical assisting. Sending documents out without proofreading them may lead to confusion on the part of the recipient, or even to possible misdiagnosis or treatment of a patient.

Materials

- Computer document to be proofread
- Computer with word-processing software

Competency

(**Conditions**) With the necessary materials, you will be able to (**Task**) proofread a written document (**Standards**) correctly within the time limit set by the instructor.

1. Open the document using the word-processing software.
2. Use the word processor's spelling and grammar checking functions.
3. Save any changes.
4. Starting at the top, read the entire document to verify that all spelling, punctuation, and grammatical errors were corrected.
5. Save any changes.
6. Print the document.
7. Review the entire document to verify that all spelling, punctuation, and grammatical errors were corrected. If changes were made, reprint the document.
8. Give the document to the physician for signature.

TABLE 6-7 MEDICAL ABBREVIATIONS TO AVOID

Abbreviation	Potential Problem	Preferred Replacement(s)
U (unit)	Mistaken for "0" (zero), the number "4" (four), or "cc."	"unit"
IU (International Unit)	Mistaken for IV (intravenous) or the number 10 (ten).	"International Unit"
Q.D., QD, q.d., qd (daily); Q.O.D., QOD, q.o.d., qod (every other day)	Mistaken for each other. The period after the Q is mistaken for "I" and the "O" is mistaken for "I" (q.i.d. is four times a day dosing).	"daily" or "every other day"
Trailing zero (X.0 mg) Lack of leading zero (.X)	Decimal point is missed.	X mg or 0.X mg
MS	Can mean morphine sulfate or magnesium sulfate.	"morphine sulfate"
MS04 and MgS04	Confused for one another.	"magnesium sulfate"

Source: Joint Commission on the Accreditation of Healthcare Organizations.

Mailing Written Communication

Standard paper size is 8½″ × 11″, while standard business envelope size is 4⅛″ × 9½″. Professional business letters should be mailed in business-sized or "Size 10" envelopes. Such envelopes easily accommodate business letters that are folded in thirds (Figure 6-13 ◆).

The envelope's upper left corner should carry the office's address (Figure 6-14 ◆). Many offices buy envelopes preprinted with this information. The recipient's name and address should appear in the envelope's center and the stamp or postage-meter mark in the far upper right. When mail is personal, the word "Personal" or "Confidential" should appear below the recipient's address.

Some medical offices place their required registration forms on their Web site. By directing patients to access the Web site to download, print, and fill out the needed forms, the medical office saves the cost of printing the packets and mailing them to the patient ahead of time.

Window Envelopes

For certain types of mail, like insurance billing forms or patient billing statements, medical offices often use window envelopes. Before such envelopes are sealed, however, medical assistants should ensure that addresses appear in the windows (Figure 6-15 ◆).

HIPAA Compliance

Regardless of size or type, for personal patient information medical offices must use security envelopes. Security envelopes have internal patterns that keep the contents of documents obscured. Figure 6-16 ◆ shows a security envelope.

Running and Resetting Postage Meters

Many medical clinics have **postage meters**, which weigh mail pieces, determine correct postage and print postage on en-

MEMORANDUM

Date: _____

To: _____

From: _____

Figure 6-12 ◆ Sample opening of an interoffice memo.

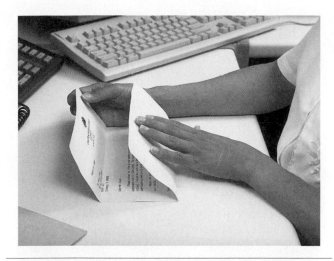

Figure 6-13 ◆ When folded into thirds, the letter will easily fit within the standard business envelope.

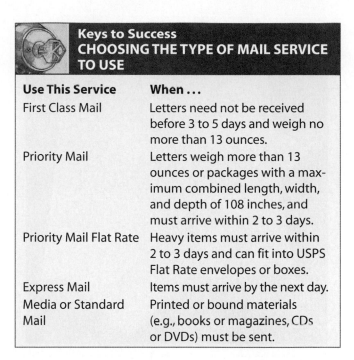

Keys to Success CHOOSING THE TYPE OF MAIL SERVICE TO USE	
Use This Service	**When . . .**
First Class Mail	Letters need not be received before 3 to 5 days and weigh no more than 13 ounces.
Priority Mail	Letters weigh more than 13 ounces or packages with a maximum combined length, width, and depth of 108 inches, and must arrive within 2 to 3 days.
Priority Mail Flat Rate	Heavy items must arrive within 2 to 3 days and can fit into USPS Flat Rate envelopes or boxes.
Express Mail	Items must arrive by the next day.
Media or Standard Mail	Printed or bound materials (e.g., books or magazines, CDs or DVDs) must be sent.

velopes or labels (Figure 6-17 ◆). Basic models simply weigh pieces of mail and print postage, while advanced versions accept stacks of mail, insert documents into envelopes, seal envelopes, and affix proper postage. Postage meters are extremely useful to the medical office because they are generally user friendly and reduce wasted postage as well as time spent at the post office.

Most medical offices lease their postage meters from companies that supply the meters as well as corresponding supplies (e.g., ink cartridges, ribbons, labels). Once offices have arranged payment for their postage, medical assistants facilitate meter use by calling the postage companies' customer service departments and providing their user identification numbers, office passwords, and meters' serial numbers and access codes.

Classifying Mail, Size Requirements, and Postage

The United States Postal Service (**USPS**) varies its services for mailing letters and packages according to urgency and value. A standard postage stamp facilitates first-class mail service, which is available for items weighing no more than 13 ounces. Mail that weighs over 13 ounces must be sent via Priority Mail or Parcel Post.

After Express Mail, which is the fastest USPS service (with a guaranteed next-day delivery 7 days a week), Priority Mail is the U.S. government's fastest mail service. For most destinations in the U.S., Priority Mail arrives within 2 to 3 days. However, Priority Mail items must weigh no more than 70 pounds, and packages cannot exceed a combined length, width, and depth of 108 inches. When senders use envelopes and packages provided by USPS that clearly state "Flat Rate," Priority Mail is available at a flat rate (Figure 6-18 ◆).

Media Mail, or Standard Mail, is strictly for printed or bound materials, such as books or magazines, sound recordings, videotapes, or CDs and DVDs. This service is more economical than the other services, but it tends to take longer, usually 2 to 10 days. Advertising cannot be sent by Media Mail.

In addition to its base services, the USPS offers a variety of optional services for added costs. Certified mail, for example, provides a mailing receipt and a record of the mailing at the local post office, but it is available only for First-Class and Priority Mail packages and letters. Confirmation receipts are

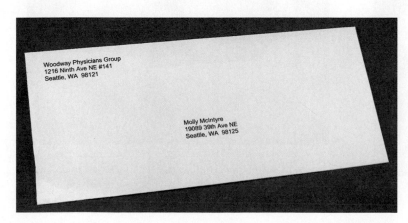

Figure 6-14 ◆ Example of a properly addressed business envelope.

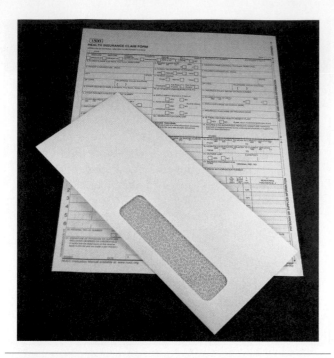

Figure 6-15 ◆ Example of a window envelope.

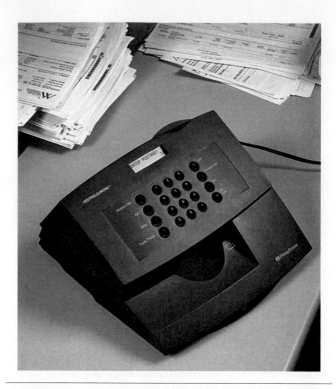

Figure 6-17 ◆ An electronic postage meter.

another, added service (Figure 6-19 ◆). Delivery confirmation allows senders and receivers to track pieces of mail or packages online. Registered mail, another option available for only First-Class and Priority Mail, offers the ability to purchase insurance up to $25,000 for the value of the item. A return receipt can also be added to this service. Insurance can be purchased for any item shipped via the USPS, but the cost of the insurance rises with the value of the item.

Buying Postage Online

The USPS now sells postage online to any consumer with a computer and a printer. This service is available for both

domestic and international shipments and includes such options as insurance (up to a $500 value) and delivery confirmation.

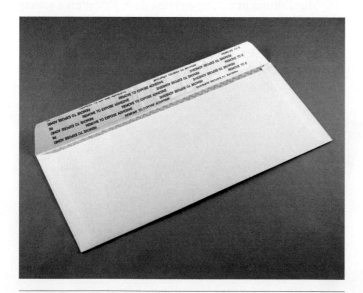

Figure 6-16 ◆ Example of a security envelope.

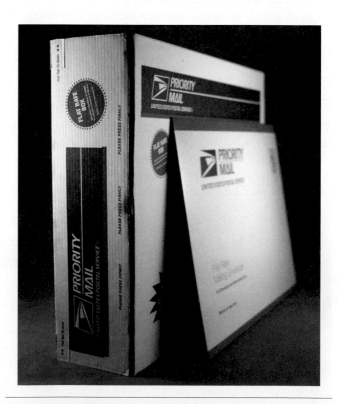

Figure 6-18 ◆ The USPS charges one flat rate to use their flat rate envelopes and boxes, regardless of where the item is being shipped within the United States or how much it weighs.

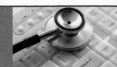

PROCEDURE 6-5 Fold Documents for Window Envelopes

Theory and Rationale

When documents are folded properly before they are placed in window envelopes, post-office machinery can read addresses correctly and deliver mail in a timely manner.

Materials

■ Document to be mailed
■ Window envelope

Competency

(**Conditions**) With the necessary materials, you will be able to (**Task**) fold a document for use with a window envelope (**Standards**) correctly within the time limit set by the instructor.

1. Locate the mailing address on the document.
2. Compare the location of the mailing address to the location of the window on the envelope.
3. Fold the document such that the mailing address will be viewable through the envelope's window once the document has been inserted in the envelope.
4. Insert the document in the envelope.
5. Verify that the address is viewable through the window.
6. Seal the envelope.

Using Multiline Optical Character Readers

The USPS uses multiline optical character readers (**MLOCRs**), which use optical character recognition (**OCR**) to determine how to route mail through its systems. MLOCRs capture images of the fronts of pieces of mail, look up postal codes, print barcodes, and perform mail sorts.

MLOCRs cannot read all mail, however. Some handwriting is hard to read and addresses may sometimes appear in incorrect locations. This type of mail is either sent to another, more powerful computer for scanning or to a human operator.

"ZIP + 4" Codes

The ZIP code is the USPS system of using five digits to indicate mail's intended destination. Since 1983, the USPS has been using "ZIP + 4" codes to expedite postal service by directing mail to more precise locations. These codes, which as their name suggest extend traditional ZIP codes by four digits, appear on the USPS Web site at http://zip4.usps.com/zip4/welcome.jsp.

USPS-Approved Abbreviations in Addresses

Mail that follows USPS recommendations reaches its destination far more quickly than mail that does not. Some of these recommendations, approved abbreviations for mailing addresses, appear in Table 6-8.

Restricted Materials

The USPS will mail no item that is outwardly or of its own force dangerous or injurious to life, health, or property. Similarly, it will not transport most hazardous material. The following items are also subject to certain restrictions:

■ Intoxicating liquors
■ Firearms
■ Knives or other sharp instruments
■ Odor-producing chemicals
■ Liquids and powders
■ Controlled substances

When in doubt about the mailability of an item, the medical assistant should call or visit the USPS.

Other Delivery Options

Some services compete with the USPS by offering package tracking, insurance, and delivery services that include Federal Express, United Parcel Service (**UPS**), and DHL. Federal Express (FedEx) offers overnight courier, ground, heavy freight, and document copying services. FedEx services are available

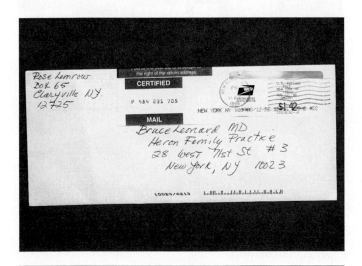

Figure 6-19 ◆ Important items should be sent via certified mail.

TABLE 6-8 USPS-APPROVED ABBREVIATIONS

For Streets and Towns

Alley	ALY	Hill	HL
Annex	ANX	Island	IS
Avenue	AVE	Junction	JCT
Boulevard	BLVD	Lake	LK
Bridge	BRG	Lane	LN
Brook	BRK	Manor	MNR
Bypass	BYP	Meadow	MDW
Canyon	CYN	Mountain	MTN
Cape	CPE	Orchard	ORCH
Causeway	CSWY	Parkway	PKWY
Center	CTR	Place	PL
Circle	CIR	Plaza	PLZ
Cliff	CLF	Point	PT
Club	CLB	Port	PRT
Common	CMN	Ridge	RDG
Corner	COR	River	RIV
Court	CRT	Road	RD
Cove	CV	Route	RTE
Creek	CRK	Shore	SHR
Crossing	XING	Spring	SPG
Drive	DR	Square	SQ
Estate	EST	Station	STA
Expressway	EXPY	Street	ST
Forest	FRST	Terrace	TER
Freeway	FWY	Throughway	TRWY
Garden	GDN	Trail	TRL
Gateway	GTWY	Tunnel	TUNL
Grove	GRV	Turnpike	TPKE
Harbor	HBR	Valley	VLY
Heights	HTS	View	VW
Highway	HWY	Village	VLG

For Secondary Unit Designators

Apartment	APT	Office	OFC
Basement	BSMT	Penthouse	PH
Building	BLDG	Room	RM
Department	DEPT	Space	SPC
Floor	FL	Suite	STE
Front	FRNT	Trailer	TRKR
Lobby	LBBY	Upper	UPPR
Lower	LOWR		

both to home and business customers, and FedEx offers shipping services via Express, Ground, Freight, and International services. The United Parcel Service (UPS), much like FedEx, offers shipping services both within the United States and worldwide via various shipping speeds and methods. Both of these companies offer package pickup, which alleviates the need to take a package to a FedEx or UPS retail location. The Deutsche Post World Net (DHL) offers shipping services worldwide at a variety of shipping speeds. In 2003, DHL purchased Airborne Express—then the third largest private express delivery company in the United States.

Using E-Mail to Communicate

Electronic mail, or e-mail, is an electronic means of communication. Many medical offices use e-mail to communicate with patients. As a general rule, patients who give medical offices their e-mail addresses authorize those offices to send them e-mail. However, it is crucial that medical staff remember that e-mail is far from secure. For example, e-mail addresses can be misspelled, causing incorrect parties to receive messages. Also, employers have the right to view any e-mail their employees send on company systems. Because confidentiality is not guaranteed, all medical staff, including the medical assistant, should only use e-mail to send patients such nonconfidential information as appointment reminders.

Managing Mail and Correspondence

Administrative medical assistants are typically in charge of sorting and distributing medical office's incoming mail (Figure 6-20 ◆). Because many such items, such as pathology reports or consultation letters, are time sensitive, assistants should sort and distribute incoming mail daily.

Many times, the person who sorts and distributes the mail is also asked to stamp the date the mail was received. Many offices also require the person sorting the mail to open each piece so recipients can easily access the contents. Items marked "personal" or "confidential" should be left unopened, however.

To avoid confusion, each office should have a mail sorting and distribution policy that includes a list of the items each staff member should receive. For example, the physician may

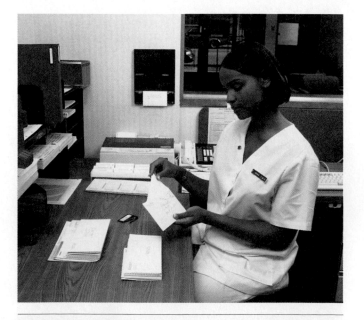

Figure 6-20 ◆ The medical assistant is commonly the person to open and sort the mail.

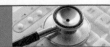

PROCEDURE 6-6 Open and Sort Mail

Theory and Rationale

The medical office receives various kinds of mail daily. Some mail contains important, private patient information, whereas other is considered "junk." The medical assistant will likely need to learn to sort mail properly.

Materials

- A stack of incoming mail, including payments from insurance companies and patients, advertisements, drug samples, magazines, professional journals, bills for office services, a letter to the physician marked "Personal and Confidential," and consultation reports from other physicians
- Date stamp
- Letter opener

Competency

(**Conditions**) With the necessary materials, you will be able to (**Task**) open and sort the office mail (**Standards**) correctly within the time limit set by the instructor.

1. Using a date stamp, stamp the date on each received item.
2. Sort the mail into the appropriate files according to the following:
   - Physician—correspondence from other physicians, hospitals, or laboratories, as well as any professional journals
   - Office manager—bills for office services, drug samples, advertisements for supplies or services
   - Receptionist—magazines
   - Billing office—payments from patients or insurance companies, correspondence from insurance companies
3. Open each piece of mail, except for the piece marked "Personal and Confidential."
4. Distribute the mail appropriately. Leave the mail piece marked "Personal and Confidential" on the physician's desk.

receive all communications or reports regarding patients, any professional journals, and literature from professional organizations. The office manager, by contrast, may receive all bills, advertisements for services or supplies, and samples from drug or supply companies.

HIPAA Compliance

Because many of the items sent to the medical office contain private patient information, mail should never be left where other people can access it, even when unopened.

Annotation

To abbreviate their reviews of the information they receive, some physicians charge their administrative medical assistants with **annotation,** a process that involves reading, highlighting, and summarizing information. Medical assistants who annotate should clarify the information physicians consider pertinent before they undertake the task (Figure 6-21 ◆). Typically, the physician will ask the medical assistant to highlight the patient's name, any pertinent information about the patient, such as a diagnosis or treatment plan, and the name of the sender of the letter.

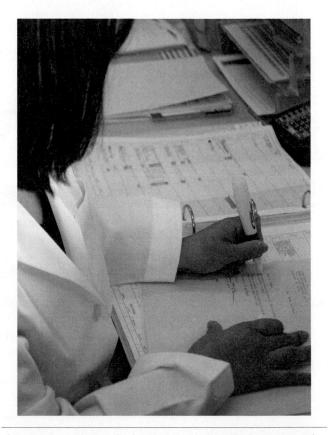

Figure 6-21 ◆ The medical assistant may be asked to open and annotate portions of the physician's incoming mail.

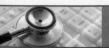

PROCEDURE 6-7 Annotate Written Correspondence

Theory and Rationale

In a busy medical office, the physician may want the medical assistant to scan and annotate medical reports to save time. Medical assistants who know what information to look for save time for the physician and can point out key pieces of information.

Material

- Written correspondence
- Highlighter pen
- Letter opener

Competency

(**Conditions**) With the necessary materials, you will be able to (**Task**) annotate a written correspondence (**Standards**) correctly within the time limit set by the instructor.

1. Open the envelope with the document to be annotated.
2. Read the document once in its entirety.
3. Using the highlighter pen, review the document again, highlighting such pertinent information as:
   - Patient's name
   - Findings of any examination or laboratory work
   - Dates for followup appointments
   - Diagnosis
4. Read the document a third time to ensure all pertinent information has been noted.
5. Place the annotated document on the physician's desk for review.

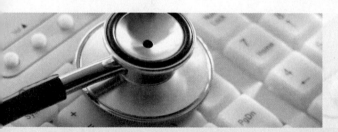

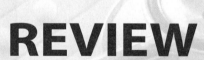

REVIEW

Chapter Summary

- Proper grammar, spelling, and punctuation are all paramount to a medical office's positive image.
- Medical assistants should follow a defined process when composing letters to patients and other members of the health care team.
- Medical assistants must be familiar with the use of a medical dictionary.
- The proofreading of business letters, which involves attention to detail as well as a solid understanding of English essentials, is a means by which the medical assistant can help support a positive professional image for the office.

- In all correspondence, medical assistants should use only abbreviations that are accepted in the health care industry.
- Memos are one vehicle health care staff can use to communicate with other team members.
- The U.S. mail system is governed by a set of rules and restrictions the medical assistant should be familiar with to function as part of the health care team.
- E-mail is governed by its own unique set of rules and policies.
- The medical assistant is responsible for managing incoming mail and correspondence according to office policy.
- The medical assistant may be called upon to annotate the physician's mail correspondence.

Chapter Review

Multiple Choice

1. Which of the following USPS mail types is appropriate for mailing a DVD?
   a. Media
   b. Priority
   c. Express
   d. Ground

2. Which of the following mail types is appropriate for sending a letter that must arrive the next day?
   a. Media
   b. Priority
   c. Express
   d. Ground

3. A piece of mail marked _____ should be left unopened and given directly to the intended recipient.
   a. "Open Immediately"
   b. "Personal"
   c. "Important"
   d. All of the above

4. Which of the following substances may be prohibited by the USPS for mailing?
   a. Alcoholic beverages
   b. Firearms
   c. Flammable material
   d. All of the above

5. In the medical office, it is appropriate to use a memo when the:
   a. Office manager wishes to notify staff of a holiday party
   b. Medical assistant must notify a patient of a missed appointment
   c. Physician would like to contact a patient with test results
   d. All of the above

True/False

T F 1. Any written correspondence in the medical office reflects on the physician and the office.

T F 2. As a general rule, numbers from one to ten should be written out when writing letters.

T F 3. The rules for making medical terms plural confuse the medical office.

T F 4. "Miss" is the appropriate title to use when addressing a woman of unknown marital status.

T F 5. The most common salutation in professional letters is "Yours Truly."

T F 6. E-mail is a secure way to send patients test results.

Short Answer

1. What is the purpose of the subject line in a professional letter?

2. What is a typical closing in a professional letter?

3. What are the reference initials for Mark S. Stevens, MD, who authors a letter, and medical assistant Sarah Ellen Parker, who types it?

4. Which three fonts appear most often in a business letter?

5. Explain the process of annotation.

6. Describe the function of spell-check software.

7. Give several examples of words in English that sound the same yet have different meanings.

8. What is a logo, and why is it used?

Research

1. What classes could you take at your local community college to help improve your written communication skills?

2. Looking at the USPS Web site, how would you calculate postage to various locations throughout the United States? Outside the United States?

3. Review the Web sites for both FedEx and UPS. Compare their services. Does either offer a service the other does not?

Externship Application Experience

When Dr. Yi asks office manager Marnie Glaser, CMA, to open and distribute the day's mail, Marnie accidentally opens a piece to Dr. Yi marked "Personal." What is the proper way to handle this situation?

Resource Guide

United States Postal Service
Phone: (800) 275-8777
www.usps.com

Federal Express
www.fedex.com
Phone: 1-800-GO-FEDEX

United Parcel Service
www.ups.com
Phone: 1-800-PICK-UPS

DHL
www.dhl-usa.com
Phone: 1-800-CALL-DHL

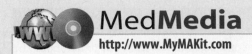

Med**Media**

http://www.MyMAKit.com

More on this chapter, including interactive resources, can be found on the Student CD-ROM accompanying this textbook and on http://www.MyMAKit.com.

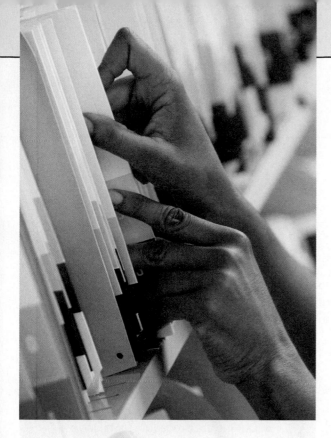

SECTION II

Administrative Responsibilities of the Medical Assistant

My name is Kae Montgomery. When I first started working in a clinic during my externship, there was so much to learn. I had been taught all the basics in school, but now I had to apply this knowledge to the real world. One area I had to perfect was calling patients. On the electronic medical record (EMR) system we used, calling patients was referred to as phone notes. A patient would call in with a request, such as a referral or a prescription refill from the doctor. This would generate a phone note. Handling the phone notes was the easy part; calling the patient was sometimes tricky. We always called the home phone number, and since most people work, this would mean leaving a message on their answering machine. I had to be careful when leaving the message so that no specific details were given. I learned to leave just a general message such as "This is Kae calling from Dr. Yap's office. Your request is ready to be picked up."

If a spouse answered and I had no signed consent form for that person, I could not leave detailed information, even if they knew what the call was about. The spouse did not always understand why I could not leave a message since they were not aware of the fact that due to HIPPA privacy regulations, we were not allowed to share any of the patients' information with them, no matter what! One of the first things I learned in the EMR was where to look to find the patients' signed consent form.

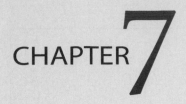

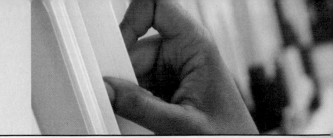

CHAPTER 7

Telephone Procedures

Case Study

Martha Hagen, one of the medical office's established patients, calls to notify the office that she is having chest pains. Martha is not sure if she should make an appointment to come into the office or if she should go to the emergency room.

Objectives

After completing this chapter, you should be able to:

- Define and spell the key terminology in this chapter.
- Describe the main features of telephone systems.
- Outline the benefits of an answering service.
- Explain how to perform telephone triage, including a list of the steps to take when triaging patients this way.
- Describe how to handle emergency calls and calls with difficult patients.
- Outline the procedure for taking a proper telephone message.
- Respond to telephone prescription requests.
- Describe the steps to take when calling patients via telephone.
- Use a telephone directory effectively.
- Discuss how the medical assistant can protect patient confidentiality when using the telephone.

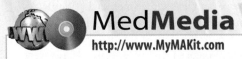

MedMedia
http://www.MyMAKit.com

Additional interactive resources and activities for this chapter can be found on http://www.MyMAKit.com. For a video, tips, audio glossary, legal and ethical scenarios, on-the-job scenarios, quizzes, and games related to the content of this chapter, please access the accompanying CD-ROM in this book.

Videos: *Patient Reception; Telephone Etiquette*
Legal and Ethical Scenario: *Telephone Procedures*
On the Job Scenario: *Telephone Procedures*
Tips
Multiple Choice Quiz
Audio Glossary
HIPAA Quiz
Games: Spelling Bee, Crossword, and Strikeout

MEDICAL ASSISTING STANDARDS

CAAHEP ENTRY-LEVEL STANDARDS	ABHES ENTRY-LEVEL COMPETENCIES
■ Identify styles and types of verbal communication (cognitive) ■ Recognize communication barriers (cognitive) ■ Identify techniques for overcoming communication barriers (cognitive) ■ Recognize the elements of oral communication using a sender-receiver process (cognitive) ■ Identify resources and adaptations that are required based on individual needs, i.e., culture and environment, developmental life stage, language, and physical threats to communication (cognitive) ■ Recognize the role of patient advocacy in the practice of medical assisting (cognitive) ■ Discuss the role of assertiveness in effective professional communication (cognitive) ■ Identify time management principles (cognitive) ■ Use reflection, restatement, and clarification techniques to obtain a patient history (psychomotor) ■ Report relevant information to others succinctly and accurately (psychomotor) ■ Explain general office policies (psychomotor) ■ Instruct patients according to their needs to promote health maintenance and disease prevention (psychomotor) ■ Demonstrate telephone techniques (psychomotor) ■ Demonstrate empathy in communicating with patients, family, and staff (affective) ■ Apply active listening skills (affective) ■ Demonstrate sensitivity appropriate to the message being delivered (affective) ■ Demonstrate recognition of the patient's level of understanding in communication (affective)	■ Adapt to change ■ Maintain confidentiality at all times ■ Use appropriate guidelines when releasing records or information ■ Project a positive attitude ■ Be cognizant of ethical boundaries ■ Evidence a responsible attitude ■ Conduct work within scope of education, training, and ability ■ Professional components ■ Monitor legislation related to current health care issues and practices ■ Orient patients to office policies and procedures ■ Adapt what is said to the recipient's level of comprehension ■ Adaptation for individualized needs ■ Instruct patients with special needs ■ Locate resources and information for patients and employers ■ Use proper telephone techniques ■ Be courteous and diplomatic ■ Serve as a liaison between the physician and others ■ Exercise efficient time management ■ Receive, organize, prioritize, and transmit information expediently

COMPETENCY SKILLS PERFORMANCE

1. Answer the telephone in a professional manner.
2. Take a telephone message.
3. Call a pharmacy with prescription orders

Key Terminology

automatic dialer—telephone feature that dials numbers programmed into the system using codes; see also *speed dialer*

automatic routing unit—telephone equipment that allows callers to self-select their call destinations via an automated, electronic prompt system

call forwarding—telephone feature that forwards incoming calls to other numbers

conference call—telephone feature that allows parties in different locations to participate in one call

direct telephone lines—telephone number that reaches a person directly rather than an operator or a receptionist

established patient—patient whom the medical office has seen previously

generic message—telephone answering message that fails to identify the receiver specifically

hands-free telephone device—headset or headphones with a speaker and microphone that allow users to participate in calls without picking up the telephone's receiver

hold feature—telephone feature that allows the user to place one call on hold and take another

last number redial—telephone feature that dials the last number dialed from that telephone

route—to direct telephone calls to other numbers

speaker phone—telephone feature that broadcasts the speaker's voice

speed dial—telephone feature that dials numbers programmed into the system using codes; see also *automatic dialer*

triage notebook—notebook the administrative medical assistant uses to properly handle calls from patients with potentially life-threatening conditions

triaging—process of prioritizing patients based on need

Abbreviations

ADA—Americans with Disabilities Act

HIPAA—Health Insurance Portability and Accountability Act

TTY—teletypewriter system

Introduction

Professional telephone skills are essential for the administrative medical assistant. Often, the telephone is the first contact a patient has with the physician's office and can set the tone of the patient's relationship with the clinic. Allowing the telephone to ring too long before answering or placing a patient on hold for extended periods are two examples of poor telephone procedure. One disadvantage to using the telephone is that neither party can use nonverbal communication to determine the attitude or sincerity of the other party. For this reason, it is important for medical assistants to keep their voice pleasant, polite, and professional while on the telephone. Handling telephone calls courteously and efficiently is the best way to make a good first impression on callers.

Telephone System Features

Today's telephone systems are sophisticated, multifeature units that require training for new administrative employees, including medical assistants.

Making Calls with Hands-Free Devices

For staff who answer telephone calls often throughout the day, **hands-free telephone devices** not only free the hands, they place little stress on the body. Wireless versions of these devices also allow medical assistants to conduct calls away from the telephone system, a feature that is particularly helpful when patient files must be pulled or assistants must move to different workstations (Figure 7-1 ◆). Assistants can wear wireless headsets all day throughout the office.

Dialing Numbers Automatically

Many telephone systems today have **automatic dialer** or **speed dial** functions that allow medical assistants to dial up to 100 programmed numbers with the push of a few buttons instead of several (Figure 7-2 ◆). Such features save medical assistants a great deal of time when contacting insurance companies, pharmacies, hospitals, laboratories, and physicians via the phone.

Redialing Last Numbers Called

The **last number redial** telephone feature, common today in home and office systems, dials the last number called from the phone with one button. Some systems offer a feature that will redial the last number called until there is an answer.

Making Conference Calls

The **conference call** feature allows two or more parties to speak on the same phone line at once. Conversation flows more easily and misunderstandings between parties diminish when all parties involved are on the line at the same time. In the medical office, the physician may use this feature to speak with a patient and another member of the health care team, like the physical therapist.

As the parties to a conversation increase, however, so does the potential for confusion. Therefore, when conference calls

have more than three parties, all parties should identify themselves before commenting.

Conversing via Speaker Telephone

The **speaker telephone** feature, which broadcasts the speaker's voice from the unit, helps when more than one party at the same location wishes to participate in a telephone conversation. In the medical office, the physician may use this feature to broadcast the voice of another health care professional while a patient is in the office, for example. Medical professionals can work hands free, which means they can do things like write in patients' charts while taking part in the conversation. When-

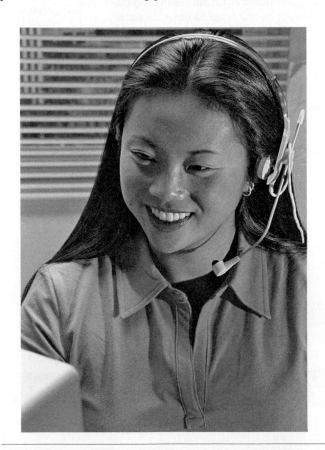

Figure 7-1 ◆ Using a hands-free headset makes the medical assistant's job easier.

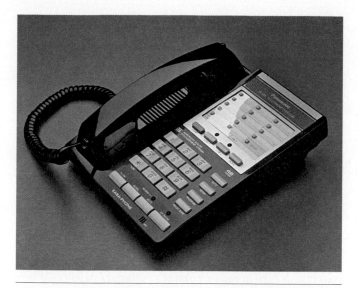

Figure 7-2 ◆ Most telephone systems in the medical facility have features such as speed dial.

ever the speaker phone feature is used, however, it is important and courteous to advise speakers that they are being broadcast and to advise them of all other listeners in the room.

HIPAA Compliance

Patient confidentiality is an important part of Health Insurance Portability and Accountability Act (**HIPAA**) compliancy. The speaker-phone feature must only be used to discuss confidential patient information when parties unauthorized to have the patient's information are unable to overhear the conversation.

Call Forwarding

Call forwarding automatically routes incoming calls to other telephone numbers. In the medical office, this feature is most commonly used after business hours to direct incoming calls to an answering service.

Recording Telephone Calls

The medical office, like other businesses, may wish to record incoming calls. Recorded calls support both quality-assurance efforts and training initiatives.

Direct Telephone Lines

Many medical offices use **direct telephone lines** that **route** to select members of the staff. Patients can call the billing department, for example, or staff in charge of appointment scheduling. While direct lines can eliminate the need for hold times, they require patients to have multiple telephone numbers for the office.

Automatic Routing Units

In many medical offices, callers can use **automatic routing units** to choose the parties they wish to reach by dialing the

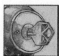

Keys to Success
RECORDING CALLS

Recording telephone calls without the callers' consent is illegal. Medical offices that wish to record calls should do one of the following:

■ Prerecord a message that plays before the medical assistant takes the line. Such a recording may say, "This call may be recorded to maintain quality customer service."
■ Have the medical assistant advise callers that calls may be recorded.

Callers can choose to avoid participating in recorded calls. When they do, medical offices cannot record calls.

main line and choosing extensions. Automated instructions direct callers to the parties they wish to reach. While such systems can be beneficial, they can also have drawbacks. For example, such systems may impose long wait periods on callers or require multiple steps to reach desired extensions.

Placing Callers on Hold

The **hold feature** of telephone systems places callers on hold so users can complete other tasks. With this feature, staff can juggle multiple telephone lines or handle calls while assisting patients in person. Callers cannot see who is in the medical office when they call, however, so medical assistants must use the hold feature judiciously. Improper use can extend wait times and give the impression that the patient on hold is not important. Medical assistants should verify that callers have only nonemergency issues before placing those callers on hold. In general, all members of the health care team should use the hold function in such a way that minimizes wait times and treats all patients equally.

Even the simplest telephone systems can play music or recorded information during hold times. The most rudimentary systems connect the telephone system to a radio, while more advanced units allow callers to choose the type of information they will hear. Many medical offices record or buy messages for this purpose. Such messages can be specific to the practice, such as messages about well-child check ups for pediatric offices, or informational, like those about seasonal allergies for allergists' offices. Some physicians use **generic messages** and some will even record their own messages in their own voices. Messages like these add a personal touch that can both reassure patients and fortify their trust in the practice. However, only physicians with warm, pleasant-sounding, and clear voices should record messages like these. As mentioned earlier, the telephone is usually the patient's first contact with the medical office. Unpleasant-sounding physicians may unnerve new patients. Medical assistants with proper speaking voices can sometimes record such messages effectively.

Like the recorded information that is played during hold periods, hold music should be used with some stipulations. First, the music must be clear and generally pleasant. Callers are a captive audience that may become irritated by music that is broken

Keys to Success
PLACING CALLERS ON HOLD

Never place a caller on hold without first asking for and receiving permission. When callers agree to hold, they should wait no more than 20 to 30 seconds before a member of the health care team checks in with an update. Long periods of hold time give the impression that patients are forgotten or unvalued when callers should instead feel that the medical office values them and their time.

Keys to Success
DISCLOSING PERSONAL INFORMATION ABOUT COWORKERS

Never give callers the personal telephone numbers of physicians or other members of the health care team. When physicians are unavailable and callers express an urgent need to speak with them, the medical assistant should take the caller's name, number, and call purpose and call the physician with the information. It is illegal to disclose any personal information about coworkers without the coworker's permission.

by static or considered offensive. Religious music, for example, should be avoided, because it could offend followers of different faiths. So that they may better understand their callers' experiences, it is good practice for medical assistants periodically to call the offices where they work and assess the offices' recordings.

Critical Thinking Question 7-1

If the medical office uses an automated system where callers are greeted by a recording, how can the medical assistant best serve a patient who has a possible emergency?

Other Special Features

Large medical offices may have the funds to purchase special telephone features, such as programs that call patients with electronic appointment reminders or requests. "Automatic redial in reverse," which prevents long wait periods, is another such feature. With this feature, patients call the medical office and choose a number for the type of service they need, such as "1 to schedule an appointment." The patients then record their names, enter their telephone numbers, and hang up. When a medical assistant becomes available, the system automatically redials the patient and connects the call. Patients are free to go about other tasks, and office staff need not retrieve messages.

Using an Answering Service

When they are closed, perhaps during lunch or after conventional business hours, most medical offices use professional answering services to handle their calls. Such services forward calls to appropriate parties and thereby eliminate the need for the call forwarding feature mentioned earlier. Some telephone systems are designed to forward any calls not answered by the fourth ring to an answering service.

To ensure patients always receive high-quality customer service, medical offices should only use answering services experienced in health care. In addition, answering services should always have the contact information for the physicians on call. This way, the service can reach the physicians in the event of patient emergency. To retrieve any of the messages the service has taken, the medical office usually must call the service once the office reopens. Some answering services send messages via fax or e-mail.

Using the Voicemail Feature

Most medical offices use voicemail within their system. Often, voicemail is used at each employee's personal extension. When a patient calls the office after hours via the main office telephone line, the patient will typically reach an answering service. If the call comes through to an internal extension within the medical office, for example, the billing office, a voicemail may be reached after hours.

When using the voicemail feature, each employee should leave their name, their department name, and information to let the caller know when they should expect a return telephone call. An example might be: "This is Debra Meyers in the billing office at Martha Lake Family Practice. I am away from my phone right now. If you will leave me a message, including your name and telephone number, I will return your call within 24 hours."

Patient Telephone Use

Some medical offices provide telephones for patient use, often in the reception area or at the front desk, although growing cellular-phone use is eroding this practice. Offices that do provide patient phones will typically install a separate line that does not interfere with incoming calls, as well as restrict the phone to local calls only.

In Practice

Established patient Josie Welton often arrives early for her appointments. While she waits in the reception area, Josie uses the patient phone to make a call during which she details her health care problems and other personal information. The other patients in the reception area overhear the entire conversation. How should the medical assistant address this situation?

Answering the Telephone

Answering calls professionally is an art form that medical assistants should master, because telephone work is a large part of medical assisting. Before answering any calls, the medical assistant should obtain a pen and paper and prepare a cheerful yet professional greeting. Many assistants find practicing before a mirror, or even placing a "smile" symbol near the telephone, to be helpful when preparing for telephone work.

When medical assistants answer calls, they should speak clearly as they identify their office and themselves. Some offices identify themselves by physician names, while others use the names of their offices. Some offices even use original greetings, such as, "It's a great day at Mountain View Clinic. This is Sara."

As customer-service representatives are trained to do, medical assistants should answer calls within two to three rings. Any longer period gives a negative impression, perhaps that staffing in the office is inadequate or the office is overburdened. Once the caller begins speaking, the medical assistant should try to match their rate of speech, although the assistant should always strive for a moderate pace.

As soon as the caller gives their name, the assistant should write the name down. Throughout patient calls, the medical assistant should refer to the caller by name, reinforcing that the caller is important. When the call is complete, the medical assistant should always say goodbye and allow the caller to hang up first. This reinforces the impression that the caller remains important and that the medical assistant is in no hurry to move on.

In terms of call content, medical assistants should be familiar enough with their office location to be able to give most callers directions, as well as such related information as parking fees and availability. In addition to office location, medical assistants should be familiar with the insurance plans their office participate in so they are armed to answer patient questions in that arena. Printed lists near the phone serve as good reference. Figure 7-3 ◆ identifies some behaviors to avoid while on the phone.

Screening Telephone Calls

As part of their telephone duties, medical assistants are charged with screening calls, which involves determining a call's purpose and whether that purpose is an emergency. To give assistants solid guidelines, every medical office should have a written policy for screening calls. ∞ Chapter 13 provides more information on creating office policies.

Directing Patient Calls to Physicians

Often, the calls medical assistants take are from parties who ask to speak with the physician directly. As a result, physicians

should outline criteria for when they will accept patient calls (Figure 7-4 ◆). In addition to meeting physicians' needs and desires, such policies give medical assistants guidelines for telephone use. Many physicians accept no telephone calls, even when not with patients.

When patients ask physicians return their calls, the medical assistant should place the message with the patient's chart on the physician's desk. In offices with several physicians, typically only one physician will be "on call" after hours, a role the physicians serve on a rotating basis. Any physician who is on call after hours must have some way of being reached. Due to the nature of the occupation, physicians must be available at all times, whether by telephone or pager. In addition to being readily available to the medical assistant, such numbers must be readily available to the office's answering service. When physicians do accept calls, the medical assistant should gather a caller's name and reason for calling before transferring the call to the physician.

Prioritizing Telephone Calls

In general, it is most efficient to address short telephone calls before longer ones. Short calls include those that simply need to be routed to staff or that derive from **established patients** needing to make appointments. Long, time-consuming calls include those from new patients or patients with elaborate questions. Calls from angry or agitated patients take precedence above all others, however. Hold periods, even short ones, could worsen

- Acting with no authority or out of the scope of training (e.g., reducing fees, agreeing to refill prescriptions without the physician's consent, making diagnoses).
- Arguing with callers. Medical assistants must remain professional and calm.
- Violating patient confidentiality. Medical assistants must never release any patient information without the patient's permission, including the fact that the patient patronizes the medical office.
- Answering telephone calls where other patients can hear them.
- Taking inaccurate or incomplete messages.
- Eating or drinking while using the telephone.
- Allowing callers on hold for more than 30 seconds with no contact.

Figure 7-3 ◆ Improper telephone procedures.

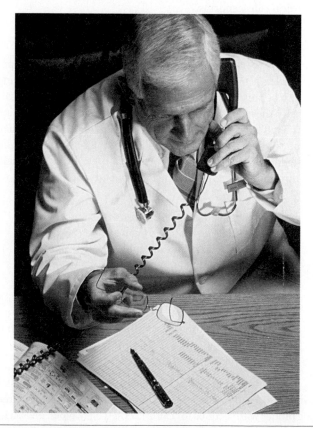

Figure 7-4 ◆ A physician takes a telephone call at his desk.

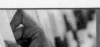

PROCEDURE 7-1 Answer the Telephone

Theory and Rationale

One of the administrative medical assistant's main duties, which is critical to the medical office, is to answer the office telephone. To complete this task, the assistant must have attention to detail, as well as the ability to multitask.

Materials

- Pen
- Paper
- Telephone

Competency

(**Conditions**) With the necessary materials, you will be able to (**Task**) answer the medical office telephone (**Standards**) correctly within the time limit set by the instructor.

1. Answer the telephone between the second and third rings.
2. State the office's name, followed by your name.
3. If the caller fails to provide a personal name, ask for it and write it down.
4. Determine the reason for the call.
5. If the caller is having a medical emergency, ask if someone can come to the phone to speak about it. If not, motion a coworker to dial for emergency services while keeping the patient on the line.
6. If the patient is calling to speak with another member of the health care team, transfer the call to that person if available.
7. When a requested party is unavailable, record a message. Include the name of the caller, the date and time of the call, the telephone number where the caller can be reached, the reason for the call, and the name of the person the caller wishes to reach.
8. When taking a message, inform the caller when the call will likely be returned.
9. Clarify information (e.g., appointment time) as appropriate.
10. Allow the caller to hang up before hanging up.
11. Route any message to the proper staff member.
12. Chart any health care–related information into the patient's chart as appropriate.

---

the situation. The sooner medical assistants provide for patient needs, the happier patients are. Figure 7-5 ◆ outlines some common call scenarios.

Telephone Triage

The ability to **triage** patient telephone calls, or place them in priority order, is important not only for patient safety and well being, but also because it cultivates a positive office image. To triage calls properly, the medical assistant must know the types of complaints considered emergencies and, of those, which demand immediate attention. Calls from patients with potentially life-threatening emergencies must be handled before all other calls. Potentially life-threatening emergencies include, but are not limited to:

- Complaints of chest pain
- Complaints of heavy bleeding due to an injury
- Bleeding in a pregnant woman
- High fever in an infant or child
- Severe asthma attack
- Severe shortness of breath
- Possible poisoning or allergic reaction
- Obvious broken bone
- Sudden confusion, loss of consciousness, or change in mental status
- Mention of suicide or harm to themselves or others.

When triaging calls, a **triage notebook** at the front desk is invaluable (Figure 7-6 ◆). The triage notebook is typically a three-ring binder with sections for call and emergency types. Physicians should participate in these notebooks' construction so they can

dictate the actions medical assistants and other staff must take. Figure 7-7 ◆ explains how a triage notebook might be used.

— Critical Thinking Question 7-2—

If the medical office mentioned in the case study lacks a triage notebook, how should the medical assistant go about creating one?

Taking Emergency Telephone Calls

When patients need immediate transport to the hospital, the medical assistant may be asked to call for emergency services. If the emergency has occurred in the medical office, the medical assistant will need to direct emergency services to the office to pick up the patient (Figure 7-8 ◆). The medical assistant should have the patient's name, age, and gender before making the call, as well as the problem type and type of care the physician is requesting. The medical assistant will need to be sure to give any specific directions, such as the office or suite number, and then advise the physician of the estimated time of arrival of the emergency services team.

Being Professional on the Telephone

When using the telephone, the medical assistant must be professional. Professionalism includes never chewing gum or eating while using the telephone and being careful to pronounce words, including names, correctly. Assistants should avoid using unfamiliar words or slang, especially when speaking to people who use

❑ **Line 1:** A mother is calling to schedule her 4-month-old child for a well-child checkup and vaccines. The office has not seen this child as a patient previously.

❑ **Line 2:** An equipment salesperson wants to speak with someone about equipping the office with new billing software.

❑ **Line 3:** An extremely angry patient states that she has been placed on hold twice by the "billing person" and has been disconnected both times.

❑ **Line 4:** A patient is calling to confirm the preoperative instructions he was given last week. His surgery appointment is for tomorrow morning.

❑ **Line 5:** A patient is calling for the results of her laboratory work done yesterday.

The medical assistant should address Line 3 first, because the patient is very angry. To minimize the damage, the medical assistant should apologize for the patient's inconvenience, secure the patient's return number, and advise the patient to expect a return call within an hour. The assistant should contact the billing department immediately upon handling all other calls and make the request for a return call.

After the angry caller, the callers on Lines 4 and 5 take priority. The assistant should route both to a clinical medical assistant or the nurse on staff. Line 2 is the next call in priority order. The medical assistant should route this call to the office manager, and then turn to the caller on Line 1. The Line 1 caller comes last in this situation, because a new-patient call takes the longest to resolve.

Figure 7-5 ◆ Prioritization of telephone calls.

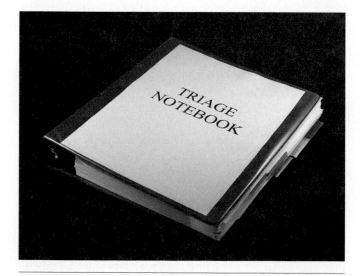

Figure 7-6 ◆ A triage notebook.

English as a second language. The medical assistant's voice should be calm and pleasant and its tone polite and warm. Callers should feel they have the medical assistant's complete attention.

In addition to using proper words and a soothing voice, medical assistants must be organized and prepared to answer the telephone properly. They should have a pen or pencil and paper ready before picking up the line. Never should assistants be rushed or anxious to end patient calls. When the time callers need exceeds the time medical assistants have, those assistants

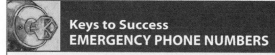

Keys to Success
EMERGENCY PHONE NUMBERS

Every medical office should keep a list of emergency telephone numbers near every office telephone. This list should include number for police nonemergency services, the sheriff's department, and poison control, among others.

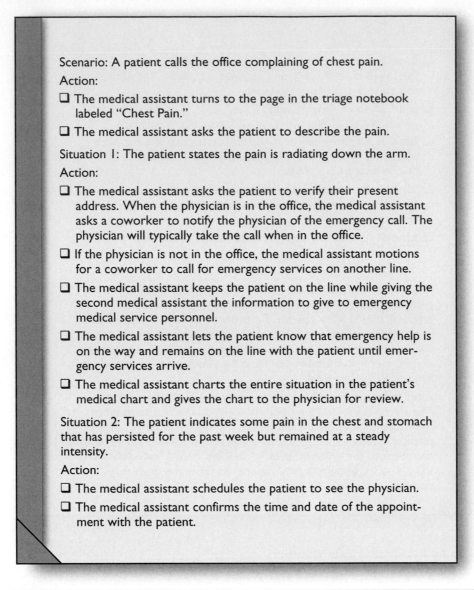

Scenario: A patient calls the office complaining of chest pain.

Action:

❑ The medical assistant turns to the page in the triage notebook labeled "Chest Pain."

❑ The medical assistant asks the patient to describe the pain.

Situation 1: The patient states the pain is radiating down the arm.

Action:

❑ The medical assistant asks the patient to verify their present address. When the physician is in the office, the medical assistant asks a coworker to notify the physician of the emergency call. The physician will typically take the call when in the office.

❑ If the physician is not in the office, the medical assistant motions for a coworker to call for emergency services on another line.

❑ The medical assistant keeps the patient on the line while giving the second medical assistant the information to give to emergency medical service personnel.

❑ The medical assistant lets the patient know that emergency help is on the way and remains on the line with the patient until emergency services arrive.

❑ The medical assistant charts the entire situation in the patient's medical chart and gives the chart to the physician for review.

Situation 2: The patient indicates some pain in the chest and stomach that has persisted for the past week but remained at a steady intensity.

Action:

❑ The medical assistant schedules the patient to see the physician.

❑ The medical assistant confirms the time and date of the appointment with the patient.

Figure 7-7 ◆ Sample triage notebook use.

should take the callers' names and numbers and get permission to call them back.

Especially over the telephone, many people get into habits of using phrases or terminology that fail to work in health care. Figure 7-9 ◆ provides some examples with proposed improvements.

Communicating with Hard-to-Understand Callers

Part of acting like a professional includes listening to patients speak without interruption. When patients have speech impediments or English that is unclear, medical assistants may have to ask those patients to repeat themselves. When confusion persists, the medical assistant should try repeating what they heard to verify the patient's message was understood correctly.

Handling Difficult Callers

Occasionally, patients call the office while very upset. With calls like these, the most important thing the medical assistant can do is to remain calm and professional and avoid both attacking the patient personally and taking the patient's emotions personally. Medical assistants must always speak politely and courteously, whatever the callers' attitudes. While the medical assistant's job is not to take verbal abuse, most angry callers will calm quickly when the medical assistant remains calm and polite. Any calls like this, however, must be documented in patients' files.

To resolve matters involving difficult callers, the medical assistant should apologize for whatever the patient is angry about and determine how to correct the situation. Any calls from patients that cannot be resolved must be brought to the physician's attention. The physician may choose to call the patient in the hope of finding resolution.

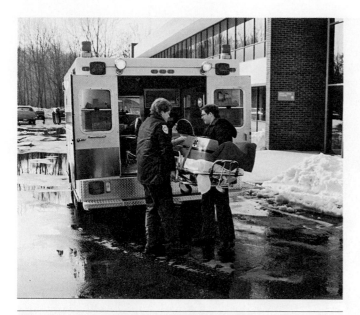

Figure 7-8 ◆ In the event of a medical emergency, an ambulance may be called to the medical office to transport the patient to the hospital.

- When a caller asks for a staff member who is not in the office, inappropriate phrases include, "He isn't in yet," "She's in the restroom right now," or "I don't know where she is." An appropriate substitution is, "He's unavailable at the moment. May I take a message?"
- When a caller requests information or help with something, improper phrases include, "That isn't my job," "The computer is down," or "You'll need to talk with someone in billing." Instead, the medical assistant should take the caller's name and number, commit to checking with another member of the health care team, and promise to call the patient with the desired information.
- When a new patient calls to schedule an appointment, the medical assistant should not say things like, "We don't accept that insurance," "We don't take patients with your condition," or "I've never heard of the doctor who referred you." Instead it is appropriate to say, "We are not preferred with your insurance plan, but let me find out who is and call you back," or "Our office doesn't specialize in conditions such as yours, but let me check with the doctor to see who she would refer you to and call you back." Another appropriate response is, "Will you please spell the referring doctor's last name, and do you have that office telephone number?" These statements are unlikely to offend the caller.
- The habit of asking patients, "How are you?" is an undesired one. Although common in American culture as a generic opener, some patients take the question literally and provide personal information. As has been discussed before, personal patient information must be guarded, especially at an office's busy front desk.
- Medical assistants should anticipate how terms may be interpreted. For example, the term "waiting room" implies an area where patients wait, but a more positive term is "reception room," because it means patients are received into the office.

Figure 7-9 ◆ Appropriate telephone phrases.

Receiving Calls from Emotional Patients

Emotional patients, such as those who are grieving or have been in accidents, will likely need more of the medical assistant's time. If the patient is emotional and calling to schedule an appointment, the medical assistant will need to determine if the patient needs to be seen right away. In a situation like this, the medical assistant should chart in the patient's medical record what happened during the telephone call and bring the situation to the physician's attention. It may be appropriate for the physician to call the patient back.

Documenting Calls from Patients

While not all patient calls must be documented in the patients' chart, any related to the patients' health care should be charted. Figure 7-10 ◆ outlines which calls should and should not be charted. Every medical office should have a policy about when and how to chart telephone calls, and medical assistants should be familiar with their offices' policies. In most offices, the administrative medical assistant makes the entry in the patient's chart and places the chart on the physician's desk for review or possible followup action.

Taking Telephone Messages

Taking a telephone message properly saves time for the member of the health care team who is returning the call. Most offices have message pads for this purpose (Figure 7-11 ◆). Such pads, which serve as reminders to the medical assistant, have spaces for all the information needed from patients.

Calling in Prescriptions and Refill Requests

Guidelines for prescription refills vary from one office to another. Generally, most offices require at least 24 hours' notice to refill prescriptions. Medical assistants should forward these calls, which may come from patients or pharmacists, to the clinical

---

Calls That Typically Must Appear in Patients' Charts
- Patients who cancel appointments and fail to reschedule
- Patients who say they are in the hospital
- Relatives of patients who say the patient has died
- Patient who indicates they are not returning to the office for care
- Patient who contends they cannot afford to keep their appointments, fill their prescriptions, or see specialists

Calls That Typically Require No Charting
- Patients confirming appointment times
- Patients rescheduling appointments
- Patients complaining about their bills

Figure 7-10 ◆ Charting telephone calls in patient charts.

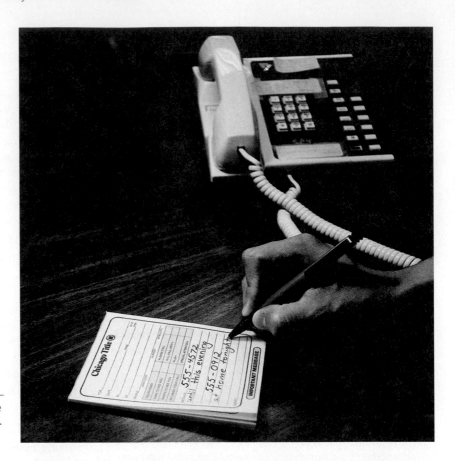

Figure 7-11 ◆ Telephone message pads should be located near every office telephone in the administrative portion of the medical office.

medical assistant or nurse. Alternatively, the medical assistant can check with the physician to see if the physician wishes to see the patient before allowing their refill. When office policy requires the medical assistant to check with the physician on all prescription refill requests but the physician is unavailable when the call comes in, the assistant must take the patient's name; the medication requested, including dosage; and the number where the patient or pharmacist can be reached. The medical assistant

must then pull patient's file and place it, with the corresponding message, on the physician's desk (Figure 7-12 ◆).

Calling Patients

Before making telephone calls, medical assistants should have all materials and information at hand, including the patients' medical charts. Assistants who are calling patients to schedule appointment should be well versed in the time each procedure takes, as well as any special patient instructions, such as not eating for 12 hours before a particular visit. Any patient calls that are medically relevant must be charted in the patients' charts.

Leaving Messages

To remain HIPAA compliant, medical assistants must maintain confidentiality at all times, including while on the telephone. When leaving messages, for example, assistants must remember that the people taking those messages, such as the patients' spouses or parents of minors seeking treatment for pregnancy, sexually transmitted diseases, mental illnesses, or drug and alcohol counseling, may lack the patients' permission to know the nature of the calls. ∞ Chapter 4 provides more information on the legalities of releasing information for minors.

When medical assistants must leave messages for patients, those assistants should leave their names, the physicians' names, and the appropriate telephone numbers. When an office's name self-identifies, such as "Marysville Oncology

---

Keys to Success
TAKING A TELEPHONE MESSAGE

Capture all the following information when taking telephone messages:

- Date and time of telephone call
- Name of person with whom the caller wishes to speak
- Name of the caller (verify the spelling when unsure)
- Telephone number, including area code, where the caller can be reached
- Nature or reason for the call
- Your name

Advise the caller when to expect a return call. If, for example, the caller is calling for Jane in the billing department but Jane is out, tell the caller when to expect a return call. This way, the caller can avoid wasting time waiting for the call. Also, be sure to route messages to appropriate parties in a timely manner.

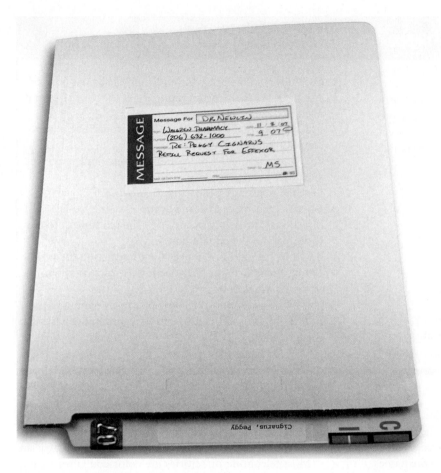

Figure 7-12 ◆ When prescription refill requests come into the office, the medical assistant should pull the patient's file and give both to the physician.

PROCEDURE 7-2 Take a Telephone Message

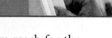

Theory and Rationale

Administrative medical assistants often take telephone messages for other members of the health care team. In this task, accuracy is paramount. A simple numeric transposition, for example, can make a message useless.

Materials

- Pen
- Telephone message pad
- Telephone

Competency

(**Conditions**) With the necessary materials, you will be able to (**Task**) take a telephone message (**Standards**) correctly within the time limit set by the instructor.

1. Answer the telephone call by the second ring.

2. Once the caller identifies the desired party, reach for the message pad.
3. Ask for the caller's full name, verify the spelling, and document it on the pad.
4. Verify the name of the party the caller is trying to reach, and document on it the pad.
5. Ask for the reason for the call, and document it on the pad.
6. Ask for the caller's telephone number, including area code, and document it on the pad.
7. Repeat the telephone number to the caller to verify it was documented correctly.
8. Write the date and time of the call on the pad.
9. Write your name or initials on the pad.
10. Tell the caller when to expect a return call.
11. Bid goodbye to the caller, and allow the caller to hang up before hanging up.
12. Route the message to its intended recipient.

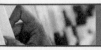

PROCEDURE 7-3 Call a Pharmacy with Prescription Orders

Theory and Rationale

As part of their duties in the medical office, administrative medical assistants often call pharmacies with new or refill prescriptions. To complete this task properly and ensure patient safety, assistants must demonstrate strict attention to detail.

Materials

- Telephone
- Patient's chart
- Pen
- Prescription information
- Pharmacy telephone number

Competency

(**Conditions**) With the necessary materials, you will be able to (**Task**) call a pharmacy with a new or refill prescription order (**Standards**) correctly within the time limit set by the instructor.

1. Carefully read the prescription the physician has ordered.
2. Ask the physician any questions about the prescription if needed.
3. Call the pharmacy where the patient would like the prescription filled.
4. Give the pharmacist the patient's name, and verify the spelling.
5. Give the pharmacist the patient's birth date.
6. Give the pharmacist the medication's name, dosage, and directions per the physician. Alert the pharmacist to any drug allergies the patient has.
7. Ask the pharmacist to repeat the information for verification, and inform the pharmacist if the patient is en route to the pharmacy.
8. Note the prescription, including pharmacy name and telephone number, on the medication record in the patient's medical chart.

Specialists" or "Monroe Women's Care and Family Planning Clinic," the medical assistant should not leave the office's name, because doing so discloses some of the patient's confidential information. Instead, medical assistants should leave the names of physicians only, as in, "This is Christine calling from Dr. Wilson's office. I'm leaving a message for Jose. Please call me at 555-123-4567."

Calling Other Health Care Facilities

Medical assistants often will be asked to call other health care facilities involved in the care of mutual patients, whether to schedule appointments with specialists or obtain information from patients' primary care providers. Whatever the reason for the call, the medical assistant will need to maintain patient confidentiality at all times. This means disclosing only absolutely necessary information to the other office staff when placing the call. If the medical assistant is scheduling a patient with a specialist, for example, that assistant will need to provide the patient's contact and insurance information. Other private patient information, like lifestyle habits and payment history, should remain undisclosed. Figure 7-14 ◆ provides tips on patient-related exchanges via telephone.

Using a Telephone Directory

In the past, a "telephone directory" usually meant a "telephone book," but today several different companies produce telephone books. The medical office may have one book for white pages and one for yellow pages, for example. When a medical office is in a large metropolitan area, it may have several books to cover its surrounding areas. Listings in the white pages are alphabetical by the person's name and alphabetical by business type in the yellow

pages. Most telephone books create sublistings for business types, as well. For example, under the directory for physicians may be an alphabetical listing of physicians by type, such as pediatrician.

Most telephone directories are color coded for ease of use. Many precede their white pages with business sections in different colors. Directories typically have listings for local ZIP codes at their beginnings and a government section that includes listings for federal, local, and state agencies. These pages are typically colored differently, sometimes blue.

Using an Online Directory

Many medical offices today use the Internet to look up telephone numbers. Many Web sites, including www.Yahoo.com, www.anywho.com, www.dexknows.com, www.yellowpages.com, www.superpages.com, and www.bigbook.com, search for both local and national telephone numbers for both personal and business information.

Using a Rolodex System

Every medical office should keep a directory of commonly called telephone numbers on the computer or in a Rolodex card file (Figure 7-15 ◆). Such tools make it easier to locate the number for the cardiac specialist the physician refers patients to, for example.

Keys to Success
LONG DISTANCE CALLS

Factor in time zones before making long-distance calls (Figure 7-13 ◆). When calling California from New York, for example, the medical office must factor in a 3-hour time difference.

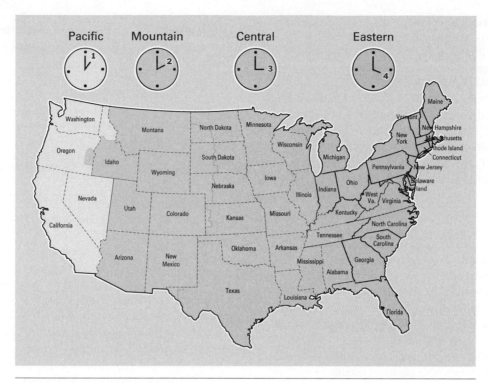

Figure 7-13 ◆ A time zone map.

Long Distance or Toll-Free Calls

The medical assistant may frequently make long-distance telephone calls on behalf of the medical office. Some offices require staff to log any long-distance telephone calls with the call's purpose, as well as the name and number of the party being called. To comply with such requests, medical assistants should familiarize themselves with their offices' policies.

Most suppliers and businesses the medical office buys from will have toll-free telephone numbers, which typically begin with 1-800, 1-888, or 1-866, and impose no charges on callers.

Patient Confidentiality

Maintaining patient confidentiality is extremely important. Violations of patient privacy are serious offenses punishable by fines under HIPAA. Patients must know that their private information will be kept confidential. One of the best ways to do this is for the medical assistant to refrain from discussing any patient information within hearing distance of other patients. When patients hear office staff discussing other patients, they may assume that their private information is similarly discussed. Keeping conversations professional, and never resorting to gossip about other

- If your physician is running behind on appointments or has been delayed getting to the office, call patients who will be impacted. Offer to reschedule when a delay is unacceptable.

- When the physician cannot do so, have the medical assistant make followup calls to patients after surgical procedures. When patients report anything unusual, transfer the call to the physician.

- Give new patients all administrative information, such as parking and preferred manner of dress, medications and foods to avoid for certain tests and procedures.

- Advise patients of important policies (e.g., pay at the time services are rendered) before they visit the office.

- Remind all patients to bring necessary information to visits (e.g., insurance cards or lists of medications).

- Stagger staff lunch hours so a live person always answers the telephone.

Figure 7-14 ◆ Ways to show patient importance through telephone use.

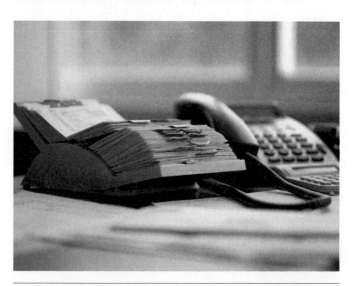

Figure 7-15 ◆ A Rolodex card system next to the telephone allows the administrative medical assistant to quickly locate commonly called numbers.

staff members or patients, is one way to reinforce to patients that the medical assistant is trustworthy and professional.

HIPAA Compliance

The medical office must treat all callers requesting patient information cautiously. Because callers' identities cannot be determined via telephone, the office should disclose no confidential information over the telephone. Instead, members of the health care team should advise callers to send any requests via fax or mail and to accompany those requests with a signed authorization from the patient or a court order.

Personal Telephone Calls

Studies on businesses across America have found that the average employee spends 65 hours per year on personal calls while at work. Because personal calls are very expensive for employers, they are generally frowned on. Some employers feel that employees who spend time on personal telephone calls during work hours are stealing from them.

To avoid ill will, medical assistants should review and abide by their offices' policies for personal telephone use. Making or receiving personal telephone calls is unprofessional, and it ties up a business's telephone line (Figure 7-16 ♦). Most offices allow employees to receive only emergency telephone calls during work hours. When medical assistants must make personal calls, they should do so on break or during lunch and out of patients' hearing range.

Telecommunication Relay Services

Patients who are hearing or speech impaired may use a telecommunication relay system to contact the medical office. The Americans with Disabilities Act (**ADA**) requires that telephone companies have telecommunication relay systems available 24

- The caller types a message into a special telephone.
- The message transmits to the relay service.
- An operator calls the medical office.
- When the medical assistant answers, the operator self-identifies and identifies the caller.
- The operator mediates between the medical assistant and the caller, reading messages to the assistant and typing responses to the caller.
- When the call is complete, the medical assistant bids the patient goodbye, awaits the interpreter's response, and then hangs up.

Figure 7-17 ♦ How a telecommunication relay system works.

hours per day, 365 days per year. Figure 7-17 ♦ describes how a telecommunication relay system works.

A medical office with a large number of hearing-impaired patients, perhaps an audiology practice, may have a teletypewriter (**TTY**) system (Figure 7-18 ♦). TTY systems connect to the telephone, allowing both parties to the call to type their responses and thereby eliminate the need for a telecommunication relay service.

When using services like these, it is important to note that conversations be aimed at the caller, not the operator. The operator is charged with typing every spoken word, not serving as the call's recipient. In other words, the medical assistant should not say, "Tell Sharon the physician can see her at 10 A.M." Instead, the assistant should say, "Sharon, the physician can see you at 10 A.M. Will that time work?"

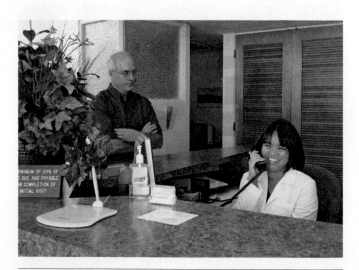

Figure 7-16 ♦ Making or receiving personal telephone calls is unprofessional. When medical assistants must make personal calls, they should do so on break and out of patients' hearing.

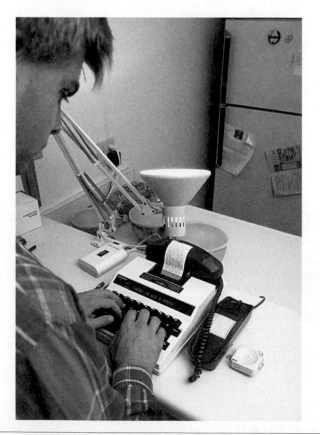

Figure 7-18 ♦ A patient using a teletypewriter (TTY) system.

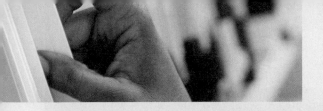

REVIEW

Chapter Summary

- Like the medical assistant, an answering service serves a crucial role in handling telephone calls efficiently and professionally.
- To triage the medical office's incoming calls properly, medical assistants need a distinct skill set, including a good understanding of any procedure's time requirements.
- Emergency calls dictate special telephone attention, as do callers who are angry or otherwise upset.
- When answering calls in the medical office, the medical assistant should follow all office policies for taking messages properly.

- Prescription requests must be made using proper, professional telephone procedure.
- When calling patients on medical offices' behalf, it is crucial that medical assistants remain calm and professional at all times.
- Telephone directories, both electronic and conventional hard-copy versions, are helpful tools in the office's search for telephone numbers.
- While conducting telephone procedures in the medical office, the medical assistant's most crucial task is to maintain patient confidentiality.

Chapter Review

Multiple Choice

1. Which of the following telephone features dials a number with the push of just one button?
   a. Last number redial
   b. Speed dialer
   c. Automatic dialer
   d. All of the above

2. Which of the following pieces of information need not be included when taking a message?
   a. Caller's name
   b. Call date
   c. Patient's insurance information
   d. Medical assistant's name

3. Which of the following is an appropriate way to handle an angry caller?
   a. Hang up the phone
   b. Remain calm
   c. Use the hold feature
   d. None of the above

4. Which of the following calls should be handled first?
   a. Patient calling for lab results
   b. Doctor's college roommate calling for the doctor
   c. Patient complaining of shortness of breath
   d. Patient confirming an appointment time

5. Which of the following is the best choice for patients on hold?
   a. Generic message thanking callers for holding
   b. Local news station with slight static
   c. Physician's gruff voice
   d. Any of the above

6. For a caller with a life-threatening emergency who needs emergency medical services, the medical assistant should:
   a. Ask the caller to hold while dialing emergency medical services on another line
   b. Ask the caller to hang up and immediately dial 9-1-1
   c. Ask the caller to hold while transferring the call to a clinical medical assistant
   d. Hang up on the caller and dial 9-1-1

7. To find the telephone number for a medical supplier, the medical assistant could:
   a. Use an Internet directory
   b. Check a telephone book
   c. Search Rolodex card file
   d. All of the above

True/False

T F 1. Telephone triage is the ability to transfer calls to voicemail.

T F 2. When patients call to cancel their appointments and but fail to reschedule, the calls should be charted in the patients' medical charts.

T F 3. When leaving messages for a patient, it is acceptable to tell the patient's spouse the purpose for the patient's visit.

T F 4. When calling other health care facilities to schedule appointments for patients, the medical assistant should disclose only needed patient information.

T F 5. Before answering the office telephone, medical assistants should know the insurance plans the office participates with.

Chapter Review (continued)

T F 6. Because medical terminology is unfamiliar to most patients, layman's terms are best when speaking with patients.

T F 7. Unidentified callers should be routed directly to the physician.

Short Answer

1. Why is it important to speak clearly on the telephone?

2. Explain why taking personal telephone calls during office hours is problematic.

3. Explain how a telephone relay system works.

4. What is the purpose of a telephone triage notebook?

5. Explain how a medical office can legally record patient telephone calls.

6. Differentiate between screening and prioritizing telephone calls.

Research

1. Look online for companies that sell multi-line telephone systems. What kind of features do they offer?

2. What local companies can you find in your area that offer answering services to medical offices? What services do they offer?

3. How many local telephone directories are there in your local area? Why would a person choose one over another?

Externship Application Experience

When Sofie Pouillon calls the office, she says wants to cancel her upcoming appointment because she is very unhappy with the physician. What can the medical assistant say to this pa-tient? What is the proper way to chart this call and notify the physician?

Resource Guide

**Amateur Radio Research
and Development Corporation**
Telecommunications for the Deaf
Post Office Drawer 6148
McLean, VA 22106-6148
www.amrad.org

Online Yellow Pages
http://www.yellowpages.com

SkillPath Seminars
"The Secrets to Being a Front Desk Superstar" Seminar
P.O. Box 2768
Mission, KS 66201-2768
Phone: (800) 873-7545
Fax: (913) 362-4241
http://www.skillpath.com

MedMedia

http://www.MyMAKit.com

More on this chapter, including interactive resources, can be found on the Student CD-ROM accompanying this textbook and on http://www.MyMAKit.com.

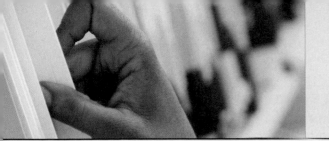

Objectives

After completing this chapter, you should be able to:

- Define and spell the key terminology in this chapter.
- Describe the steps to opening and closing the office efficiently.
- List the steps to prepare files for patient arrivals.
- Describe appropriate ways to greet and register both new and established patients.
- Identify means of maintaining patient confidentiality in all front-desk activities.
- Describe techniques for persuading patients to provide information.
- Communicate with patients regarding scheduling delays and cancellations.
- Manage difficult patients effectively in the reception area.
- List the types of patients who should not be left in the reception room.
- Discuss how to maintain a safe and pleasant reception-room environment.
- Name appropriate reading materials for the reception room.
- Describe safe and effective ways to incorporate a children's area in the reception room.

Front Desk Reception

Case Study

When Marilyn Peterson enters the medical office for a new patient appointment, the medical assistant greets her and gives her paperwork to complete. In response, Marilyn frowns and says, "I don't want to fill all of that out. I'm only here to see the doctor about a sore throat. I don't have time for paperwork."

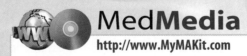

MedMedia

http://www.MyMAKit.com

Additional interactive resources and activities for this chapter can be found on http://www.MyMAKit.com. For a video, tips, audio glossary, legal and ethical scenarios, on-the-job scenarios, quizzes, and games related to the content of this chapter, please access the accompanying CD-ROM in this book.

Video: *Patient Reception*
Legal and Ethical Scenario: *Front Desk Reception*
On the Job Scenario: *Front Desk Reception*
Tips
Multiple Choice Quiz
Audio Glossary
HIPAA Quiz
Games: Spelling Bee, Crossword, and Strikeout

Key Terminology

Americans with Disabilities Act (ADA)—federal law that outlines appropriate treatment or accommodations for patients or employees with disabilities

checklist—list of activities or steps to take to perform a task

copayment—a pre-determined amount of money a patient must pay for each physician's visit

front desk—place in a medical office where the receptionist welcomes patients as they enter

hazard—something that is dangerous or possibly dangerous

HIPAA compliant—in line with federal patient confidentiality laws

office policy—agreed-upon standard for handling a situation or procedure in the office

reception area—waiting area for patients in the medical office

receptionist—medical staff member who greets patients, answers the telephone, and directs office flow

service animal—animal that has been trained to assist a person with a handicap

sign-in sheet—paper or electronic document on which patients sign their names upon entering the office

Abbreviations

ADA—Americans with Disabilities Act

HIPAA—Health Insurance Portability and Accountability Act

✚ MEDICAL ASSISTING STANDARDS

CAAHEP ENTRY-LEVEL STANDARDS	ABHES ENTRY-LEVEL COMPETENCIES
■ Identify styles and types of verbal communication (cognitive) ■ Identify nonverbal communication (cognitive) ■ Recognize communication barriers (cognitive) ■ Identify techniques for overcoming communication barriers (cognitive) ■ Recognize the elements of oral communication using a sender-receiver process (cognitive) ■ Identify resources and adaptations that are required based on individual needs, i.e., culture and environment, developmental life stage, language, and physical threats to communication (cognitive) ■ Identify the role of self boundaries in the health care environment (cognitive) ■ Recognize the role of patient advocacy in the practice of medical assisting (cognitive) ■ Discuss the role of assertiveness in effective professional communication (cognitive) ■ Recognize the role of patient advocacy in the practice of medical assisting (cognitive) ■ Identify time management principles (cognitive) ■ Use reflection, restatement, and clarification techniques to obtain a patient history (psychomotor) ■ Report relevant information to others succinctly and accurately (psychomotor) ■ Explain general office policies (psychomotor) ■ Instruct patients according to their needs to promote health maintenance and disease prevention (psychomotor) ■ Respond to nonverbal communication (psychomotor) ■ Advocate on behalf of patients (psychomotor) ■ Develop and maintain a current list of community resources related to patients' health care needs (psychomotor) ■ Demonstrate empathy in communicating with patients, family, and staff (affective) ■ Apply active listening skills (affective)	■ Adapt to change ■ Maintain confidentiality at all times ■ Project a positive attitude ■ Show a responsible attitude ■ Conduct work within scope of education, training, and ability ■ Instruct patients with special needs ■ Be courteous and diplomatic ■ Serve as a liaison between the physician and others ■ Orient patients to office policies and procedures ■ Adapt what is said to the recipient's level of comprehension ■ Adaptation for individualized needs ■ Exercise efficient time management ■ Receive, organize, prioritize, and transmit information expediently

✚ MEDICAL ASSISTING STANDARDS (CONTINUED)

CAAHEP ENTRY-LEVEL STANDARDS	ABHES ENTRY-LEVEL COMPETENCIES
■ Use appropriate body language and other nonverbal skills in communicating with patients, family, and staff (affective) ■ Demonstrate awareness of the territorial boundaries of the person with whom communicating (affective) ■ Demonstrate sensitivity appropriate to the message being delivered (affective) ■ Demonstrate awareness of how an individual's personal appearance affects anticipated responses (affective) ■ Demonstrate recognition of the patient's level of understanding in communication (affective) ■ Analyze communications in providing appropriate responses/feedback (affective) ■ Recognize and protect personal boundaries in communicating with others (affective) ■ Demonstrate respect for individual diversity, incorporating awareness of one's own biases in areas including gender, race, religion, age, and economic status (affective)	

✓ COMPETENCY SKILLS PERFORMANCE

1. Open the office, following office guidelines and procedures.
2. Greet and register patients.
3. Collect payments at the front desk.
4. Close the office, following office guidelines and procedures.

Introduction

The adage "There is no second chance to make a good first impression" holds as true for the medical office as it does for any other business. In the medical office, the person who answers the telephone, often the medical assistant, plays a substantial role in patients' first impressions. Because poor impressions can prompt patients to seek care in other facilities, the medical assistant who is serving as **receptionist** at the **front desk** must treat all patients with a high level of customer service. That level of service should carry through from the telephone, into the **reception area** when patients arrive, and beyond into the clinical and treatment areas. The visual impressions made by the presentation of the reception area, in conjunction with the appearances and professional manners of the health care staff, greatly impact a patient's first impression of the office.

Characteristics of the Front Desk Receptionist

While people can learn the skills they need to be adequate front-desk receptionists, they must exhibit positive personality traits to excel at the job. When receptionists excel, they can positively impact the medical office's bottom line. Studies have shown that patients will continue to seek treatment with physicians they do not really like just because they feel well cared for by the rest of the health care team. Conversely, many patients will not return to the office when they feel the staff lack caring about their needs (Figure 8-1 ◆).

In short, front desk receptionists should really enjoy interacting with people. Successful front-desk receptionists remember patients' names. Remarkable receptionists remember the names of patients' children or spouses. Superior front-desk receptionists also remain calm, even with the rudest of patients or in the busiest of circumstances. Because receptionists can rarely start and finish their tasks without interruption, they must be open to constantly shifting their focus. The best front-desk receptionists are happy, kind people who genuinely care about patients and who have the utmost faith in the clinical staff and physicians on their health care teams.

— Critical Thinking Question 8-1—

How can the medical assistant demonstrate caring and concern to Marilyn?

Opening the Office

The task of opening and closing the medical office usually falls to the front-desk receptionist. A policy that outlines the steps to opening and closing the office helps train new staff and ensures that other, established staff can follow the proper procedures when serving in a cross-functional capacity. A printed **checklist** helps ensure that all staff follow all necessary steps.

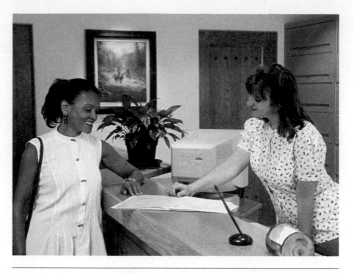

Figure 8-1 ◆ The front desk receptionist must be kind and professional with all patients.

While opening and closing procedures vary from office to office, most offices follow some basic steps. In general, staff should arrive at the office 30 or more minutes before patients are expected to arrive to ensure the facility is ready for business. Scrambling to find supplies or searching for files while patients are in the office is unprofessional and gives the impression that the health care team is unprepared.

Upon entering the office, the receptionist should turn on the lights and disarm the alarm system. Next, he should check the office answering system to identify patients who need visits that day or who have canceled their appointments. Calls should be handled in order of importance.

After making necessary calls, the front-desk receptionist should ensure that the reception room is ready to receive patients. This means making sure the room is tidy and free of litter. When the office provides coffee or water, the receptionist should ensure that related supplies are adequate.

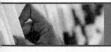

PROCEDURE 8-1 Open the Office

Theory and Rationale
When a medical office documents its standard opening procedures in a list, that list can help ensure that all members of the health care team have the tools to perform those procedures fully, accurately, and consistently.

Materials
■ Checklist of office opening procedures

Competency
(Conditions) With the necessary materials, you will be able to **(Task)** open the medical office **(Standards)** correctly within the time limit set by the instructor.

1. Arrive in the office at least 30 minutes before the first patient appointment.
2. Turn off the office alarm system.
3. Turn on all appropriate lights and equipment.
4. Retrieve messages from the office answering system, and return telephone calls as appropriate.
5. Verify that all patient charts needed for the morning were pulled the night before and that all needed information is attached to those charts.
6. Check the office for safety and cleanliness issues. For example, be sure all garbage cans are empty.
7. When the office is ready, unlock the door for patients to enter.

Preparing Patient Files

Before the office closes for the night, staff should pull all patient files needed for the next morning. Any new patient files should be started, which means inserting all appropriate paperwork. Figure 8-2 ◆ depicts a new patient file folder with various paperwork the patient and healthcare professionals will fill out. The amount and type of paperwork contained within the patient file depends upon the type of practice and the policies regarding necessary forms in that particular facility. Figure 8-3 ◆ is an example of a new patient history form. These forms may be purchased from a variety of medical office supply retailers, though many medical facilities create their own. Figure 8-4 ◆ shows an example of a HIPAA authorization agreement. This form is necessary in any medical setting where private patient information will be gathered and kept on file.

HIPAA Compliance

There are some patients who will refuse to sign the HIPAA authorization agreement form in the medical office. This is an infrequent event. When this happens, the medical assistant should simply write "refused to sign" where the patient's signature is indicated, along with the date. The fact that the patient has refused to sign the form should be brought to the physician's attention and the form, with the medical assistant's notation, should be filed in the patient's medical record.

Before patients arrive, the receptionist must verify that all patient files have all necessary paperwork, such as laboratory results reports (outlining the findings of a patient's blood tests, urine tests, or analysis of secretions taken from the patient) and pathology reports (a report outlining the findings of

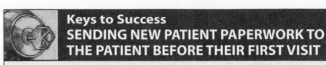

Keys to Success
SENDING NEW PATIENT PAPERWORK TO THE PATIENT BEFORE THEIR FIRST VISIT

When patients' first visits are scheduled at least a week after those patients call to schedule, administrative medical assistants may mail those patients new patient history forms to complete before arriving at the office. This system has one potential drawback, however: Patients may forget to bring their paperwork to their first visit.

any gross or microscopic tissue examination). When the billing office asks to see patients about their accounts, notes should be placed on the patients' files so those patients can be routed to the billing office before seeing the physician. To ensure patient confidentiality, all patient files must be kept out of sight of nonessential staff and other patients.

—Critical Thinking Question 8-2—
Thinking back to the case study at the beginning of the chapter, how can the medical assistant argue to the physician or office manager that sending new patient history forms before patients' first visits will in fact benefit the office?

Greeting and Registering Patients

The front-desk receptionist is the host or hostess of the medical office. As such, the receptionist should welcome all patients upon arrival, even when busy with other tasks. If, for example,

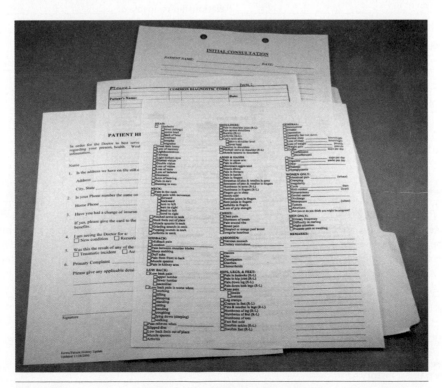

Figure 8-2 ◆ A new patient medical record with various forms.

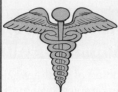

Victory Medical Center

4100 SW Highway 6
Victorville, WA 12345
(509) 555-9832

Patient Name: _____
　　　　　　　　Last Name　　　　　　　　　First Name　　　　　　　　Middle Initial

Address: _____
　　　　　　Street　　　　　　　　City　　　　　　　State　　　　　　Zip

Home Phone: _____ Work Phone: _____

Mobile Phone: _____ Birthdate: _____

Social Security Number: _____ Age: _____

Sex: _____ Marital Status: S M D W Children: _____

How do you prefer to be addressed? _____

Spouse's Name: _____

Primary Care Physician: _____ Phone No.: _____

Name of Person Responsible for Bill: _____

Relationship to Patient: _____ Phone No.: _____

Address of Person Responsible for Bill: _____

Patient's Employer: _____ Phone No.: _____

Occupation: _____

Spouse's Employer: _____ Phone No.: _____

Occupation: _____

INSURANCE INFORMATION

Primary Insurance: _____ Policy No.: _____

Name of Policyholder: _____ Birthdate: _____

SS#: _____ Relationship to Insured: _____

Secondary Insurance: _____ Policy No.: _____

Name of Policyholder: _____ Birthdate: _____

If Injured: Date: _____ Place: _____

Claim Number: _____ Nature or Cause of Injury: _____

Employer at Time of Injury: _____ Phone No.: _____

EMERGENCY INFORMATION

In case of emergency, local friend or relative to be notified (not living at same address)

Name: _____ Relationship to Patient: _____

Address: _____ Phone No.: _____

I hereby authorize the health care professionals in this clinic to diagnose and treat my condition. I clearly understand and agree that all services rendered me are charged directly to me and that I am personally responsible for payment. I agree that I am responsible for all bills incurred at this clinic. I hereby authorize assignment of my insurance rights and benefits directly to the provider for services rendered. I also authorize the health care professionals to discuss my care with other health care providers who I am currently treating with.

_____　　_____

Patient's Signature　　　　　　Date　　　　Parent or Guardian Signature　　　　　Date

---

Figure 8-3 ◆ Sample new patient history form.

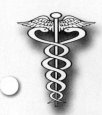

Martin Country Medical Clinic
2413 NW Greenlake Ave.
Westford, CA 12745

AUTHORIZATION TO RELEASE INFORMATION

ACKNOWLEDGMENT OF RECEIPT of the Notice of Privacy Practices of the Martin County Medical Clinic (MCMC)

I acknowledge that I have received or been offered the Notice of Privacy Practices of the Martin County Medical Clinic. I understand that the Notice describes the uses and disclosures of my protected health information by the Covered Entities and informs me of my rights with respect to my protected health information.

_____
Name of Patient

_____
Patient Date of Birth

_____
Signature of Patient or Personal Representative

_____
Printed Name of Patient or Personal Representative

_____
Date

If Personal Representative, indicate relationship:

_____

Declinations

_____ The Individual declined to accept a copy of the Notice of Privacy Practices.

_____ The Individual received a copy of the Notice of Privacy Practices but declined to sign an Acknowledgment of Receipt.

_____
Signature of MCMC Healthcare Representative

_____
Name of MCMC HealthCare Representative

Figure 8-4 ◆ Sample HIPAA authorization form.

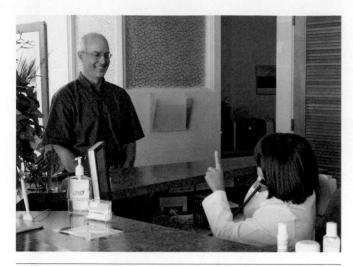

Figure 8-5 ◆ If the receptionist is on the telephone when a patient comes in, she should look up and make eye contact with the patient immediately.

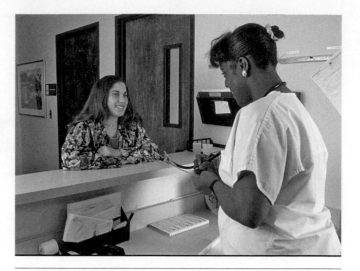

Figure 8-7 ◆ The receptionist must maintain patient confidentiality at the front desk by keeping her voice low.

the receptionist is on the telephone when a patient arrives, the receptionist should look up and smile at the patient and hold up an index finger to indicate a slight delay in service (Figure 8-5 ◆).

Years ago, a window separated the receptionist's desk and the reception room to keep conversations behind the front desk private. Today, most medical offices have adopted a friendlier, more open system in the reception room (Figure 8-6 ◆). Now when medical assistants must have private conversations with patients, they must either lower their voices or move the patients to private areas of the office. In modern times, the window is seen as a barrier to effective customer service.

As part of greeting new patients, medical assistants should orient patients to the office with such information as the locations of the rest room and coat rack and where to find reading

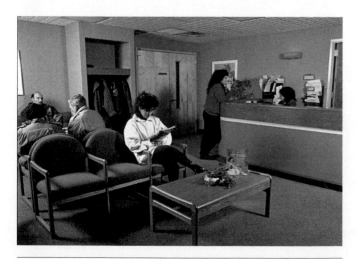

Figure 8-6 ◆ Many reception rooms in medical offices today have adopted a friendlier, more open system.

materials. When greeting established patients, assistants should confirm that all information on file (e.g., address, telephone number, and insurance carrier) remains the same as the last visit. When patients' insurance information has changed, the medical assistant should photocopy both sides of new insurance cards.

Patient confidentiality at the front desk is essential to the medical office. Whenever the medical assistant must discuss confidential health or financial information with a patient, all exchanges must occur out of the hearing range of other patients (Figure 8-7 ◆).

Using Sign-in Sheets Effectively

Some medical offices require patients to sign in upon arrival. Before the Health Insurance Portability and Accountability Act (**HIPAA**) was enacted, **sign-in sheets** were typically sheets of paper that patients signed when entering the office. Such sheets alerted the medical assistant to a patient's arrival and served as proof of the patient's visit. Today, any office sign-in sheets must be **HIPAA compliant**, which means that a patient's signature must be invisible to the next patient who signs the sheet. Offices often use separate sheets for physicians, although this is not a legal requirement.

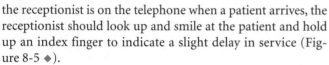

HIPAA Compliance

Simply covering a sign-in sheet or blacking out patients' names after check-in fails to meet HIPAA standards, because signatures can still easily be viewed. Several other sign-in methods, however, are HIPAA compliant. One convenient method stores patient signatures electronically, much like department stores do (Figure 8-8 ◆). Another method keeps individual sign-in sheets in patients' files.

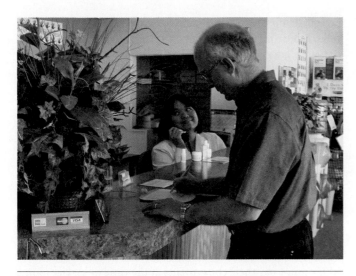

Figure 8-8 ◆ A patient signs an electronic sign-in sheet.

Administering Patient Paperwork

When patients arrive at the office, the medical assistant must give them any necessary forms to complete and identify any important landmarks, such as where signatures are needed. At this time, the assistant should also copy new patients' identification and insurance cards.

The patient registration form (Figure 8-3) is one of the medical office's most important forms, because it contains all information needed to bill for patient care. To ensure billing processes remain up to date, this form should be verified at every visit but no more than once every month. When working with patient paperwork, medical assistants must keep all information confidential. For example, assistants should only ask patients to verify their birth dates or addresses when other patients cannot overhear. Similarly, the reasons for patients' visits should only be disclosed when other patients cannot overhear.

Sometimes, patients will refuse to disclose certain information. Patients most commonly balk at providing their Social Security numbers and birth dates, often because they fear identity theft. When medical assistants encounter patients like these, they should gently remind the patients that all information in medical files is confidential and is only released with the patients' written consent or a court order. When these facts fail to persuade a patient, the medical assistant should note on the

PROCEDURE 8-2 Greet and Register Patients

Theory and Rationale

As patients enter the medical office, each needs to be greeted by the administrative medical assistant and then registered according to their needs.

Materials
■ Patient history form
■ Pen
■ Clipboard

Competency

(**Conditions**) With the necessary materials, you will be able to (**Task**) greet and register patients (**Standards**) correctly within the time limit set by the instructor.

1. As the patient arrives at the front desk, look up and make eye contact right away. If you are on the telephone, make a motion to the patient with your index finger to indicate you will be with the patient in one moment. If you are not on the telephone, smile and ask the patient for his or her name.
2. Once you have obtained the patient's name, check the appointment schedule to verify the patient is there at the right time and to verify the type of appointment the patient is scheduled to have.
3. If the patient is new to the office, give him or her the appropriate new patient forms to fill out on a clipboard, along with a pen.
4. Ask the patient to take a seat in the reception area and provide the patient with an approximate amount of time he or she can expect to wait before being taken back to see the provider.
5. Alert the clinical medical assistant to the patient's arrival.

**Keys to Success
OBTAINING BIRTHDATES
FROM PATIENTS**

Because insurance carriers use birth dates to help identify their members, they will not process claims when that information is missing. When patients refuse to disclose their birth dates, they may have to forego insurance coverage and self-fund their charges.

patient's chart the information that was refused and give the chart to the clinical staff. Ultimately, the physician must decide whether to accept the patient for treatment.

Notifying Patients of Delays

Once a patient has completed all necessary paperwork, the medical assistant must notify the clinical staff of that patient's arrival. Delays happen in the medical office regularly, often due to unforeseen circumstances with emergencies or competing priorities. When delays occur, it is important for the assistant to keep patients apprised. Such consideration demonstrates sound customer service, because it lets patients know that the medical assistant and the physician value patients' time.

Some offices use electronic signs at the front desk to broadcast physicians' schedules, but such signs are only as good as the staff updating them. Therefore, whenever electronic signs are used, the medical assistant must ensure they accurately depict wait times. Whatever system is used, when delays start to

exceed 20 minutes the medical assistant should try to reach patients before they arrive at the office and suggest that they visit the office later or even reschedule.

Collecting Payments at the Front Desk

Part of greeting patients at the front desk includes collecting patients' **copayments** as those patients register. Most offices have signs at their front desks that state, "Copayments are due at the time of service." Patient files should clearly list any copays that are expected. For patients' convenience, the medical office should accept multiple forms of payment (e.g., cash, personal check, credit/debit card). To ensure payments are somehow procured, offices should have policies for addressing patients who cannot pay their copayments at the time of service. Some offices allow patients to mail their copayments or to discuss payment with the billing office.

To track fees, most offices use preprinted fee slips, also called encounter forms or superbills. Fee slips follow patients through the office. The physician and/or clinical medical assistant circles the services or procedures that were performed, as well as any diagnoses the physician assigns to the patient (Figure 8-9 ◆). While medical office supply companies sell standard fee slips, many medical offices customize fee slips to include the diagnoses and procedures they commonly use. Because procedural and diagnosis codes change every year, fee slips should be reviewed for accuracy annually and reprinted as needed.

Typically, the medical assistant who is working at the front desk when the patient arrives prepares the patient's fee

---

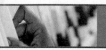

PROCEDURE 8-3 Collect Payments at the Front Desk

Theory and Rationale
Most medical insurance plans today require the patient to pay an out-of-pocket amount at the time of each visit. This payment, known as a co-pay, should be collected from the patient upon arrival in the medical office.

Materials
- Pen
- Cash receipt book
- Credit card machine
- Check endorsement stamp

Competency
(**Conditions**) With the necessary materials, you will be able to (**Task**) collect payments at the front desk (**Standards**) correctly within the time limit set by the instructor.

1. As the patient arrives at the front desk, check the computer or chart to verify the patient's co-payment amount.
2. After registering the patient, let the patient know the amount of the expected payment.
3. Ask the patient if he or she would prefer to make the payment via cash, check, or credit card.
4. If the patient pays via cash, write a receipt from the cash receipt book.
5. If the patient pays via check, endorse the check with the bank endorsement stamp. Ask the patient if he or she would like a written receipt. If so, write a receipt from the cash receipt book.
6. If the patient pays via credit card, process the card on the credit card machine, have the patient sign the slip, and provide the patient with their portion as a receipt.

UROLOGIC GYNECOLOGY
GENERAL GYNECOLOGY
OBSTETRICS

WINDY CITY CLINIC
Beth Williams, M.D.
123 Michigan Avenue, Chicago, IL 60610
(312) 123-1234

ID.# 20-1342846
No. 4815

PATIENT INFORMATION

PATIENT'S LAST NAME		FIRST		INITIAL	BIRTHDATE		SEX ☐ MALE ☐ FEMALE		TODAY'S DATE / /
ADDRESS	CITY	STATE	ZIP		RELATION TO SUBSCRIBER		REFERRING PHYSICIAN		
SUBSCRIBER or POLICY HOLDER					INSURANCE				
ADDRESS	CITY	STATE	ZIP		INSURANCE ID.#		COVERAGE CODE		GROUP

OTHER HEALTH COVERAGE?
☐ NO
☐ YES   IDENTIFY

DISABILITY RELATED TO:
☐ ACCIDENT   ☐ PREGNANCY
☐ INDEPENDENT   ☐ OTHER

DATE SYMPTOMS APPEARED, INCEPTION OF PREGNANCY, OR ACCIDENT OCCURED: / /

ASSIGNMENT and RELEASE: *I hereby assign my insurance benefits to be paid directly to the undersigned physician. I am financially responsible for noncovered services. I also authorize the physician to release any information required to process this claim.*

SIGNATURE OF PATIENT (or Parent, if Minor) _____ DATE / /

PROCEDURES	CPT-Mod	AMOUNT	PROCEDURES	CPT-Mod	AMOUNT	PROCEDURES	CPT-Mod	AMOUNT
A. OFFICE VISITS			31 Post-Partum	59430		60 PG Test, Urine	86006	
1 New GYN, Limited	90010		**F. GYN PROCEDURES**			61 Antigen Test	86006	
2 New GYN, Intermediate	90015		32 Irrigation of Vagina	57150*		62 Cytopathology Smear	88155	
3 New GYN, Extensive	90017		33 Insert Pessary	57160*		63 Specimen Handling	99000	
4 New GYN, Comprehensive	90020		34 Pessary Supplies	99070		**I. MISCELLANEOUS**		
5 Return GYN, Minimal	90030		35 Colposcopy	57452		64 Surgical Tray	99070	
6 Return GYN, Brief	90040		36 Biopsy, Cervix	57500		65 Therapeutic Injection	90782	
7 Return GYN, Limited	90050		37 Biopsy, Vagina	57100		66 Injection, Kenalog	J1870	
8 Return GYN, Intermediate	90060		38 Biopsy, Vulva	56600		67 Injection, Xylocaine	J3480	
9 Return GYN, Extended	90070		39 Biopsy, Endometrium	58100		68 Injection, Estrogen	J2655	
10 Return GYN, Comprehensive	90080		40 Biopsy, Skin			69 Injection, Progesterone	J2675	
11 Return GYN, Post-Operative	99024		0.5 cm.	11420		70 Injection, Vitamin B12	P4320	
B. CONSULTATION			0.6 to 1.0 cm.	11421		71 Special Reports	99080	
12 GYN Consultation, Limited	90600		1.1 to 2.0 cm.	11423				
13 GYN Consultation, Intermed.	90605		41 Cryotherapy, Cervix	57511				
14 GYN Consultation, Compreh.	90620		42 Destruct. Condyloma	56501				
15 GYN Consultation, Complex	90630		43 Diaphragm Fitting	57170				
16 Second Opinion Surgery	90653		44 Diaphragm Supplies	99070				
C. TELEPHONE CONSULTATION			45 IUD Insertion	58300				
17 Telephone Consult., Simple	99013		46 IUD Supplies	99070				
18 Telephone Consult., Intermed.	99014		47 IUD Removal	58301				
19 Telephone Consult., Compreh.	99015		**G. UROLOGIC PROCEDURES**					
D. SPECIAL SERVICES			48 Urethral Dilation	53660				
20 ER Service after Office Hrs.	99064		49 Urethral Dilation, Repeat	53661				
21 ER Service during Office Hrs.	99065		50 Bladder Instillation	51700				
22 Night Call before 10 pm	99050		51 Periurethral Injection	53665				
23 Night Call after 10 pm	99052		52 Simple Catheterization	53670				
24 Sunday or Holiday Service	99054		53 Manual Electric Stimulation	97118				
25 Office Non-Schedule	99058		**H. LAB**					
E. OB CARE			54 Urine Analysis	81000				
26 Prenatal Dx, Consultation	90620		55 Urine Culture	87068				
27 Initial OB, NOrmal	59400		56 Hematocrit	85015				
28 Initial OB, High Risk	59400.22		57 Hemogram	85021		**TODAY'S TOTAL FEE**	$	
29 Return OB, Normal	59420		58 Commercial-Lat.	87087				
30 Return OB, High Risk	59420.22		59 Wet Mount	87210				

DIAGNOSIS	CODE	DIAGNOSIS	CODE	DIAGNOSIS	CODE	DIAGNOSIS	CODE
Abortion:		Breasts	216.5	Galactorrhea	676.6	Pregnancy Postpartum	V24.2
Threatened	640.0	Vulva	221.2	Hemorrhoids	455.0	Rectocele	618.0
Incomplete	637.1	Breast Disorder (Mass)	611.72	Hypertension	401	Retention of Urine	788.2
Habitual	646.3	Bronchitis	491	Incontinence of Urine	788.3	Stress Incontinence	625.6
Abnormal Urination	788.6	Carcinoma In Situ:		Interstitial Cystitis	595.1	Urethral Stricture	598
Abnormal PAP Smear	795.0	Cervix	233.1	Irritable Colon	564.1	Urethral Syndrome	597.81
Adenomyosis	617.0	Uterus	233.2	Irregular Menstrual Cycle	626.4	Uterine Leiomyoma	218
Adnexal MAss	625.8	Female Genital Organs	233.3	Malignant Neoplasm:		Uterine Prolapse:	
Amenorrhera	626.0	Cervical Dysplasia	622.1	Cervix	180.9	Incomplete	618.2
Anemia	285.9	Cervicitis	616.0	Uterus	182.0	Complete	618.3
Arthritis	716.9	Contraceptive Management	V25.0	Ovary	183.0	Vaginal Discharge-Non Specific	623.5
Artificial Menopause	627.4	Cystocele	618.0	Vagina	184.0	Vaginal Enterocele	618.6
Asthma-Hayfever	493.0	Cystourethritis	595.0	Vulva	184.4	Vaginal Prolapse	618.0
Atrophic Vaginitis	627.3	Diabetes Melliuts	250.0	Menopausal Syndrome	627.2	Vaginal Vault Prolapse Post	
Bartholin Abscess	616.3	Thyroid Disorder	246.9	Menometrorrhagia	626.2	Hysterectomy	618.5
Benign Neoplasm:		Dysmenorrhea	625.3	Oligomenorrhea	626.1	Vulvovaginitis:	
Cervix	219.0	Dyspareunia	625.0	Obesity	278.0	Non Specific	616.1
Uterus	219.1	Dysuria	788.1	Ovarian Cyst	620.2	Candida	112.1
Ovary	220	Ectopic Pregnancy	617.0	Pelvic Inflammatory Disease	614.9	Trichomonas	131.01
Vagina	221.1	Endometriosis	617.9	Pelvic Peritoneal Adhesions	614.6		
Vulva	221.2	Enuresis-Unstable Bladder	788.3	Polycystic Ovaries	256.4		
Benign Neoplasm of Skin:		Frequency of Urination	788.4	Postmenopausal Bleeding	627.1		
Buttocks	216.5	Functional Disorder:		Post-Op Wound Infection	998.5		
Abdomen	216.5	Bladder Instability	596.5	Pregnancy Prenatal	V22		

MISCELLANEOUS DIAGNOSIS

DOCTOR'S SIGNATURE _____ DATE / /

SERVICES PERFORMED AT: ☐ Office ☐ Emergency Room
☐ **WINDY CITY CLINIC**
123 Michigan Avenue, Chicago, IL 60610
(312) 123-1234
☐ Hospital Calls at $_____ per Visit

ADMITTED / /
DISCHARGED / /

RETURN VISIT INFORMATION
15 • 30 • 45 • 60
____ DAYS ____ WEEKS ____ MONTHS ☐ WILL CALL
Procedure: _____

ACCEPT ASSIGNMENT
☐ YES
☐ NO

INSTRUCTIONS TO PATIENT FOR FILING INSURANCE CLAIMS

1. Complete patient information portion of this form.
2. Sign and date.
3. Mail this form directly to your insurance company with your own insurance company's form.
4. Patients with health care insurance please remember:
   A. Professional services are charged to the patient, and not to the insurance company.
   B. Insured patients are expected to take care of their fees as services are rendered.
   C. This office cannot accept responsibility for collecting your insurance claim or for negotiating a settlement on a disputed claim.
   D. You are responsible for payment of your account.

TODAY'S FEE	$
OLD BALANCE	$
ADJUSTMENTS	$
TOTAL DUE	$
AMOUNT RECEIVED TODAY	$
☐ CASH ☐ CHECK ☐ C.C.	
NEW BALANCE	$

Figure 8-9 ◆ Sample medical office fee slip.

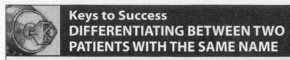

Keys to Success
DIFFERENTIATING BETWEEN TWO PATIENTS WITH THE SAME NAME

Because patients may sometimes have the same first and last names, medical assistants must verify files for all patients. Patient birth date is one way to differentiate files.

slip for that date of service. The medical assistant attaches the slip to the patient's file and routes the file to the clinical medical assistant.

Escorting Patients

Almost always, a medical assistant or clinical medical assistant should escort patients to the examination room after verifying the patients' identities. To do this, the assistant should open the door to the reception area and call out a patient's first name. When more than one patient stands, the assistant should then call out the patient's last name. Once in the back office area, the assistant should confirm the patient's birth date using the patient's file.

Managing Difficult Patients in the Reception Area

As the hub of the reception area, the front desk is on display for the rest of the office. Occasionally, the front-desk receptionist must manage difficult patients in the reception area. Many difficulties can be avoided by keeping patients apprised of expected delay times. Medical assistants who remain calm and professional are best equipped to function in and defuse patient interactions.

When the medical assistant encounters a difficult patient in the reception area, the first goal is to remove the patient from the area. Patients who are out of the sight and hearing ranges of other patients tend to have less leverage. Once an angry patient is in another location, the medical assistant should work to address the patient's issue or find someone who can.

? — Critical Thinking Question 8-3—
How should the medical assistant respond to Marilyn? What is appropriate for facial expression and tone of voice?

Keeping Only Appropriate Patients in the Reception Area

In general, patients visit their physicians when they are ill. Depending on the type of practice, medical assistants may help support patients with contagious diseases or life-threatening conditions. As a rule, any patients with contagious conditions

should not be left in the reception room. This includes children suspected of having chicken pox and anyone with a high fever (Figure 8-10 ◆).

Any patient who is exhibiting signs of a condition that may make other patients in the reception room uncomfortable should also be moved. This includes patients who are coughing continuously, are bleeding or visibly ill, or have conditions that may cause other patients to stare. Moving these patients out of the reception room addresses those patients' comfort, as well as the comfort of the other patients. Any emergency patient must be brought back to see the physician right away.

Maintaining the Reception Room

The reception room should be quiet and peaceful. Patients who are waiting for appointments should be able to sit calmly, undisturbed by loud noises and other distractions. In addition to being quiet, the reception room must be kept clean and free of **hazards.** To attain this goal, medical assistants must check the reception room throughout the day to remove any garbage and retrieve any lost or forgotten items. To keep control of the room, the assistant must do things like ask children to be quiet and instruct patients to take food outside. Many offices play relaxing music in the reception area.

Providing Adequate Seating and Decoration

To ensure patient comfort, the reception room should have an adequate amount of comfortable, easy-to-clean furniture. Experts in medical office space planning believe medical offices should have enough seating to accommodate at least 1 hour's worth of patients per physician, as well as the friends or relatives who accompany those patients. The furniture should be at a level from which most patients can rise easily and without assistance. Many offices have coat racks for patients' coats or umbrellas.

Practice type dictates the reception room's décor. A pediatric practice has a very different reception room than a women's health care practice, for example. A pediatric practice

---

- ■ A patient who is bleeding
- ■ A patient who is visibly ill
- ■ A patient who has broken out in a contagious rash, such as chicken pox
- ■ A patient who states they feel they may vomit
- ■ A patient who is complaining of shortness of breath
- ■ A patient who is complaining of chest pain
- ■ A patient who states he is feeling very dizzy or lightheaded

Figure 8-10 ◆ Examples of patients who should not be kept waiting in the reception area.

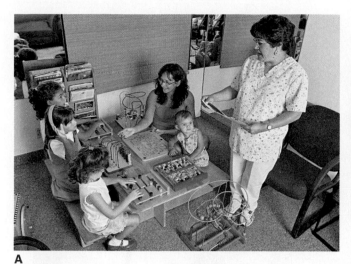

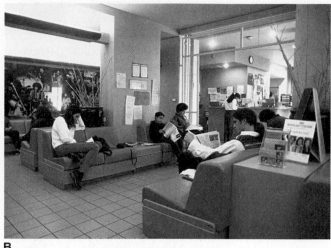

A

B

Figure 8-11 ◆ (a) A pediatric reception room will typically have child-size furniture and toys; (b) a family practice reception room will cater to patients of all ages.

should have videos and toys, whereas a practice that caters to geriatric patients might have a fish tank or other soothing decorations (Figure 8-11 ◆).

Choosing Reading Material for the Reception Room

Like décor, reading material in the reception area is dictated by practice type. Reading material that is current and tailored to office clientele is a nice customer service touch. For example, a practice that specializes in prostate problems might have magazines about fishing, hunting, or sports activities, while a practice that specializes in women's breast surgery might have magazines about women's fashion (Figure 8-12 ◆).

Managing Children in the Reception Room

Pediatric offices or family practices often have reception areas geared toward children. In offices where children are not the primary patient population, reception areas may have small areas devoted to children. All child-geared areas should have toys and books and other items of interest to children. In all cases, child-geared reception areas and materials must be safe and clean. For example, any toys must be checked regularly to confirm they are safe and in good working order. Young children may place small items, including toys, in their mouths. Most states have laws that dictate how to clean toys for public settings. In Washington State, for example, the law dictates that toys must be cleaned with a 10 percent bleach solution after every use.

At no time, including when parents see physicians, should children be left unattended in the reception room. Medical assistants who allow children to be unattended give unspoken consent and assume responsibility for those children on behalf of the office. To ensure safety, children must remain with their parents throughout the parents' office visits. To be

proactive, medical assistants might speak with parents before scheduling those parents' next appointments. To underscore the message, an office might post a sign in the reception area that states, "Children May Not Be Left Unattended in the Reception Area."

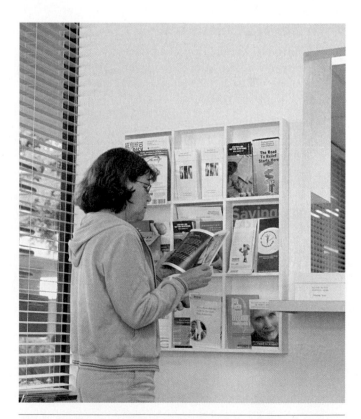

Figure 8-12 ◆ Having educational materials available to the patients in the reception area is very common.

The small physician's office where Jenny works as a front-desk medical assistant is on the first floor of a building where cars are parked outside the door. When Marion Wilson arrives for her appointment, she approaches the front desk and tells Jenny that she is going to leave her 2-year-old son sleeping in his car seat because Jenny can see the car from her desk. How should Jenny respond to Marion? What are some appropriate suggestions?

Accommodating Patients with Disabilities

The **Americans with Disabilities Act (ADA)** stipulates that patients with disabilities must be able to access all public buildings, including medical facilities. Medical offices must therefore be able to accommodate people who are in wheelchairs or otherwise unable to use stairs. Ramps and elevators can render medical offices accessible.

Any entrance door must be at least 36 inches wide to accommodate a wheelchair. Any interior door, such as to a restroom or treatment room, must also be accessible by wheelchair. Any carpeting in the facility must be no more than ½ in. high, because wheelchair users find deeper carpeting difficult to navigate. In addition, all restrooms must be clearly marked and all doorknobs operational with a closed fist.

Serving Patients with Service Animals

Service animals, usually easy identifiable by their collars or harnesses, must accompany their owners throughout those owners' office visits. Service animals of all kinds assist their owners by doing such things as:

■ Pulling wheelchairs
■ Carrying or picking up items
■ Alerting to hazards

While dogs serve as service animals most often, some patients enlist cats, monkeys, or even ferrets in this role (Figure 8-13 ◆).

Caring for Patients as They Leave the Office

In most medical offices, patients pass the reception desk as they exit. Offices are designed this way to ensure that patients complete any final activities, such as scheduling followup appointments. In some large offices, staff in the back office may

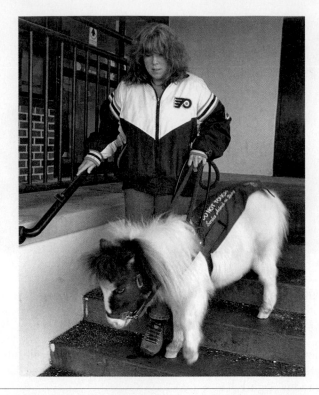

Figure 8-13 ◆ A woman is guided down a flight of stairs by her seeing eye miniature horse.

schedule followup appointments. In small offices, the front-desk receptionist makes such appointments. In all cases, exiting patients should be instructed to give the receptionist their super bills or fee slips. On these forms, the physicians should have noted any followup appointments they would like scheduled. Only with this information in hand should the front-desk receptionist schedule the followup appointment. In some offices, the fee slip is kept with the patient's chart to go to billing, rather than carried to the front desk by the patient.

The receptionist should bid goodbye to all patients exiting the office, even those who need no follow up. This small act not only reinforces that the office staff care about their patients, it promotes a friendly, warm environment.

Closing the Office

To ensure the medical office is closed consistently, properly, and comprehensively, offices should document their desired procedures in **office policies**. Any member of the health care team who is charged with closing the office should complete such tasks as pulling charts for patients scheduled for the following morning, transferring telephone lines to the office answering system, turning off all machinery and lights, locking the doors, and enabling the office alarm system.

PROCEDURE 8-4 Close the Office

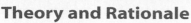

Theory and Rationale

Medical assistants are often tasked with closing the medical office. Just as it supports the office-opening procedure, a checklist helps ensure that medical staff complete this procedure correctly.

Materials

■ Checklist of office closing procedures

Competency

(**Conditions**) With the necessary materials, you will be able to (**Task**) close the medical office (**Standards**) correctly within the time limit set by the instructor.

1. Ensure all patients have exited the office. Check treatment rooms and restrooms.

2. Verify that all the day's patient files have been routed to the appropriate area (e.g., billing, physician, clinical medical assistant).
3. Pull all files for patients scheduled for the following morning.
4. Confirm that all information needed for the morning's patients (e.g., lab reports or consultations) is available.
5. Attach needed information to patient files.
6. Call to confirm any patient appointments made prior to 3 days ago.
7. Forward the telephones over to the answering system.
8. Turn off all appropriate equipment and lights.
9. Activate the alarm and lock the doors when leaving the building.

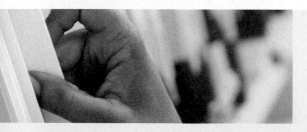

REVIEW

Chapter Summary

■ Office policies are invaluable tools for ensuring medical offices are closed and opened properly by all members of the health care team.
■ When patients arrive, office staff should be prepared with all necessary information and paperwork.
■ Both new and established patients deserve the highest level of customer service from the medical office.
■ It is paramount that the entire health care team safeguard patient confidentiality at the front desk and throughout the medical office.
■ Medical assistants should learn to professionally persuade patients to provide necessary information and to handle unavoidable delays in nondisruptive ways.

■ When patients are difficult, medical assistants must strive to remain calm and diffuse the situation.
■ Medical assistants should ensure that the reception area is used only for patients who may be left alone and is always in a condition that is appropriate both for the patients and the overall image and goals of the office.
■ When patients have special needs, medical assistants should strive to provide them appropriate care.
■ It is particularly important that children and other unique populations receive the care and attention that is appropriate for their needs.

Chapter Review

Multiple Choice

1. Staff members should arrive in the office _____ minutes before the first patient appointment.
   a. 10
   b. 15
   c. 30
   d. 40

2. Which of the following patients should not be left alone in the reception room?
   a. Child with symptoms of chicken pox
   b. Adult with HIV
   c. Patient with eczema
   d. Patient with a sight impairment

Chapter Review (continued)

3. When a physician is running 30 minutes behind schedule, the medical assistant should:
   a. Notify patients of the delay as they enter the office
   b. Avoid eye contact with patients in the waiting area
   c. Ask a clinical medical assistant to notify the patients in the reception area
   d. All of the above

True/False

T F 1. Studies have shown that patients will stay with physicians they do not really like when they feel the rest of the staff care about their needs.

T F 2. A window between the reception room and the receptionist's desk is the best way to keep patients from overhearing the receptionist's conversations.

T F 3. Copayments should never be collected at the front desk.

T F 4. An electric sign that relays the physician's scheduling delays precludes staff from having to communicate those delays verbally.

T F 5. HIPAA prevents staff from calling patients' names in the reception room.

T F 6. When patients refuse to disclose all necessary information, medical assistants should ask them to leave.

T F 7. Patients who are bleeding visibly should not be left in the reception room.

T F 8. Reading materials in the reception room should be geared toward the type of patients receiving services.

T F 9. Educational materials that are specific to the type of practice make good reading materials for the reception room.

Short Answer

1. Describe how, while on the telephone, the front-desk receptionist should greet patients entering the office.

2. Explain how to render a sign-in sheet HIPAA compliant.

3. Why is it important to notify patients of any delays in the office?

4. What does it mean to escort a patient?

5. Why may patients become irritable in the reception room?

6. What is the best way to handle a loud, angry patient in the reception room?

7. Why is it important regularly to inspect children's toys in the reception room?

8. Why is it important to have a policy that states no children may be left unattended in the reception room?

Research

1. What classes could you take at your local community college that would help you to communicate better with patients at the front desk?

2. What are the laws in your state that pertain to how often toys in the office must be cleaned?

3. Interview someone who works in a medical office. Ask the person how their reception staff deal with difficult patients.

Externship Application Experience

When Mrs. Rundholz calls to make an appointment for a complete physical examination, she says she can make the appointment but will not have child care for her 2-year-old and 6-month-old children. She asks if she can bring her children to her hour-long appointment. How should the medical assistant respond to Mrs. Rundholz? What are some appropriate suggestions?

Resource Guide

The Americans with Disabilities Act (ADA) Homepage
www.ada.gov

Microsoft Office Online
Work Essentials
http://office.microsoft.com/en-us/workessentials/

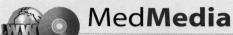

Med**Media**

http://www.MyMAKit.com

More on this chapter, including interactive resources, can be found on the Student CD-ROM accompanying this textbook and on http://www.MyMAKit.com.

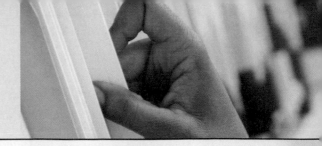

CHAPTER 9

Patient Scheduling

Case Study

When Glenn Jenson calls the office to set up an appointment, he says he has never been in to see the physician before. When the medical assistant asks him why he must see the physician, he responds, "I'd rather not go into that with you. I'll tell the doctor when I see her."

Objectives

After completing this chapter, you should be able to:

- Define and spell the key terminology in this chapter.
- Create guidelines for scheduling patient appointments.
- Differentiate between paper and electronic scheduling systems.
- Chart patient no-shows accurately.
- Follow up on patients who miss their appointments.
- Manage the physician's appointment calendar for professional travel.
- Schedule patients for hospital services and admissions.
- Arrange for language interpreters for non–English-speaking patients.
- Arrange for patient transportation.

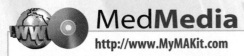

MedMedia
http://www.MyMAKit.com

Additional interactive resources and activities for this chapter can be found on http://www.MyMAKit.com. For a video, tips, audio glossary, legal and ethical scenarios, on-the-job scenarios, quizzes, and games related to the content of this chapter, please access the accompanying CD-ROM in this book.

Video: *Scheduling Patients*
Legal and Ethical Scenario: *Patient Scheduling*
On the Job Scenario: *Patient Scheduling*
Tips
Multiple Choice Quiz
Audio Glossary
HIPAA Quiz
Games: Spelling Bee, Crossword, and Strikeout

✚ MEDICAL ASSISTING STANDARDS

CAAHEP ENTRY-LEVEL STANDARDS	ABHES ENTRY-LEVEL COMPETENCIES
■ Identify styles and types of verbal communication (cognitive) ■ Identify nonverbal communication (cognitive) ■ Recognize communication barriers (cognitive) ■ Identify techniques for overcoming communication barriers (cognitive) ■ Recognize the elements of oral communication using a sender-receiver process (cognitive) ■ Identify resources and adaptations that are required based on individual needs, i.e., culture and environment, developmental life stage, language, and physical threats to communication (cognitive) ■ Discuss pros and cons of various types of appointment management systems (cognitive) ■ Describe scheduling guidelines (cognitive) ■ Recognize office policies and protocols for handling appointments (cognitive) ■ Identify critical information required for scheduling patient admissions and/or procedures (cognitive) ■ Identify time management principles (cognitive) ■ Use reflection, restatement, and clarification techniques to obtain a patient history (psychomotor) ■ Report relevant information to others succinctly and accurately (psychomotor) ■ Explain general office policies (psychomotor) ■ Instruct patients according to their needs to promote health maintenance and disease prevention (psychomotor) ■ Respond to nonverbal communication (psychomotor) ■ Advocate on behalf of patients (psychomotor) ■ Management appointment schedule, using established priorities (psychomotor) ■ Schedule patient admissions and/or procedures (psychomotor) ■ Use office hardware and software to maintain office systems (psychomotor) ■ Implement time management principles to maintain effective office function (affective)	■ Adapt to change ■ Maintain confidentiality at all times ■ Project a positive attitude ■ Be cognizant of ethical boundaries ■ Show a responsible attitude ■ Orient patients to office policies and procedures ■ Adapt what is said to the recipient's level of comprehension ■ Instruct patients with special needs ■ Manage physician's professional schedule and travel ■ Use proper telephone technique ■ Application of electronic technology ■ Schedule and monitor appointments ■ Apply computer concepts for office procedures ■ Be courteous and diplomatic ■ Serve as a liaison between the physician and others ■ Exercise efficient time management

Key Terminology

buffer time—an appointment scheduling method of leaving certain times of day open to accommodate situations such as patients who call for same-day appointments or physicians who need to catch up on charting

cluster scheduling—scheduling method that groups patients with similar appointments around the same time of day

double booking—scheduling more than one patient for the same appointment time

established patient—patient whom the medical office has seen previously

fixed-appointment scheduling—scheduling system that assigns every patient a specific appointment time

matrix—process of blocking out times in the appointment schedule when the provider is unavailable or out of the office

modified wave scheduling—a scheduling system where two or three patients are scheduled at the beginning of each hour, followed by single patient appointments every 10 to 20 minutes for the rest of that hour

new patient—patient whom no provider of the same specialty in the office has seen for 3 or more years

new patient checklist—list of information new patients must provide when calling to schedule appointments

office brochure—pamphlet outlining an office's staff and services

open hours—scheduling method that allows patients to seek treatment without appointment times

preapprovals—the process of calling a patient's insurance carrier prior to a service in order to obtain preapproval or authorization for the service to be performed

slack time—an appointment scheduling method of leaving certain times of day open to accommodate situations such as when patients call for same-day appointments or physicians who need to catch up on charting

Key Terminology *(continued)*

triage notebook—notebook kept near the administrative medical assistant answering incoming telephone calls that out-

lines questions and steps to follow in the event callers have potentially life-threatening conditions

wave scheduling—a scheduling system where patients are scheduled only during the first half of each hour.

Abbreviations

EKG—Electrocardiogram

✓ COMPETENCY SKILLS PERFORMANCE

1. Schedule a new patient.
2. Establish an appointment matrix.
3. Schedule an established patient appointment.
4. Use patient reminder cards.
5. Reschedule a missed patient appointment.
6. Manage the physician's professional schedule and travel.
7. Schedule a hospital procedure.
8. Schedule an inpatient admission.

Introduction

While the specifics of appointment scheduling vary from one medical office to another, the basic concepts remain the same. Patients may call to schedule their first visit or routine followup appointments. They may also call with medical emergencies. Administrative medical assistants must know how to best handle each of these situations.

Scheduling New Patient Appointments

When a **new patient** calls the medical office to schedule an appointment, it is important to collect all needed information (Figure 9-1 ◆) while remaining professional, objective, and consistent. A patient's financial information should not command special attention from the medical assistant and should not be the first question the medical assistant asks of the caller. A **new patient checklist** (Figure 9-2 ◆) can help ensure that medical assistants ask appropriate questions, cover all bases, and gather information from all new patients consistently.

— Critical Thinking Question 9-1—
If Glenn fails to state his reason for requesting a physician visit, how can the medical assistant determine the time to allot for the appointment?

Because most health care providers are members of several managed care plans as preferred providers, it is important that medical assistants ask for patients' insurance information

before scheduling appointments. When patients refuse to provide this information, assistants should let the patients know that this information is needed for patients to receive the highest benefits from their plans and that the patient may need to

☐ Correct spelling of the patient's full name
☐ When mailing paperwork for completion before the appointment, the patient's address
☐ Patient's home and work or mobile telephone numbers
☐ Reason for the patient's visit
☐ Name of the referring physician, when applicable
☐ Patient's insurance type
☐ Whether the patient need directions

Figure 9-1 ◆ Information to gather from new patients over the telephone.

- ❑ Full name, correctly spelled
- ❑ Home telephone number
- ❑ Work telephone number
- ❑ Mobile telephone number
- ❑ Reason for the visit
- ❑ Length of condition
- ❑ Type of insurance
- ❑ Referring party, correctly spelled
- ❑ Appointment date and time
- ❑ Treating physician
- ❑ Directions provided or not

Figure 9-2 ◆ Sample new patient checklist.

pay in full for their visit if the physician is not participating with their plan. When the medical office requires payment at the time of the visit, the medical assistant must also apprise patients of this policy.

— Critical Thinking Question 9-2—
How should the medical assistant respond if Glenn refuses to disclose his insurance information?

In addition to obtaining information, the medical assistant may need to provide the patient with information. Patients sometimes need directions to the office or information regarding bus routes that reach the office. Preprinted directions near the office telephone can serve as clear guides. The medical assistant will also need to inform patients of any special parking arrangements and costs.

— Critical Thinking Question 9-3—
Assume Glenn will be taking the bus to the office. What steps can the medical assistant take to ensure Glenn obtains correct route information?

Many offices choose to mail new patients information before those patients' first visits. This practice is especially beneficial when patients must complete several forms. As added information, offices should expand their mailings to include their **office brochure** and information about the physicians or office policies (Figure 9-3 ◆).

When medical assistants will be mailing forms to patients, they must advise the patients that they will be receiving the forms and should complete them before arriving for their first appointment. When offices do not send forms as a practice, assistants will need to ask patients to arrive early for their ap-

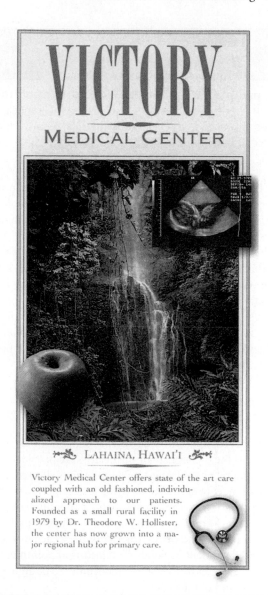

Figure 9-3 ◆ Sample medical office brochure.

pointments so they can complete their paperwork before seeing the physician. The number of forms drives how much time patients will need for this task, but in general, 10 to 20 minutes will suffice. When other health care providers have referred new patients to the office, medical assistants may want to ask those patients to bring their referral forms and any other relevant materials (e.g., X-rays or laboratory reports) to their visits. Sometimes, however, referring providers send such information separately.

New and Established Patients

Medical offices have varying policies on what constitutes "new" and "established" patients. In general, a new patient has not been seen in the medical office by any of the health care providers of the same specialty within the past 3 years. Conversely, an **established patient** has seen one of the health care providers of the same specialty in the medical office within the past 3 years. This rule especially applies when billing patients'

Keys to Success
ACCIDENTAL INJURY FILES

Keep patients' accidental injury files separate from those patients' general medical files. Then, when insurance companies request copies of patients' medical records due to the accidental injury, the copying task is far easier.

Keys to Success
CONSIDERING PATIENT REQUIREMENTS

Every office has a few patients who need extended appointment times due to disability or complex health issues. Staff should note these unique requirements on the patients' hard-copy or electronic records so that the medical assistant who is scheduling appointments can allot appropriate amounts of time.

health insurance plans. When patients have been seen in the medical office, even by practitioners different from the one they are seeing on their next visit, those patients are considered established by their insurance carriers.

Patients who have been involved in accidents, such as car or on-the-job injuries, may be considered "new" when seeking care for related injuries because they will likely need to provide accidental-injury information and undergo evaluations as if the office has never seen them before. Therefore, it is important for medical assistants to know their offices' policies for "new" and "established" patients and to follow those policies consistently.

Allowing Appointments Adequate Time

The time patient appointments require depends on the type of practice and the preferences of the health care providers. Table 9-1 lists general appointment types and times allowed. In typical offices, new patients are seen for longer periods than established ones. For example, a new patient appointment may be scheduled for 30 minutes, whereas an established patient appointment may extend only 10 or 15 minutes. Each medical office should document its policy for allotting appointment time and review it regularly to ensure it continues to be appropriate for patients and physicians.

Many physicians prefer to limit certain types of appointments in any given day. For example, a pediatrician may only want to see one or two sports physicals in a day. An OB/GYN physician may only want to see one or two new maternity patients in a day. Again, documented policies are beneficial, because they can clarify physicians' preferences and help the medical assistant schedule appointments properly. If, for example, the pediatrician will only allow two sports physicals a day, the office may schedule those appointments for 10 A.M. and 3 P.M. Once those appointments are filled, the medical assistant can easily see that the schedule will support no more sports physicals that day.

Creating an Appointment Matrix

The process of scheduling medical office appointments begins with an appointment **matrix**. An appointment matrix, which can be applied to paper and computerized appointment schedules alike, depicts the appointment times available in the medical office. Medical assistants block out the times on the matrix when physicians are unavailable due to hospital rounds, vacations, or holidays. When appointment matrices are paired with appointment systems, medical assistants can also block times for certain pieces of equipment so equipment conflicts do not arise.

Depending on the type of practice or the specialties of the physicians, medical assistants use certain abbreviations in their matrix notations. Within an office, however, these abbreviations must be standard so that all members of the health care team can interpret the abbreviations accurately. For example, an office may use the abbreviation "NP" for a new patient.

Balancing Patient and Office Needs in Scheduling

When medical assistants schedule appointments, they must pay attention to patients' needs. For example, assistants should schedule patients who need fasting blood draws at the beginning of the day. Just as assistants should heed patient needs, they should factor in what is appropriate for the office. For example, if the office has only one electrocardiogram (**EKG**) machine, it would be inappropriate for the medical assistant to schedule two patients who need the machine at once. When only one staff member performs a certain procedure or test, the medical assistant must keep that person's availability in mind when scheduling appointments.

Paper and Electronic Scheduling

Today, most large medical offices use computer software to manage their patient appointments (Figure 9-4 ◆). Electronic appointment scheduling offers many advantages. With computerized systems, several staff members can access the appointment schedule at once and from different locations in the office. Some computerized systems allow staff and/or physicians to access the appointment schedule from outside the office.

Offices that use paper appointment books should choose books that support their number of physicians and patients. In multiphysician practices, appointment books, whether paper or electronic, might be color coded by provider (Figure 9-5 ◆).

TABLE 9-1 TIME ALLOTTED FOR PATIENT APPOINTMENTS

Appointment Type	Allotted Time (in Minutes)
New patient	30
Physical exam	60
Routine checkup	15
Well child checkup	15
Blood pressure check	5

PROCEDURE 9-1 Establish an Appointment Matrix

Theory and Rationale
With an appointment matrix, the administrative medical assistant is able to create time slots for the various appointment types in the medical office. Using this method, the medical assistant is better able to accurately schedule patients for the necessary amount of time and facilitate efficient flow in the office.

Materials
- Pen
- Appointment book

Competency
(**Conditions**) With the necessary materials, you will be able to (**Task**) establish an appointment matrix (**Standards**) correctly within the time limit set by the instructor.

1. Determine the amount of time the providers want patients to have for each appointment type.
2. Within the appointment book, block out the time when the providers will be out of the office for lunch or other appointments.
3. Highlight or create blocks of time in the appointment book for appointments the provider specifies as those he or she would like only a limited number of, such as physical exams.
4. Go over the created appointment matrix with the providers to determine where any adjustments need to be made.

Even in one-physician practices, different columns of the appointment book may be used for different procedures. For example, all new patients might be scheduled in the far left column and all followup appointments in the far right one. In some offices, appointment types are highlighted in different colors to indicate type of patient or procedure. For example, patients undergoing laboratory work might be highlighted in orange while patients having X-rays might be highlighted in blue. Each office devises a system that works for it.

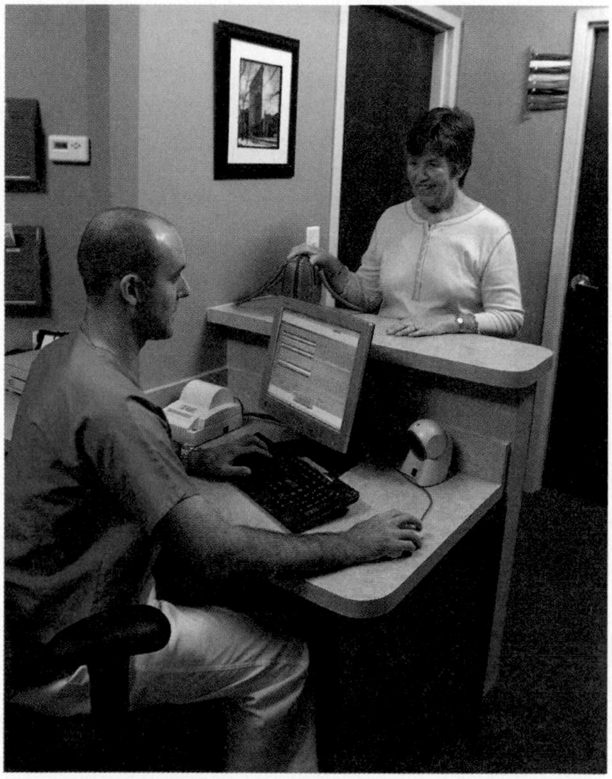

HIPAA Compliance
The appointment book, whether hard copy or electronic, is considered a legal document. Paper appointment books, like all hard-copy medical records, must be kept in a safe location. Computerized appointment schedules must be protected just like any other item that contains private patient information. Computerized schedules are secured through secure computer systems and password use by all administrative staff. At the end of the day, any prints of the computerized system should be shredded to protect patient confidentiality.

Figure 9-4 ◆ Scheduling appointments on the computer saves time over using a manual scheduling system.

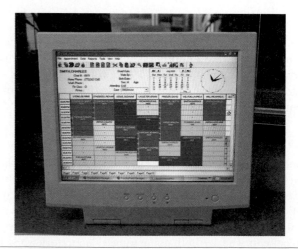

Figure 9-5 ◆ Using a color-coded scheme is easier in a multi-physician practice.

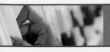

PROCEDURE 9-2 Schedule a New Patient

Theory and Rationale

Most patients who schedule appointments in the medical office do so over the telephone. The administrative medical assistant must know the information needed from each new patient and be able to answer any questions professionally.

Materials

- Telephone
- Blue or black pen
- Appointment book
- New patient checklist

Competency

(**Conditions**) With the necessary materials, you will be able to (**Task**) schedule a new patient who calls the medical office (**Standards**) correctly within the time limit set by the instructor.

1. Using a professional, friendly voice, answer the telephone by the second ring.
2. State the office name followed by your name.
3. When the caller does not self-identify as a new patient, ask the caller if he or she has been in to the office previously.
4. Ask the patient to spell his or her first and last names.
5. Write the patient's full name on the checklist.
6. Ask the patient for work and home telephone numbers, and home address.

7. Ask the patient how he or she was referred to the office.
8. Ask the patient to identify the type of health insurance he or she will be using.
9. Confirm that your physician participates in the patient's health care plan.
10. If the physician does not participate in the patient's health care plan, advise the patient that he or she may fail to receive preferred benefits or may need to pay in full for their services.
11. Ask the patient to state the condition prompting the visit.
12. Ask the patient to define the length of the condition.
13. Offer the patient appointment times to see the physician.
14. Schedule the patient.
15. If mailing paperwork to the patient to complete before the appointment, direct the patient to complete the paperwork before the visit.
16. If the patient will need to complete the paperwork at the first visit, direct him or her to arrive 15 minutes before the appointment's scheduled start time.
17. Document the patient's information in the manual or electronic appointment schedule.
18. Ask the patient if directions to the office are needed.
19. Give the patient any needed parking information.
20. Confirm the appointment's date and time with the patient.
21. Allow the patient to hang up the telephone before hanging up yourself.

Methods of Appointment Scheduling

Ambulatory health care uses several different methods to schedule patient appointments. Practice type and physician preference determine which method is used.

Cluster Scheduling

Cluster scheduling is a system of booking several patients around the same block of time. This method is normally used when the patients all need the same type of service, such as laboratory work or consultations. By clustering similar appointments, the office can serve patients most efficiently.

Double Booking

Double booking is done when two or more patients are scheduled to see the same health care provider at once. This method serves when an emergency patient must be seen that day, or it may be used to accommodate patients who need added services while in the office. For example, if the medical office has two patients who are both going to need laboratory work, the medical assistant might schedule both patients for the same appointment time. This option works, because the clinical medical assistant can perform laboratory work with one patient while the physician sees the other. This system uses the treatment rooms as well as the clinical staff's time effectively.

Fixed Appointment Scheduling

The most common method of scheduling patients is **fixed appointment scheduling**. In this method, the office gives each patient a specific appointment time.

Scheduling with Open Hours

The **open hours** scheduling method works for patients who do not need specific appointment times. This system is used in walk-in clinics, laboratories, and X-ray facilities where patients are normally seen on a first-come, first-served basis.

Wave Scheduling

Medical clinics with large numbers of procedure rooms and clinical staff may use something called **wave scheduling**. In wave scheduling, patients are scheduled only for the first half of each hour. The first patient to arrive is seen first. If two or more patients arrive at once, the clinical medical assistant will need to triage the patients to make the decision on who to take first.

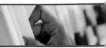

PROCEDURE 9-3 Schedule an Established Patient Appointment

Theory and Rationale
Patient scheduling, which constitutes a large portion of the administrative medical assistant's job, is vital to proper time management in the medical office. Therefore, the assistant must be properly trained to perform this task.

Materials
- Appointment schedule
- Blue or black pen
- Patient's chart

Competency
(**Conditions**) With the necessary materials, you will be able to (**Task**) schedule a patient appointment (**Standards**) correctly within the time limit set by the instructor.

1. Locate the chart of the patient to be scheduled.
2. Determine the type of appointment that is needed.
3. Determine the patient's schedule.
4. Determine the physician's schedule.
5. Enter the patient in the appointment schedule.
6. Restate the appointment date and time to the patient. If the patient is in the office, provide a written reminder card. Remind the patient to bring any needed items to the appointment or to follow any procedures (e.g., fasting before the visit).

Modified Wave Scheduling
The **modified wave scheduling** method is a variation on the wave method just discussed. With modified wave scheduling, two or three patients are scheduled at the beginning of each hour, followed by single patient appointments every 10 to 20 minutes for the rest of that hour. Complicated cases are generally scheduled at the beginning of the hour, while minor cases are usually scheduled toward the end.

Leaving Slack or Buffer Time
Most medical offices that use scheduling systems for patient appointments leave certain times of day open to accommodate things like patients who call for same-day appointments or physicians who need to catch up on charting. Such open periods, called **slack** or **buffer time**, are generally 15- to 30-minute slots at the end of the morning and the end of the afternoon or evening.

Conducting Triage and Appointment Scheduling
Patients with medical emergencies will sometimes call their physicians' offices for assistance. When they do, administrative medical assistants should have clearly written protocols for handling the

situations. A **triage notebook,** detailed in ∞ Chapter 8, outlines these protocols, as well as questions to ask patients who call with possible medical emergencies. Such a notebook, which should be clear, concise, and written under the physicians' direction, should be left near the telephone where patient calls are answered. ∞ See Chapter 8 for more information on the triage notebook.

Using Appointment Reminder Systems
Typically, patients are given appointment reminder cards as they leave the office (Figure 9-6 ◆). These reminder cards are normally the size of a business card and contain the date, day, and time of the patient's next appointment, as well as the office's name and telephone number.

Keys to Success
CHRONICALLY LATE PATIENTS

When patients are habitually late for their appointments, the medical office should give those patients "dummy" times that precede scheduled appointment times by 15 minutes. When a chronically late patient is scheduled for a 2:15 P.M. appointment, for example, the office should advise the patient to arrive at 2:00 P.M.

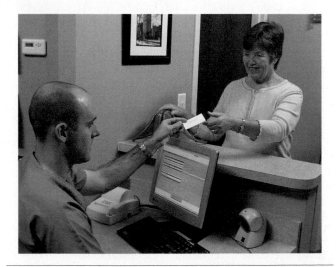

Figure 9-6 ◆ Typically, patients are given appointment reminder cards when they leave the office.

Even with reminder cards, patients may forget their appointments. For this reason, many offices call patients the day before their appointment to remind them. Such calls must remain confidential. When leaving messages, staff should disclose no patient information. Instead, the assistant can leave a message like, "This is Jared calling from Dr. Barker's office to remind Kaneesha of her appointment tomorrow at 2 P.M. If you have any questions, please call me back at 201-555-6000."

For patients who schedule followup appointments a month or more in the future, many offices choose to send reminder cards. These cards can be postcards only when they contain no personal patient information such as the reason for the visit. If the name of the office discloses the reason for the patient's visit, the office should not use postcard reminders. For example, if the office is called "Woodland Oncology Center," someone who sees a postcard with this name may assume the patient has cancer. Offices like these should either mail appointment reminders in envelopes or call patients with reminders. Some form of reminder card or call has been proven to reduce dramatically the number of no-show appointments.

Correcting the Appointment Schedule

White correction fluid, as with patients' medical records, is disallowed from the appointment book. When an appointment is changed in the appointment book, it should not be obliterated or erased or blacked out with a marker. Instead, the medical assistant should draw one line through the patient's name and note why the patient failed to keep the appointment (Figure 9-7 ◆). Some medical offices use color-coded systems to indicate schedule changes. For example, a red "X" next to a patient's

name might indicate an appointment cancellation. Electronic schedules accept notations, cancellations, and rescheduled or missed appointments.

Documenting No-Show Appointments

Patients who fail to arrive for their appointment and do not call to reschedule are considered "no-shows." The medical office must try to reach all no-shows. Typically, this is done via telephone 15 to 30 minutes after a patient's appointed time. When medical assistants reach such patients, they should try to reschedule the appointment. When they cannot reach patients, however, they should leave messages requesting return calls to reschedule. When assistants can neither reach patients nor leave messages, they may mail notes requesting rescheduling.

Following Up on No-Show Appointments

Missed patient appointments, for whatever reason, must be documented in the patients' medical records. Any steps the medical office staff takes to try to reschedule those patients must be documented as well. When patients refuse to reschedule or remain unreachable, medical assistants must make notes in those patients' medical records and submit those records to the physician for review.

Well-documented patient medical records become particularly important when patients experience adverse outcomes due to missed appointments. Medical offices with clear, comprehensive patient records are better able to defend against malpractice suits. Some offices take the extra step of sending patients certified letters when they miss important followup

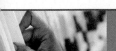

PROCEDURE 9-4 Use Patient Reminder Cards

Theory and Rationale

Many patients, as they leave the medical office, will require a follow-up appointment. The medical assistant will need to schedule that appointment for the patient and provide the patient with a reminder card.

Materials

- Pen
- Appointment book
- Appointment reminder card

Competency

(**Conditions**) With the necessary materials, you will be able to (**Task**) use patient reminder cards (**Standards**) correctly within the time limit set by the instructor.

1. As the patient arrives at the reception desk, look at the fee slip to verify when the provider wants the patient to return for an appointment.
2. Ask the patient if there is a day or time that works best for their schedule for the appointment.
3. Check the appointment book to find an appointment time that fits with the patient's schedule.
3. After verifying that the appointment will work with the patient's schedule, write or type the appointment into the appointment schedule.
5. Write the patient's appointment on a reminder card and give the card to the patient.

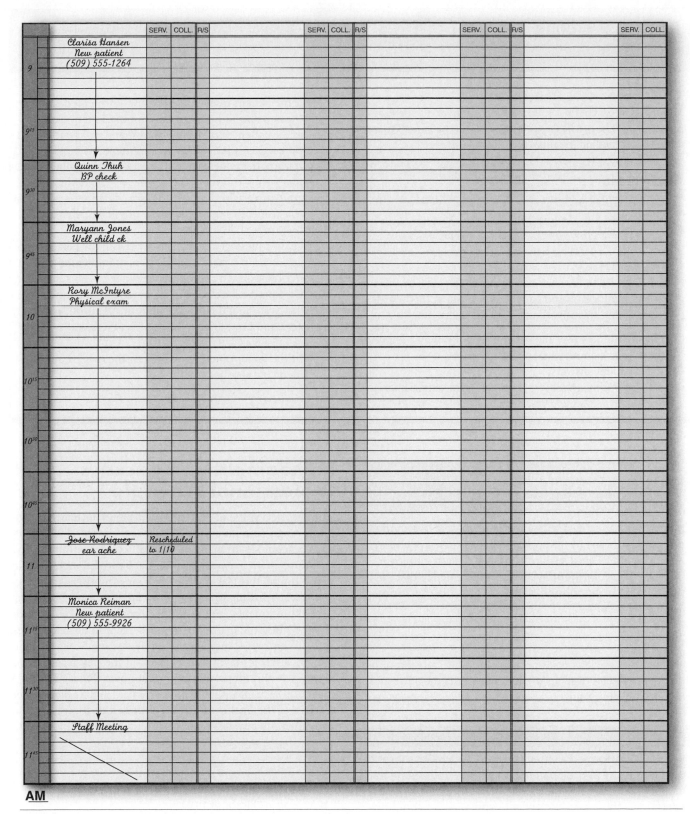

Figure 9-7 ◆ Sample appointment book indicating patients who have changed appointments.

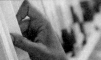

PROCEDURE 9-5 Reschedule a Missed Patient Appointment

Theory and Rationale

The medical office must follow up on all missed patient appointments. The medical assistant must call the patient to attempt to reschedule the missed appointment.

Materials

- Appointment schedule
- Pen
- Patient's chart

Competency

(**Conditions**) With the necessary materials, you will be able to (**Task**) reschedule a missed patient appointment (**Standards**) correctly within the time limit set by the instructor.

1. Fifteen minutes after the patient's appointment time, call the patient's home telephone number.
2. If the patient answers:
   - Point out the missed appointment time and ask for an appropriate time to reschedule.
   - If the patient reschedules the appointment, document the new appointment in the appointment book as well as the patient's chart. Also chart that the patient missed the originally scheduled appointment.
   - If the patient does not wish to reschedule, politely state that you will inform the physician. Chart the missed appointment and refusal to reschedule in the patient's chart, and give the chart to the physician.
3. If the patient fails to answer:
   - Leave a message on voice mail or with the person who answers. Be certain to disclose no confidential patient information. An appropriate message is, "This is Juan at Dr. Saunders's office. I'm calling for Mrs. Banfield. We had you scheduled for an appointment today at 9:00 A.M., and I'm calling to reschedule. Please call me back at 715-555-6789."
   - In the patient's chart, document the missed appointment and the message.

Keys to Success
AUTOMATED TELEPHONE REMINDER SYSTEMS

Many medical offices today use automated telephone reminder systems to remind patients of their upcoming appointments. These systems, typically paired with computerized appointment systems, automatically dial patients' contact telephone numbers and play recorded reminder messages.

appointments, such as postoperative appointments. Proof of the patients' receipt of such letters demonstrates the office took every step possible to encourage patients to obtain needed care.

In Practice

Dr. Brosnan performed a vasectomy on William Grissom and asked him, as he asks all patients who have undergone this procedure, to have a followup evaluation and laboratory work to determine the procedure's effectiveness. Mr. Grissom, however, failed to show for his followup appointment. Three months later, Dr. Brosnan received a notice that Mr. Grissom has filed a malpractice suit. According to the notice, Mr. Grissom is alleging that Dr. Brosnan was negligent because Mr. Grissom's wife is newly pregnant. How could Dr. Brosnan's office have protected itself against this situation?

Managing the Physician's Professional Schedule

Many physicians attend professional meetings outside the office. These range from lunches with colleagues to traveling to out-of-state seminars. In many medical offices, the administrative medical assistant manages the physician's professional schedule. At minimum, this task includes blocking out times in the appointment schedule when the physician is unavailable for patient appointments. The assistant may also be asked to book airline flights or hotel rooms, or to reserve seats at conferences.

To ensure accuracy and efficiency, medical assistants should clearly write all information on the physician's travel plans, including any confirmation numbers (Figure 9-8 ◆). A copy of all such information should remain in the office to keep the rest of the health care team apprised of the physician's schedule. The physician can retain any original documents.

- Leaving on United Airlines Flight #12 at 7:10 P.M. Thursday.
- Arriving in Chicago at 10:02 P.M.
- Reservations with Hertz car rental, Confirmation #1298745.
- Reservations at the Red Lion hotel, Confirmation #LEN987.
- Seminar starts in the Capital Boardroom at 9 A.M. Friday.
- Return on United Airlines Flight #81 at 9:10 A.M. Sunday.

Figure 9-8 ◆ Sample physician's travel schedule.

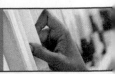

PROCEDURE 9-6 Manage the Physician's Professional Schedule and Travel

Theory and Rationale

Many physicians travel out of town for speaking engagements or seminars while gaining continuing education credits for relicensure. The medical assistant will often be asked to coordinate the physician's schedule and make all necessary travel arrangements for these trips.

Materials

- A telephone
- A list of the physician's travel needs, including dates and times of the meeting or seminar, place of the seminar, and physician preference for airline and hotel arrangements.
- Paper and pen

Competency

(**Conditions**) With the necessary materials, you will be able to (**Task**) manage the physician's professional schedule and travel (**Standards**) correctly within the time limit set by the instructor.

1. Call the physician's preferred airline and book the appropriate flight.
2. Make a note of the date, time, airline, and flight number for the departure time and arrival time for both the outgoing flight and the return flight.
3. Call the physician's preferred hotel and book the appropriate room.
4. Make a note of the confirmation number for the hotel room.
5. Arrange for any necessary transportation to or from the hotel and airport.
6. Create a list of all arrangements made and give the list to the physician.
7. Give a copy of the list of arrangements to the office manager and to the receptionist.
8. Verify the receptionist has blocked out the dates the physician will be away, if applicable.

Keys to Success
PREPARING THE PATIENT FOR THE MEDICAL PROCEDURE

Medical procedures make many patients nervous. Medical assistants can help make patients' experiences positive ones by letting them know exactly what to expect before, during, and after their procedures. Assistants should include any dietary or activity restrictions before or after procedures, specify how long the procedures are expected to take, and provide information on warning signs.

When the physician attends a seminar or conference that awards continuing-education credits, the medical assistant should track that information, as well.

Scheduling Hospital Services and Admissions

Many physicians care for or perform procedures on patients in hospital settings as well as in ambulatory clinics. For this reason, administrative medical assistants must be well versed in the procedures for scheduling patients for hospital services.

To facilitate the hospital scheduling process, the medical office should keep all hospital and related telephone numbers near the telephone or program them into speed dial. Most health insurance plans require physicians to obtain **preapprovals** for surgical procedures. Unless the procedure is an emergency, the medical assistant should call the patient's insurance carrier to obtain authorization for the procedure before scheduling the patient. Whenever possible, medical assistants should schedule patients for hospital services while those patients are in the office. With patients present, assistants are better able to coordinate patients' schedules.

Every office should have guidelines for scheduling patients for hospital services. Such guidelines should list the type of procedure, the physician, the time the physician needs, and any information that must be relayed to the patient, such as fasting presurgery. The medical office should also have preprinted informational forms from the hospital or outpatient facility that gives such specifics as directions to the facility and check-in procedures. Patients should receive such forms before they leave the office.

Specialty Referral Appointments

Many patients in the medical office will need to be scheduled for an appointment with a specialist. When this happens, the physician will notify the medical assistant of the patient's need for a specialty referral. The physician will also state the name of the specialist the patient is to be referred to, information regarding the condition for which the patient needs to be seen, and a time frame within which the appointment should be made.

Depending upon the policy in the medical clinic, the medical assistant may call to schedule the referral for the patient directly. In other offices, the medical assistant may supply the information about the referral to the patient and the patient makes the telephone call directly. Either way, the medical

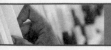

PROCEDURE 9-7 Schedule a Hospital Procedure

Theory and Rationale

When procedures cannot be performed in the medical office or patients would be better served in hospitals, physicians ask the medical assistant to schedule patients for hospital procedures.

Materials

- Patient's chart
- Hospital/surgery scheduling form
- Scheduling guidelines
- Calendar
- Telephone
- Notepad
- Pen

Competency

(**Conditions**) With the necessary materials, you will be able to (**Task**) schedule a patient for a hospital procedure (**Standards**) correctly within the time limit set by the instructor.

1. Obtain information from the physician or clinical medical assistant about the needed surgery or procedure and the desired hospital.
2. Call the patient's insurance carrier to obtain preauthorization for the procedure.

3. Document the preauthorization number in the patient's chart along with the name of the insurance company customer service representative spoken to.
4. If the patient is in the clinic, ask what date or time would be most convenient for the procedure. If the patient is not in the clinic, call the patient to determine scheduling needs.
5. Call the hospital to communicate the procedure the physician has planned, the amount of time needed for the procedure, and the date preferred for the procedure.
6. Provide the hospital staff the patient's information, including name, birth date, address, telephone number, insurance information, and preauthorization number. Also relay all pertinent health information, such as allergies or disabilities.
7. After agreeing on a date and time, give the information to the patient and enter it in the physician's appointment schedule.
8. Advise the patient that the hospital will likely call to provide instructions and verify the check-in date and time.
9. Schedule the patient for a postoperative appointment in the physician's office, if needed.
10. Chart all information in the patient's medical record, and give the chart to the physician for review.

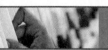

PROCEDURE 9-8 Schedule an Inpatient Admission

Theory and Rationale

When patients require inpatient procedures or observations, physicians will ask medical assistants to schedule those patients for inpatient hospitalizations. Medical assistants who know the proper procedure help ensure that the scheduling process goes smoothly.

Materials

- Patient's chart
- Inpatient scheduling guidelines
- Calendar
- Telephone
- Notepad
- Pen

Competency

(**Conditions**) With the necessary materials, you will be able to (**Task**) schedule an inpatient admission (**Standards**) correctly within the time limit set by the instructor.

1. Call the patient's insurance carrier to obtain preauthorization for the procedure, the needed followup, and the allowable number of hospital days.
2. Document the preauthorization number in the patient's chart along with the name of the insurance company customer service representative spoken to.
3. Call the hospital admissions office with the patient's name, physician's name, and reason for admission.
4. Let the admissions office know when the physician would like the patient to be admitted.
5. Give the admissions office the patient's contact information, birth date, insurance information, and preauthorization number.
6. Instruct the patient when to arrive at the hospital and where to go once there.
7. Give the patient any specifics on what to bring (or not) to the hospital.
8. Chart all information in the patient's medical record, and give the chart to the physician for review.

assistant must supply the patient with the needed information regarding the need for the additional appointment.

Arranging for Language Interpreters

Occasionally, the medical office will treat patients who are not fluent in English or who cannot communicate due to a disability. Typically, these patients visit the office with family members or friends who can translate for them. When patients cannot arrange for interpreters, the medical office must arrange interpreter services. Many states offer translation services for their Medicaid-covered patients. When translation services are needed, offices should keep interpreters' telephone numbers at the front desk. When using a translator, the medical assistant must document the name and contact information of the translator in the patient's chart.

To bring translation services in house, many medical offices, especially those in communities with large non–English-speaking populations, seek employees who are fluent in other languages. Members of the health care team who can translate for patients are valuable assets to the medical office.

Arranging Transportation for Patients

Many medical offices treat patients who cannot drive themselves to the office. Patients may have disabilities or offices may be in challenging locations. As a courtesy to patients, administrative medical assistants should keep telephone lists of transportation services. Such lists should include taxicab services as well as local services for the elderly or disabled.

Achieving Efficiency in Scheduling

All medical offices at some point realize that their appointment scheduling procedures could be improved. Physicians may routinely exceed scheduled appointment times, or extended delays may regularly irritate patients. When flaws like these become apparent, it is important for the health care team as a whole to re-evaluate how the office schedules appointments. Every member of the team should participate in improvement efforts, because scheduling affects every staff member (Figure 9-9 ◆).

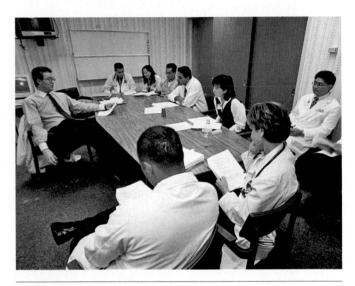

Figure 9-9 ◆ Regular staff meetings keep the lines of communication in the medical office open.

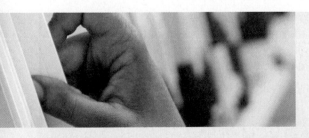

REVIEW

Chapter Summary

- Guidelines for scheduling patient appointments are invaluable tools for medical offices intent on providing effective, efficient patient service.
- Today, medical offices can choose between paper and electronic scheduling systems.
- Both paper and electronic scheduling systems accommodate patient no-shows, which always must be documented properly for legal and other purposes.
- Whenever patients miss their appointments, the medical assistant should follow up to attempt rescheduling.

- The physician's professional schedule, which includes travel, is part of a medical office's overall scheduling scheme.
- Like the physician's travel, the medical assistant must be able to accommodate patients' hospital appointments in the office's scheduling system.
- Effective medical assistants arrange appropriate transportation services or language interpreters for patients in need.

Chapter Review

Multiple Choice

1. At _____ minutes after a patient has missed an appointment, the medical assistant should call to reschedule.
   a. 5
   b. 10
   c. 15
   d. 60

2. A new patient is defined as someone who has:
   a. not been seen in the medical office for more than 1 year
   b. not been seen by any physician in the office for more than 3 years
   c. been seen by another physician in the office within the last year but is now seeing a new provider in the office
   d. all of the above

3. A new patient checklist is worthwhile when scheduling new patient appointments to ensure the medical assistant:
   a. gathers all necessary information from the new patient
   b. provides directions to the office, if needed
   c. gives information on parking arrangements
   d. all of the above

4. The medical office should ask new patients to arrive _____ minutes before their scheduled appointments to complete new patient paperwork.
   a. 5
   b. 15
   c. 25
   d. 35

5. Which of the following scheduling methods books several patients around the same time?
   a. Cluster booking
   b. Stream scheduling
   c. Set appointment time scheduling
   d. None of the above

True/False

T F 1. The time allowed for patient appointments remains constant from practitioner to practitioner.

T F 2. The appointment book is a legal document.

T F 3. Double booking is the process of allowing patients to arrive for appointments at their leisure.

T F 4. It is appropriate to tell chronically late patients that their appointments are 15 minutes before the times scheduled in the appointment book.

T F 5. It is unnecessary to chart a no-show appointment in a patient's chart.

T F 6. Medical offices that chart patients' missed appointments can help avoid losing malpractice lawsuits.

T F 7. When scheduling patients for procedures, it is important to disclose everything to expect.

T F 8. Administrative medical assistants do not arrange transportation services.

T F 9. A medical office's appointment scheduling system should be reviewed periodically to determine its efficiency.

Short Answer

1. What is one way to prepare the appointment schedule to allow appointments for patients who call and want same-day appointments?

2. Describe a triage notebook and its role in the medical office.

3. How can administrative medical assistants help patients remember to keep their appointments?

4. What is meant by a "no-show" appointment?

5. What can medical assistants do when they find that patients are waiting long periods for their appointments?

6. Describe how an appointment matrix is used in the medical office.

Research

1. Research online for companies that sell medical office appointment scheduling software. How do these companies compare to one another?

2. Interview someone who works in a medical office. Do the physicians in this office travel for out-of-town events related to their practice? If so, who in the office handles the scheduling arrangements?

3. What local resources are available in your area for arranging for medical language interpreters?

Externship Application Experience

When Shawn Guthmein calls to schedule a new patient appointment with Dr. Gootkind, he mentions that he will be bringing his service animal to his appointment because he is legally blind. Because Shawn is a new patient, he will need to complete several forms once he is in the clinic. How can the medical assistant best handle this patient?

Resource Guide

MicroWiz Medical Appointment Scheduling Software
http://www.microwize.com/ohpro.htm

MedStar Medical Appointment Scheduling Software
http://www.medstarsystems.com

NewMedia Medicine Medical Appointment Scheduling Software
http://www.newmediamedicine.com/

ScheduleView Medical Appointment Software
http://www.scheduleview.com/

 # Med**Media**

http://www.MyMAKit.com

More on this chapter, including interactive resources, can be found on the Student CD-ROM accompanying this textbook and on http://www.MyMAKit.com.

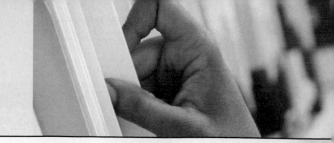

CHAPTER 10

Medical Records Management

Case Study

When Melissa begins working for Dr. Kingsley, Caroline, one of the physician's longtime medical assistants, is charged with training her. One day, as Caroline pulls charts for patients scheduled for that afternoon, she points out a note on the outside of Robert Olson's chart that reads, "Problem." Caroline explains that the note alerts the medical assistants and the physician to patients who are "hard to work with." She says these patients complain, are late to their appointments, or are just generally unpleasant.

Objectives

After completing this chapter, you should be able to:

- Define and spell the key terminology in this chapter.
- List information contained in the medical record.
- Explain various charting styles.
- Discuss how to chart patient communication.
- Define cross-referencing and how it should be used.
- List the steps to take to find a missing file.
- Discuss color-coded filing systems.
- Describe why an office would choose to use numeric filing.
- Name the common types of file storage systems.
- Differentiate between active, inactive, and closed patient files.
- Distinguish electronic medical records from paper ones.
- Name ways to store inactive patient files.
- Identify the steps to take to destroy a medical record.
- Describe how to correct an error in a patient chart.
- List the steps to take when patients want to make changes to their medical records.

MedMedia

http://www.MyMAKit.com

Additional interactive resources and activities for this chapter can be found on http://www.MyMAKit.com. For a video, tips, audio glossary, legal and ethical scenarios, on-the-job scenarios, quizzes, and games related to the content of this chapter, please access the accompanying CD-ROM in this book.

Videos: *The Lost File; Getting Along with Coworkers*
Legal and Ethical Scenario: *Medical Records Management*
On the Job Scenario: *Medical Records Management*
Tips
Multiple Choice Quiz
Audio Glossary
HIPAA Quiz
Games: Spelling Bee, Crossword, and Strikeout

MEDICAL ASSISTING STANDARDS

CAAHEP ENTRY-LEVEL STANDARDS	ABHES ENTRY-LEVEL COMPETENCIES
■ Identify systems for organizing medical records (cognitive) ■ Describe various types of content maintained in a patient's medical record (cognitive) ■ Discuss pros and cons of various filing methods (cognitive) ■ Describe indexing rules (cognitive) ■ Discuss filing procedures (cognitive) ■ Identify types of records common to the healthcare setting (cognitive) ■ Organize a patients' medical record (psychomotor) ■ File medical records (psychomotor) ■ Maintain organization by filing (psychomotor) ■ Document accurately in the patient record (psychomotor) ■ Apply HIPAA rules in regard to privacy/release of information (psychomotor) ■ Consider staff needs and limitations in establishment of a filing system (affective)	■ Maintain confidentiality at all times ■ Use appropriate guidelines when releasing records or information ■ Be cognizant of ethical boundaries ■ Evidence a responsible attitude ■ Application of electronic technology ■ Apply computer concepts for office procedures ■ Prepare and maintain medical records ■ File medical records

✓ COMPETENCY SKILLS PERFORMANCE

1. Prepare the medical chart.
2. Chart patient telephone calls.
3. File documents usng the alphabetic filing system.
4. File manually using a subject filing system.
5. File documents in patient medical records.
6. Use the numeric system to file medical records.
7. Correct errors in the patient medical record.

Introduction

Medical records play an important role in health care delivery, so they must be accurate and complete. Health care providers rely on patients' medical records as accurate depictions of patients. With patients' consent, medical records are often sent between physicians and hospitals to give physicians complete pictures of patients' medical histories.

As legal documents, medical records are often the single most important tools health care providers can use to defend against medical malpractice lawsuits. Risk management and quality improvement programs rely on medical records to catch errors in patient care. Insurance companies often request copies of patient medical records to determine the appropriateness of billing codes and reimbursement levels. Medical records that are incomplete or **indecipherable** may cause problems in patient care.

Key Terminology *(continued)*

personal information—information such as patient's name, birth date, gender, marital status, occupation, next of kin, and any other items collected for personal identification

Problem-oriented medical record (POMR) charting—type of medical record charting that focuses on patients' health care problems and addresses those problems at each visit

progress notes—notes in patients' medical charts outlining those patients' progress or complaints

purge—to remove closed or inactive patient medical records from the medical office

shingling—process of attaching small pieces of paper to standard-size sheets of paper so the small items are easy to locate in patients' charts

SOAP note charting—type of charting that considers the patient's subjective and objective findings, the provider's assessment of the patient's condition, and the prescribed plan of action for treatment

social information—information about a patient's social habits, such as tobacco, drug, or alcohol use

standard of care—legal term that describes the type of care a reasonable health care provider is expected to provide under the same situation

statute of limitations—period within which a patient must file a lawsuit after an injury

subpoena—court order demanding that a party appear in court or copies of the medical record be sent to a third party

Abbreviations

FDA—Food and Drug Administration

HIPAA—Health Insurance Portability and Accountability Act

NKA—No Known Allergies

POMR—Problem-Oriented Medical Record

SOAP—Subjective, Objective, Assessment, and Plan

Information Contained in the Medical Record

Medical records have four types of **patient information:** (1) **personal information,** (2) **financial information**, (3) **medical information**, and (4) **social information.** Personal information is the information patients supply when first seeing physicians for care. Such information includes a patient's name, birth date, gender, marital status, occupation, next of kin, and any other items collected for personal identification. Personal information may also include any comments the medical assistant might write in the patient's file regarding the patient's language or cultural background, if such information pertains to the patient's health care.

A patient's financial information includes a patient's ledger and insurance information, which includes policy and identification numbers and insurance-plan contact information, as well as any other information needed to bill the insurance company for the patient's care. In many medical offices, some portion of the patient's financial information is kept in a separate file from medical information. Financial information also includes copies of insurance company correspondence, and signed authorizations from the patient allowing the medical provider to release information to the insurance company.

Medical information includes the **chief complaint,** or the main reason a person seeks care; any family medical history; the patient's medical history; the results of examinations; the physical examination form; the prescribed course of treatment, including any medications or referrals; and the patient's diagnoses, progress notes, operative reports, radiology reports, laboratory reports, and any other reports or information that pertains to the patient's health care (Figure 10-1 ◆).

Social information is any personal information on the patient, such as race and ethnicity, hobbies, and regular sports participation. Social information also includes such lifestyle choices as smoking, alcohol consumption, drug use, and sexual habits.

In addition to personal, financial, medical, and social information, other documents are routinely part of the patient's medical record. These documents include the **HIPAA** understanding form, which indicates the patient has been notified of the office's privacy policies; the HIPAA release form ∞ (see Chapter 8), which authorizes the medical provider to discuss the patient's care with other parties; documents from hospitalizations; and any items the patient brings to the appointment, such as a list of current medications or copies of information from other medical providers' files.

The Purpose of the Medical Record

A patient's medical record documents a patient's treatment plan and goals in paper or electronic form. The medical record must contain a full account of all patient treatment, including what treatment was given and why it was given or if treatment was withheld and why.

In whatever form, medical records must be complete, accurate, organized, concise, timely, and factual. They should never contain opinions or judgments about patients. Whenever medical records are **subpoenaed** for trials, physicians may

OPERATION DATE: 8/11/10

PATIENT: ADAM PARCHER

SURGEON: MARIA FERNANDEZ-RAUL, MD

PREOPERATIVE DIAGNOSIS;
Congenital external nasal deformity.

POSTOPERATIVE DIAGNOSIS:
Congenital external nasal deformity.

PROCEDURE:
Aesthetic rhinoplasty

DESCRIPTION OF PROCEDURE:
The patient is a 33-year-old male who presented with concerns for nasal airway obstruction and discontent with the external appearance of his nose. Examination confirms the above-noted concerns with a widened nasal base, palpable and visible dorsal cartilage and nasal bones.

Correction of the external deformity by open rhinoplasty, lowering of the dorsum, lowering of the cartilaginous dorsum, narrowing of the nasal bones, resection and narrowing of the nasal tip, excision of caudal septum and nasal spine were discussed. The nature of the procedures and risks, including bleeding, hematoma, infection, poor wound healing, scarring, asymmetry, airway difficulties, palpable or visible nasal structures and possible need for secondary procedures were all discussed. The patient understands and wishes to proceed as outlined.

FINDINGS:
The patient underwent open rhinoplasty through a columellar chevron incision. The nose was copiously infiltrated with 1% lidocaine with epinephrine prior to incision. The chevron incision was incised and carried to bilateral rim incisions. The nasal skin was then degloved using sharp dissecting scissors. This was opened over the nose up to the root of the nose to allow full exposure. The irregular nasal bones were initially smoothed with a rasp. Excision of the dorsal nasal bone was then carried out using a straight guarded osteotome. Approximately 1 mm thickness of bone was removed. After osteotomy was completed from a low to high position, infracture of the nasal bones was carried out. This provided good narrowing of the nasal base. A small piece of septal cartilage was crushed and flattened using the cartilage crusher and this was placed over the nasal dorsum. Hemostasis was assured. The skin was redraped and closure was carried out using interrupted 6-0 Prolene for the columellar and stab incisions. Interrupted 5-0 plain gut sutures were used to close the rim incisions and the septal transfixion incision. Xeroform packs were removed and nasal splints were placed. A second set of Xeroform packs was placed lateral to the nasal splints. The dorsum of the nose was taped and a dorsal thermoplast splint was also placed. The procedure was well tolerated. The posterior throat was suctioned and a throat pack that had been placed at the beginning of the procedure was removed. The patient was awakened and extubated and discharged to the recovery room in stable condition.

Maria Fernandez-Raul, MD

Figure 10-1 ◆ Sample operative report.

have to explain notations. A jury who thinks a physician is judgmental or unkind could hand down an unfavorable verdict. In addition, unprofessional notations may predispose other health care professionals to treat patients differently. The best way to keep medical charting professional is to always write as if the patient will be reading the comments. Anything the medical assistant would not say to the patient should remain out of the patient's medical record.

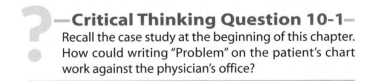

?—Critical Thinking Question 10-1—
Recall the case study at the beginning of this chapter. How could writing "Problem" on the patient's chart work against the physician's office?

Risk management departments use medical records to determine if the **standard of care** has been met. The standard of care states that a health care provider must use reasonable and necessary skill when caring for patients, the same care another provider with the same training would use in the same circumstances. The best defense against malpractice claims are well kept, accurate medical records. Some civil cases have held health care providers liable for their failure to maintain proper records. ∞ Chapter 4 provides more detail on medical malpractice.

Some health care providers may review patient medical records as part of consultation visits or "second opinions." Others will review medical records when patients transfer to other offices.

When patients have completed **advance directives**, a copy of that document should be placed in the patient's medical record.

Medical records are frequently used to determine reimbursement. The coding professionals who work in the medical office will often review the medical record in order to determine the proper code to use for billing purposes. This is another reason why proper documentation in the medical record is so important.

Signing Off on Medical Records

Any entry in a patient's medical record must have an identifying mark indicating the person who made the entry. Policies on this will vary from one medical office to the next, but the minimum should be no less than the initials and credentials of the person making the entry. Some medical offices require a complete signature along with credentials; others allow a first initial, last name, and credentials (Figure 10-2 ◆).

Keys to Success
THE FIVE C'S OF MEDICAL CHARTING

Medical charting must adhere to the following "Five Cs rule," which means patient charts must be

- **Concise**—Patient charts must be to the point and contain no entries that fail to relate to the patient's health care in some way.
- **Complete**—Medical records must be complete and objective. All pertinent information must be included while opinions and judgments are excluded.
- **Clear**—When handwritten, patient information should be printed, not written in cursive, and delivered in a clear, easy-to-read manner.
- **Correct**—Medical records must be error free. Errors are both improper additions and omissions. When errors are made, their creators must correct them as soon as possible.
- **Chronologic**—Medical records should be in chronologic order, with the latest entries on top.

Keys to Success
DOCUMENTING THE PATIENT'S MEDICAL RECORD

There is a phrase in health care, "If it wasn't charted, it wasn't done," which means anything that is not documented in a patient's medical record did not happen as far as the law is concerned. Similarly, anything that is charted in a record did happen from a legal standpoint. Therefore, ensure medical records are comprehensive and accurate, because even the smallest omission or incorrect statement can cause a host of problems, including malpractice lawsuits, incorrect patient care, patient injury, and miscommunication between health care providers.

Any time a medical record contains a signature with initials rather than the full name, the medical office must keep a permanent record of the signer. In Figure 10-2, for example, Sara Mendoza's full signature must be on file in the administrative office so that her initials "SPM" or partial name "S. Mendoza" can be easily mapped to Sara Mendoza.

An office that uses **electronic medical records** may use an **electronic signature.** In offices where medical notes are dictated and printed for patient files, an electronic signature or rubber-stamp signature may replace handwritten signatures. Again, there must be a permanent record of the signer, as well as an original version of the signature on file.

Forms of Charting

Just as medical offices vary, so, too, do the methods of inserting information into medical records.

The Narrative Style

Narrative notes are simply written descriptions of patients' visits. As one of the oldest forms of medical charting, narratives are chronological. Findings of the visit appear with the doctor's instructions or prescriptions. Many physicians dictate their narrative notes about patient care, have their notes transcribed, and place their typewritten notes in the patients' files, although narratives can be manual or electronic. In some offices, physi-

Initials only—*SPM, CMA (AAMA)*
Full signature—*Sara P. Mendoza, CMA (AAMA)*
Variation—*S. Mendoza, CMA (AAMA)*

Figure 10-2 ◆ Sample Sign-Off Signatures

PROCEDURE 10-1 **Prepare the Medical Chart**

Theory and Rationale

Every patient in the medical office must have a medical chart. In many ambulatory clinics today, paper medical charts are more common than electronic versions. Until paper charts become obsolete, administrative medical assistants must be able to prepare them.

Materials

- Medical chart
- Metal file clips
- Medication record sheet
- Progress notes record
- Color-coded alphabet stickers
- File label
- Two-hole punch
- Patient's name

Competency

(**Conditions**) With the necessary materials, you will be able to (**Task**) prepare a patient medical chart (**Standards**) correctly within the time limit set by the instructor.

1. Print the patient's name on a file label, with the last name followed by first name and middle initial. For example, print "Smith, John R." on the file label.

2. Verify the spelling of the patient's name.

3. Using the color-coded alphabet stickers, place the first two letters of the patient's last name on the file near the file label. In the preceding example, "SM" stickers would appear near the file label.

4. One space after the stickers in the preceding step, place a color-coded alphabet sticker for the first letter of the patient's first name. Building on the preceding example for John R. Smith, the file stickers would read "SM [space] J."

5. Add metal file clips to both sides of the file.

6. Using the two-hole punch, punch holes in the top of the documents to be filed in the patient's chart. These documents include the patient's history form, the Health Insurance Portability and Accountability Act (HIPAA) notification form, and the patient's consent to be examined.

7. Place the medication record sheet on one side of the chart.

8. Place the progress report sheet on the other side of the chart.

9. On the front of the chart in red ink, note any of the patient's known allergies. When the patient has no known allergies, write "**NKA**" (i.e., no known allergies) on the front of the chart.

---

cians underline or outline certain terms in narrative notes to add emphasis (Figure 10-3 ◆).

Charting with SOAP

Soap note charting is a method that tracks the subjective, objective, assessment, and plan (SOAP) for a patient's visit. Subjective findings include patient statements, including any

Keys to Success
OBTAINING SENSITIVE PATIENT INFORMATION

Patients sometimes refuse to divulge such private information as Social Security number or birth date or such lifestyle information as smoking, drinking, or drug habits. Let such patients know that anything in their medical records is confidential and cannot be released to anyone without the patients' written consent or a court order. When patients remain uneasy, notify the physician. Notification gives physicians an opportunity to discuss issues with patients and decide if they wish to treat those patients if those patients continue to refuse to provide the requested information.

information about the chief complaint. This section would include any quotes the patient may make about his condition ("My back feels as if I have a heavy weight on it"), and any other information provided by the patient regarding the duration and intensity of the complaint.

Objective findings are observations by the medical assistant and the health care provider, examination findings, and patient vital signs. This section would include the results of any tests performed, such as orthopedic or neurological tests, as well as any visual examination findings made by the physician, such as rashes the patient is exhibiting or the fact that the patient winces when the physician touches a certain body part.

The assessment of the patient is the doctor's diagnosis, possible diagnosis, or the diagnosis that the physician wishes to rule out for that visit. In the event that the diagnosis is one the physician can make at the time of the visit, the assessment will include that information. An example would be an assessment of "eczema" when the physician can clearly see this condition on the patient. If the physician must access certain test results before she can make a definitive diagnosis, the assessment might list "possible pneumonia" while the physician waits to see the patient's chest x-ray to make a definitive diagnosis.

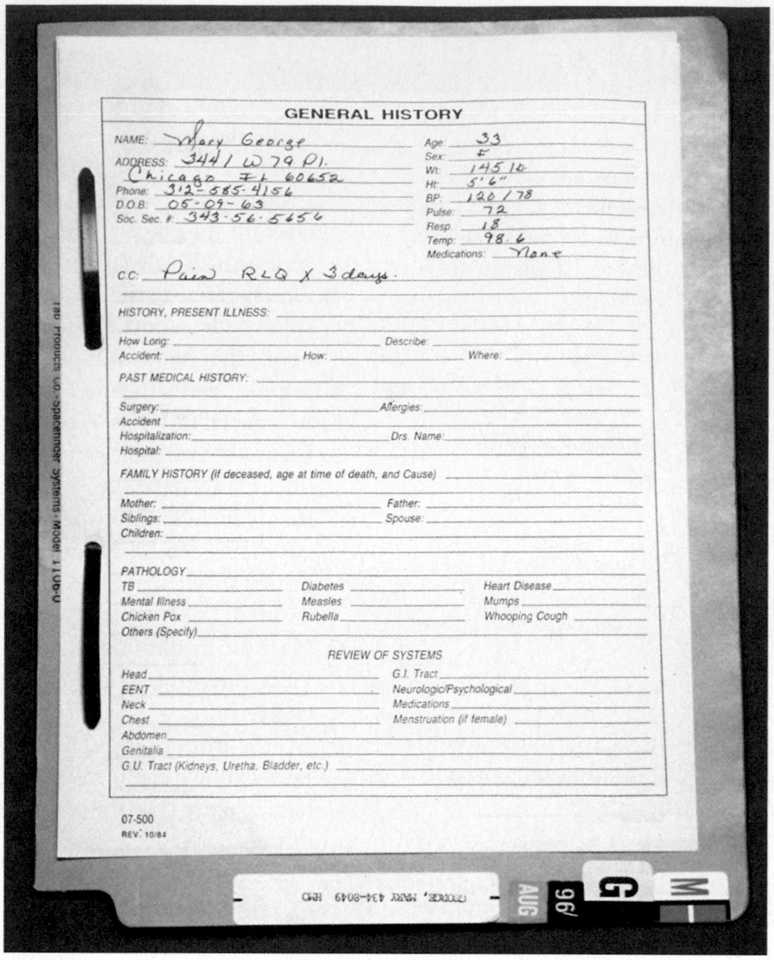

Figure 10-3 ◆ Sample handwritten chart documentation.

The plan is the health care provider's prescribed plan of action, which includes any prescriptions, tests, instructions, or referrals to other providers or therapies. This section will include any information about both prescription and over-the-counter medications, herbal remedies, or diet plans the physician has recommended for the patient.

The SOAP method of charting is extremely popular and easy to use. By clearly identifying the four areas in the SOAP format, anyone reading the notes can easily locate information within the patient medical record notes (Figure 10-4 ◆).

Problem-Oriented Medical Record Charting

Problem-oriented medical record (POMR) charting tracks a patient's problems throughout medical care. Each problem is assigned a number, and that number is referenced when the patient comes in for care (Figure 10-5 ◆). Advocates for POMR charting believe that charting according to patients' problems renders health care providers less likely to overlook previous problems. For example, assume Horatio Black arrives for an initial appointment with Dr. Stella Bartlett. When Horatio ar-

rives, he mentions he has had trouble with back pain for the past year or so. He also states that he has been diagnosed as "borderline diabetic." The main reason for today's visit, however, is for Horatio to discuss problems with depression and sleeplessness.

Using the POMR method of charting, Dr Bartlett would assign a number to each of the problems Horatio mentioned. She might assign the main reason for the visit, depression and sleeplessness, the number 1, Horatio's back pain number 2, and possible diabetes number 3. Each of these problems would have its own page in the medical chart so Dr. Bartlett can easily reference the problems at each visit. Once a condition is resolved, a notation is made so the doctor need not reference the problem on subsequent visits. As new problems arise, new numbers are assigned, and new pages are allotted for tracking the problems.

Inserting Flow Charts in Medical Records

Flow charts are visual tools that help track certain information in patients' medical records. Take the growth of children, for example. Each time the physician sees an infant, the clinical

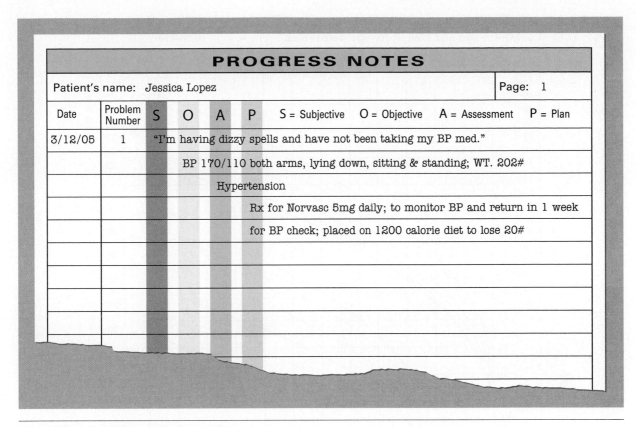

PROGRESS NOTES

| Patient's name: Jessica Lopez | | | | | | Page: 1 |

Date	Problem Number	S	O	A	P	S = Subjective O = Objective A = Assessment P = Plan
3/12/05	1					"I'm having dizzy spells and have not been taking my BP med."
						BP 170/110 both arms, lying down, sitting & standing; WT. 202#
						Hypertension
						Rx for Norvasc 5mg daily; to monitor BP and return in 1 week
						for BP check; placed on 1200 calorie diet to lose 20#

Figure 10-4 ◆ Sample SOAP note charting.

medical assistant will measure the child's weight, length, and head circumference and make notations on a flow chart that the physician can then use when discussing any concerns with the child's parent or guardian (Figure 10-6 ◆).

Progress Notes

Progress notes are daily chart notes made during patient visits to document patients' progress or status with certain conditions. Assume a patient arrives for an appointment complaining of fatigue. On the patient's subsequent visits, progress notes would outline the patient's current condition, any treatment recommendations, and outcomes. Depending on the office, progress notes may be made in SOAP, POMR, or narrative format. The notes may also be handwritten or electronic.

Using Abbreviations in Charting

Given that abbreviations can lead to confusion in health care, or even errors in patient care, medical assistants must be extremely careful when using abbreviations in patients' charts and ensure that the abbreviations are accepted by their facilities. Because different facilities may use different abbreviations for medical terms, when in doubt assistants should write out rather than abbreviate words. For example, one office may use the abbreviation "cx" to mean appointment cancellation. Another office may use the same abbreviation to indicate a cancer diagnosis.

Confusion among abbreviations can be avoided with a standard list of abbreviations between facilities. ∞ Chapter 6 lists abbreviations that are common in health care, as well as abbreviations that should never be used.

Problem #1: Fatigue
Problem #2: Low blood pressure
Problem #3: Right shoulder pain
Problem #4: Headaches

Figure 10-5 ◆ Sample POMR charting.

?—**Critical Thinking Question 10-2**–
What are the potential implications of abbreviations for "problem" patients? How does this approach compare to full notes on patient charts, as described in the chapter-opening case study?

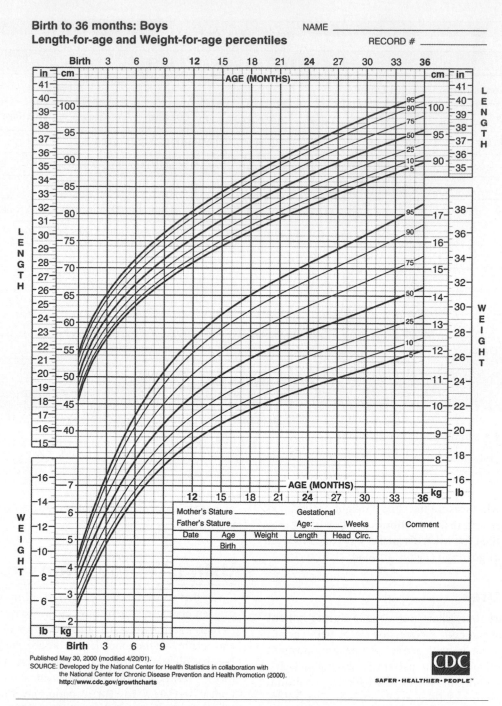

Birth to 36 months: Boys
Length-for-age and Weight-for-age percentiles

NAME _____

RECORD # _____

Published May 30, 2000 (modified 4/20/01).
SOURCE: Developed by the National Center for Health Statistics in collaboration with
the National Center for Chronic Disease Prevention and Health Promotion (2000).
http://www.cdc.gov/growthcharts

CDC
SAFER • HEALTHIER • PEOPLE™

Figure 10-6 ◆ Sample growth chart.
Source: www.cdc.gov.

Charting Patient Communication

Communications with patients, outside of office visits, must be documented in patients' charts when it is medically relevant. Such communications include telephone calls or e-mails from patients that relate to those patients' medical care, missed or cancelled appointments, or pharmacy requests to refill pre-scriptions. It is important to accurately chart all such exchanges in patients' medical records. Each office should have a policy regarding the type of communication that requires charting, and all members of the health care team should closely follow that policy. Such chart notes help to safeguard the medical office from malpractice claims or misunderstandings.

While thoroughness is important, not all patient conversations merit charting. Medical assistants should use their best judgment to determine if conversations are medically relevant.

PROCEDURE 10-2 Chart Patient Telephone Calls

Theory and Rationale

Patient telephone calls are frequently noted in patients' medical records. Chart notes such as these help to safeguard the medical office from malpractice claims and/or misunderstandings. Medical offices should have clear policies for charting patient calls, and medical assistants should understand their offices' policies.

Materials

- Notepad and pen
- Patient's chart

Competency

(**Conditions**) With the necessary materials, you will be able to (**Task**) chart a telephone call from a patient (**Standards**) correctly within the time limit set by the instructor.

1. While answering an incoming patient call, determine if the call is medically relevant to the patient's care in the office.

2. When the call is medically relevant to the patient's care, note the call's time and date, the patient's complete name and telephone number, and the nature of the message.
3. When the call ends, pull the patient's chart.
4. In the progress notes section of the patient's chart, note the current date and time.
5. Write the medically relevant portion of the call in the patient's medical record, using quotation marks to indicate any direct quotes from the patient.
6. Sign your name and credentials at the end of the chart entry.
7. When the call requires the physician's attention, leave the chart on the physician's desk. When the call does not require the physician's attention, file the chart.
8. After transferring all relevant information to the chart, shred any notes from the call that contain personal patient information.

In Practice

Dylan McElvaney, RMA, has taken a telephone call from Lynn Kinney, a patient in the office. Lynn states she is very unhappy with the office because she has been waiting for three days for her laboratory results to be conveyed to her. She says she won't be coming back to the office and will be calling to have copies of her medical file sent to another facility. What should Dylan say to Lynn? How should Dylan chart this telephone call in Lynn's medical record?

Filing Systems

Most medical offices use one of two types of filing systems: (1) alphabetic or (2) numeric. While alphabetic is far more common overall, numeric filing is more common in facilities where patient treatment records must be kept extremely confidential, such as in facilities specializing in mental health, HIV or AIDS treatment, or reproductive health care.

Alphabetic Filing

In alphabetic filing, patient information is filed alphabetically by last name. Some offices file according to the first two letters of the patient's last name; others use the patient's first and last name initials. Still others use a portion of the patient's last name and the first initial of the first name. Offices that use alphabetic filing place color-coded alphabetic stickers on the outside of patients' charts (Figure 10-7 ◆). Color coding helps misfiled charts stand out.

Patients with hyphenated last names can confuse filing practices in medical offices. When a patient's last name is Morris-Davidson, for example, some staff may file the patient's chart under the first part of the hyphenated name, Morris, while other staff may file according to the latter part, which is Davidson. To avoid confusion, medical offices should have clear policies for filing the charts of patients with hyphenated names and strictly follow those policies.

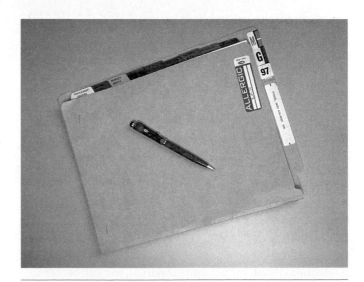

Figure 10-7 ◆ Using color coded labels enables the medical assistant to quickly locate a misfiled chart.

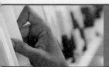

PROCEDURE 10-3 File Documents Using the Alphabetic Filing System

Theory and Rationale

Most medical facilities use the alphabetic method for filing patient medical record files. The medical assistant must pay close attention to detail and be certain files are filed accurately in order to assure the file will be easily found when needed. Color coding helps misfiled charts stand out.

Materials

- Patient medical records
- Color-coded alphabetic file letter stickers

Competency

(**Conditions**) With the necessary materials, you will be able to (**Task**) file documents using the alphabetic filing

system (**Standards**) correctly within the time limit set by the instructor.

1. Using the color-coded alphabetic file letter stickers, apply stickers to each medical record using the patient's first two letters from the last name.
2. Arrange the medical records in alphabetical order by last name.
3. File the medical records accurately in the filing cabinet.

Unfortunately, even with clear policies, hyphenated names can still be confusing. A patient with the last name Morris-Davidson may go by Morris on some occasions yet use Morris-Davidson or even Davidson at others. **Cross-referencing** files with cards that direct staff to proper files can help address such variations. In the case of Morris-Davidson, for example, the patient's original medical record would be filed under the correct full name of Morris-Davidson and a blank patient file, labeled with the name's other combinations, would be filed under Morris and Davidson. Under this system, if the patient called

and identified herself as "Mrs. Ann Davidson," the medical assistant would look in the "Davidson" file and find a blank file that said "Ann Morris-Davidson's file is under Morris-Davidson."

Shingling Items for Medical Records

Many medical offices file such small items in patients' medical records as written telephone messages or half-size sheets containing patient progress notes. To keep these small items from

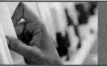

PROCEDURE 10-4 File Manually Using a Subject Filing System

Theory and Rationale

Medical facilities will often keep documents relating to various diseases or illnesses on file in the office. These documents may be given to patients as part of the education process.

Materials

- Documents to be filed by subject
- Alphabetic card file
- Index card listing subjects

Competency

(**Conditions**) With the necessary materials, you will be able to (**Task**) file manually using a subject filing system (**Standards**) correctly within the time limit set by the instructor.

1. Organize the documents by subject matter.
2. Match the subject of the document to the appropriate category on the index cards.
3. Underline the subject title on the document.
4. File the document under the appropriate category.
5. If the document fits into more than one category, create an index card as a cross-reference listing the name of the document and the category under which it is filed.

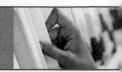

PROCEDURE 10-5   File Documents in Patient Medical Records

Theory and Rationale

A patient's medical record expands as new documents, test results, and consultations from other health care facilities are added to it. Often, the administrative medical assistant is responsible for filing documents in patients' medical records.

Materials

- Patient medical record
- Documents to be filed
- Two-hole punch

Competency

(**Conditions**) With the necessary materials, you will be able to (**Task**) file documents into a patient medical record (**Standards**) correctly within the time limit set by the instructor.

1. Using the two-hole punch, punch holes in the top of each document to be filed.
2. Verify that the physician has viewed any report to be filed (e.g., laboratory or pathology report) by locating the physician's initials on the report.
3. Verify that the patient file matches the name on the documents to be filed.
4. Using the metal clips in the file, place the documents in the patient medical record with the most recent documents on top.
5. Fasten the metal clips.

---

being lost in the records, offices employ **shingling,** which is the process of simply taping the small items to an 8½″ × 11″ sheet of paper and then filing the paper in the patient's chart (Figure 10-8 ◆).

Numeric Filing

Some patient files, such as those in offices devoted to HIV or AIDS–related care, mental health, pregnancy or family planning, or alcohol and drug rehabilitation, may demand a higher

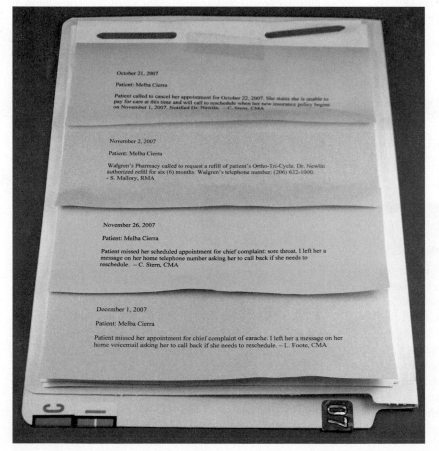

Figure 10-8 ◆ Sample shingled chart note.

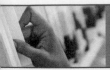

PROCEDURE 10-6 Use the Numeric System to File Medical Records

Theory and Rationale

Some medical facilities use the numeric method for filing patient medical record files. These facilities are typically ones where the patient medical information is considered of a highly sensitive nature. The medical assistant must pay close attention to detail and be certain files are filed accurately in order to assure the file will be easily found when needed.

Materials

- Patient medical records
- Color-coded numeric file stickers

Competency

(**Conditions**) With the necessary materials, you will be able to (**Task**) use the numeric system to file medical records

(**Standards**) correctly within the time limit set by the instructor.

1. Using the color-coded numeric file stickers, attach the first two numbers of the patient's medical record number to the patient's medical record.
2. After verifying that the patient's numeric identification number is accurately recorded on a master sheet kept away from the patient files, organize the records in numerical order.
3. File the medical records in numerical order into the medical records filing cabinet.

---

level of security. Numeric filing is often used in these types of offices. Because the numeric system masks the identity of patients, it is difficult to retrieve filed information without the proper number. In offices that file with numeric systems, lists of patient names and corresponding numbers must be kept in a secure location for the systems to work.

File Storage Systems

Most medical office filing systems consist of metal cabinets that hold paper patient charts in alphabetical order. Old-style filing cabinets were designed in a tower shape, with drawers that pulled out to reveal the files within. Other styles of freestanding filing cabinets have drawers that pull out to reveal the sides of files. These cabinets are useful for identifying files by their color-coded alphabetic or numeric tabs (Figure 10-9 ◆).

Large medical offices often require large file storage systems. These offices use filing systems that allow the entire filing cabinet to move to access files (Figure 10-10 ◆). These types of filing systems take up less space than stationary models and are ideal for large facilities that must accommodate large numbers of paper files.

Keys to Success
MISFILED MEDICAL INFORMATION

When medical records are misplaced, look first under the patients' first names instead of their last. When the file for Krystle Shawger is not filed under "S" for "Shawger," for example, look under "K" for Krystle. If the file is not there, next determine when Krystle was last in the office. Identify the other patients who were in the office at the same time, and determine if Krystle's file was accidentally filed with one of those patient's files. Apply the same method to misfiled medical information. If, for example, Krystle's lab results are missing, check the files of patients who had lab work around the same time.

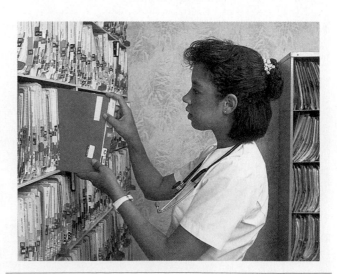

Figure 10-9 ◆ A medical office filing system.

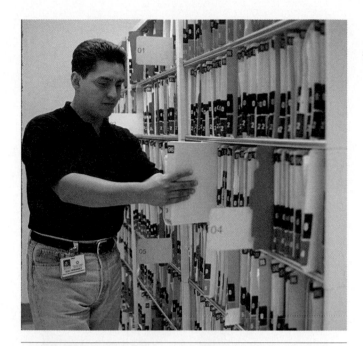

Figure 10-10 ◆ A space-saving filing system allows the user to move the entire cabinet to access files.

Active, Inactive, and Closed Patient Files

Paper medical charts take up a lot of space, especially in large offices or offices where physicians have been in practice for long periods. Keeping all patient charts in the same filing system can be overwhelming and increases the time it takes to find patients' files. For these reasons, many clinics **purge** inactive or closed patient files. This process entails moving medical files to other locations or perhaps scanning the documents in the files and then digitally storing the data on microfilm, microfiche, CD, DVD, or other electronic storage system. Once this process is done, the paper medical records can be destroyed. To purge properly, however, a clear policy on what constitutes a closed or inactive file must be written.

Most offices would agree that files for patients who actively have appointments or who have been in to see the physician recently are considered **active patient files. Inactive patient files** are normally those for patients who have not been in to see the physician for a period between 2 and 5 years depending on the type of practice, the number of files the practice must store, and the office policy. Removing inactive patient files leaves room for new patient files and makes it easier to find active patient files.

The term "closed" is normally reserved for the files of patients who have moved and will not be continuing to treat with the physician or facility. It is also used to describe files for patients who are deceased or files for patients who have stated they will be discontinuing treatment in that facility. **Closed patient files** are normally moved to other storage systems, leaving the space available for active patient files. Patient files fluctuate among active, inactive, and closed status. A file that is considered active today may be closed tomorrow if the patient contacts the office to report an out-of-state move. That same file may return to active status if the patient moves back and resumes care in the medical office.

Converting Paper Records to Electronic Storage

Paper records can be converted to an electronic format for long-term storage. When this happens, the paper records are typically no longer needed. Paper records that are no longer needed must be destroyed so their information cannot be related to patients. Typically, paper records are shredded after copying or scanning (Figure 10-11 ◆). All medical offices should have paper shredders to destroy confidential information. Shredding companies can complete large projects. Such companies will shred documents and provide certifying notices to the medical office.

Retaining Medical Records

State and federal regulations dictate how long medical records must be kept. To comply with those regulations, medical assistants should know the **statute of limitations** in the state where they practice and help their offices keep medical records at least as long as those statutes require. Patients can bring malpractice lawsuits during the statute of limitations, which typically begins when the injury occurs. In many states, however, the discovery rule can greatly alter the statute of limitations. The discovery rule states that the statute of limitations starts on the day the injury was discovered or should have been discovered. Take a patient who has had surgery during which the surgeon leaves a surgical sponge in the surgical site. This patient may fail to realize

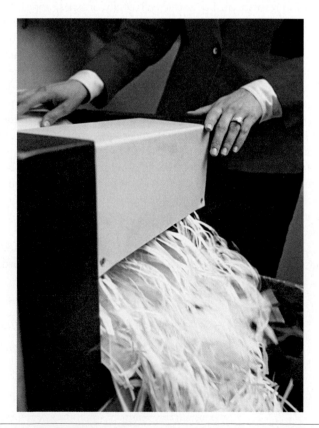

Figure 10-11 ◆ Using a paper shredder ensures patient confidentiality.

the medical error for some time. In states where the discovery rule applies, the statute of limitations would begin when the injury, the sponge in this case, is discovered, even if it is many years later. This rule can also apply to minors by beginning the statute of limitations on the day the minor child turns 18. ∞ Chapter 4 lists the statutes of limitations for each state.

Medicare guidelines state that medical records must be retained for at least 5 years. Because the statute of limitations may exceed 5 years in some states, and because medical records are an extremely important part of defending any claim of medical negligence, it is a good idea to keep medical records for as long as possible. Once an office is out of room for storing medical record files, records can be scanned and kept on CDs, DVDs, microfilm, or any other safe electronic format. In all forms, medical records must be stored in a secure environment, safe from any water or fire damage, and easily accessible by the health care team as needed.

HIPAA Compliance

HIPAA states that medical records must be kept confidential. A record can only be disclosed with a patient's consent or a court order. When it is determined appropriate to destroy a medical record, HIPAA dictates that the record must be shredded beyond recognition. It cannot be in a condition such that it can be put back together to reveal personal patient information.

Correcting Medical Records

Medical records must be corrected lawfully, or it may appear the medical office is trying to conceal an error in patient care. When errors do happen, they must be corrected as soon as possible. The correct way to address an error is to draw one line through the error, initial and date the correction, and write the correct information above or beside the inserted line (Figure 10-12 ◆).

When an error is an entire line or several lines in the patient chart, the entire portion of the entry that is in error should be struck with a line. When an entire entry is in error, which can happen if the medical assistant accidentally charts in the wrong patient's chart, the assistant should draw a line through the entire entry, make a notation such as "wrong patient's chart," and include the date and the medical assistant's initials and credentials. Only the person who made the error should correct the medical chart (Figure 10-13 ◆).

Errors in medical charts should never be **obliterated**, scribbled out, or covered with correction fluid, because records

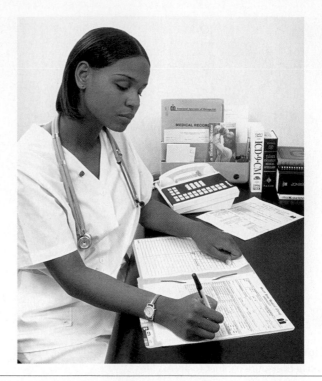

Figure 10-13 ◆ The medical assistant must chart accurately.

with such effects are viewed as attempts to hide the truth or cover wrongdoing. One line through an incorrect entry leaves no doubt as to the information being corrected.

?—Critical Thinking Question 10-3—

Imagine that the medical office has decided to discontinue notes like "Problem" on patient charts. How should the office go about removing such notes from patient files?

Adding to Medical Records

When an error in a medical chart is one of omission, information may be added to the medical record after the fact by beginning the entry with the date the addition is being added, followed by the words "Late Entry," the date of the visit the late entry pertains to, the notes that were originally omitted, and the signature of the person making the entry. When a correc-

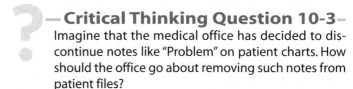

Figure 10-12 ◆ Sample correction of a charting error.

TABLE 10-1 ADDITIONS TO THE MEDICAL RECORD

Addition Type	Example
Late entry	Oct. 3, 2007 LATE ENTRY for Sept. 25, 2007: Patient stated she was unable to fill her prescription due to cost. *S. Nguyen*, CMA
Addendum	Oct. 2, 2007 ADDENDUM for Sept. 25, 2007: Ms. Manfredo stated she had been involved in an automobile accident on Sept. 24, 2007. She was seen in the emergency room of Brattleboro Community Hospital. Ms. Manfredo stated, "The pain in my right arm was so bad I could not put on my jacket." *S. Nguyen*, CMA

tion exceeds the space where the error is, the medical assistant can insert an addendum to the medical record. This insertion should read "ADDENDUM to [date of the visit]" just before the entry. The use of all capitals is significant in such entries. Table 10-1 provides examples.

Charting Conflicting Orders

Every member of the health care team is obligated to take reasonable action to ensure patient safety. Medical assistants should follow no orders they feel may harm patients. Instead, they should consult the physicians out of patients' hearing range. When physicians insist that their orders be followed according to their instructions and they explain why the orders will not cause patient injury, the medical assistants should chart the

events, including the fact that they questioned the doctor as to the accuracy of the orders. They should also include the physicians' responses.

"Owning" the Medical Record

Medical records belong to the physicians or facilities where they are created. The information inside, however, belongs to the patients. Patients have a right to access their medical records and to correct those records when they feel errors have been made. Patients should not, however, be left alone to peruse their chart. When patients request corrections to their medical records, the health care team must determine whether errors exist. If the physician agrees an error has been made, the correction should be made as described earlier in this chapter. If the physician feels the entry was not in error, the physician cannot be forced to treat the entry as an error. In this case, patients must be allowed to create their own version of the event, and copies of those written statements must be placed in the medical records (Figure 10-14 ◆). Such statements become permanent parts of the patients' medical records.

Documenting Prescription Refill Requests

Pharmacies call in prescription refill requests to the medical office. Each medical office should have a policy that requires at least 24 hours for refill requests so physicians have time to review patients' files.

When a pharmacy calls with a prescription request, the medical assistant must pull the patient's file and place the request and patient file on the physician's desk for review. If the physician feels the patient should be seen in the office before a prescription refill, the medical assistant should first call the pharmacy to notify them of the physician's request and then

---

PROCEDURE 10-7 Correct Errors in the Patient Medical Record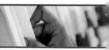

Theory and Rationale
Medical assistants regularly make notations and entries in patients' medical records. When assistants make errors, they must follow legal protocol to correct those errors.

Materials
■ Patient medical record
■ Blue or black ink pen

Competency
(**Conditions**) With the necessary materials, you will be able to (**Task**) correct an error in the patient medical record

(**Standards**) correctly within the time limit set by the instructor.

1. Locate the error in the patient's medical record.
2. Draw a straight line through the error.
3. Initial and place the date above the line.
4. When the corrected entry will fit above the line, write the correction there. Include the date of the new entry and your initials. When the corrected entry will not fit above the line, add a new entry to the progress notes with the day's date and the word "ADDENDUM" in all capitals. Include the date of the addendum, enter the corrected entry, and initial the entry.

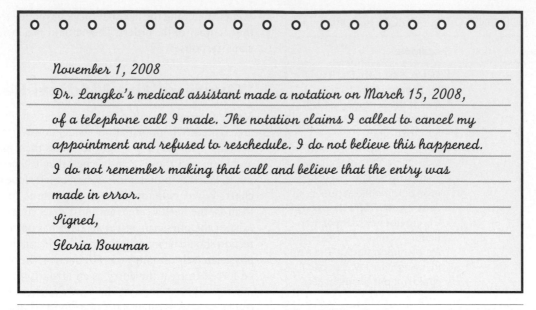

November 1, 2008

Dr. Langko's medical assistant made a notation on March 15, 2008, of a telephone call I made. The notation claims I called to cancel my appointment and refused to reschedule. I do not believe this happened. I do not remember making that call and believe that the entry was made in error.

Signed,

Gloria Bowman

Figure 10-14 ◆ Sample addition to the medical record from the patient.

call the patient to schedule an appointment. If the physician authorizes the refill request, the medical assistant should call the pharmacy back with the appropriate information. All information about the refill request, authorized or not, must be charted in the patient's medical record. ∞ Chapter 7 lists the steps to calling in and charting prescription refills.

Releasing Medical Records

Requests for copies of the patient's medical record are common. These requests may come from insurance companies, other health care facilities, or from the patient. Any request for copies of the patient's medical record must be accompanied by a signed authorization from the patient or a court order.

Copies of the medical record cannot be released to anyone, including the patient's spouse, without the patient's consent. HIPAA legislation allows for the medical facility to obtain a signature from the patient allowing the medical office to discuss the patient's care with anyone listed on the list. Frequently, patients will use this form to indicate they wish to have their spouse or adult child be given access to the patient's medical record.

When copies of the chart are needed right away, some insurance companies or other entities may request the copies be faxed. It is important to note that faxing personal patient information should never be done unless it is absolutely necessary as use of the fax in this manner is not considered

to be an appropriate way to safeguard patient confidential information.

Releasing Information When a Medical Practice Closes

When a medical practice closes and no other facility takes responsibility for the patient's medical records, notices must be sent to all patients with medical files at the facility. Such notices should give patients a reasonable timeline within which to contact the office to request file transfers. Whether transfer requests are made or not, the physician or the physician's estate will be responsible for the original files for the period outlined by the state's statute of limitations.

Conducting Research with Medical Records

When patients participate in **medical research programs,** their medical records must be kept indefinitely. If adverse affects arise, even in other generations, the medical office must be able to prove the physician had the patient's consent to participate in the research. Medical research involves patients taking experimental medication or patients involved in **nontherapeutic research**.

In nontherapeutic research, a pharmaceutical company develops a new drug to combat a certain disease or disorder. Before that company can market the drug, however, it must receive approval from the Food and Drug Administration (**FDA**). The FDA requires extensive testing before drugs are considered safe and effective enough to be released. Part of FDA testing usually includes a nontherapeutic research trial in which companies pay physicians to dispense the drug to healthy patients who do not have the disease or disorder the drug is targeting so as to identify any side effects. Patients in these types of research programs must be fully aware of the risks and must sign consent forms to that effect.

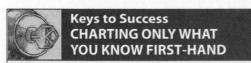
Keys to Success
CHARTING ONLY WHAT YOU KNOW FIRST-HAND

Make entries to patient charts only after direct contract with patients. Do not chart what is shared or requested by other members of the health care team.

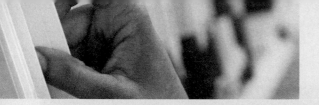

REVIEW

Chapter Summary

- Medical records are an integral piece in the health care process, so it is crucial that they are complete, accurate, and effective.
- Medical offices should have systems in place to find missing files.
- Color-coded filing systems are one efficient way for offices to find patient information.
- Offices desiring a high level of security might choose a numeric filing system, as it masks patient identity.

- Depending on their size and intent, medical offices may choose varying file storage systems.
- Patient files fluctuate between active, inactive, and closed status as patients traverse the health care system.
- Medical offices should correct errors in patient charts according to accepted protocol.

Chapter Review

Multiple Choice

1. Which of the following is NOT one of the four types of patient information contained in medical records?
   a. Personal information
   b. Social information
   c. Geographic information
   d. Social information

2. Which of the following describes the patient's chief complaint?
   a. The main reason the patient is seeking care that day
   b. The most significant finding on the patient's exam
   c. The highest level diagnosis code assigned to the patient
   d. The most noticeable symptom the patient has

3. Which of the following describes a reason why a "late entry" might be made in a patient's chart?
   a. The medical assistant realizes he forgot to add a relevant fact into the patient's medical chart. He makes that entry the following day.
   b. The patient asks the medical assistant to make a correction in the medical record.
   c. The medical assistant realizes she has charted something in the wrong patient's file.
   d. The medical assistant doesn't chart in the patient's chart until the end of her shift.

4. Which of the following type of medical record keeping is the oldest form of medical charting?
   a. SOAP format
   b. POMR
   c. Narrative style
   d. None of the above

True/False

T F 1. Flow charts are used to note patients' progress relative to others in the population.
T F 2. Numeric filing systems are more secure than alphabetic filing systems.
T F 3. All medical facilities use the same medical abbreviations.
T F 4. Nontherapeutic studies do not benefit the patient/subject.

T F 5. Inactive patient files are typically those patients who have not been in to see the physician for a period of 2 to 5 years.
T F 6. Health care facilities in all states must keep patient medical records on file for the same period of time.
T F 7. The term "closed" patient files typically describes patients who have moved or will not be continuing treatment with the physician or facility.

Short Answer

1. What is the most common reason for a cross-referencing system in the medical office?
2. Medical records should be faxed only under what circumstances?
3. What does the acronym POMR stand for?
4. Describe how a prescription refill request should be handled.
5. What are the "Five Cs" of medical charting?
6. What does the acronym SOAP stand for?
7. What is another term for "electronic medical record (EMR)"?
8. Describe how a late entry should be charted in a patient's medical chart.
9. Outline the steps to take to locate a missing patient chart.

Research

1. Interview a person who works in a medical office. How does that office file patient files? Alphabetically or numerically? How are the files labeled? Are color-coded labels used?
2. Research online for local companies that offer shredding services. How much do they charge for their services? How do they guarantee confidentiality?
3. Look online for companies that sell filing systems to medical offices. What type of systems can you find? What type of system is more expensive?

Externship Application Experience

Sylvia Bissey, a patient of Dr. Borshack's for over 20 years, tells the medical assistant that she would like to get a copy of her husband's current lab results. The medical assistant explains that she will need a signed authorization from Mr. Bissey in order to release the information to his wife. Sylvia becomes upset and says, "I have *always* been given copies of his lab results in the past." How should the medical assistant respond to Sylvia?

Resource Guide

Health Insurance Portability and Accountability Act (HIPAA) Web site
http://www.hhs.gov/ocr/hipaa/

The Institute of Medicine
http://www.iom.edu

iHealth Record Web site
http://www.ihealthrecord.org/

This Web site allows users/consumers to house their medical records online.

Med**Media**

http://www.MyMAKit.com

More on this chapter, including interactive resources, can be found on the Student CD-ROM accompanying this textbook and on http://www.MyMAKit.com.

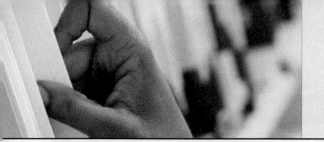

Objectives

After completing this chapter, you should be able to:

- Define and spell the key terminology in this chapter.
- Distinguish between the use of electronic medical records and paper medical records.
- Understand how to convert from paper to electronic medical records.
- Identify the steps to complete an electronic medical record.
- Describe the steps to correct a mistake in the electronic medical record.
- Identify the steps to take to properly destroy a paper medical record after it has been converted to electronic format.
- Understand HIPAA compliance with regard to the use of electronic medical records.
- Describe the use of personal digital assistants with electronic medical records.
- Know the benefits of using electronic medical records.

Electronic Medical Records

Case Study

Walter Reardon is an 80-year-old patient in Dr. Rand's office. Dr. Rand has recently converted his patient files from paper medical records to electronic medical records. David is Dr. Rand's medical assistant. David escorts Mr. Reardon to the examination room and then begins to perform his initial assessment using the electronic medical record he accesses from the computer in the examination room. When he notices this, Mr. Reardon becomes upset, saying he doesn't trust computers and doesn't want his private medical information "out there for everyone to see."

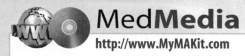

MedMedia
http://www.MyMAKit.com

Additional interactive resources and activities for this chapter can be found on http://www.MyMAKit.com. For a video, tips, audio glossary, legal and ethical scenarios, on-the-job scenarios, quizzes, and games related to the content of this chapter, please access the accompanying CD-ROM in this book.

Video
Legal and Ethical Scenario: *Electronic Medical Records*
On the Job Scenario: *Electronic Medical Records*
Tips
Multiple Choice Quiz
Audio Glossary
HIPAA Quiz
Games: Spelling Bee, Crossword, and Strikeout

Key Terminology

electronic medical records— medical records kept via computer; also called electronic health records

electronic signature— electronic version of a person's signature to be used in electronic medical records (see preceding entry)

indecipherable—unreadable

Abbreviations

EHR—electronic health record

EMR—electronic medical record

HIPAA—Health Insurance Portability and Accountability Act

MEDICAL ASSISTING STANDARDS

CAAHEP ENTRY-LEVEL STANDARDS	ABHES ENTRY-LEVEL COMPETENCIES
■ Organize technical information and summaries (cognitive) ■ Document patient care (cognitive) ■ Document patient education (cognitive) ■ Identify systems for organizing medical records (cognitive) ■ Describe various types of content maintained in a patient's medical record (cognitive) ■ Discuss principles of using Electronic Medical Record (EMR) (cognitive) ■ Identify types of records common to the healthcare setting (cognitive) ■ Discuss the importance of routine maintenance of office equipment (cognitive) ■ Execute data management using electronic healthcare records such as the EMR (psychomotor) ■ Use office hardware and software to maintain office systems (psychomotor) ■ Use Internet to access information related to the medical office (psychomotor) ■ Document accurately in the patient record (psychomotor) ■ Apply HIPAA rules in regard to privacy/release of information (psychomotor)	■ Maintain confidentiality at all times ■ Use appropriate guidelines when releasing records or information ■ Be cognizant of ethical boundaries ■ Evidence a responsible attitude ■ Application of electronic technology ■ Apply computer concepts for office procedures ■ Prepare and maintain medical records

✓ COMPETENCY SKILLS PERFORMANCE

1. Correct an electronic medical record.

Introduction

Electronic medical records, sometimes called electronic health records, are part of health care's future. Although electronic medical records have been around since the Mayo Clinic began using them in the 1960s, the technology has been slow to move into ambulatory care. As today's health care providers strive to make health care safer and allow for efficient team communication, electronic records are playing a more prominent role.

In his 2004 State of the Union address, President George W. Bush stated, "By computerizing health records, we can avoid dangerous medical mistakes, reduce costs, and improve care." Shortly after this speech, President Bush outlined a plan to ensure that most Americans have electronic health records by 2014.

Electronic Medical Records Are Easily Accessible

Electronic medical records are simply the portions of patients' medical records that are kept on a computer's hard drive or a medical office's computer network rather than on paper. While physicians must retrieve paper files from separate and often large rooms, electronic records are easily accessible on a computer. In large offices where patients may see several different providers, electronic medical records allow physicians easily to locate patients' laboratory results, consultations, X-rays, and examination findings from other providers.

Using electronic health records (**EHRs**), medical offices are able to access any one patient's file from more than one networked computer in the office. For example, the billing office might have the patient's medical record open on a computer screen while they are accessing information needed for coding a specific procedure. At the same time, the physician might have the same patient's file open on a separate computer screen while she inputs treatment notes.

Charting patient information, such as telephone calls, is easily done within the electronic medical record. Typically the software will contain a section for adding information, such as telephone calls or personal conversations that are related to the patient's medical care.

Many medical offices have computer terminals in each examination room, allowing the medical personnel to add information to the patient's electronic medical record, download test results, or research past medication records while the patient is in the room. In some offices, the physician or medical assistant uses a portable electronic tablet to enter patient data into the computer system (Figure 11-1 ◆).

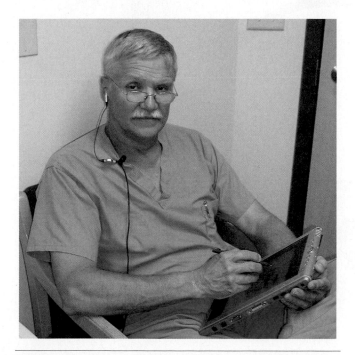

Figure 11-1 ◆ A physician uses a TabletPC to enter patient data while in the examination room.

How Does Paper Charting Differ from Electronic Charting?

With paper charting, the patient's chart is only available to one staff member at a time. The following example illustrates the steps an office using paper charting might take:

1. The patient telephones the medical office and schedules an appointment to see the physician. The receptionist writes down the information the patient gives her, such as the patient's name, address, telephone numbers, insurance information, and the patient's current complaint.
2. Sometime before the patient's appointment, the receptionist or the billing office may call the patient's insurance carrier to verify the patient's benefits.
3. The day before the patient's appointment, the receptionist may call the patient to remind him of his appointment for the next day.
4. The day before the patient's appointment, the receptionist will prepare the new patient's chart. This is typically done by gathering a paper file folder, color-coded labels to identify the patient's last name, and any other paper forms the patient and the medical staff will fill out on that first visit.
5. When the patient arrives for his visit, the receptionist will give the patient the necessary papers to fill out.
6. When the patient is taken back to the examination room, the clinical medical assistant will begin taking vital signs, such as blood pressure, pulse, and temperature, and begin noting this information by writing in the patient's paper medical chart.
7. When the physician sees the patient, she will review the information the patient has filled out along with the information the medical assistant has filled out and begin making notes of her own into the patient's paper chart. If the physician writes a prescription, she will make a note of this in the patient's chart, along with writing the actual prescription on a paper for the patient to take to the pharmacy. In some offices, the physician does not make written notes in the patient's chart and instead dictates her findings into a tape recorder. Those notes will be transcribed by an assistant or a transcription service, then added to the patient's paper chart.
8. If the physician orders X-rays or laboratory tests, the patient's paper chart will be pulled once those reports are returned to the office in order for the physician to review the results along with the patient's chart (Figure 11-2 ◆). Figure 11-3 ◆ shows the workflow in a medical office using paper charts.

In contrast, here are the steps an office using electronic charting might take:

1. A patient calls the office to schedule a new appointment. The receptionist begins an electronic chart while she has the patient on the telephone, adding information about telephone numbers, insurance information, and symptoms into the software program.

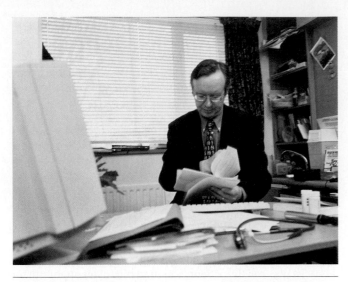

Figure 11-2 ◆ The physician will pull the patient's paper charts to review the results of tests alongside the patient's chart.

2. Sometime before the patient's appointment, the software may be programmed to confirm electronically the patient's health insurance coverage.
3. The day before the patient's appointment, the software may be programmed to call and remind the patient of his appointment the next day. If not, it may send a reminder for office personnel to make this phone call.
4. When the patient arrives in the office, he may be escorted to an examination room, where a medical assistant will fill out the patient information form on the computer while the patient is present to answer any questions.
5. The medical assistant will then take the patient's vital signs, entering all gathered information into the electronic medical record as she goes.
6. When the physician comes into the room, he will review the patient's information in the electronic medical record and make his own notes there while interviewing and

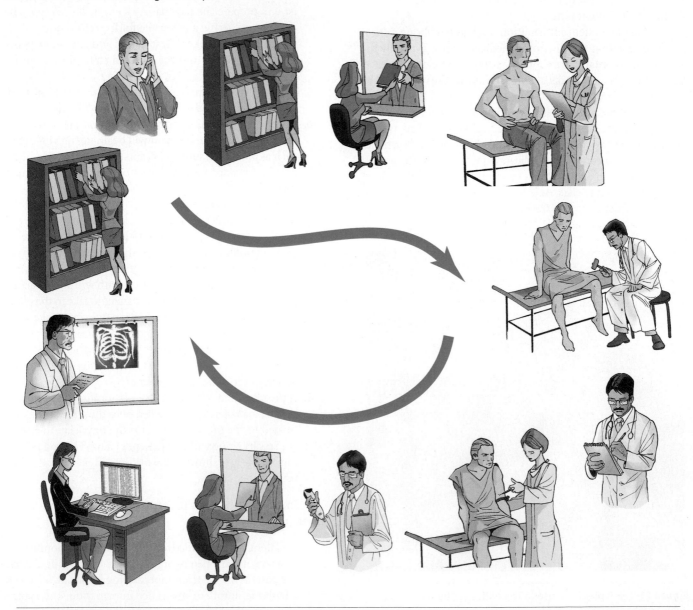

Figure 11-3 ◆ Workflow in a medical office using paper charts.

examining the patient. If a prescription is written, the physician will fill this information out in the electronic medical record, including faxing the prescription to the pharmacy the patient chooses. If any laboratory work or X-rays are ordered, the physician or medical assistant will fill this out within the electronic medical record. If the physician wishes to give the patient any educational materials, such as information on reducing cholesterol, this information may be quickly printed from within the computer system, including making a notation within the patient's electronic medical record that the information was given.

7. If laboratory work or X-rays were ordered, the physician will need only to review the patient's electronic medical record on the computer, which may be done from any computer terminal within the clinic (Figure 11-4 ◆). Figure 11-5 ◆ shows the workflow in a medical office using electronic medical records.

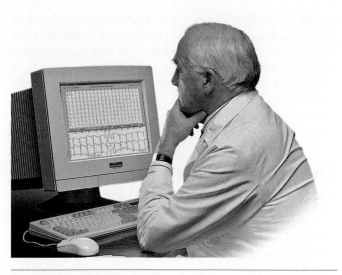

Figure 11-4 ◆ A physician uses a computer to access a patient's electronic medical record.

IQ mark™ Advanced Holter. Courtesy of Midmark Diagnostic Group.

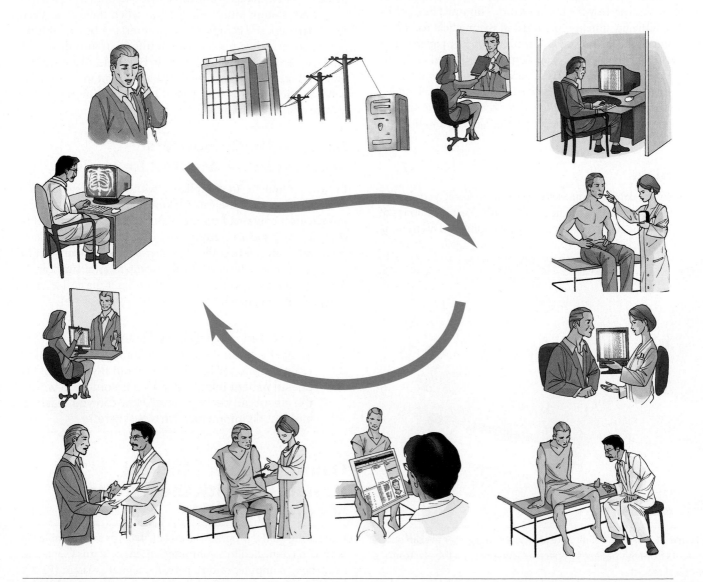

Figure 11-5 ◆ Workflow in a medical office using electronic medical records.

Making the Conversion from Paper to Electronic Medical Records

Though many health care providers and clinical support staff find that the process of changing from paper to electronic medical records format is time consuming, most would agree that once the **EMR** have been implemented, using the computer rather than writing in the patient's chart by hand saves a great deal of time.

The conversion from paper to electronic medical record format is typically done over a period of time. Some clinics are able to use a scanner to scan documents from the patient's paper medical record to the electronic record. Other clinics may need to enter information from the paper chart to the electronic record manually. The process depends on the type of electronic medical record software being used and the preferences of the medical staff (Figure 11-6 ◆).

Once the information from the paper medical record has been transferred to the electronic medical record, the clinic staff may choose to destroy the paper record. This must be done by shredding the documents contained in the medical record. In some offices, the staff chooses to simply store the paper record in a secure location rather than destroy the file. When documents such as written reports or consultations from other facilities come into the office, these documents are typically added to the electronic medical record using a scanner. If the original document is no longer needed, it can be shredded in order to protect patient privacy.

Training

Any software company that sells electronic medical records software should supply the medical office with a certain amount of training for the staff to learn to use the equipment. This training

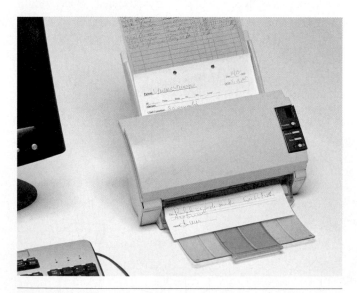

Figure 11-6 ◆ Some clinics are able to use a scanner to scan documents from the patient's paper medical record to the electronic medical record.
ImpactMD Document Scanner. Courtesy of Allscripts LLC.

should be attended by anyone within the office who will be using the software, including the physicians. In addition, a training manual should be supplied for use in training future staff members. Software companies that sell electronic medical record software should also supply the office with contact information to reach a technical support person in the event a question or concern with the new software should arise within the medical clinic.

Electronic Health Records and HIPAA Compliance

Just as with paper medical records, electronic medical records must be kept private. In order to assure patient privacy and compliance with **HIPAA** legislation, all computer users must have their own password to access the patient medical records. With each person having login information, the software can track each entry or deletion and who made it. With paper records, it is not always obvious who last had a record and who made the latest changes if the user is not identified.

Each station must be logged off when the user is away from their desk and computer screens must not be viewable by other patients while private patient information is displayed on the screen. Given the regulations in HIPAA legislation, computerized medical records are just as safe, if not more so, than paper medical records with regard to possible improper disclosure of information.

Backing Up Computers and Electronic Medical Records

In order to remain in compliance with HIPAA regulations, medical offices must use data backup systems to safeguard the information contained on the office computer systems, including patient medical records. This is typically done on a daily basis and in most offices the computer backup system is set to work automatically. By having daily backup files, the medical office will not likely lose computer data, even if the entire computer system goes down.

?—Critical Thinking Question 11-1—
Recall the case study at the beginning of this chapter. What can you tell Mr. Reardon about the safety of his private patient information as it is contained within the electronic health record? How can you reassure him that his information isn't "out there"?

Using Personal Digital Assistants with Electronic Medical Records

Depending on the program, electronic records are available via keyboard connected to a computer system or stylus tapped on a notebook computer or on a personal digital assistant (PDA). These devices have many of the same functions as a full-size computer and have the added benefit of being small enough for physicians to carry with them from patient to patient. Most electronic medical records systems can be configured to work according to an office's specific needs. Figure 11-7 ◆ lists the functions many of these systems provide. One of the many benefits of such systems is the ability to access medical record information from many locations in the health care facility and to quickly search for and retrieve information in the patient's medical record (Figure 11-8 ◆).

In Practice

Dr. Jonas runs a private practice and makes rounds in two local hospitals. He uses one type of electronic medical records software in his private office and two other packages in the two hospitals. Not only must Dr. Jonas learn three software systems, he may at times be unable to move patient information between those systems due to incompatibility. What might Dr. Jonas do to address these issues?

Other Benefits of Electronic Medical Records

There are additional benefits to using electronic medical records, which are discussed in the following sections.

Electronic Signatures

An office that uses **electronic medical records** may use an **electronic signature.** In offices where medical notes are dictated and printed for patient files, an electronic signature or

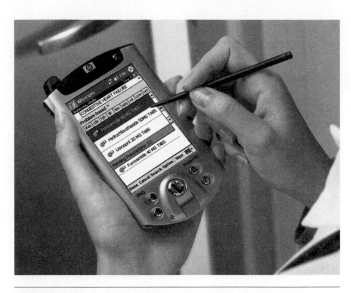

Figure 11-8 ◆ A handheld PDA.
Courtesy of Allscripts LLC.

rubber-stamp signature may replace handwritten signatures. In these offices, there must be a permanent record of the signer, as well as an original version of the signature on file.

Avoiding Medical Mistakes

Electronic medical records can be used to alert health care providers to possible medication reactions. This is especially helpful when treating patients who are cotreating with several specialists. The EMR software will typically have a safeguard mechanism built in that alerts the prescribing physician to any contraindicated medications a particular patient may have (Figure 11-9 ◆).

One of the most convincing arguments for converting paper medical records to an electronic format is based on patient safety. In 1999, the Institute of Medicine published a report called "To Err Is Human: Building a Safer Health System." This report stated, "At least 44,000 people, and perhaps as many

---

❑ Time-stamp recordings in the EMR/EHR

❑ Prescriptions printed or faxed to the pharmacy

❑ Printed patient education information that directly relates to the patient's care

❑ Search for a certain type of condition or certain age or geographic location of a group of patients

❑ Digital photos or X-rays attached in the patient's EMR/EHR

❑ Electronically ordered lab results, imaging items, or medical tests

❑ Electronic graphs of lab results of height, weight, or blood pressure data

❑ Letters to or about patients

❑ Electronic data transmission to other health care providers

Figure 11-7 ◆ Functions of an EMR/EHR.

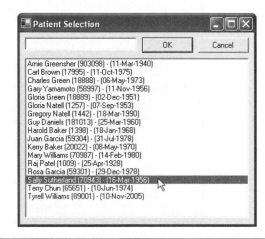

Figure 11-9 ◆ Selecting the right patient is easy with electronic medical records.
Courtesy of Medcin.

as 98,000 people, die in hospitals every year as a result of medical errors that could have been prevented." One of the Institute's recommendations was to move to electronic medical records. Their conclusions suggested that some medical errors are caused by **indecipherable** handwriting, a problem that would be eliminated if providers made their entries electronically rather than in handwritten form.

Some states have enacted legislation to address the issue of illegible handwriting and medical errors. In March 2006, Washington State passed a law that requires all prescriptions written by physicians to be submitted electronically to pharmacists or to be printed rather than written in cursive.

?—Critical Thinking Question 11-2—

Recall the case study at the beginning of this chapter. What might you say to Mr. Reardon to convince him the change from paper to electronic medical records is in his best interest?

Saving Time

The time saved by electronic medical records may be better invested in patient care. Many health care providers believe they spend a great deal of time charting, far more time than they spend on actual patient care. With the cost of health care rising, it makes sense to free up the health care provider's time while decreasing avoidable patient injuries (Figure 11-10 ◆).

Most electronic medical records programs have "drop-down menus" that allow the user to choose information or symptoms from a preprogrammed list. For example, when the user inserts a diagnosis of "diabetes," the software may display a list of possible symptoms the patient may be having, such as excessive thirst or frequent urination. Many EMR programs also include lists of possible diagnoses for the physician to choose from based on the symptoms the patient lists. For example, if the patient complains of excessive thirst and frequent urination, the program may offer "diabetes" as a possible diagnosis for the physician to choose from.

Electronic medical records allow medical staff easily to transmit patient information to patients' health insurance companies when requested, rather than having to photocopy the paper records and send them via the postal service. It is just as important to follow HIPAA guidelines for releasing medical records electronically as it is for releasing photocopies of the patient's paper medical record.

Health Maintenance

Many medical offices send reminder cards or letters to patients regarding the need for upcoming services. These are typically used to remind patients of the need for a dental exam, a mammogram, a yearly physical, immunizations, or well child checkups. Using electronic medical records, the administrative medical assistant can ask the software program to print these reminders.

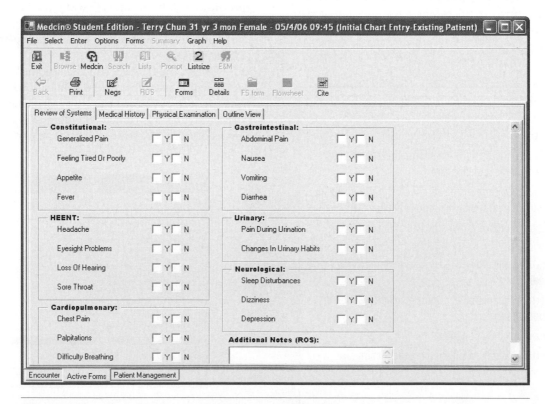

Figure 11-10 ◆ An intake screen in an electronic medical record.
Courtesy of Medcin.

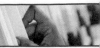

PROCEDURE 11-1 Correct an Electronic Medical Record

Theory and Rationale

As with a paper medical record, mistakes may be made within an electronic medical record. The medical assistant must be aware of how to make appropriate corrections to the electronic medical record in an accurate manner. Corrections must be made in an accurate manner to avoid lawsuits or other legal issues.

Materials

■ Computer with electronic patient medical record

Competency

(**Conditions**) With the necessary materials, you will be able to (**Task**) correct an electronic medical record (**Standards**) correctly within the time limit set by the instructor.

1. Identify the correct patient electronic medical record where the error was made.
2. Locate the error within the record.
3. Using the rules associated with the software you are using, make the appropriate correction within the medical record.
4. Sign off on the changes as necessary, according to the steps required within the software program.
5. Verify that the change is correct before closing the patient's electronic medical record.

Using Electronic Medical Records with Diagnostic Equipment

With electronic medical records software, the medical office is able to perform many tests in the office and have the results show immediately within the electronic medical record. This can also be done with digital X-rays, Holter monitors, spirometers, and a number of laboratory tests on blood and urine samples (Figure 11-11 ◆).

?—Critical Thinking Question 11-3—

Referring back to the case study at the beginning of the chapter, what sort of health maintenance reminders do you think a patient such as Mr. Reardon might benefit from receiving?

Marketing Purposes

Many medical clinics send informational flyers to patients on a regular basis. An example would be a flyer that is sent during flu season and describes the signs and symptoms of the flu along with prevention tips. Part of the prevention tips would be to encourage readers to come into the physician's office for a flu vaccine.

With electronic medical records, the administrative staff is also able to create a list of patients according to specific parameters. For example, if the office has recently welcomed a physician who specializes in allergies to the office, the administrative staff can create a list of patients who have been treated for allergies and use that list to send a letter to patients to let them know of the availability of the new physician.

Communicating Between Staff Members

There are times in the medical office when one member of the staff needs to communicate with another staff member about a particular patient. An example would be a patient who has an outstanding balance owing in the medical office. The billing staff member may need to see the patient when he comes into the office for his visit with the physician. Using the electronic medical record, the billing staff member can post an alert that will be seen by the receptionist when she checks the patient in. The alert allows the billing staff member to have the receptionist direct the patient to the billing office prior to his visit with the physician.

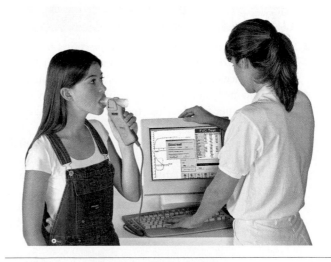

Figure 11-11 ◆ A medical assistant performs a spirometry test using electronic medical record software.
Courtesy of Midmark Diagnostic Group.

Putting Medical Records Online

Some clinics, like Group Health in Washington State, allow patients to look up portions of their electronic medical records via the Internet. Using this password-protected system, patients can access a company's network or intranet for their lab results, dates of immunizations, or medication levels, which can help when patients travel or need to seek emergency care with someone other than their primary care provider. Several Internet-based businesses now offer individuals online storage of medical information, such as immunizations, medications, and surgeries.

—Critical Thinking Question 11-4—
Recall the case study at the beginning of this chapter. Do you think you could convince Mr. Reardon that having access to his medical records online might be helpful to him?

Making Corrections in the Electronic Medical Record

Just as with paper medical records, medical staff entering data into the electronic medical record may make mistakes in their entries. When this happens, the mistake must be corrected as soon as possible. With electronic health records, the steps to take to make the correction will depend upon the software. Most often, the user will make the correction by crossing out the error and entering the correct information. The original entry will still be viewable, though it may show on a separate screen or it may show as having a line drawn through the entry (Figure 11-12 ◆).

Patient complains of ~~right~~ left leg pain.

Figure 11-12 ◆ Mistakes in the electronic medical record must be corrected as soon as possible. Most often, the user will cross out the error and enter the correct information, as shown in this example.

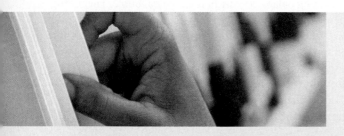

REVIEW

Chapter Summary

- Electronic medical records are the portions of a patient's medical record that are kept on a computer's hard drive or a medical office's computer network rather than on paper.
- Electronic medical records are gaining popularity over conventional paper files because they offer enhanced ease, efficiency, and accessibility.
- With paper charting, the patient's chart is only available to one staff member at a time. Electronic medical records make the patient's chart available to many healthcare team members at the same time.
- The conversion from paper to electronic medical record format is typically done over time. Once paper medical records

are converted to electronic versions, those paper records must be appropriately destroyed.
- Medical offices should correct errors in a patient chart according to accepted protocol.
- By using electronic medical records, a medical office is able to perform tasks such as sending reminder post cards more easily than performing these same tasks with paper medical records.
- Other benefits of electronic medical records include using electronic signatures, avoiding medical mistakes, saving time, and communicating between staff members.

Chapter Review

Multiple Choice

1. A PDA is often used in the medical office. What does PDA stand for?
   a. Professional desk assistant
   b. Personal digital assistant
   c. Progressive digital assistant
   d. None of the above

2. Which of the following is a reason the medical office would send post card reminders to patients?
   a. Yearly physical examination
   b. Mammogram
   c. Immunizations
   d. All of the above

3. Using EMR, the medical staff will typically be able to do which of the following?
   a. Locate possible contraindications with prescribed medications
   b. Allow two or more staff members to access the same patient file at the same time
   c. Fax medical records to other medical offices
   d. All of the above

4. Which of the following is a reason a patient may want to access their own medical records on line?
   a. View their current medications
   b. View the date of their vaccination
   c. Read a current lab report
   d. All of the above

True/False

T F   1. Electronic medical records do not have to comply with HIPAA regulations.

T F   2. Electronic medical records are the same thing as electronic health records.

T F   3. Converting from paper to electronic medical records is a quick and easy process.

T F   4. Correcting charting errors in an electronic medical record is much the same as correcting an error in a paper chart.

T F   5. Electronic medical records allow one staff member to communicate with another staff member via electronic notes.

T F   6. Using PDAs, physicians can transfer data about their patients from one computer system to another.

Short Answer

1. Explain how the use of EMR can help to avoid medication prescription errors.

2. Why would it be important for all staff members, even those with extensive computer experience, to attend a training session for new electronic medical records software?

3. Explain how a medical office might enter a letter from an outside medical facility into a patient's electronic medical record.

4. How would a medical office use the information contained within their electronic medical records software for marketing purposes?

5. Who is quoted as saying "By computerizing health records, we can avoid dangerous medical mistakes, reduce costs, and improve care"?

6. Explain how an electronic signature is used.

7. What is a drop-down menu?

8. How would using electronic medical records save time over using paper medical records?

9. What was the first medical clinic to begin using electronic medical records?

10. Why should a medical office shred papers that contain patient information once those records have been entered into an electronic format?

Research

1. Interview a person who works in a medical office that is using electronic medical records. How does that person feel about working with the electronic medical record as opposed to using paper records?

2. Research the various personal digital assistants (PDAs) that are available for medical personnel to purchase. What kinds of features do they offer?

3. Search the Internet for companies that offer an electronic medical record. How do the services offered compare?

Externship Application Experience

Dr. Shelley Fredrich is a physician working in a busy family practice clinic. When the office begins the conversion from paper to electronic medical records, Dr. Fredrich says she does not think she needs to attend the orientation and training session scheduled for the remainder of the staff. She believes that she is "computer-savvy" and that the training session will be a waste of her time. How could Dr. Fredrich be convinced to attend the training session?

Resource Guide

Epic (a computerized electronic health record system)
1979 Milky Way
Verona, WI 53593
Phone: (608) 271-9000
Fax: (608) 271-7237
http://www.epicsystems.com

Health Insurance Portability and Accountability Act (HIPAA) Web site
http://www.hhs.gov/ocr/hipaa/

The Institute of Medicine
http://www.iom.edu

Medical Records Institute
425 Boylston Street, 4th Floor
Boston, MA 02116-3315
Phone: (617) 964-3923
Fax: (617) 964-3926
http://www.medrecinst.com/

PowerMed (a computerized electronic health record system)
48 Free Street
Portland, Maine 04101
Phone: (207) 772-3920
Fax: (207) 772-3281
http://www.powermed.com/

 MedMedia

http://www.MyMAKit.com

More on this chapter, including interactive resources, can be found on the Student CD-ROM accompanying this textbook and on http://www.MyMAKit.com.

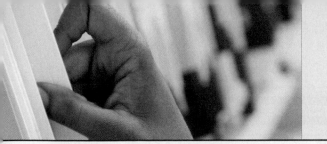

Objectives

After completing this chapter, you should be able to:

- Define and spell the key terminology in this chapter.
- Describe the functions and uses of computers in the medical office.
- List the steps to researching the purchase of a new computer system.
- Name the components of a computer system.
- Explain how properly to maintain computer equipment.
- Describe ways to secure office computers.
- Use the Internet to search for information.
- Create a policy for personal computer use in the office.
- Describe a personal digital assistant and how it works with computers.
- Explain the basic principles of computer ergonomics.

Computers in the Medical Office

Case Study

D r. Crates has asked the medical assistant to research options for adding a new computer terminal to the office. The physician wants to ensure that the chosen system can run all the latest software in addition to the practice management and electronic health record software used in the office.

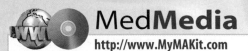

MedMedia
http://www.MyMAKit.com

Additional interactive resources and activities for this chapter can be found on http://www.MyMAKit.com. For a video, tips, audio glossary, legal and ethical scenarios, on-the-job scenarios, quizzes, and games related to the content of this chapter, please access the accompanying CD-ROM in this book.

Video
Legal and Ethical Scenario: *Computers in the Medical Office*
On the Job Scenario: *Computers in the Medical Office*
Tips
Multiple Choice Quiz
Audio Glossary
HIPAA Quiz
Games: Spelling Bee, Crossword, and Strikeout

Key Terminology

bar-code scanners—devices that scan or view bar codes for transfer to attached computers

battery backup systems—systems that protect computers in the event of power surges or power outages

computer peripherals—devices that connect to computers to add function or use

computer viruses—programs written to disrupt computer function

electronic sign-in sheets—computer programs that display the names of those who sign in

ergonomic—designed for proper body posture

flash drives—small, external computer storage devices; see *thumb drives*

health-related calculators—computer programs that quantify health-related conditions (e.g., target body weight)

Internet search engines—Web sites that search the Internet for information based on set criteria

malware—computer programs that can destroy computer programs

medical management software—software medical offices use to perform day-to-day functions (e.g., billing, appointment scheduling)

personal digital assistants (PDAs)—small, portable devices that store and transmit data

scanners—devices that copy documents or pictures for transfer to computer systems

thumb drives—small, external computer storage devices; see *flash drives*

✚ MEDICAL ASSISTING STANDARDS

CAAHEP ENTRY-LEVEL STANDARDS	ABHES ENTRY-LEVEL COMPETENCIES
■ Discuss the importance of routine maintenance of office equipment (cognitive) ■ Perform routine maintenance of office equipment with documentation (psychomotor)	■ Maintain confidentiality at all times ■ Use appropriate guidelines when releasing records or information ■ Be cognizant of ethical boundaries ■ Conduct work within scope of education, training, and ability ■ Monitor legislation related to current healthcare issues and practices ■ Application of electronic technology ■ Apply computer concepts for office procedures ■ Perform medical transcriptions ■ Exercise efficient time management ■ Receive, organize, prioritize, and transmit information expediently ■ Fundamental writing skills

✓ COMPETENCY SKILLS PERFORMANCE

1. Use computer software to maintain office systems.
2. Use an Internet search engine.
3. Verify preferred provider status on an insurance company Web site.

Introduction

Most medical offices use computer systems for some form of operations. From appointment scheduling to bookkeeping and electronic charting, computers have become integral to medical offices. To function most effectively, medical assistants should understand the components of the computer system, as well as how to maintain parts and update software. Computer systems and software programs advance quickly, so it is important to maintain skills and attend training classes as needed.

Components of the Computer System

Computer systems have three main components:

1. **Hardware**—the equipment itself
2. **Software**—programs in the system
3. **Peripherals**—extras that can attach to or be installed in the hardware

Each computer component is intricately intertwined with the others. An office can have the most powerful hardware available yet be limited by software. Similarly, an office can have top-of-the-line software that fails to work due to old, outdated systems. Table 12-1 discusses main computer-system types.

Abbreviations

AMA—American Medical Association
CD—compact disc
CDC—Centers for Disease Control
CPU—central processing unit
DPI—dots per square inch
DVD—digital versatile/video disc
FDA—Food and Drug Administration

HIPAA—Health Insurance Portability and Accountability Act
JAMA—Journal of the American Medical Association
JCAHO—Joint Commission for the Accreditation of Healthcare Organizations
PDA—personal digital assistant
PHI—patient health information

RAM—random access memory
ROM—read-only memory
URL—universal resource locator
USB—universal system bus
VIPPS—Verified Internet Pharmacy Practice Site

TABLE 12-1 MAIN COMPUTER SYSTEM TYPES	
Supercomputers	Introduced in the 1960s; have the fastest processing capacity of today's computers
Mainframe computers	Used for large-volume applications (e.g., government statistics)
Minicomputers	Multiuser computers that fall between mainframe computers and microcomputers in size and capabilities
Microcomputers	Generally small, ranging from desktop models to handheld versions; commonly used in health care facilities

Computer Hardware

Computer hardware consists of several parts. For example, firewalls, which allow or deny computer access, may sometimes be considered hardware, but they can be software as well. All computers have a central processing unit (**CPU**), which is the computer's brain. The CPU enables the computer to process data and run software. All CPUs function in the same basic way but differ in speed and capabilities. Generally, the faster the CPU, the higher the computer's cost.

Virtually all computers have ports that serve as keyboard, monitor, mouse, printer, and speaker connections (Figure 12-1 ♦). Other ports may be used for such add-on items as scanners or backup drives.

?—Critical Thinking Question 12-1—

What must the medical assistant know about the medical office's computer needs? How does office need dictate computer choice?

The Keyboard

Computer keyboards may be standard or **ergonomic** (Figure 12-2 ♦). Ergonomic keyboards reduce typing stress by supporting the hands and wrists comfortably. Keyboards typically attach to computers via cords, but many offices now have wire-

less models that work from any spot within the computer's range, typically 15–30 feet.

The Monitor

Computer monitors come in various sizes and qualities. To conserve desk space, many offices opt for flat-screen models. Monitor display is based on the number of dots per square inch (**DPI**). The higher a monitor's DPI, the clearer its picture. Much like with the CPU just discussed, cost increases as DPI increases.

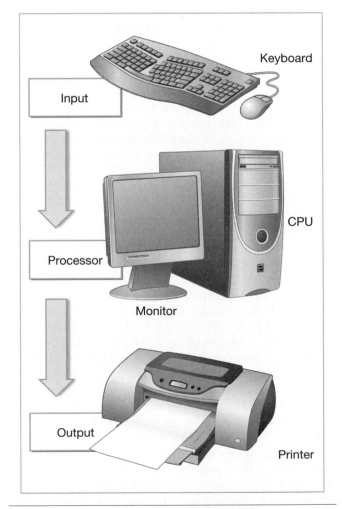

Figure 12-1 ♦ Components of a computer system.

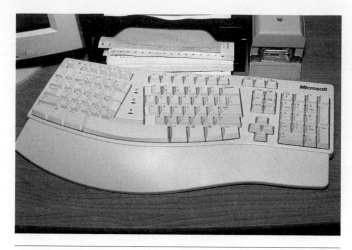

Figure 12-2 ◆ Ergonomic keyboard.

?—Critical Thinking Question 12-2-
What factors would justifiably influence the medical office to fund a flat-screen monitor?

The Computer Hard Drive
A computer's hard drive houses the computer's files and programs as a read/write device. The term read/write refers to the computer's ability to read data that is introduced from other sources and its ability to write (save) data to its own hard drive. Because hard drives can fail, jeopardizing critical data, medical offices should back up their hard drives regularly. This is typically done with a backup system, such as using a separate computer to save data to, or using some form of external device designed to save the computer data. Again, the larger the hard drive, the more expensive the computer.

Types of Computer Drives
Computers have varied types of drives. Most systems come with compact disc (**CD**) drives that allow computers to access files and programs on CDs. CDs are plastic discs used to store data or programs. Digital versatile disc (**DVD**) drives, an option for most contemporary computers, provide access to files on DVDs. DVDs, like CDs, are plastic discs that are used to store data or programs. DVDs have the ability to hold approximately 6 times the amount of information than a CD can hold. Floppy drives, for their part, provide a route to information on floppy disks. Floppy discs are data storage devices composed of a thin flexible magnetic sheet enclosed in a square or rectangle plastic shell. As technology advances, floppy disks are becoming obsolete. Apple® computers, for example, no longer come with floppy disk drives.

Flash drives are small memory devices with no moving parts. These devices, sometimes called **thumb drives**, vary in size from 8 megabytes to 64 gigabytes and are used to store files for transport between computer systems. These drives are small enough to carry in a pocket; many attach to neck chains for

convenience. Flash drives usually connect to computers via a universal system bus (**USB**) port. The USB port may be located on the back or side of the computer and consists of a plug-in for the USB device. Just as with other computer components, the greater the storage capability, the higher the price.

Like flash drives, Zip drives and Jaz drives store data. These devices are slightly larger than floppy drives and hold much more data. Because they are portable, Zip and Jaz drives can be used to transport data between computers. They are also commonly used for file backup.

Computer Memory
A computer's memory consists of read-only memory (**ROM**) and random access memory (**RAM**). ROM is a class of storage media that is not easily modified. It is used mainly to hold permanent data: programs that do not change or alter with use. RAM is a type of storage media that allows the data contained to be accessed in any order. The computer manufacturer writes permanent instructions on ROM chips, which are installed on the computer's motherboard. The amount of RAM, which varies according to users' needs, is also in chip form on the motherboard. Information stored in RAM erases when the computer shuts down or experiences a power failure. When a computer's RAM is insufficient, the computer typically runs more slowly.

The Printer
When a printer is attached to a computer, the user can print information housed on the computer. Printers come in varied types, sizes, and speeds. Some, called inkjet printers, use liquid ink, whereas laser printers use toner to print. Offices may sometimes need to order printer supplies from manufacturers. Other printer supplies may be found at office supply stores. Because the cost of printing supplies can vary greatly, offices should factor in these costs when selecting printers.

?—Critical Thinking Question 12-3-
What type of information can the medical assistant gather to give the physician an accurate idea of printer costs?

Surge Protection
Computers should be protected against damage caused by power outages or electrical surges. All computers in the medical office should be connected to an uninterruptible power supply or **battery backup systems.** All computer power supplies should also have surge protection to prevent voltage surges, which can be very damaging to computer components.

Backing Up Computer Systems
To avoid critical data loss, computers in the medical office should be backed up regularly. Offices can use the various tapes or drives discussed earlier in this chapter, or they can back up data from one computer system to another. Whatever backup

system the medical office uses, the backup tape, drive, and computer should be housed in a location separate from the originating computer so fire, flood, or theft cannot threaten the data.

HIPAA Compliance

Health Insurance Portability and Accountability Act (**HIPAA**) regulations require medical offices to prevent unauthorized users from accessing office computers. Virus-detection and elimination software, firewall technology, and intrusion-detection tools all serve this purpose by keeping unauthorized users from violating office computers and patient information.

Computer Peripherals

Computer peripherals connect to computer systems to offer useful functions. Examples include scanners, digital cameras, bar-code readers, and electronic sign-in sheets (Figure 12-3 ◆).

Scanners

Scanners are similar to photocopiers in that they copy documents. Unlike photocopiers, however, scanners can transfer electronic versions of documents or images to computers.

Digital Cameras

Digital cameras take pictures without film. Images store electronically in the camera until the user downloads them to a computer. Typically, images are downloaded from the camera to the computer via a USB cable. Digital cameras range from inexpensive models designed for home use to expensive models capable of high-quality images. In the medical office, these cameras typically are used to document patient injuries, such as a patient who presents with visible signs of abuse. Other medical offices might use these cameras to create office brochures or other marketing materials.

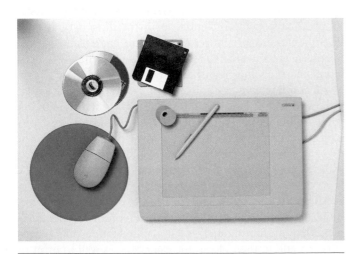

Figure 12-3 ◆ Various computer peripherals.

Figure 12-4 ◆ Bar-code scanner.

Bar-Code Readers

Many modern medical offices use bar coding to manage information. Some offices use bar codes to identify patient files or enter patient data in computers. Others use the technology to track inventory or supplies. **Bar-code scanners,** one type of reader, vary in size and type. Some models work via trigger, while others use what look like an ink pen (Figure 12-4 ◆).

Electronic Sign-in Sheets

Electronic sign-in sheets, which work like the devices department stores use at checkout, arose because HIPAA deemed paper sign-in sheets insufficient for safeguarding patient information. With **electronic sign-in sheets,** patients enter their names electronically on tablets or pads, and the sheets display the resulting signatures on receptionists' computer screens (Figure 12-5 ◆).

Maintaining Computer Equipment

Because computer equipment is expensive and fragile, the medical office should strive to maintain it. To start, office policies should disallow food and drink near computers. One liquid spill can irreversibly damage a computer or destroy a keyboard. In addition, computer systems, as well as CDs, DVDs, and other discs, should be kept in cool, dry places, out of direct sunlight and away from potentially damaging items. Discs should be handled carefully and cleaned only with static-free, soft cloths and appropriate chemicals. All parts of the computer, including the keyboard and mouse, should be dusted regularly. A trained professional should perform any maintenance.

Computer Software

Most medical offices use some form of **medical management software** that performs such functions as appointment scheduling, patient charting, electronic medical record management,

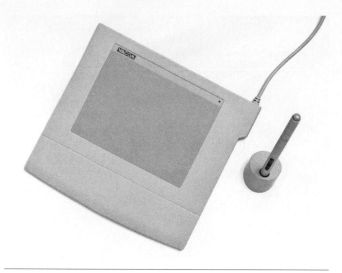

Figure 12-5 ◆ Electronic sign-in sheet.

bookkeeping, insurance billing, and task and prescription managing. An office's needs determine which software it uses. Demonstrations by the software salesperson can help medical offices ensure that they buy programs that are appropriate for their needs. Following the trend in other areas of technology, feature-rich management software tends to cost more than simple programs. Figure 12-6 ◆ names common features in medical management software. Figure 12-7 ◆ identifies medical software companies.

❏ **Patient accounting**—enter patient charges and payments and track accounts receivables

❏ **Coding**—choose codes for patients' procedures and diagnoses

❏ **Appointment scheduling**—track patient appointment times and send reminder cards

❏ **Insurance billing**—print medical insurance claims

❏ **Electronic billing**—submit medical insurance claims electronically

❏ **Verify insurance coverage**—verify patients' insurance benefits via insurance companies' Web sites

❏ **Credit card authorization**—authorize patients' credit-card payments

❏ **Accounts payable**—track the medical office's finances and pay bills

❏ **Payroll**—process and track payroll functions and complete such tasks as printing paychecks and running quarterly reports

❏ **Transcription**—transcribe documents via dictation equipment or voice recognition

Figure 12-6 ◆ Common features in medical management software.

❏ AccuMedic Computer Systems, Inc.
http://www.accumedic.com

❏ Advanced Data Systems (ADS)
www.adsc.com

❏ Lajolla Digital
http://www.lajolladigital.com

❏ MediPro
www.medipro.com

❏ Medisoft Practice Software
www.medisoft.com

❏ MedStar
www.medstarsystems.com

❏ NuMD
http://www.numd.com

❏ Per-Se Technologies
http://www.per-se.com

❏ Practice Partner
www.pmsi.com

❏ TheraManager
http://www.theramanager.com

Figure 12-7 ◆ Medical software companies.

Training Staff on Medical Software

Medical office management software should come with an on-site training option that includes telephone customer service support and manuals or demos for future training needs. All staff who will be working with the software should attend training. Because such training may incur costs, medical offices should explore that possibility before making any software purchases.

Types of Software Packages

Most medical offices use word-processing software, most commonly Microsoft Word.® Using such software, medical assistants can type patient letters, print mailing lists, format documents and brochures, and create charts and forms. Spreadsheet software like Microsoft Excel® completes calculations statistics and creates corresponding graphs and charts. Medical offices may use spreadsheet software to track statistics on patient care and personnel management. Presentation software like PowerPoint® helps when medical offices plan educational meetings or seminars for patients. Not only can presenters create slides for projection, they can print those slides as note-taking tools for attendees (Figure 12-8 ◆).

Several software programs currently on the market, such as Microsoft Outlook®, keep electronic calendars, which can be invaluable to medical offices trying to coordinate staff schedules. Many such programs send e-mail invitations that recipients can add to their electronic calendars, as well as print in daily, weekly, or monthly slices.

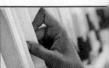

PROCEDURE 12-1 Use Computer Software to Maintain Office Systems

Theory and Rationale
The computer software used in the medical office is capable of performing a multitude of tasks. One such task is to maintain the office systems. An example of such a task would be to keep track of the equipment used in the medical office. By performing this task, the medical assistant can keep track of information pertaining to needed maintenance, such as the name of the company that performs the repairs, and the schedule for which the equipment must be maintained.

Materials
- Computer with spreadsheet software
- List of equipment to enter into the computer

Competency
(**Conditions**) With the necessary materials, you will be able to (**Task**) utilize computer software to maintain office sys-

tems (**Standards**) correctly within the time limit set by the instructor.

1. Launch the spreadsheet software.
2. Using the list of equipment, enter each piece of equipment onto a separate line on the spreadsheet.
3. Enter the date each piece of equipment was purchased or leased by the medical office.
4. Enter the name of the manufacturer that supplied the piece of equipment.
5. Enter the type of maintenance the piece of equipment needs on a regular basis.
6. Enter information about the needed maintenance, such as the name of the company that performs the repairs, and the schedule for which the equipment must be maintained.

Computer Security

To safeguard computer systems, staff members should be required to use alphanumeric passwords to access them. To thwart hackers, users should choose unobvious passwords, taking care to avoid initials, birthdates, and telephone numbers. Users should also be careful to avoid sharing their passwords and leaving their passwords in plain view. It is good practice for users to log off whenever leaving their computer workstations unattended. Figure 12-9 ◆ outlines HIPAA standards for safeguarding patient health information.

Computer Viruses

Computer viruses are programs designed to perform mischievous functions. **Malware**, a twist on the computer virus, is designed to damage computer programs by infiltrating computers. Malware includes spyware, adware, Trojan horses, and worms. These programs can damage or corrupt hard drives, as well as infect other computers without users' knowledge. Because these types of programs exist, every computer in the medical office should have virus-protection software that is updated

Figure 12-8 ◆ A physician giving a PowerPoint presentation.

> ❑ Patient health information (PHI) must be backed up periodically.
> ❑ An audit trail must exist for backed-up data that leaves the medical facility.
> ❑ Access to backed-up data must be restricted to authorized parties.
> ❑ A backup plan and disaster recovery plan must be in place.
> ❑ Data must be a retrievable, exact copy.
> ❑ All computers must be password protected.

Figure 12-9 ◆ HIPAA standards for safeguarding patient health information.

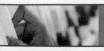

PROCEDURE 12-2 Use an Internet Search Engine

Theory and Rationale

The Internet has a vast amount of information the medical office can use to educate patients, research new technologies and equipment, and contact patients. Search engines can quickly locate desired information and resources.

Materials

- A computer with Internet access

Competency

(**Conditions**) With the necessary materials, you will be able to (**Task**) use the computer to search for a topic via an Internet search engine (**Standards**) correctly within the time limit set by the instructor.

1. Turn on the computer.
2. Launch an Internet browser.
3. Visit the uniform resource locator (**URL**) of the search engine.
4. Enter the search keywords.
5. Visit retrieved Web sites to obtain the desired information.
6. To refine the search, enter more or different key words.

---

regularly. The two most commonly used antivirus software programs are made by McAfee and Norton.

Internet Search Engines

Internet search engines use key words and phrases to retrieve information from the Internet. Popular search engines are Yahoo, Google, Dog Pile, and Ask.com. Contemporary health care providers often search the Internet for medical information. Medical offices often need source material for patient brochures or presentations, and the Internet can be a valuable resource in this area.

In Practice

Dr. Victor is giving a presentation on a new procedure she is performing for scar-tissue removal. Dr. Victor has asked Jamie, her medical assistant, to use the Internet to find information on other, similar procedures for comparison. How should Jamie begin, and where? What key words would be appropriate for the search engine?

Keys to Success
USING THE COMPUTER FOR
WORK-RELATED PURPOSES ONLY

Because the computer systems in a medical office belong to the physician or the office, they should only be used for private use when employers grant permission. Even with permission, staff should download no screen savers or other, similar files. Most computers get viruses and malware when users open malicious e-mails or visit certain Web sites. Therefore, to protect computers, medical assistants should open no attachments from unknown sources or Web sites.

Finding Appropriate Web Resources

When newly diagnosed with conditions or illnesses, patients often have many questions for their health care providers. Many such providers find it helpful to give patients lists of reputable Web sites for further information. When patients have long-term or chronic illnesses or conditions and may be seeking support groups, such lists can be especially beneficial.

Professional medical Web sites are the sites physicians visit when seeking up-to-date information on conditions, illnesses, or pharmaceuticals. Figure 12-10 ◆ lists some reputable examples. Many physicians subscribe to online journals that charge for access but offer the latest information on research, medications, and techniques. Seminars and conferences can be informative, but Web sites serve as ongoing resources as topics arise.

Many Web sites have **health-related calculators** that aid both patients and health care staff. Such calculators address such factors as basal metabolic rate, body mass index, preg-

❑ American Medical Association (AMA)
(www.ama-assn.org)
❑ Joint Commission for the Accreditation of Healthcare Organizations (**JCAHO**) (www.jcaho.org)
❑ Journal of the American Centers for Disease Control and Prevention (**CDC**) (www.cdc.gov)
❑ Lancet (www.lancet.org)
❑ Medical Association (**JAMA**)
(www.jama.ama-assn.org)
❑ New England Journal of Medicine (www.nejm.org)

Figure 12-10 ◆ Medical Web sites.

Keys to Success
OBTAINING PHYSICIAN APPROVAL
BEFORE DISTRIBUTING MATERIAL
TO PATIENTS

Before giving Web site information to patients, be sure to obtain the physician's permission. Give patients only information from reputable Web sites.

Keys to Success
KEEPING INFORMATION
ON THE PDA CONFIDENTIAL

When a physician's PDA contains private patient information, it must be kept inaccessible to unauthorized parties. Passwords protect PDAs just like computers.

nancy due date, ovulation, target heart rate, children's adult height predictions, smoking costs, and seafood mercury intake.

Often, major health insurance carriers maintain their own, comprehensive Web sites that allow subscribers and physicians alike to access a wide span of information. Some sites even give physicians access to patients' benefit information, although direct contact with the insurance companies is often still needed, especially when authorizations are required. Such sites are particularly helpful for offices wishing to verify that patients have active policies at the time of visit.

Buying Medications Online

Patients who lack prescription drug coverage may leverage the Internet as an economical way to obtain medications. Online medication purchase can be dangerous, however, so medical offices should encourage patients to use only sites certified by the Verified Internet Pharmacy Practice Site (**VIPPS**). VIPPS certification ensures that the National Association of Boards of Pharmacy has reviewed the online pharmacy for safety and compliance. Certified online pharmacies provide information on prescribed medications, including possible adverse reactions or side effects and any safety concerns.

Patient Education

Medical offices should advise patients never to purchase medications from Internet sites outside the United States. Direct patients to the U.S. Food and Drug Administration (**FDA**) (www.fda.gov) Web site for tips on buying medications online.

Allowing Personal Computer Use in the Office

All medical offices should write policies for personal use of office computers and ensure that all members of the health care team follow those policies strictly. Patients who feel office computers are being used for personal reasons may develop negative impressions of the office. As a result, some offices forbid all personal computer use, while others allow personal use during breaks or the periods before and after shifts. Policies should reflect an office's approach. For example, personal computer use may be allowed, but not within sight of patients.

Personal Digital Assistants

Many physicians today use **personal digital assistants** (**PDAs**) to do things like quickly check medication dosages or research drug interactions. *Personal digital assistant* is a term used to describe any small, mobile hand-held device that provides computing and information storage retrieval capabilities for

---

PROCEDURE 12-3   Verify Preferred Provider Status on an Insurance Company Web Site

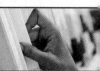

Theory and Rationale

Insurance company names can change when companies merge. Administrative medical assistants must keep abreast of the insurance plans their offices participate with. The ability to verify preferred provider status is a valuable function for both the physician and the patient.

Materials

■ Computer with Internet connection
■ Insurance company's URL
■ Name of target physician

Competency

(**Conditions**) With the necessary materials, you will be able to (**Task**) verify a provider's preferred status on an insurance company Web site (**Standards**) within the time limit set by the instructor.

1. Using the computer, launch an Internet browser.
2. Enter the URL of the insurance company.
3. Navigate to the provider page or section.
4. In the search field, enter the provider's name and/or location.
5. Verify if the physician is preferred with the target insurance company.

personal or business use, often for keeping schedule calendars and address book information handy. Outside the medical office, PDAs can serve to record patients' hospital visits or the calls physicians take while on call (Figure 12-11 ◆).

Because PDAs can connect to computer systems, information can transfer between the two. For example, physicians can enter patient information into their PDA and then later download that information to their desktop computers. PDAs especially benefit physicians who wish to review patient charts outside the office. Rather than remove patient charts from the office, physicians can record the necessary information in their PDA.

Computer Ergonomics

Long-term computer use has prompted a number of recommendations that help address health concerns. For example, members of the health care team can avoid eye strain by fre-

quently looking away from the computer screen. Antiglare screens are another option, as is placing the monitor at an angle to avoid glare. Carpal tunnel syndrome is associated with repeated use of the wrists, such as when typing on a keyboard. Many computer users find that the ergonomic keyboards mentioned earlier in this chapter alleviate this syndrome's symptoms. Keyboard wrist supports are also helpful.

Proper posture and equipment placement are crucial to avoiding computer-related injuries. Users should sit straight in chairs that support the lower back (Figure 12-12 ◆). Chairs should have armrests, but users should only use those features when not typing. Keyboards should be placed to allow a 90-degree angle at the elbows and close enough so users need not reach forward. Monitors should be at eye level, with a viewing angle of 5 to 30 degrees. Users should not have to twist to see their monitors. Users' feet should be flat on the floor, and legs should be uncrossed.

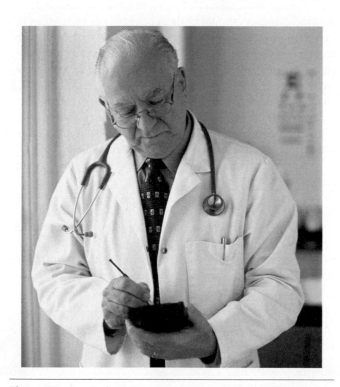

Figure 12-11 ◆ A physician using a personal digital assistant (PDA).

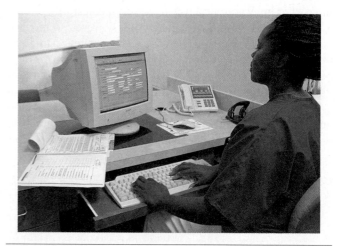

Figure 12-12 ◆ The medical assistant should have an ergonomically correct desk, chair, and keyboard.

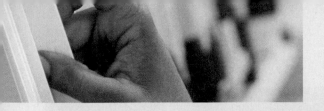

REVIEW

- Computers serve varied functions and uses in the medical office, all of which the medical assistant should be familiar with.
- The purchase of a new computer system entails careful, informed research to ensure that the needs of the medical office are met.
- The components of a computer system include hardware, software, and peripherals.
- Office staff can take steps to maintain computer equipment, but repairs should be left to professionals.

- Security is an important part of office computing, because it helps ensure the confidentiality of patient information.
- The Internet can serve as a resource for nearly infinite medical information.
- When using computers, medical offices should instate clear policies for the computers' use.
- Personal digital assistants can help bridge the computing gap when out of the office.
- Ergonomically designed computer equipment helps ensure that all members of the health care team work safely.

Chapter Review

Multiple Choice

1. Computer peripherals include:
   a. Printers
   b. Scanners
   c. External hard drives
   d. All of the above

2. Another term for flash drive is _____ drive.
   a. Star
   b. Thumb
   c. Media
   d. Small

3. An electronic sign-in sheet is designed to:
   a. Maintain patient confidentiality
   b. Ensure HIPAA compliance
   c. Track patients in the office
   d. All of the above

4. A medical office may use a scanner to:
   a. Copy photos into a patient's chart
   b. Photocopy documents to give to patients
   c. Track insurance correspondence
   d. Maintain patient confidentiality

5. Which brand of computer no longer comes with floppy disc drives?
   a. Apple
   b. Dell
   c. Hewlett-Packard
   d. All of the above

True/False

T F 1. The CPU is considered the computer's brain.
T F 2. Flat-panel monitors are often used when desk space is at a premium.
T F 3. Computer passwords should be easy to remember, such as birth date or addresses.

T F 4. Medical management software companies should provide onsite training of staff.
T F 5. A trained professional should perform any maintenance on office computers.
T F 6. Bar-code scanners are used in health care to track supplies, among other things.

Short Answer

1. What is PowerPoint software used for?
2. What is the importance of an external battery backup system?
3. What is a thumb drive used for?
4. What is the difference between a computer virus and malware?
5. What is the main danger in downloading files to an office computer?
6. Name Internet search engines for finding information online.
7. Name some functions of a health-related calculator.
8. What is an "ergonomically correct keyboard"?
9. Describe the functions of medical practice management software.

Research

1. Search the Internet for computer retailers. What type of system do you think would be a typical set up for a medical office computer station? What components do you believe would be included?
2. Interview a person who works in a medical office. How does that facility back up its data? How often is the back up done?
3. Research online for information on computer ergonomics. What kind of information did you find about posture and working at a computer?

Externship Application Experience

As Monica Friedenrich is training the medical assistant on the medical office's computer systems, she explains the HIPAA regulations for passwords, which includes a unique password for every staff member. Monica then directs the medical assistant to use her own password during training. Should the medical assistant comply? If the assistant chooses to comply, what issues could result?

Resource Guide

AltaVista Translation Services
www.altavista.com

CSGNetwork and Computer Support Group Health-Related Calculators
http://www.csgnetwork.com

Occupational Safety and Health Administration (OSHA) Web site
www.osha.gov

 MedMedia

http://www.MyMAKit.com

More on this chapter, including interactive resources, can be found on the Student CD-ROM accompanying this textbook and on http://www.MyMAKit.com.

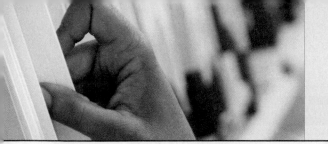

CHAPTER 13

Equipment, Maintenance, and Supply Inventory

Objectives

After completing this chapter, you should be able to:

- Define and spell the key terminology in this chapter.
- Write an office equipment maintenance manual.
- Research the best options for purchasing supplies and equipment.
- Explain the pros and cons of leasing and purchasing office equipment.
- Maintain patient confidentiality while faxing.
- Discuss the functions of a photocopier in health care.
- Describe how to use a ten-key adding machine.
- Name the functions of a transcription machine in a medical office.
- Identify transcription services outside the medical office.
- Create an inventory control manual.
- Explain the steps involved in receiving and logging drug samples.
- Discuss how supplies are stocked in a medical office.
- Explain how scanners are used in supply ordering.

Case Study

During a medical office's weekly staff meeting, several staff members voice their frustration over frequently running out of clerical supplies before new supplies are received. As the person in charge of inventory and supply ordering in the administrative office, the office manager asks the medical assistant to devise a system to address the situation.

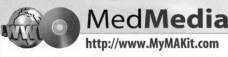

MedMedia

http://www.MyMAKit.com

Additional interactive resources and activities for this chapter can be found on http://www.MyMAKit.com. For a video, tips, audio glossary, legal and ethical scenarios, on-the-job scenarios, quizzes, and games related to the content of this chapter, please access the accompanying CD-ROM in this book.

Video
Legal and Ethical Scenario: *Equipment, Maintenance, and Supply Inventory*
On the Job Scenario: *Equipment, Maintenance, and Supply Inventory*
Tips
Multiple Choice Quiz
Audio Glossary
HIPAA Quiz
Games: Spelling Bee, Crossword, and Strikeout

Key Terminology

expiration date—date on which something loses full strength or validity

inventory—supplies on hand

maintained—kept in good working order

packing slip—list of supplies ordered and included in a shipment

scanner—piece of equipment that takes an exact image of a photo or document and transfers that image to a computer

transcribe—to type words as they are spoken

transcription machine—piece of equipment that allows the user to listen to and type taped words

user manual—document that describes how something (e.g., equipment) is used

warranty—period within which a piece of equipment is repaired without cost to the buyer

Abbreviations

EPA—Environmental Protection Agency

HIPAA—Health Insurance Portability and Accountability Act

OSHA—Occupational Safety and Health Administration

WHO—World Health Organization

✚ MEDICAL ASSISTING STANDARDS

CAAHEP ENTRY-LEVEL STANDARDS	ABHES ENTRY-LEVEL COMPETENCIES
■ Discuss the importance of routine maintenance of office equipment (cognitive) ■ Perform routine maintenance of office equipment with documentation (psychomotor) ■ Perform an office inventory (psychomotor)	■ Conduct work within scope of education, training, and ability ■ Dispose of controlled substances in compliance with government regulations ■ Application of electronic technology ■ Maintain records for accounting and banking purposes ■ Serve as a liaison between the physicians and others ■ Exercise efficient time management ■ Receive, organize, prioritize, and transmit information expediently ■ Maintain physical plant ■ Operate and maintain facilities and equipment safely ■ Inventory equipment and supplies ■ Evaluate and recommend equipment and supplies for practice

✓ COMPETENCY SKILLS PERFORMANCE

1. Take inventory of administrative equipment.
2. Perform routine maintenance of a computer printer.
3. Fax a document.
4. Prepare a purchase order.
5. Receive a supply shipment.

Introduction

In medical offices that run smoothly, equipment is well **maintained** and supplies and **inventory** are effectively managed. While some large offices track their supplies and inventories electronically, others opt for manual processes. Medical assistants who are adept at equipment use in the medical office are both efficient at their jobs and competitive in the job market.

Working with Medical Office Equipment

Every piece of equipment a medical office buys or leases comes with a **user manual**. A new piece of equipment typically also comes with a **warranty**, a guarantee from the vendor that certain defects or problems will be repaired for a predetermined period. Many companies sell extended warranties that cover equipment for longer periods. To track warranty periods and expedite repairs or replacement, the date a piece of equipment was leased or purchased should be written on the equipment's user manual. When possible, any receipts should be included. User manuals should be kept in a central location, like a file cabinet, so they can quickly and easily be found when needed.

Training employees on the use of the photocopier.

Familiarize employees with:

❑ On/off switch
❑ Paper placement on glass
❑ Paper replacement
❑ Use of enlarge/reduce feature
❑ Toner replacement
❑ Location of telephone number for repairs
❑ Location of telephone number for supplies

Signature of Employee:

Signature of Trainer:

Date:

Figure 13-1 ◆ Sample page from a office equipment training manual.

Training Employees to Use Medical Office Equipment

Every employee who is asked to use a piece of office equipment must be trained on that equipment's proper use and care. Many suppliers train employees when equipment is purchased, but often just once, which means staff who have been trained must document their training if future employees are to be trained, as well.

Training manuals can be invaluable tools for documenting training content in the medical office. Manuals should devote one page to each piece of equipment. In addition to explaining how to use and maintain the equipment, each page should provide a place for employees to sign and date once properly trained (Figure 13-1 ◆). In addition to furthering training objectives, such manuals keep the medical office in compliance with Occupational Safety and Health Administration (**OSHA**) safety regulations. ∞ Chapter 21 details OSHA safety regulations in the medical office.

Keeping a Maintenance Log for Medical Office Equipment

For each piece of equipment that requires regular maintenance, the medical office should keep a log of the maintenance requirements, schedule, and responsible party. When equipment must be maintained by the manufacturer or another professional repair person, the log should include those parties' contact information. Anyone who performs maintenance should sign and date the maintenance log. A complete maintenance log helps the medical office prove that its equipment has been well maintained, which can in turn help expedite warranty work (Figure 13-2 ◆).

Replacing or Buying Medical Office Equipment

When the time comes to replace or acquire equipment, the physician may ask the medical assistant to research options. For small, easy-to-transport pieces, assistants may ask sales representatives to bring samples to the office for review. Assistants may also research equipment online or visit stores where equipment is displayed. For high-dollar purchases, sales representatives should give medical assistants references of customers who are using the products. In turn, the assistants should take the time to call those references and poll them on customer service and ease of the equipment's use.

When calling other medical offices for equipment references, the medical assistant should be sure to talk to the staff members who actually use the equipment. Those staff will accurately depict how that equipment works.

Weighing Equipment Leasing Against Buying

Leasing and buying have distinct advantages when it comes to equipment. Leasing does not award ownership, but it typically requires no down payment. In the event the equipment breaks or malfunctions, the manufacturer usually replaces or repairs it as part of the lease. Purchased equipment generally requires

Office Equipment Maintenance Log				
Equipment name	Maintenance to be performed	Maintenance schedule	Name of person performing the maintenance	Signature and date
Photocopier	Clean spilled toner inside the machine	Once monthly	Louise Glaser, CMA (AAMA)	*L. Glaser, CMA (AAMA) 9/4/10*

Figure 13-2 ◆ Sample office equipment maintenance log.

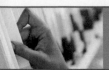

PROCEDURE 13-1 Take Inventory of Administrative Equipment

Theory and Rationale
An up-to-date list of a medical office's administrative equipment helps determine the equipment's age in the event the equipment needs repair, or if fire, flood, or theft occurs.

Materials
- Paper
- Pen
- Computer with word-processing or spreadsheet software

Competency
(**Conditions**) With the necessary materials, you will be able to (**Task**) perform an inventory of administrative equipment

(**Standards**) correctly within the time limit set by the instructor.

1. Locate all administrative equipment in the medical office.
2. List each piece of equipment with manufacturer name, serial number, and date of purchase, when known.
3. Include information about the company maintaining the equipment.
4. Include information about the supplies needed to maintain the equipment, including where those supplies are purchased.
5. Using word-processing or spreadsheet software, create an inventory sheet of all equipment information.
6. Update the inventory sheet as needed when new equipment is purchased or older equipment is replaced.

---

full funding up front or a down payment and financed balance. Buying, however, confers ownership. Once the equipment is paid for, the owner need only cover the costs associated with maintenance or repairs. Physician's preference, price, and intended use all help drive the lease/buy decision.

Using Fax Machines in the Medical Office

Facsimile or fax machines are common pieces of medical office equipment that come in varied sizes and prices (Figure 13-3 ◆). Via telephone lines, fax machines make it possible to send and receive printed documents anywhere in the world where other fax machines are located. Simple, relatively inexpensive models simply fax documents from one location to another. Higher end versions also serve as photocopiers and **scanners**.

To guard patient confidentiality, fax machines must be kept in areas of the office that are inaccessible to patients. Such machines should not reside on the counter at the front desk or in a hallway, for example. While medical offices commonly use fax machines to send and receive confidential patient information, the Health Insurance Portability and Accountability Act (HIPAA) dictates that fax machines only be used in the event other modes of transmission fail to suffice. Therefore, when

---

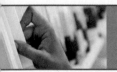

PROCEDURE 13-2 Perform Routine Maintenance of a Computer Printer

Theory and Rationale
While most equipment in the medical office requires trained technicians to provide maintenance, the medical assistant performs basic maintenance on many pieces, such as the computer printer.

Materials
- Paper
- Pen
- Computer printer
- Maintenance logbook

Competency
(**Conditions**) With the necessary materials, you will be able to (**Task**) perform routine maintenance of a computer printer

(**Standards**) correctly within the time limit set by the instructor.

1. Review the maintenance logbook for the computer printer.
2. Following the manufacturer's directions, open the printer cover and remove the toner cartridge.
3. Using the manufacturer-provided cleaning tool, clean any dust and spilled toner from within the printer.
4. Replace the cleaning tool and the toner cartridge.
5. Close the printer cover.
6. In the maintenance logbook, enter information about the maintenance, including the date and your signature.

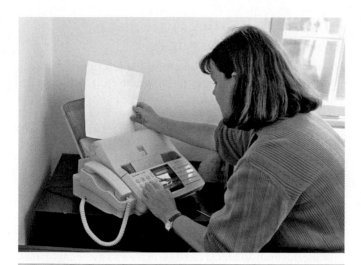

Figure 13-3 ◆ The fax machine in the medical office must be located outside of areas frequented by patients.

medical offices must transmit information on patients' behalf, medical assistants should use conventional mail when there is time. Some medical offices use courier services in lieu of faxing, especially for such highly confidential information as HIV status or reproductive health care decisions. Any faxed documents

Keys to Success
EQUIPMENT MALFUNCTION

Medical office equipment may sometimes malfunction. When it does, report the malfunction to the office manager or physician immediately. Malfunctions in some equipment, especially clinical equipment, can injure patients or medical staff.

must be accompanied by a HIPAA-compliant fax cover sheet like the one shown in Chapter 4. ∞ Such cover sheets include disclaimers that the faxed information cannot be disclosed to any party without the patient's written consent or a court order.

Using Copy Machines in Health Care Facilities

Copy machines, like fax machines, come in all sizes and price levels. Medical offices should have high-quality copiers that are maintained and serviced regularly. Because medical offices tend to use their copiers heavily, unreliable machines can severely impede office functioning. Like fax machines, office copiers should be placed where patients cannot access them. Copiers are best placed behind the front desk or near the billing office, as staff in those areas use copiers the most. See Chapter 6 for a procedure on preparing a document for photocopying.

When researching copiers, medical offices should consider various factors. While price and warranty items are of obvious concern, the cost of supplies is also an important consideration. Some copiers require difficult-to-find or expensive parts.

Adding Health Care Data with Machines

Upon hearing "adding machine," many people envision ten-key calculators. Such calculators are normally electronic, and most have tape for printing (Figure 13-4 ◆). Through consistent use, most administrative staff in the medical office become able to use ten-key calculators by touch. This skill is especially helpful when adding long columns of numbers, like those on pegboard day sheets, deposit slips, or patient ledgers. Medical staff also often use handheld calculators. These machines come in all shapes and sizes, typically run on battery power, and are convenient when ten-key systems are impractical. Some

---

PROCEDURE 13-3 **Fax a Document**

Theory and Rationale
Faxing documents from the medical office requires strict attention to HIPAA regulations for safeguarding private patient information.

Materials
- Document to be faxed
- HIPAA-compliant fax cover sheet
- Pen
- Fax machine

Competency
(**Conditions**) With the necessary materials, you will be able to (**Task**) fax a document using a fax machine (**Standards**) correctly within the time limit set by the instructor.

1. Complete the fax cover sheet with personal name, phone number, and clinic contact information.
2. Fill in the name and fax number of the fax recipient.
3. List the number of pages in the fax, including the cover sheet.
4. Properly orient the fax cover sheet and document to be faxed in the fax machine.
5. Dial the target fax number.
6. When the fax has fully transmitted, remove the documents and file them with the fax confirmation sheet in the patient's file.

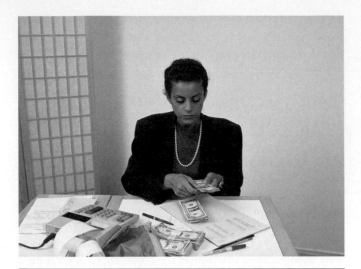

Figure 13-4 ◆ The administrative medical assistant will use a ten-key calculator for tasks such as totaling the daily deposit.

handheld calculators are small enough to fit in the pocket of a clinic jacket.

Medical Transcription

In years past, **transcription machines** were common in medical offices (Figure 13-5 ◆). Physicians would dictate patient information into these tape recorder–devices and give the tapes to administrative staff, who would **transcribe** the spoken words to printed form. Staff would use headphones to hear the tapes and foot pedals to control the tapes. Volume and speed buttons would control those functions.

Physicians must be afforded the opportunity to review the transcripts of transcribed tapes before the tapes are erased. Physicians may verify wording or correct errors. Once physicians have approved transcriptions, the tapes can be erased and reused.

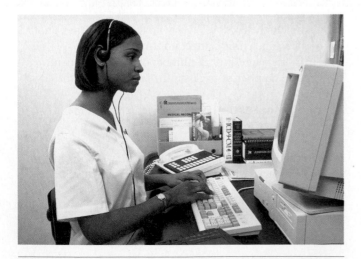

Figure 13-5 ◆ A medical assistant using a transcription machine.

Finding Outside Transcription Services

Most medical offices today use outside transcription services. Such services typically require physicians to call a recorded telephone line to dictate their information. The corresponding printed documents arrive via fax, e-mail, or postal service.

For a number of reasons, thorough research is important when choosing outside transcription services. Many transcription services are based outside the United States, where patient privacy laws can vary and fail to meet U.S. **HIPAA** regulations. Research should reveal companies' reputations as well as prices and services. While the Internet can be a valuable research tool in this realm, the best way to find an outside transcription service is to identify which services other medical offices in the area use. Medical assistants can then delve into those companies' patient confidentiality policies, costs, and turnaround times. Armed with this type of information, medical assistants can give informed, comprehensive presentations to the physician on recommended services.

Logging Medical Office Supplies

To effectively manage office inventory and supplies, the medical office should create a master list of all regularly purchased items. This list should include all disposable supplies; separate lists should detail clinical and clerical supplies. All such lists should include the supply, the order or part number, the name of the company, and the typical quantity and frequency of ordering (Figure 13-6 ◆).

Inventorying Supplies

To ensure that the medical office remains at fully functioning status, one member of the health care team should regularly inventory all supplies to ensure they remain in stock (Figure 13-7 ◆). Out-of-stock items force offices to reschedule procedures or incur high next-day reordering expenses. Offices use supplies at different rates, and their reorder schedules should reflect those differences. Most offices inventory supplies weekly, while others adhere to monthly or daily schedules. Because medical assistants' vacation schedules and days off vary, the inventory task works best when shared by more than one staff member.

?—**Critical Thinking Question 13-1—**
How does rotating the person in charge of inventory each week benefit the medical office's inventory process?

The key to effective supply management is to have enough supplies to efficiently run the office but not so much as to risk expiration or storage issues. Many of the supplies used in the clinical part of the office, such as laboratory collection containers or medications and vaccines, have expiration dates.

Inventory Supply Log				
Supply	**Order or Part Number**	**Supplier**	**Number in Order**	**Frequency of Order**
Fee slips	N/A	Minuteman Press (425) 555–9000	5,000	Twice annually
Fax toner cartridges	HP6545	Office Depot (800) 345-3000	2	Once monthly

Figure 13-6 ◆ Sample inventory supply log.

Keys to Success
TAKING OFFICE SUPPLIES

Medical office staff should have a high level of integrity, which means office and medical supplies must stay in the office. Employees who take office pens, notepads, or even bandages without permission steal and place the office in jeopardy of running out of supplies sooner than expected, which can impede procedure scheduling. Taking office supplies without permission may result in termination or loss of trust in the offender.

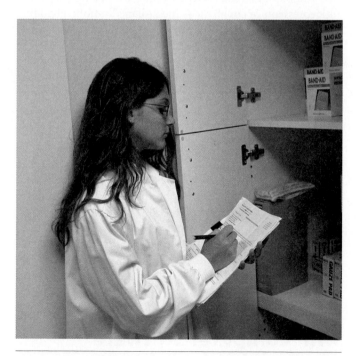

Figure 13-7 ◆ Medical supplies must be inventoried on a regular basis.

Some supplies, especially medications, have expiration dates of no more than one year from the date of manufacture. A medical office might get a good price on gloves by ordering 500 boxes at once, for example, but if the staff will take 2 years to use those gloves and storage space is at a premium, the savings is not likely worth the inconvenience. Many offices devise systems to remind themselves when certain supplies must be ordered. If, for example, staff know to reorder gloves when only ten boxes are left in stock, a reorder reminder note can be attached to the tenth box of gloves.

Some medical offices use purchase orders for ordering supplies or equipment needed in the office. In some facilities, these purchase orders must be authorized by the office manager or the physician; in other facilities they are filled out by the person in charge of ordering supplies and sent directly by that person to the supplier.

In Practice

Before the medical assistant was hired, the medical office lacked a system for ordering supplies. Members of the health care team simply ordered supplies as they felt necessary. As a result, the office now has cupboards full of supplies that will expire in a month. As a new employee, the medical assistant is charged with devising a system for tracking office inventory. Where should the assistant start? What steps will help ensure all supplies are counted correctly?

Checking for the Next Day's Supplies

At the end of the workday, one member of the health care team should ensure that the office has enough supplies for all procedures scheduled the next day. Rescheduling due to supply deficiencies reflects poorly on the office as well as impedes efficient office operation. The medical office should develop a good relationship with other, nearby offices so that supplies can be borrowed in the event of unexpected shortages.

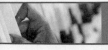

PROCEDURE 13-4 Prepare a Purchase Order

Theory and Rationale
The use of purchase orders is one way the medical office can accurately keep track of the supplies that are needed and used in the clinic, as well as how often these supplies are being ordered.

Materials
- List of needed supplies
- Purchase order form
- Pen
- Fax machine or telephone

Competency
(**Conditions**) With the necessary materials, you will be able to (**Task**) prepare a purchase order (**Standards**) correctly within the time limit set by the instructor.

1. Review the list of needed supplies, grouping them according to the vendor they will be ordered from.

2. Fill in the name and fax number of the company the supplies are to be ordered from.
3. List each supply individually on the purchase order, taking care to note the quantity needed and the part number associated with each item.
4. If the physician's signature is required, obtain his or her signature. If it is not required, sign and date the form with your own signature.
5. If the purchase order can be faxed to the supplier, fax the document and make a note of the date and time the fax went through.
6. If the purchase order cannot be faxed to the supplier, call the supplier and place the order over the telephone. Document the name of the person you spoke to and the date and time of the call.
7. File the purchase order in a folder for pending orders.

Storing Supplies Upon Arrival

When supplies arrive in the medical office, one staff member must locate the **packing slip** and check to ensure all supplies are included. Usually, this slip is sealed in a plastic envelope and attached to the outside of the box, or it may be in the box with the supplies. The packing slip lists the supplies that were ordered and the supplies in the shipment. This slip may also serve as an invoice. If so, it must be routed to the accounts payable office after the order is checked for completeness. When part of an order is missing or backordered, the medical assistant must make a notation and keep the packing slip until the remaining supplies arrive in the office.

Except for clerical supplies, all newly arrived medical office supplies should be stored behind older inventory so older supplies are used first. Because many medical supplies have **expiration dates**, this procedure helps eliminate waste.

Handling Drug Samples

Many medical offices welcome the pharmaceutical representatives who supply them drug samples, which are normally small amounts of the drugs pharmaceutical companies sell. Usually, samples are name-brand, costly drugs new to the market. Companies give physicians drug samples in the hope those physi-

cians will prescribe the drugs to their patients. Typically, physicians set aside short periods to meet with drug-company representatives. In most states, medical assistants may sign for the drug samples which sales representatives leave. Not all medical offices permit pharmaceutical representatives access to the physicians or other clinical staff.

In medical offices, drugs should be grouped according to type. Antibiotics should be kept together, for example, as should antidepressants or cough medicines. All medications, including drug samples, must be kept out of patient access areas. Medications, including drug samples, have expiration dates and must be discarded once those dates have passed. In some states, sample drugs must also be tracked. Medical offices should track samples even when the law does not require it. Tracking discourages staff from taking drugs and supplies for personal use.

Stocking Clerical Supplies

Clerical supplies are easier to stock than clinical supplies because most medical offices know how many envelopes, stamps, and forms they regularly use. In addition, clerical supplies do not expire and most such items, except for preprinted business cards or letterhead (Figure 13-8 ◆), are readily available at local supply stores. While an abundance of clerical supplies can present a storage problem, many suppliers offer volume discounts.

Tracking Supplies with Computer Software

Many medical offices today use barcode-equipped computer software to ensure that they have adequate supplies. When members of the health care team take items from the supply

Keys to Success
EXPIRED MEDICAL SUPPLIES

It is illegal to use expired medical supplies. Once supplies have passed their expiration dates, discard them.

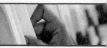

PROCEDURE 13-5 Receive a Supply Shipment

Theory and Rationale
Medical office supplies are ordered and received regularly. To ensure that all ordered supplies have been received, the medical assistant must carefully check the supplies' packing slip.

Materials
- Box of supplies
- Packing slip
- Supply inventory logbook
- Pen

Competency
(**Conditions**) With the necessary materials, you will be able to (**Task**) receive a supply shipment (**Standards**) correctly within the time limit set by the instructor.

1. Open the box of supplies, and locate the packing slip.
2. Remove each item from the box, checking it on the packing slip.
3. On the packing slip, circle any missing supplies.
4. Put the supplies away, newer ones behind older ones.
5. Note in the supply log that the supplies have been received.
6. When any supplies on the packing slip are absent from the shipment, notify the supplier.
7. When any supplies on the packing slip are on back order, retain the slip until the backordered supplies arrive.
8. When the packing slip also serves as an invoice, route it to the accounts payable department.
9. Discard packing materials appropriately.

Keys to Success
DISCARDING MEDICATIONS

The Environmental Protection Agency (**EPA**) and World Health Organization (**WHO**) recommend discarding expired medications by wrapping those medications in plastic or sealing them in plastic bags before disposal. Flushing medications is not recommended because it exposes people, pets, and the environment to potential harm.

room, they use the software to scan those items' bar codes and note the departments using the supplies. When supplies drop below a preprogrammed level, the staff member in charge of ordering supplies is notified to order more of that supply. Software ordering systems are only as accurate as the staff members who use them, however. When supplies are scanned inaccurately, they cannot be tracked and supplies may not be adequately stocked.

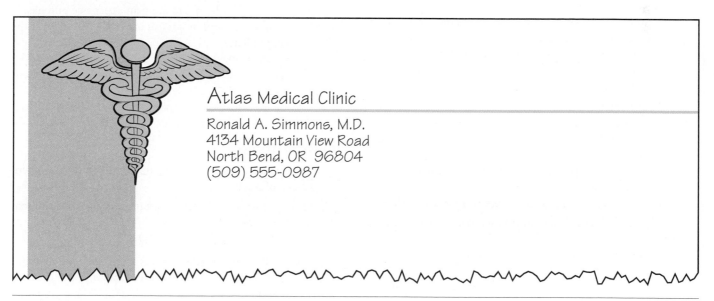

Figure 13-8 ◆ Sample of medical office letterhead paper.

REVIEW

Chapter Summary

- For the medical office, an equipment maintenance manual serves to ensure all needed equipment is in working order and able to support business initiatives.
- At the physician's request, the medical assistant is often charged with researching the best options for buying supplies and equipment.
- Depending on factors like need, cost, and long-term objectives, medical offices may choose to lease or buy their business equipment.
- Fax machines are just one common piece of equipment that require all members of the health care team to remain vigilant to patient confidentiality.
- A photocopier in the medical office functions to provide copies of documents for patient and office use.

- Staff in the medical office often become adept at using ten-key calculators to manipulate numbers.
- Transcription machines, once predominant in health care, are still sometimes used today to convert spoken words to written ones.
- When researching transcription services outside the medical office, the medical assistant should be conscious of such factors as location and cost.
- An inventory control manual helps a medical office ensure that it is always fully equipped with needed supplies.
- Medical supplies may have expiration dates and should be ordered with the goal of using all supplies before they expire.
- Drug samples must be tracked and notice must be taken of any expiration dates on these samples.

Chapter Review

Multiple Choice

1. When investigating options for replacing medical equipment, it is acceptable to:
   a. Have a salesperson bring the equipment to the office to demonstrate it
   b. View the equipment online
   c. Visit a local supplier and view the item in person
   d. All of the above

2. In the medical office, fax machines:
   a. Should be used to send patient information between offices because it saves postage
   b. Can be placed anywhere where most convenient for office staff
   c. Come in all sizes and prices
   d. All of the above

3. The best way to dispose of expired medications is to:
   a. Donate them to an agency that will use them outside the United States
   b. Give them to patients who might want them
   c. Sell them on eBay
   d. Wrap them in plastic and place them in the garbage

4. It is important to keep a maintenance log for medical office equipment to:
   a. Prove the equipment has been maintained in the event warranty work is needed
   b. Ensure the equipment is being maintained so it will work properly
   c. Avoid having to purchase a replacement piece
   d. All of the above

5. When looking to purchase a new copy machine for the medical office, staff should consider the:
   a. Cost of supplies
   b. Features of the machine
   c. Availability of supplies
   d. All of the above

True/False

T F 1. It is always a good idea to call for references with any new supplier before making an expensive purchase.

T F 2. Many transcription services use employees outside the United States.

T F 3. Clinical inventory in the medical office should be taken weekly, whatever the practice type or patient load.

T F 4. Taking office pens and paperclips for home use is stealing, and should not be done.

Short Answer

1. Give one advantage to leasing a piece of office equipment instead of buying it.

2. Name one advantage to buying a piece of office equipment instead of leasing it.

3. Explain the use of a scanner in the medical office.

4. When calling other medical offices to get references for supply companies, why speak with the staff who use the supplies or equipment?

5. Explain why the medical office should keep an employee training manual for office equipment.

Chapter Review

6. What should be the medical office's main consideration when researching outside transcription services, and why?

7. Why separate the inventory list of clerical supplies from the list for clinical supplies?

8. Explain why expiration dates on medical supplies are important to track.

9. Why is it important to check the packing slip for supplies shipment?

10. Why do pharmaceutical companies give medical offices free drug samples?

11. What clerical supplies are usually ordered with an office's name, address, and telephone number preprinted?

Research

1. Interview a person who works in a medical office. How does that office keep track of the various supplies needed and used?

2. Research various office supply companies online for information about photocopiers. What type of machine do you think would be appropriate for a medical office?

3. Call a medical office supply company. How quickly are orders typically shipped? Are there discounts offered for higher quantity purchases?

Externship Application Experience

A package of medical office supplies arrives at the medical office. While checking off the supplies received on the packing slip, the medical assistant notices five items on the packing slip are not in the box. How should the medical assistant handle the situation?

Resource Guide

Child Family Health International (this agency takes donated, unused medical supplies)
995 Market Street, Suite 1104
San Francisco, CA 94103
Phone: (415) 957-9000 or (866) 345-4674
Fax: (415) 840-0486
http://www.cfhi.org

Par Inventory Management System (manufactures bar code scanning software for inventory control management)
Phone: (800) 272-7537
Fax: (440) 266-7400
http://www.parker.com

Visual Supply Pro (manufactures bar code scanning software for inventory control management)
2689 Danforth Terrace
Wellington, FL 33414
Phone: (561) 792-1477
Fax: (561) 792-1677
http://www.decisionsw.com

World Health Organization
Avenue Appia 20
CH - 1211 Geneva 27
Switzerland
Phone: +41 22 791 2111
Fax: +41 22 791 3111
http://www.who.org

 Med**Media**

http://www.MyMAKit.com

More on this chapter, including interactive resources, can be found on the Student CD-ROM accompanying this textbook and on http://www.MyMAKit.com.

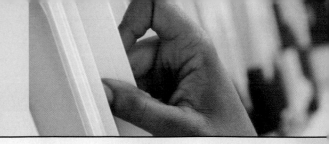

CHAPTER 14

Office Policies and Procedures

Case Study

Monte Taylor recently passed the medical assisting registration exam and has just obtained his first job as a registered medical assistant. Dr. Radcliff, an internist who shares her office space with several other physicians, has hired Monte. On Monte's first day, he asks the office manager if there is a manual that outlines office procedures. The office manager tells Monte that office staff have never taken the time to compose a procedures manual. She asks Monte if he would be willing to take on such a task.

Objectives

After completing this chapter, you should be able to:

- Define and spell the key terminology in this chapter.
- Create patient information pamphlets.
- Develop a personnel manual.
- Create a policies and procedures manual for the medical office.

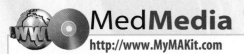

MedMedia
http://www.MyMAKit.com

Additional interactive resources and activities for this chapter can be found on http://www.MyMAKit.com. For a video, tips, audio glossary, legal and ethical scenarios, on-the-job scenarios, quizzes, and games related to the content of this chapter, please access the accompanying CD-ROM in this book.

Video: *Coping with Sales Calls*
Legal and Ethical Scenario: *Office Policies and Procedures*
On the Job Scenario: *Office Policies and Procedures*
Tips
Multiple Choice Quiz
Audio Glossary
HIPAA Quiz
Games: Spelling Bee, Crossword, and Strikeout

⊕ MEDICAL ASSISTING STANDARDS

CAAHEP ENTRY-LEVEL STANDARDS	ABHES ENTRY-LEVEL COMPETENCIES
■ Recognize elements of fundamental writing skills (cognitive) ■ Organize technical information and summaries (cognitive) ■ Describe the process to follow if an error is made in patient care (cognitive) ■ Explain general office policies (psychomotor) ■ Use office hardware and software to maintain office systems (psychomotor) ■ Use Internet to access information related to the medical office (psychomotor) ■ Maintain organization by filing (psychomotor) ■ Incorporate the Patients' Bill of Rights into personal practice and medical office policies and procedures (psychomotor) ■ Apply ethical behaviors, including honesty/integrity in performance of medical assisting practice (affective)	■ Maintain confidentiality at all times ■ Be cognizant of ethical boundaries ■ Conduct work within scope of education, training, and ability ■ Orient patients to office policies and procedures ■ Adapt what is said to the recipient's level of comprehension ■ Adaptation for individualized needs ■ Apply computer concepts for office procedures ■ Exercise efficient time management ■ Fundamental writing skills

✓ COMPETENCY SKILLS PERFORMANCE

1. Create an office brochure.
2. Create a procedure for the office procedure manual.

Introduction

Every business needs written policies and procedures to ensure that employees know how to perform their jobs correctly, and health care is no exception. Policies and procedures are perhaps even more important in the medical field than in others because they may contribute to patient safety and risk reduction. A **policy** is a statement of guidelines or rules on a given topic. A **procedure** describes how to perform a given task or project.

Creating Patient Information Pamphlets

Every member of the health care team is responsible for educating patients. Much of the information physicians ask that patients receive may be in written form. Many medical offices buy educational **brochures** to give to patients. These documents are available on a multitude of topics, including back pain, child immunizations, and menopause (Figure 14-1 ◆).

For physicians who want to provide more detailed information, brochures may be created with the help of in-house staff or a professional printing company. However the office chooses to create patient educational pamphlets, those pamphlets must be professional. All printed material must be accurate and free of typographical errors. Depending on the cultural makeup of an office's patients, brochures may be printed in various languages (Figure 14-2 ◆).

Key Terminology

brochure—document containing information about a topic

mission statement—statement that describes the medical office's reason for existing

organizational chart—breakdown of the chain of command in a business

personnel manual—compilation of employment policies for an office; also called an employee handbook

policy—guidelines or rules for an issue

procedure—steps to perform a task or project

Acronyms

HIPAA—Health Insurance Portability and Accountability Act

OSHA—Occupational Safety and Health Administration

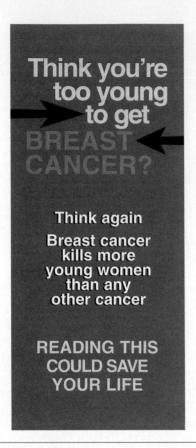

Figure 14-1 ◆ A patient education pamphlet on breast cancer.

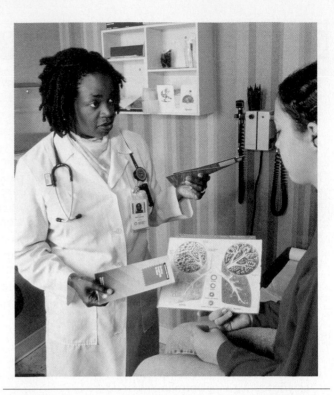

Figure 14-2 ◆ A medical assistant explains the dangers of smoking to a young patient.

Creating a Personnel Manual

A **personnel manual,** also called an employee handbook, lists the rules and regulations that apply to all staff in the medical office (Figure 14-3 ◆). This manual also breaks down the office's benefits for health, life, and disability insurance, among others. Many offices give all new employees copies of their personnel manuals upon hire. Other offices keep single copies in central locations or in an electronic format accessible to all employees.

To create a personnel manual, the office manager and/or physician should list desired manual items. For ideas, a medical

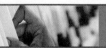

PROCEDURE 14-1 **Create an Office Brochure**

Theory and Rationale

Office brochures are a useful way to educate patients on the physician's specific types of treatment or therapy. All office brochures must be professional, accurate, and free of typographical errors.

Materials

■ Computer with word-processing software
■ List of information the physician would like in an office brochure

Competency

(**Conditions**) With the necessary materials, you will be able to (**Task**) create an office brochure (**Standards**) correctly within the time limit set by the instructor.

1. Gather information on the brochure's subject.
2. Launch the word-processing software.
3. Create a title for the brochure, such as "Living with Diabetes."
4. Add information to the brochure in an easy-to-read format. Use simple terms rather than medical terminology.
5. Add information regarding where the patient can look for further resources, such as Web sites.
6. Include the office's name, address, and telephone number.
7. Check for typographical and grammatical errors.
8. Print the brochure, and give it to the physician for review before making copies for patients.

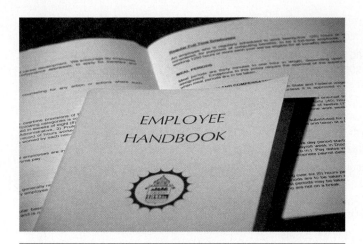

Figure 14-3 ◆ The employee handbook should be updated on a regular basis and made available to each new employee.

office might consult the personnel manuals of other offices. For all material, it is important to keep federal and state laws in mind to ensure all policies are within legal boundaries. Figure 14-4 ◆ lists items commonly found in personnel manuals.

─ Critical Thinking Question 14-1─
What type of policies and procedures should Monte start identifying for his office?

Creating Policies and Procedures for the Medical Office

The medical office's policy and procedures manual may contain both policies and procedures, or policies and procedures may be separated. Whatever the approach, each policy and procedure manual should contain the following items in separate sections:

- Mission statement
- Organizational chart
- Personnel policies
- Clinical procedures
- Administrative procedures

A table of contents should clearly direct readers to desired pages. Per Occupational Safety and Health Administra-

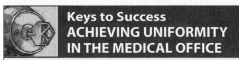

Keys to Success
ACHIEVING UNIFORMITY IN THE MEDICAL OFFICE

One of the most important reasons for having a medical office policy and procedure manual is to clarify rules and regulations and the physician's expectations for procedures. Strict adherence to policies as they are outlined achieves uniformity in the office and provides a fair method of treating staff.

tion (**OSHA**) and **HIPAA** regulations, infection control and quality improvement and risk management procedures must be kept in separate notebooks and reviewed and updated regularly.

Writing a Mission Statement

The policy and procedures manual for a medical office should begin with an office **mission statement** that is concise and communicated to all staff. For example, a mission statement might read, "To care for all patients in a compassionate and dignified manner, with a focus on patient safety and satisfaction." Many medical offices frame and hang their mission statements for patients to see.

─Critical Thinking Question 14-2─
If Monte's office lacks a mission statement, how should he go about explaining its importance to the physician?

Preparing an Organizational Chart

In addition to the mission statement, all policy and procedure manuals should break down the offices' organizational structures in **organizational charts** (Figure 14-5 ◆). Organizational charts are maps to office hierarchies, from physicians to entry-level staff. Members of the health care team should be able to use these charts to identify their supervisors, as well as their supervisors' supervisors, all the way to the top of the chain of command. In addition to reporting structure, an organizational chart might explain how employees can contact varied health care staff.

Outlining Clinical Procedures

Any clinical procedure that requires patient intervention should be documented for employee reference. Procedures should clearly list appropriate steps, as well as information on patient education, documentation, and infection control. The type of clinical procedures found in a policies and procedures manual varies according to the type of medical practice and the physician's specialty.

Outlining Administrative Procedures

Administrative procedures should be documented to include such topics as:

- Office opening and closing
- Inventory and supply ordering
- Appointment scheduling
- Patient accounting and bookkeeping
- Insurance processing
- Insurance benefit verification
- Patients' records release
- Medical records management
- Operation of administrative office machinery

Like clinical procedures, administrative procedures vary according to the type of medical practice, but the vast

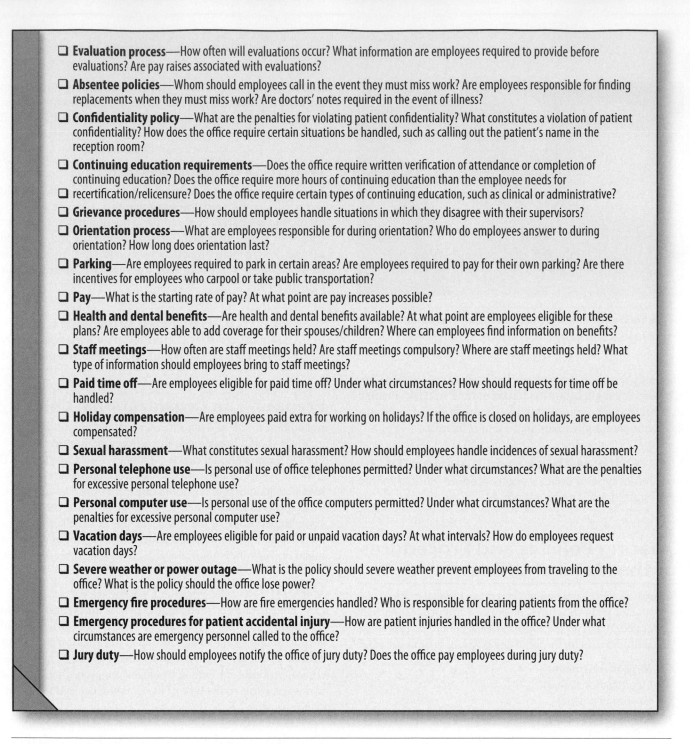

- ❑ **Evaluation process**—How often will evaluations occur? What information are employees required to provide before evaluations? Are pay raises associated with evaluations?
- ❑ **Absentee policies**—Whom should employees call in the event they must miss work? Are employees responsible for finding replacements when they must miss work? Are doctors' notes required in the event of illness?
- ❑ **Confidentiality policy**—What are the penalties for violating patient confidentiality? What constitutes a violation of patient confidentiality? How does the office require certain situations be handled, such as calling out the patient's name in the reception room?
- ❑ **Continuing education requirements**—Does the office require written verification of attendance or completion of continuing education? Does the office require more hours of continuing education than the employee needs for
- ❑ recertification/relicensure? Does the office require certain types of continuing education, such as clinical or administrative?
- ❑ **Grievance procedures**—How should employees handle situations in which they disagree with their supervisors?
- ❑ **Orientation process**—What are employees responsible for during orientation? Who do employees answer to during orientation? How long does orientation last?
- ❑ **Parking**—Are employees required to park in certain areas? Are employees required to pay for their own parking? Are there incentives for employees who carpool or take public transportation?
- ❑ **Pay**—What is the starting rate of pay? At what point are pay increases possible?
- ❑ **Health and dental benefits**—Are health and dental benefits available? At what point are employees eligible for these plans? Are employees able to add coverage for their spouses/children? Where can employees find information on benefits?
- ❑ **Staff meetings**—How often are staff meetings held? Are staff meetings compulsory? Where are staff meetings held? What type of information should employees bring to staff meetings?
- ❑ **Paid time off**—Are employees eligible for paid time off? Under what circumstances? How should requests for time off be handled?
- ❑ **Holiday compensation**—Are employees paid extra for working on holidays? If the office is closed on holidays, are employees compensated?
- ❑ **Sexual harassment**—What constitutes sexual harassment? How should employees handle incidences of sexual harassment?
- ❑ **Personal telephone use**—Is personal use of office telephones permitted? Under what circumstances? What are the penalties for excessive personal telephone use?
- ❑ **Personal computer use**—Is personal use of the office computers permitted? Under what circumstances? What are the penalties for excessive personal computer use?
- ❑ **Vacation days**—Are employees eligible for paid or unpaid vacation days? At what intervals? How do employees request vacation days?
- ❑ **Severe weather or power outage**—What is the policy should severe weather prevent employees from traveling to the office? What is the policy should the office lose power?
- ❑ **Emergency fire procedures**—How are fire emergencies handled? Who is responsible for clearing patients from the office?
- ❑ **Emergency procedures for patient accidental injury**—How are patient injuries handled in the office? Under what circumstances are emergency personnel called to the office?
- ❑ **Jury duty**—How should employees notify the office of jury duty? Does the office pay employees during jury duty?

Figure 14-4 ◆ Common personnel manual items.

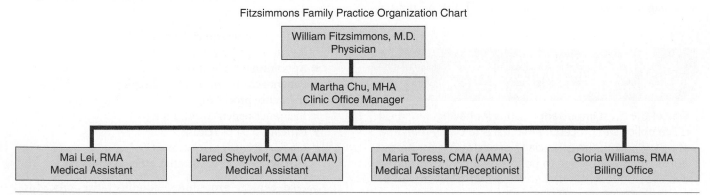

Fitzsimmons Family Practice Organization Chart

William Fitzsimmons, M.D.
Physician

Martha Chu, MHA
Clinic Office Manager

| Mai Lei, RMA Medical Assistant | Jared Sheylvolf, CMA (AAMA) Medical Assistant | Maria Toress, CMA (AAMA) Medical Assistant/Receptionist | Gloria Williams, RMA Billing Office |

Figure 14-5 ◆ Sample organizational chart for a medical office.

majority of administrative policies remain constant from office to office (Figure 14-6 ◆).

?—Critical Thinking Question 14-3—

How should Monte determine which policies should appear in his office's policy manual?

Documenting Infection Control Procedures

Infection control procedures should be written for all of a medical office's applicable procedures, including:

- Biohazardous waste disposal
- Employee needlestick injuries
- Employee exposure to infectious materials
- Employee education for infection control
- OSHA-required documentation
- Local, state, and federal reporting requirements for infectious agents

As mandated by OSHA, infection control procedures must be part of the office's exposure control plan, which must be kept separate from other procedure manuals in the office and must be made available to an OSHA inspector if needed.

In Practice

Anka is a registered medical assistant working for Dr. Radliffe. While Anka is finishing a blood draw on a patient, she accidentally sticks herself with the contaminated needle. How will Anka know what to do now that this injury has happened?

Policy: Releasing Medical Records to a Patient

Purpose: To release medical records to the patient following legal guidelines.

1. Verify the patient's identity by requesting photo identification.
2. Obtain the patient's signature on the release of records form.
3. Ensure the patient has dated the release form.
4. Check to see if the patient has made any alterations to the release form, such as restricting the records release to a limited date.
5. Check to see if the patient has checked the boxes allowing release of information regarding HIV/AIDS, reproductive health, mental health, or drug and alcohol rehabilitation.
6. Pull the patient's medical record.
7. Photocopy the appropriate parts of the medical record according to any limitations noted by the patient on the release form.
8. Send copies of the records to the patient.
9. Note in the patient's file when the records were released.
10. File the original signed release form.

Figure 14-6 ◆ Sample administrative procedure.

PROCEDURE 14-2 Create a Procedure for the Procedure Manual

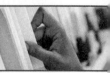

Theory and Rationale

Medical offices need clearly written policies and procedures for all members of the health care team to understand how each task is performed.

Materials

- Computer with word-processing software

Competency

(**Conditions**) With the necessary materials, you will be able to (**Task**) create a procedure for an office procedure manual (**Standards**) correctly within the time limit set by the instructor.

1. Determine the type of procedure to be created.

2. Gather the information on how this procedure is to be performed.
3. Title the procedure (e.g., "Policy: Sorting Incoming Mail"), and determine if it will be listed under administrative, clinical, infection control, personnel, or quality improvement and risk management.
4. Describe the policy's purpose (e.g., "Purpose: To describe the method of routing incoming mail to appropriate staff").
5. List each step in the procedure.
6. Print the procedure, and give it to the office manager for approval.
7. Once approved, place the procedure in the office procedure manual.

Creating Quality Improvement and Risk Management Procedures

Quality improvement and risk management procedures are designed to reduce patient or staff injury in the medical office. These policies range from information on washing children's toys in the reception room to handling life-threatening patient events in the office. While quality improvement and risk management procedures policies vary according to office needs, the vast majority apply to all office types. According to HIPAA, quality improvement and risk management procedures must be kept in a separate notebook that is clearly marked and updated regularly.

Writing Other Office Policies

To ensure ongoing compliance and relevance, all medical office policies should be reviewed and updated regularly. Many large medical offices separate their policy manuals into clinical and administrative sections. Some offices further divide their manuals according to position or department. Table 14-1 identifies policies that may be found in medical office policy and procedure manuals.

TABLE 14-1 SAMPLE POLICIES AND PROCEDURES

Policy or Procedure	Purpose
Emergency Closure Policy	Outlines the steps to take in the event the office closes due to emergency
Building Lockup Policy	Describes the steps to take to lock the building at the end of the day
Publications and Distribution Policy	Outlines the policy with regard to allowing publications or pamphlets to be distributed to patients and staff
Smoking Policy	Describes the availability of smoking areas near the office
Personal Relationships between Office Staff	Outlines the policy for personal relationships between coworkers
Personal Relationships between Staff and Patients	Outlines the policy for personal relationships between office staff and patients
Termination Policy	Describes the policy for terminating employment
Disciplinary Policy	Describes the policy for disciplining of employees. Includes an outline of the offenses justifying discipline
Grievance Policy	Describes the process staff must follow to file grievances
Continuing Education	Outlines the requirements for continuing education
Malpractice Insurance	Describes the requirements for holding malpractice insurance
Reimbursement for Seminars	Outlines the policy for reimbursing staff who attend medical-related seminars
Computers for Personal Use Policy	Describes the policy for personal use of office computers
Petty Cash Funds	Describes the policy for using petty cash, including the type of expenses that qualify as petty cash and the amount to be kept as petty cash
Parking Policy	Outlines where employees may park, as well as reimbursement for parking expenses
Dress Code Policy	Describes the dress code for each office position
Opening Office Policy	Outlines the steps to take to open the office at the beginning of the day
Disclosure of Patient Information Policy	Describes the procedure for disclosing patient information, including the forms required and the Health Insurance Portability and Accountability Act (HIPAA) regulations
Job Descriptions	Provides a job description for each office position
HIPAA Privacy Officer Duties	Outlines the duties of the HIPAA privacy officer in the medical office
Calling Patients from the Reception Room	Describes the procedure for calling patients from the reception room
Missed Patient Appointments	Describes the steps to take when patients miss their appointments. Includes proper charting technique
Termination of the Physician/Patient Relationship	Outlines the steps to legally terminate the physician/patient relationship
E-mail Policy	Describes the conditions under which the medical office may e-mail information to patients or other facilities
Obtaining Consent for a Procedure	Describes the consent forms used in the medical office and outlines the process of witnessing patient signatures
Prescription Refill Requests	Outlines the policy for taking telephone calls for prescription refills, including documentation in the patient's medical record
Jury Duty Policy	Describes the policy for employees called for jury duty
Sick Leave Policy	Describes the policy for employees who take sick leave
Personal Telephone Calls	Describes the policy for employees making and receiving personal telephone calls

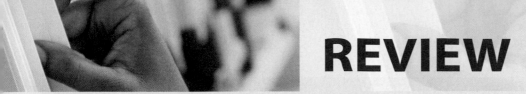

REVIEW

- Informational pamphlets are effective vehicles for educating patients.
- Office personnel manuals are needed to ensure all members of the health care team perform appropriately and to consistent standards.

- A policies and procedure manual in the medical office serves as written record of the legal, desired behavior of all health care staff.

Chapter Review

Multiple Choice

1. Any _____ procedure that requires patient intervention should be documented for patient reference.
   a. Clinical
   b. Administrative
   c. Infection control
   d. All of the above

2. Quality improvement and risk management procedures are designed to:
   a. Reduce patient injury
   b. Limit employee injury
   c. Avoid liability lawsuits
   d. All of the above

3. A procedure for filing insurance claims would be found under which policies section of the office procedure manual?
   a. Clinical
   b. Infection control
   c. Risk management
   d. Administrative

4. Once a policy and procedure manual has been written, it should be updated:
   a. Once a month
   b. Once a year
   c. Once every 5 years
   d. As the policy or procedure changes

5. The office mission statement should be shared with:
   a. Administrative staff
   b. Clinical staff
   c. Patients
   d. All of the above
   e. A and B

True/False

T F 1. Only the office manager can compose a procedure for the office manual.

T F 2. An organizational chart outlines the chain of command in the office.

T F 3. By strictly following a policy and procedure manual, medical office management gives the impression that all staff members will be treated consistently.

T F 4. Office policies for quality improvement and risk management must be kept in a separate notebook.

T F 5. Compulsory means choosing to participate.

Short Answer

1. List the sections all policy and procedure manuals should include.

2. What is the purpose of an office mission statement?

3. Give five examples of an administrative policy.

4. Give five examples of a clinical policy.

5. Give five examples of a quality improvement or risk management policy.

6. Give five examples of an infection control policy.

7. Differentiate between a policy and a procedure.

8. Describe the steps to take to create an educational brochure.

9. Why might a medical office have separate policy and procedure manuals for its administrative and clinical areas?

10. Differentiate between a clinical policy and an administrative policy.

Research

1. Search online for policy and procedure manuals for medical facilities. Describe what each of these companies has in common with the others.

2. Call a local medical office. Ask the office manager if the office has a policy and procedure manual. How often is it updated? How are employees given access to the manual?

3. Search the Internet for companies that make office educational brochures. What type of information can you get ready-made pamphlets for?

Externship Application Experience

Manuel is unsure how to handle a patient who refuses to schedule a followup appointment. He asks two other members of the health care team to explain the office policy for proceeding and receives two vastly different responses. Should Manuel follow the advice of one staff member over the other? How can he know how this situation is supposed to be handled?

Resource Guide

Employee Manual (offers downloadable and customizable employee manuals)
http://www.theemployeemanual.com/

MedMedia

http://www.MyMAKit.com

More on this chapter, including interactive resources, can be found on the Student CD-ROM accompanying this textbook and on http://www.MyMAKit.com.

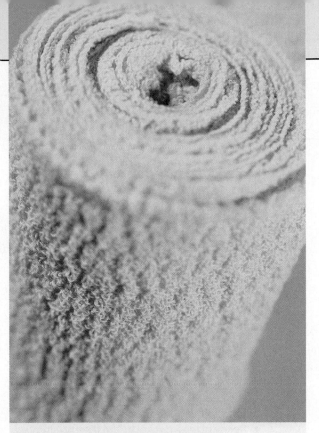

SECTION III

Responding to Emergencies in the Medical Office

Chapter 15   Handling Medical Office Emergencies

My name is Teresa Godyn. I have been working as a medical assistant for about a year. One of the things I have found when working in the medical field is that medical assistants have to remember that we are not just performing a task, but providing patients with a sense of comfort and well-being. We offer this by being conscientious about how we deliver pertinent information. Leaving phone messages plays a dominant role in patient communication when patients are out of the office. A patient may feel frustrated because a needed medication cannot be authorized through insurance, a diagnostic is not covered, or a specialist appointment may not be available in a timely fashion. The way the medical assistant handles this can dramatically change the way a patient views the quality of their health care.

Making sure the patient can hear a caring, empathetic tone is important. Though we only hear of their aches and pains, from time to time these can be all encompassing for your patient. I have found that truly listening to my patients shows them I care about them.

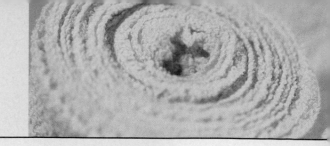

Handling Medical Office Emergencies

Case Study

Mark Whitford is a 70-year-old patient in Dr. Hardy's office. As Mark walks toward the reception desk, he stumbles, loses his balance, and falls. Mark strikes his head on a cabinet, loses consciousness, and sustains a gash on his forehead that is bleeding profusely.

Objectives

After completing this chapter, you should be able to:

- Define and spell the key terminology in this chapter.
- Describe the medical assistant's responsibilities in an emergency.
- Understand how to prevent accidents and injuries in the medical office.
- Identify supplies and equipment used in an emergency and list the contents of a crash cart.
- Describe the screening techniques for handling an emergency.
- Recognize and respond to life-threatening emergencies in the medical office.
- Recognize when to call emergency services to the medical office.
- Provide rescue breathing and perform adult cardiopulmonary resuscitation (CPR).
- Assist and monitor a patient who has fainted.
- Administer oxygen in emergencies.
- Describe how to use an automated external defibrillator.
- Know the signs and symptoms of heart attack.
- Know the signs and symptoms of choking.
- Describe the steps to stop bleeding.
- Assist patients in shock.
- Assist patients with burns.
- Describe comfort measures to take with patients with fractures.
- Discuss the potential role(s) of the medical assistant in emergency preparedness.

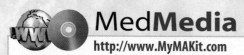

MedMedia
http://www.MyMAKit.com

Additional interactive resources and activities for this chapter can be found on http://www.MyMAKit.com. For a video, tips, audio glossary, legal and ethical scenarios, on-the-job scenarios, quizzes, and games related to the content of this chapter, please access the accompanying CD-ROM in this book.

Video: *Facing Emergencies*
Legal and Ethical Scenario: *Handling Emergencies in the Medical Office*
On the Job Scenario: *Handling Emergencies in the Medical Office*
Tips
Multiple Choice Quiz
Audio Glossary
HIPAA Quiz
Games: Spelling Bee, Crossword, and Strikeout

⊕ MEDICAL ASSISTING STANDARDS

CAAHEP ENTRY-LEVEL STANDARDS	ABHES ENTRY-LEVEL COMPETENCIES
■ Describe personal protective equipment (cognitive) ■ Identify safety techniques that can be used to prevent accidents and maintain a safe work environment (cognitive) ■ Describe the importance of Materials Safety Data Sheets (MSDS) in a healthcare setting (cognitive) ■ Identify safety signs, symbols, and labels (cognitive) ■ State principles and steps of professional/provider CPR (cognitive) ■ Describe basic principles of first aid (cognitive) ■ Describe fundamental principles for evacuation of a healthcare setting (cognitive) ■ Discuss fire safety issues in a healthcare environment (cognitive) ■ Discuss requirements for responding to hazardous material disposal (cognitive) ■ Identify principles of body mechanics and ergonomics (cognitive) ■ Discuss critical elements of an emergency plan for response to a natural disaster or other emergency (cognitive) ■ Identify emergency preparedness plans in your community (cognitive) ■ Discuss potential role(s) of the medical assistant in emergency preparedness (cognitive) ■ Comply with safety signs, symbols, and labels (psychomotor) ■ Evaluate the work environment to identify safe vs. unsafe working conditions (psychomotor) ■ Develop a personal (patient and employee) safety plan (psychomotor) ■ Develop an environmental safety plan (psychomotor) ■ Participate in a mock environmental exposure event with documentation of steps taken (psychomotor) ■ Explain an evacuation plan for a physician's office (psychomotor) ■ Demonstrate methods of fire prevention in the healthcare setting (psychomotor) ■ Maintain provider/professional level CPR certification (psychomotor) ■ Perform first aid procedures (psychomotor)	■ Adapt to change ■ Be cognizant of ethical boundaries ■ Evidence a responsible attitude ■ Conduct work within scope of education, training, and ability ■ Adaptation for individualized needs ■ Locate resources and information for patients and employers ■ Document accurately ■ Serve as a liaison between the physician and others ■ Perform telephone and in-person screening ■ Be attentive, listen, and learn ■ Recognize and respond to verbal and nonverbal communication ■ Exhibit initiative ■ Be a team player ■ Practice standard precautions ■ Recognize emergencies ■ Perform first aid and CPR

Key Terminology

anaphylaxis—severe allergic reaction
CPR mouth barrier—disposable barrier device used to prevent infection
crash cart—wheeled cart that contains emergency medical equipment
defibrillator—device that delivers an electric shock to a patient
standard precautions—infection control techniques
syncope—fainting; the sudden loss of consciousness

Abbreviations

AAMA—American Association of Medical Assistants
ABCD—airway, breathing, circulation, and defibrillation
AED—automatic external defibrillator
AHA—American Heart Association
CPR—cardiopulmonary resuscitation
FEMA—Federal Emergency Management Agency
HEPA—high efficiency particulate air filter
OSHA—Occupational Safety and Health Administration
PPE—personal protective equipment

✚ MEDICAL ASSISTING STANDARDS

CAAHEP ENTRY-LEVEL STANDARDS	ABHES ENTRY-LEVEL COMPETENCIES
■ Use proper body mechanics (psychomotor) ■ Maintain a current list of community resources for emergency preparedness (psychomotor) ■ Complete an incident report (psychomotor) ■ Recognize the effects of stress on all persons involved in emergency situations (affective) ■ Demonstrate self awareness in responding to emergency situations (affective)	

✔ COMPETENCY SKILLS PERFORMANCE

1. Perform adult rescue breathing and one-rescuer cardiopulmonary resuscitation (CPR).
2. Care for a patient who has fainted.
3. Administer oxygen to a patient.
4. Use an automated external defibrillator (AED).
5. Respond to an adult with an airway obstruction.
6. Remove an airway obstruction in an infant.
7. Control bleeding.
8. Develop an environmental exposure plan.

Introduction

Medical emergencies are rare in the medical office; however, when patients or members of the health care team become severely ill or injured in the medical office, medical assistants must be trained to respond appropriately. In fact, all members of the medical staff, including those who work in the administrative area, should have basic CPR knowledge and first aid skills. With proper first aid and/or cardiopulmonary resuscitation (**CPR**), patients may well recover completely. Instruction in CPR is offered through many medical assisting programs as a separate course. These courses can also be found through the American Red Cross or through local fire departments or hospitals.

The Medical Assistant's Role in an Emergency

When emergencies occur in ambulatory care, administrative medical assistants may be the first members of the health care team to know. In fact, when emergencies arise in offices' reception areas or hallways, medical assistants may be the first to respond. When emergencies arise in an office's clinical area, medical assistants may be asked to move patients to other areas, keep other patients or family members calm, or telephone for emergency services. ∞ Chapter 7 outlines how medical assistants should handle emergencies via telephone. To ensure that assistants are well prepared, as of 2006 the American Association of Medical Assistants (**AAMA**) requires all certified medical assistants to have CPR certification and to renew that certification every year.

**Keys to Success
PERFORMING WITHIN SCOPE
OF PRACTICE**

Medical assistants must remember to perform only those skills they have been trained to perform. In the event of medical emergencies, medical assistants should quickly alert the physician and/or emergency medical services.

Preventing Accidents and Injuries

As ∞ Chapters 4 and 21 discuss, the key to avoiding injuries and accidents in the medical office is to act proactively. For example, administrative medical assistants are likely responsible for the reception and front desk areas, places where those assistants should pick up fallen items before patients or other members of the health care team can trip and fall. Medical assistants must constantly look for potential trouble areas, such as wrinkled area rugs or outlets lacking childproof plugs.

─Critical Thinking Question 15-1─
How might the medical office have helped prevent Mark Whitford's injury?

Preparing for Medical Emergencies

In the medical office, emergency preparedness can mean the difference between chaos and ordered, effective response. As ∞ Chapter 14 describes, medical offices should have well written and complete policy and procedures manuals that identify the steps to take in the event of an office emergency. In addition to patient and staff injuries or life-threatening illnesses, office emergencies can also include severe storms, power outages, and building fires.

In most towns and cities, medical offices can reach their local emergency personnel by dialing 9-1-1. While medical offices should have all their local emergency service numbers readily available, they should also have the following numbers on hand:

- Poison Control Center (800-222-1222)
- Local fire department
- Local police department

Managing Medical Emergencies

When emergencies arise in the medical office, medical assistants must remember to stay calm so they can direct patients as needed. Patients look to medical assistants as authority figures.

Emergency intervention is called for in any situation that may be life-threatening (Table 15-1). The responder provides appropriate intervention and stays with the injured or ill person until more advanced care can be provided. Triage of emergency patients is a critical care issue.

Before assessing any patient, the medical assistant should don disposable gloves to prevent exposure to blood or other bodily fluids. The medical assistant must follow **standard precautions,** because in emergencies, all bodily fluids must be considered infectious. When the patient is nonresponsive, the medical assistant should notify the physician immediately. When the physician is unavailable, the medical assistant should ask other members of the health care team to call for emergency personnel.

After securing physician or emergency personnel assistance, the medical assistant should determine if a nonresponsive patient is breathing.

Respiratory and cardiac arrest may be caused by an occluded airway, electrocution, shock, drowning, heart attack, trauma, **anaphylaxis**, drugs, poisoning, or traumatic head or chest injury. Intervention must be immediate if resuscitation is to be succedssful. For individuals experiencing acute chest pain, loss of consciousness, or respiratory arest, follow CPR protocol.

CPR guidelines are similar for respiratory arrest, cardiac arrest, and obstructed airway but vary somewhat according to age group. Table 15-2 lists the major differences in the performance of CPR-related skills as defined by the **AHA**. Early access

TABLE 15-1 EMERGENCY INTERVENTION		
Life-Threatening Condition	**Not Life-Threatening Immediate Intervention**	**Not Life-Threatening: Intervention as Soon as Possible**
■ extreme shortness of breath (airway or breathing problems) ■ cardiac arrest ■ severe, uncontrolled bleeding ■ head injuries ■ poisoning ■ open chest or abdominal wounds ■ shock ■ severe burns, including face, hands, feet, and genitals ■ potential neck injuries	■ decreased levels of consciousness ■ chest pain ■ seizures ■ major or multiple fractures ■ neck injuries ■ severe eye injuries ■ burns not on face, hands, feet, or genitals	■ severe vomiting and diarrhea, especially in the very young and the elderly ■ minor injuries ■ sprains ■ strains ■ simple fractures

TABLE 15-2 ADULT, CHILD, AND INFANT CPR SKILLS

CPR Skill	Adult: 8+ years	Child: 1 year–puberty (approximately 12–14 years)	Infant: under 1 year
EMS access by calling 911 and giving emergency information	If sudden collapse is witnessed, immediately activate EMS and get AED. If asphyxiation (e.g., drowning, injury, overdose) suspected, first perform 2 minutes of CPR (or 5 cycles), then activate EMS.	If sudden collapse is witnessed, immediately activate EMS and get AED. Otherwise perform 2 minutes of CPR (5 cycles), then activate EMS.	If sudden collapse is witnessed, immediately activate EMS. Otherwise perform 2 minutes of CPR (5 cycles), then activate EMS.
Assessment of unresponsiveness	Shake the shoulders.	Shake the shoulders.	Snap or poke the feet. Do *not* shake the shoulders.
Rescue breathing rate of 1 second long, normal breath until chest rises	10–12 breaths per minute or one breath every 5–6 seconds	12–20 breaths per minute or one breath every 3–5 seconds	12–20 breaths per minute or one breath every 3–5 seconds
Obstructed airway foreign-body	Abdominal thrusts	Abdominal thrusts	Back slaps and chest thrusts
Pulse check location	Carotid	Carotid	Brachial or femoral
Compression technique	One hand linked over second hand, with heel of second hand on sternum	Heel of one hand on sternum	Single rescuer: two fingertips on sternum Two rescuers: two thumbs touching on sternum and hand encircling chest and back technique
Compression landmarks	Center of chest, between nipples	Center of chest, between nipples	Center of chest, just below nipple line
Compression depth	1-1/2–2"	1/2 to 1/3 depth of chest	1/2 to 1/3 depth of chest
Compression rate	100 per minute	100 per minute	100 per minute
Compression ratio to rescue breathing	Single rescuer: 30:2 Two rescuers: 30:2	Single rescuer: 30:2 Two rescuers: 15:2	Single rescuer: 30:2 Two rescuers: 15:2

to EMS is important. Access for the adult victim is initiated by calling 911 as soon as it has been determined that the victim is unconscious and not breathing. In general, "phone first" for an unresponsive adult. With children and infants, EMS access is made after two minutes of CPR. In general, perform "CPR first" for unresponsive children and infants. The sequence normally followed is airway, breathing, circulation, and defibrillation (**ABCD**).

From the crash cart, the medical assistant should secure pocket masks, also called **CPR mouth barriers** (Figure 15-1 ◆), and then give the patient two slow breaths and check for a pulse. When the patient has a pulse, the medical assistant should continue breathing into that patient every 5–6 seconds for adults and every 3–5 seconds for children. When the patient does not have a pulse, the medical assistant should begin cycles of chest compressions followed by two slow breaths. See Figures 15-2, 15-3, and 15-4 for compressions for an infant, child, and adult, respectively.

?—Critical Thinking Question 15-2–
Imagine that when Mark Whitford falls, the reception room is full of other patients waiting to see their physicians. How should the medical assistant handle this situation?

Fainting (Syncope)

Many serious disorders cause unresponsiveness. Simple fainting (**syncope**) occurs often in some people and almost never in others. Fainting or syncope, the sudden loss of

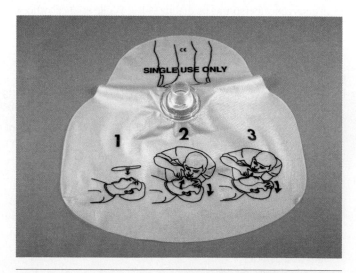

Figure 15-1 ◆ CPR mouth barrier.

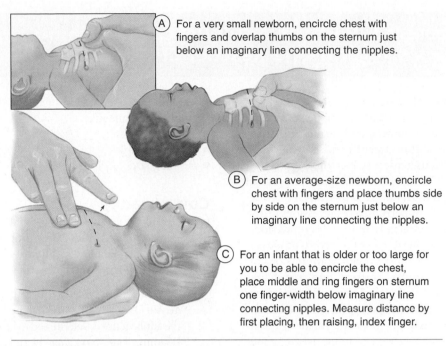

(A) For a very small newborn, encircle chest with fingers and overlap thumbs on the sternum just below an imaginary line connecting the nipples.

(B) For an average-size newborn, encircle chest with fingers and place thumbs side by side on the sternum just below an imaginary line connecting the nipples.

(C) For an infant that is older or too large for you to be able to encircle the chest, place middle and ring fingers on sternum one finger-width below imaginary line connecting nipples. Measure distance by first placing, then raising, index finger.

Figure 15-2 ◆ Compressions for an infant.

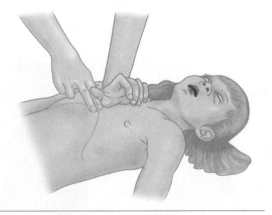

Figure 15-3 ◆ Compressions for a child.

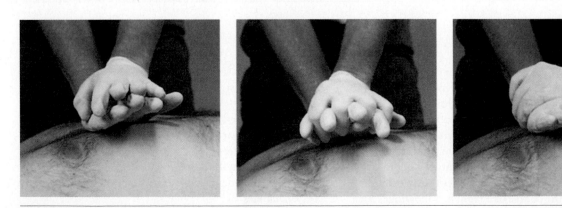

Figure 15-4 ◆ Location and position of hand during chest compressions for adult.

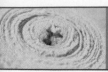

PROCEDURE 15-1 Perform Adult Rescue Breathing and One-Rescuer CPR

Theory and Rationale

Chest compressions and rescue breathing are performed in adults with an absence of respiratory and cardiac function. The American Heart Association recently revised guidelines for Cardiopulmonary Resuscitation (CPR) and Emergency Cardiovascular Care (ECC) in an effort to simplify the process. The new guidelines require healthcare providers to increase the number and quality of uninterrupted compressions delivered. Revised guidelines recommend a universal compression-to-ventilation of 30 to 2 for lone rescuers for victims of all ages (except newborns). Rescuers must provide compressions of adequate rate (approximately 100 beats/minute) and depth (1 1/2 to 2 inches) for adult victims and allow adequate chest recoil with minimal interruptions in chest compressions. Additionally, actions for Foreign Body Obstructed Airway (FBOA) were simplified. The tongue-jaw lift is no longer taught and blind finger sweep should not be performed.

Using a mouth guard with a one-way valve prevents vomit or other body fluids from contaminating the rescuer's mouth.

Materials

- approved mannequin
- gloves
- ventilator mask
- mouth guard

Competency

(**Conditions**) With the necessary materials, (**Task**) you will be able to administer rescue breathing for an adult and one-rescuer CPR for an adult (**Standards**) correctly, within the time frame designated by the instructor.

1. Assess the victim and determine if help is needed. Shout "Are you OK?" while gently shaking the victim's shoulders.
2. If the adult victim is determined to be unresponsive, activate EMS immediately by calling 911 and get an AED if available.
3. Assess the ABCs. Airway: Perform a head-tilt chin lift, or, if a neck injury is suspected, a jaw thrust (Figure 15-5 ◆). Look and feel for breath and chest movements (Figure 15-6 ◆). Attempt to get another person to call 911. If you

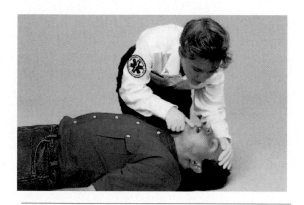

Figure 15-5 ◆ Establish an open airway.

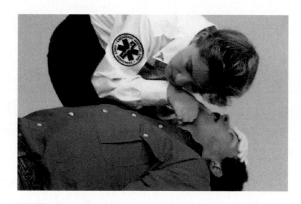

Figure 15-6 ◆ Look and feel for breath and chest movements.

consciousness, seems to be caused by a brief interruption in the body's ability to control the brain's circulation. When fainting does occur, it usually does so just after a patient has received an emotional shock of some kind. The patient usually collapses and becomes totally unresponsive, but within a minute, should awaken and return to normal function. Patients seldom become incontinent or have seizures as a result of simple fainting, but may be injured in the course of a fall. The following is a list of some serious disorders that can produce fainting:

- Airway obstruction/apnea
- Assault
- Brain infection
- Brain tumor
- Cardiac arrest
- Cardiac rhythm disturbance
- Cerebral edema
- Diabetes
- Drugs or alcohol ingestion

PROCEDURE 15-1   Perform Adult Rescue Breathing and One-Rescuer CPR *(continued)*

are alone, begin the rescue sequence for 1 minute and then attempt to call yourself. If gloves are available, put them on. If you have a ventilator mask, place it on the victim.

4. If breathing is absent, put on a mouth guard and administer two rescue breaths (Figure 15-7 ◆). If your breaths do not cause the chest to rise, look in the victim's mouth and remove an object if one is seen. If no object is seen, make a second attempt to administer a rescue breath. If the breath still does not enter the chest, proceed to abdominal thrusts for unconscious victims.

5. If the breaths cause the chest to rise, assess the patient's circulation by feeling for a pulse at the carotid artery (Figure 15-8 ◆). If you feel a pulse, begin rescue breathing. Administer 1 breath every 5 seconds, or 10–12 every minute. After 1 minute, reassess the victim for breathing and pulse.

6. If you do not feel a pulse, begin chest compressions. Kneel at the victim's side. Find the sternum and place the heel of one hand just below the nipple line.

7. Place your other hand on top of the first hand, making sure to lift your fingers off the chest, using only the heels of your hands to administer compressions.

8. Keeping your shoulders directly over your hands, compress the chest 1-1/2 to 2 inches, then allow the sternum to relax. Do not lift your hands off the chest.

9. Continue to compress the chest a total of 30 times, then administer 2 breaths.

10. Repeat this sequence for 4 total cycles. Reassess the victim.

11. If necessary, continue CPR until pulse and breathing return or you are relieved by more advanced medical personnel.

Patient Education

Advise the patient to follow up with his or her personal physician after release from the EMS.

Charting Example

08/05/XX 7:30 PM Patient found collapsed in bathroom and unresponsive. 911 call placed and CPR started. EMS arrived in approximately 10 minutes and took over care. Patient was transferred to Deaconess Medical Center. Vivian Nagle, RMA (AMT)

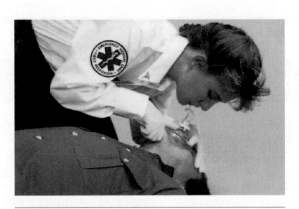

Figure 15-7 ◆ Administer two rescue breaths.

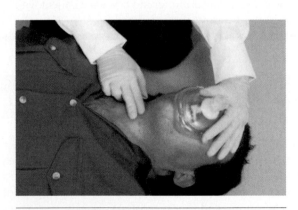

Figure 15-8 ◆ Assess the patient's circulation by feeling for a pulse at the carotid artery.

- Electrolyte imbalance
- Epilepsy
- Head trauma
- Hypoglycemia
- Hyperglycemia
- Hypovolemia
- Hypoxia
- Metabolic disorders
- Overdose
- Poisoning

- Respiratory arrest
- Seizure
- Sepsis
- Shock (any kind)
- Stroke

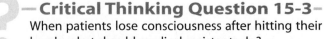

?—Critical Thinking Question 15-3—
When patients lose consciousness after hitting their heads, what should medical assistants do?

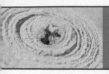

PROCEDURE 15-2 Respond to a Patient Who Has Fainted

Theory and Rationale

Patients who are ill, pregnant, or who have just received upsetting news may faint. Medical assistants must be properly trained to respond to these patients, since patients may injure themselves if they lose consciousness and fall in the medical office.

Materials

- Blanket
- Footstool or box

Competency

(**Conditions**) With the necessary materials, you will be able to (**Task**) care for a patient who has fainted (**Standards**) correctly within the time limit set by the instructor.

1. If the patient communicates a faint feeling, help the patient sit, bend forward, and place the head on the knees. If the patient collapses with no warning, do not move the patient. The patient may have sustained a neck or back injury.
2. Notify the physician.
3. Loosen any tight clothing, and cover the patient with the blanket for warmth.
4. If the physician directs, use the footstool to support the patient's legs in a raised position.
5. If the physician directs, call for emergency services.
6. Once the emergency passes, document all activities in the patient's medical record.

Patient Education

Observe the patient carefully, monitoring breathing and level of consciousness. Allow the patient to rest 10 minutes after she regains full consciousness. If the patient's vital signs are unstable or the patient does not respond quickly, notify the physician and be prepared to activate the emergency medical system.

Charting Example

Patient in exam room states that she feels faint. Patient instructed to lower her head to her knees. Instructed to and assisted with loosening of clothing. Physician notified. BP 116/62, P-82 and regular, R-20. Patient remained in position for 3 minutes until symptoms subsided. Patient transferred to exam room and physician notified and evaluated patient. Maria Jimenez, RMA (AMI)

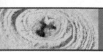

PROCEDURE 15-3 Administer Oxygen to a Patient

Theory and Rationale

A patient who is in respiratory distress may need to have oxygen administered to them in the medical office. The medical assistant should be aware of how to administer oxygen, both via nasal cannula and via oxygen mask.

Materials

- Portable oxygen tank
- Pressure regulator
- Flow meter
- Nasal cannula with connecting tubing
- Oxygen mask with connecting tubing

Competency

(**Conditions**) With the necessary materials, you will be able to (**Task**) administer oxygen via a nasal cannula or oxygen mask (**Standards**) correctly within the time limit set by the instructor.

1. Gather all equipment.
2. Wash your hands.
3. Identify the patient and explain what you are about to do.
4. Check the pressure gauge on the oxygen tank to verify the amount of oxygen in the tank.
5. Open the cylinder on the oxygen tank one full counter-clockwise turn and attach the connective tubing to the flow meter.
6. Attach either the nasal cannula or the oxygen mask to the connective tubing.
7. Adjust the administration of the oxygen to the flow ordered by the physician.
8. Verify that oxygen is flowing through the nasal cannula or oxygen mask.
9. For nasal cannula: Insert the cannula tips into the patient's nostrils and loop the tubing behind the patient's ears.
10. For oxygen mask: Place the oxygen mask over the patient's nose and mouth and slip the elastic cord over their head. Adjust the cord so that the mask fits tightly yet comfortably on the patient's face.
11. Wash your hands.
12. Document the procedure including the flow rate of oxygen being given to the patient and the method of delivery (nasal cannula or oxygen mask).

Keys to Success
EYEWASH STATIONS

OSHA Regulation {29 CFR 1910.151(c)} states, "where the eyes or body of any person may be exposed to injurious corrosive materials, suitable facilities for quick drenching or flushing of the eyes and body shall be provided within the work area for immediate emergency use."

Emergency eyewash stations are essential tools that are used when chemicals or small particles come into contact with the eye. Perform the following steps in the case of such an emergency:

1. Immediately remove contact lenses if a chemical or other substance enters the eye. If not removed, the lenses can hold the substance in the eye and cause serious damage.
2. Gently hold your eyes open and place them on the designated spot on the eyewash station.
3. The eyewash station is designed to deliver a continuous flush of water to ensure that substances are moved from the eye. While holding your eyes open, have another individual turn on the water. Irrigation should last for at least 15 minutes.
4. Never rub your eyes if dust or debris is thought to be inside as this can further irritate and possibly damage the eye.
5. Emergency response units should be called. Request that a coworker make the call for EMS while you continue to irrigate your eyes. Again, be sure to irrigate for at least 15 minutes, even after the emergency response team arrives.

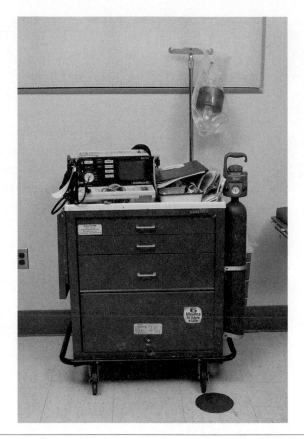

Figure 15-9 ◆ A medical crash cart.

Emergency Equipment and Supplies

Every medical office must have emergency equipment and supplies that should include an appropriately stocked **crash cart** (Figure 15-9 ◆). Figure 15-10 ◆ lists the supplies that may be found on a crash cart in the ambulatory care setting.

Emergency supplies should be easily accessible in the medical office and inventoried regularly. Staff should rotate supplies based on expiration date. In addition to items such as alcohol wipes, antimicrobial skin ointment, and cotton balls and swabs, medical offices should have elastic bandages, instant hot and cold packs, portable oxygen tanks with regulators and masks, scissors, sharps container, and steristrips or suturing materials. The office should also stock such emergency pharmaceutical supplies as activated charcoal, amobarbital, apomorphine, injectable and oral antihistamine, dextrose, diazepam, furosemide, glucose tables, syrup of ipecac, nitroglycerine tablets, injectable sodium bicarbonate, and sterile water. Every medical office should stock epinephrine, which is used for emergencies that include asthma attacks, hemorrhages, and shock.

Administering Oxygen in Emergencies

When patients require oxygen in the medical office, medical assistants must be able to administer the oxygen as well as gather necessary supplies. Oxygen may be administered via nasal cannula or face mask (Figures 15-11 ◆ and 15-12 ◆).

Automated External Defibrillator (AED)

Every medical office must have a **defibrillator** for emergency use. This machine delivers a shock to patients with no pulse in an effort to stop ventricular fibrillation. Defibrillators work by sending an electric current into the patient's heart in order to allow the heart's natural pacemaker to return to a normal rhythm. Most ambulatory settings have **automated external defibrillators** (**AEDs**), which are self-contained and portable (Figure 15-13 ◆).

Every AED has a battery, a control computer, and electrodes. To use the AED, medical personnel place the electrodes on the patient, and the control computer determines the patient's rhythm or arrhythmia. The AED then sets the appropriate power levels and signals that a shock is needed. To administer a shock, the operator must press a button, but only after ensuring that no one is touching the patient. When patients do not need defibrillation, the AED allows no shock to be administered.

- Cardiac monitor/defibrillator
- Conduction jelly
- EKG paper
- O$_2$ cylinder
- Suction catheters
- Laryngoscope
- 10 cc syringe
- O2 face mask
- Stethoscope
- IV supplies
- 1″ silk tape
- 3 cc syringes with 22 gauge needles
- Blood tubes (red tops, green tops, blue tops, and purple tops)

- Adult paddles
- Lead wires
- Suction machine
- Pocket mask
- Sterile gloves
- Endotracheal tubes
- Nasogastric tube
- Nasula cannula
- Blood pressure cuff
- Tourniquets
- 4 × 4 sterile gauze pads
- 10 cc syringes with 20 gauge needles
- Neonatal ambu bag

- Pedi paddles
- Monitor electrodes
- Suction canister
- Oral airways
- Suction tubing
- Lidocaine jelly
- 60 cc catheter-tip syringe
- Emergency trach tray
- IV solutions
- Short arm boards
- 1 cc TB syringes
- 23 gauge butterfly needles
- Pediatric ambu bag

Figure 15-10 ◆ Crash cart contents.

The Signs and Symptoms of Heart Attack

The signs and symptoms of heart attack may differ from one patient to another. Most commonly, patients complain of chest pain or pressure in the center of the chest. This pain, which patients may describe as minor, may spread to the patient's shoulder, neck, jaw, or arm. Patients experiencing heart attacks may also present with excessive sweating; nausea or indigestion; shortness of breath; or cold, clammy skin.

Women may experience different heart attack symptoms than men. Women may experience back pain or pain and aching in the biceps or forearms, dizziness or lightheadedness, or swelling in the ankles or lower legs. Medical assistants must be familiar with all these signs and immediately bring them to the physician's attention.

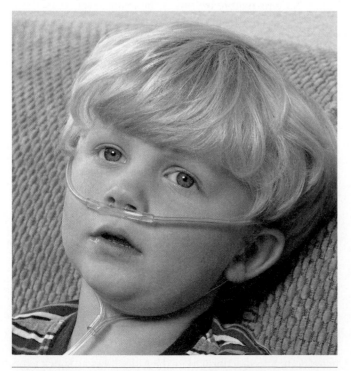

Figure 15-11 ◆ Young boy using a nasal cannula.

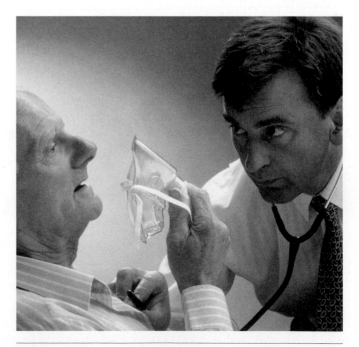

Figure 15-12 ◆ Patient with oxygen mask.

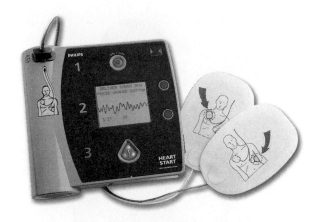

Figure 15-13 ◆ Automated external defibrillator (AED).

In Practice

When Courtney Molino enters the medical office for her physical exam, she says she feels unwell after choosing the stairs over the elevator. In fact, she says she is having chest pain and extreme dizziness. What should the medical assistant do?

The Signs and Symptoms of Choking

Choking typically results when a foreign object becomes lodged in a patient's throat. When a choking patient can speak or make any verbal sounds or is coughing, the medical assistant should encourage the patient to continue coughing until the object is dislodged. If the patient cannot make sounds or cough, the assistant should assume the airway is blocked and take appropriate action. The choking adult may

---

PROCEDURE 15-4 **Use an Automated External Defibrillator (AED)**

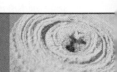

Theory and Rationale

The use of AEDs as lifesaving devices is becoming more and more common. AEDs are now found in doctors' offices, malls, airplanes, and private residences. An AED works by sending an electrical current through the myocardium of the heart, briefly causing the heart to stop and allowing the heart's natural pacemaker to take over. The goal is for the heart to resume function. All AEDs function in the same manner.

The AED is brought by a second- or third-party rescuer after the initial chest compressions and rescue breathing have begun.

Materials

- Practice AED machine
- patient chart
- mannequin

Competency

(**Conditions**) With the necessary materials, (**Task**) you will use an AED (**Standards**) correctly within the time frame designated by the instructor.

1. Place the AED next to the victim's left ear. This position allows the rescuers clear access to the chest and airway for continued rescue measures.
2. Turn the AED on and follow the voice prompts.
3. You will be prompted to attach the electrode pads to the patient's chest, on the sternum and at the apex of the heart, following the diagram for correct placement.

4. Next, you will be directed to allow the machine to analyze the heart rhythm to determine if it is a shockable rhythm. CPR should cease while the machine is analyzing.
5. The machine will begin a charging sequence prior to shocking and warn rescuers to stand back. The voice prompt will then tell you to press the "shock" button to administer the electrical current to the patient.
6. If the machine indicates "No shock is advised," assess the patient for breathing and circulation. Continue CPR as needed until advanced medical personnel arrive.

Patient Education

If a friend or family member of the patient is present at the time of rescue, you will need to help that person remain calm and out of the way so that advanced rescue personnel can treat the victim. It is also helpful if you can explain to friends or family members what is happening and to what hospital the victim will be transported. Be careful not to make comforting statements that may not be accurate, such as "He'll be all right" or "She's going to be just fine."

Charting Example

11/25/XX 3:30 PM Patient found in stairwell, unresponsive, with absence of pulse and respirations. 911 protocol initiated with 2 rescuer CPR. Third rescuer initiated AED response and patient was analyzed for shockable rhythm. CPR and AED shocks administered a total of 8 cycles prior to advanced medical support arriving. Patient released to EMS care and transferred to Sacred Heart Medical Center. Martin Cowan, CMA (AAMA)

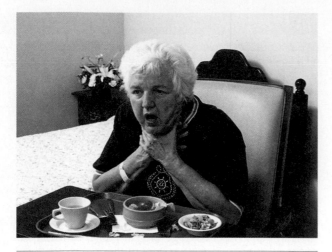

Figure 15-14 ◆ The universal choking sign.

use the universal choking sign—crossing the hands at the throat—to signal for help (Figure 15–14 ◆). Once the blockage has been removed, the patient may still be in danger of swelling in the throat, causing a decreased airway. For this reason, medical personnel should still be called after the blockage has been removed.

When Infants Are Choking Victims

When choking patients are infants up to one year of age, the medical assistant should look into the patient's mouth to see if an object is viewable. When it is, the assistant should remove the object by swiping the finger through the child's mouth. When no object is visible or the assistant cannot remove the object, the assistant should place the patient face downward, across his or her forearms or thighs, and lower than the patient's trunk. The assistant should then use the heel of the hand to administer five blows to the patient's back, between the shoulder blades (Figure 15-15 ◆). The medical assistant should also call for a coworker to dial for emergency personnel.

When an object fails to dislodge, the medical assistant should turn the patient over and use two fingers to administer five thrusts to the patient's chest, at the nipple line. The assistant should then again look in the patient's mouth to see if an object is viewable and removable. When it is not, the assistant should continue thrusting to the back and then to the front until emergency personnel arrive.

Controlling Bleeding

When medical emergencies involve patients who are bleeding, medical assistants must follow standard precautions. ∞ Chapter 4 outlines all the Occupational Safety and Health Administration (**OSHA**) standard precautions that must be observed in ambulatory care. For bleeding patients, medical assistants should don appropriate protective equipment (Figure 15-16 ◆). Personal

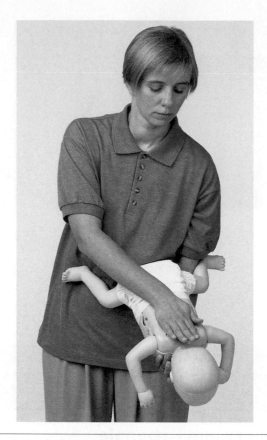

Figure 15-15 ◆ Administering back blows to a choking infant.

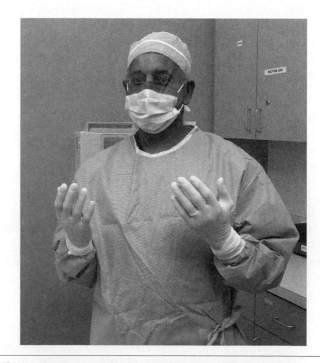

Figure 15-16 ◆ A medical assistant wearing PPE gown, face shield, and gloves.

PROCEDURE 15-5 Respond to an Adult with an Airway Obstruction

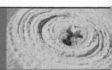

Theory and Rationale

A bolus of food is the most common object adults choke on. When the food is lodged in the upper airway, the person may put his or her hands around the throat, the universal sign of choking, to let bystanders know he or she cannot breathe properly. If the person can wheeze, make a high-pitched sound, cough, or speak, do not take any action. Instead call 911 and encourage the person to continue to cough forcefully to try to dislodge the object. If the person is unable to speak or cough, he or she is in immediate danger and action must be taken.

It is important that the rescuer call 911 even if the victim's airway is not completely blocked or the Heimlich maneuver was successful. Once the object has been expelled, the throat is likely to continue to swell as a result of the irritant, so the victim should be assessed in an emergency room.

Materials

- approved mannequin
- gloves
- ventilation mask with one-way valve for unconscious victim

Competency

(**Conditions**) With the necessary materials, (**Task**) you will administer the Heimlich maneuver to an adult (**Standards**) correctly within the time frame designated by the instructor.

1. Once it has been established that the victim is choking, with no air exchange, direct someone to call 911 and shout, "Are you choking?" or "Can you speak?" If the answer is no—as indicated by a head shake—tell the victim you are going to begin emergency treatment.
2. Stand behind the victim with your feet slightly apart, placing one foot between the victim's feet and one to the outside. This stance will give you greater stability, and if the victim should pass out, you can safely guide him or her to the ground by sliding him or her down your thigh.
3. Place the index finger of one hand at the person's navel or belt buckle. If the victim is a pregnant woman, place your finger above the enlarged uterus.
4. Make a fist with your other hand and place it, thumb side to victim, above your other hand. If the person is very pregnant, the uterus is pushing the stomach and other internal organs under the rib cage and you may have to do chest compressions.
5. Place your marking hand over your curled fist and begin to give quick inward and upward thrusts (Figure 15-17 ◆).
6. There is no set number of thrusts to give to an adult who remains conscious. Continue to give thrusts until the object is removed *or* the victim becomes unconscious.

7. If the victim becomes unconscious, gently lower him or her to the ground.
8. Activate EMS and put on gloves.
9. Immediately begin CPR with 30 chest compressions and two rescue breaths.
10. Before administering the rescue breaths, open the airway with the head-tilt chin lift and look for a foreign body in the victim's mouth and remove if visible. Blind finger sweeps are no longer recommended and should not be performed.
11. Continue with cycles of 30 compressions and two rescue breaths until the foreign body is expelled or adance medical personal arrive to relieve you.

Patient Education

If the object has been successfully removed and the patient did not lose consciousness, the patient may feel he or she no longer needs medical treatment. As a rescuer you must insist that the victim seek medical attention anyway. The lodged object may have caused swelling in the lining of the esophagus, constricting the throat and impairing the breathing.

Charting Example

10/25/XX 11:30 AM Jason Jones, CMA, exhibited signs of choking at lunch. Jason grabbed his throat and was unable to cough or make noise. Tina Muller, RMA (AMT), alerted the physician and placed a call to 911. Chest compressions and rescue breaths were given until the piece of apple was expelled. EMS arrived and checked Jason for signs of throat irritation and swelling. Janice Walker, CMA (AAMA)

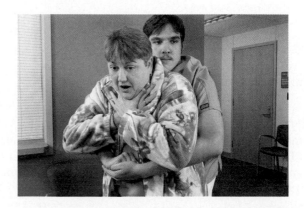

Figure 15-17 ◆ Deliver a firm thrust into the patient's abdomen in an upward direction toward you.

protective equipment (PPE) consists of an impermeable gown, goggles that completely cover the eyes, and an impermeable mask. The medical assistant should then apply several layers of sterile dressing material directly to any wounds. Direct pressure should stop or slow bleeding until emergency personnel arrive.

—Critical Thinking Question 15-4—

How should medical assistants try to control the patient bleeding?

Assisting Patients in Shock

Patients go into shock for varied reasons, including blood loss, infection, and pain. The most common signs of shock include pale, gray, or bluish skin; moist, cool skin; dilated pupils; a weak, rapid pulse; shallow, rapid respirations; and extreme thirst. When patients exhibit signs of shock, medical assistants should ensure that those patients have an open airway and proper circulation. Assistants should encourage patients to lie down with their legs elevated to return blood to the vital organs. Next, assistants should cover patients with blankets for warmth and keep them calm until emergency personnel arrive. Most emergency treatments for shock patients will need to be administered by a physician or emergency personnel. Table 15-3 outlines the cause and treatment of different types of shock.

—Critical Thinking Question 15-5—

How would a medical assistant recognize the signs of shock in Mark Whitford?

Caring for Patients with Fractures

Patients with fractures most likely require emergency room care. When patients sustain fractures in or around the medical office, they must be moved only as needed. Medical assistants should try to make these patients as comfortable as possible and notify the physician right away. The physician may ask the medical assistant to bring ice packs to the patient to reduce swelling or to apply direct pressure with sterile gauze in the event the patient is bleeding.

Keys to Success
CONTROLLING NOSEBLEEDS

Sometimes patients present in medical offices with nosebleeds due to injury or the rupture of small blood vessels in the nose. Patients with mild nosebleeds should sit up, lean forward, and apply direct pressure by pinching the nose. Pressure should continue for 10 to 15 minutes until the bleeding is controlled. If the bleeding cannot be controlled, the medical assistant should notify the physician.

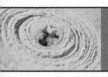

PROCEDURE 15-6 Remove an Airway Obstruction in an Infant

Theory and Rationale

When an infant has an airway obstruction, the medical assistant must be able to quickly remove the obstruction and restore the patient's airways.

Materials

■ Disposable gloves
■ Infant mannequin

Competency

(**Conditions**) With the necessary materials, you will be able to (**Task**) remove an airway obstruction from an infant (**Standards**) correctly within the time limit set by the instructor.

1. Call for a coworker to dial 9-1-1 for emergency services.
2. Open the infant's mouth and look to see if an object is visible. If so, use your finger to sweep the object from the infant's mouth. If the object is *not* visible, do not blindly sweep your finger through the infant's mouth, as you may push the object further back into the throat.
3. Place the baby face down over your forearm and across your thigh. The infant's head should be lower than the trunk, and you should support the infant's head and neck with one hand.
4. Using the heel of your free hand, administer five blows to the infant's back between the shoulder blades.
5. Turn the infant over, keeping the head lower than the trunk, and administer five thrusts to the midsternal area of the infant.
6. Look into the infant's mouth to see if the object is visible. If so, sweep your finger through the mouth to remove the object. If not, administer two rescue breaths into the infant by covering the infant's nose and mouth completely with your own mouth.
7. Repeat the above sequence until the object is dislodged or help arrives.
8. Once the emergency passes, document all activities in the patient's medical record.

TABLE 15-3 TREATMENT FOR SHOCK IN THE MEDICAL OFFICE

Cause	Treatment
Anaphylactic shock	Epinephrine
Cardiogenic shock	IV dopamine, immediate transport to the emergency room
Hemorrhagic shock	Stop bleeding, replace volume, immediate transport to the emergency room
Hypovolemic shock	Replace volume
Insulin shock	Sugar given to the patient by any means tolerated
Neurogenic shock	IV dopamine, immediate transport to the emergency room
Poisoning	Consult the poison center for treatment specific to the poison
Respiratory shock	Intubation and immediate transport to the emergency room
Sepsis	Fluids, IV dopamine, and immediate transport to the emergency room

Source: Beaman, N. and Fleming, L. Pearson's Comprehensive Medical Assisting, © 2007. Reprinted by permission of Pearson Education, Upper Saddle River, NJ.

Assisting Patients with Burns

Medical assistants may be required to assist with emergency burn victims. First, the assistants should try to determine the cause of the burn (e.g., chemical, fire, scalding). Medical staff who know the cause of a burn can provide better care. Some burns can be treated in the ambulatory care setting; others require hospital care. If possible, the medical assistant should immerse the burn in cool water, or soak sterile gauze in cool saline solution and apply the gauze to the burned area. In the event the burn was caused by a chemical, the medical assistant should attempt to flush the area with water. No matter what the cause of the burn, the medical assistant should seek the order of the physician in how to administer treatment to the patient.

Eye Treatments

Dust, dirt, chemicals, or other substances may get onto the surface of the eye and can be difficult for patients to safely remove on their own. Eye irrigations are an easy and comfortable way to remove these substances in the medical office. The procedure involves flowing a fluid across the eye and flushing the irritating substances from the surface Eyewash stations may also be used in the removal of dust, dirt, and debris.

Emergency Preparedness

The medical assistant should be knowledgeable in the area of emergency preparedness. This includes knowing how to respond in the event of a man-made disaster, such as a terrorist event, and to a natural disaster, such as a hurricane.

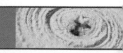

PROCEDURE 15-7 **Control Bleeding**

Theory and Rationale
Uncontrolled bleeding may lead to further injury, or even death. In such emergencies, the MA should first don appropriate protective equipment and then apply several layers of sterile dressing material directly to the wound to stop or slow the bleeding until emergency personnel arrive.

Materials
- Disposable gloves
- Personal protective equipment (gown, eye protection, mask)
- Sterile dressing
- Bandage
- Biohazard waste container

Competency
(**Conditions**) With the necessary materials, you will be able to (**Task**) control bleeding in a patient (**Standards**) correctly within the time limit set by the instructor.

1. Notify a coworker to alert the physician. If a physician is not available in the office, notify the coworker to alert emergency personnel.

2. Assemble the necessary equipment and supplies.
3. Wash your hands.
4. Don the personal protective equipment.
5. Open the sterile dressings and apply several layers directly to the wound and apply direct pressure.
6. Wrap the wound with bandage. If the wound continues to bleed, apply more sterile dressing and bandaging material. Continue to apply direct pressure.
7. If the wound continues to bleed and if it is located on an extremity, raise the extremity to a level above the patient's heart.
8. If the bleeding continues, apply pressure to the appropriate artery.
9. Once the bleeding is under control, dispose of all contaminated materials into the biohazard waste container.
10. Wash your hands.
11. Once the emergency passes, document all activities in the patient's medical record.

Earthquake

Because earthquakes can happen at any time, and without any warning, the medical assistant should know how to respond to this type of emergency. One of the first steps to preventing injury during an earthquake is to prepare before an earthquake happens. Advance preparation may save lives as well as prevent injuries.

According to the Federal Emergency Management Agency (FEMA), there are six steps involved in planning ahead for an earthquake. These steps are:

1. Check for hazards around the facility.
   - Make sure shelves are fastened securely to walls.
   - Do not place large or heavy objects on higher shelves.
   - Store any breakable items in low, closed cabinets equipped with locks.
   - Heavy items should not be hung on walls above where patients will sit or lie.
   - Overhead light fixtures should be secured.
   - Any defective electrical wiring or leaky gas connections should be repaired.
   - Water heaters should be strapped to wall studs and bolted to the floor.
   - Any deep cracks in ceilings or foundations should be repaired.
   - All flammable products should be stored in closed cabinets with locks, on the bottom shelf.
2. Identify safe places both indoors and outdoors.
   - Under sturdy furniture.
   - Against an inside wall.
   - Away from glass that could shatter.
   - Away from bookcases or furniture that could fall over.
   - In the open, away from buildings, trees, telephone or electrical lines, overpasses, or elevated expressways.
3. Educate yourself and your coworkers.
   - Contact the local emergency management office or the American Red Cross chapter for information.
   - Teach all staff members how and when to turn off gas, electricity, and water.
4. Have disaster supplies on hand.
   - Flashlight and extra batteries.
   - Portable battery-operated radio and extra batteries.
   - First aid kit and manual.
   - Emergency food and water.
   - Nonelectric can opener.
   - Sturdy shoes.
5. Develop an emergency communication plan.
   - In case staff members are separated from one another during an earthquake, develop a plan for reuniting after the disaster.
   - Define the expectations of each staff member—who will escort patients from the building, who will check the treatment rooms?
6. Help your community get ready.
   - Provide literature for patients on how to prepare for an earthquake.

Fire

Because more than 4,000 Americans die and more than 25,000 are injured in fires each year, the medical assistant should be prepared to respond to this type of disaster. Fire spreads quickly and there is typically no time to gather belongings or make a telephone call. In just two minutes, a fire can become life-threatening and in five minutes a fire can engulf a building. Heat and smoke from fire are often more dangerous than the flames.

The medical office should be equipped with properly working smoke alarms. These should be placed on every level of the building and should be placed on the ceiling or high on the walls. Every room of the office should be equipped with a smoke detector and each should be tested and cleaned once per month. The batteries should be replaced at least once per year and every smoke alarm should be replaced once every 10 years.

The medical assistant should know the escape routes to use in the event of a fire. Staff members should practice those escape routes. If the office is located above the first level, escape ladders may be used.

Fire and Electrical Safety

The medical assistant should know the location of fire exits, alarms, and fire extinguishers and should follow all emergency plans, remembering to keep all hallways and exit doors free from obstructions. *If the MA discovers a fire, he or she should pull the alarm.*

If the alarm sounds, the MA should:

- Call or direct someone to call 911 (only if it is safe to do so), or call from a safe place outside the building.
- Close all doors and windows (only if it is safe to do so).
- Check bathrooms and examination rooms to make sure all patients and staff are aware of the fire alarm.
- Evacuate with patients immediately.
- Meet at an assigned place.
- Never use the building elevator during a fire, as it can stop on the floor with the fire; use the stairs.

The only time a fire extinguisher should be used is when the fire is between you and the door. If it is necessary to use the extinguisher, use the PASS method (Figure 15-18 ◆). It is important that the MA knows how to use the appropriate kind of fire extinguisher before trying to use it. Local fire departments generally train employees regarding fire safety in the office. Practice fire drills and emergency carries.

Electrical safety requires exercising caution. The MA must be careful with all equipment and make sure it is in good condition before using it. Tell your office manager or administrator if you see:

- frayed wires or cords
- overused extension cords
- lack of ground plugs or grounded outlets
- cracked or broken switch or receptacle plates
- sparking when a plug is inserted into or removed from an outlet
- broken lights

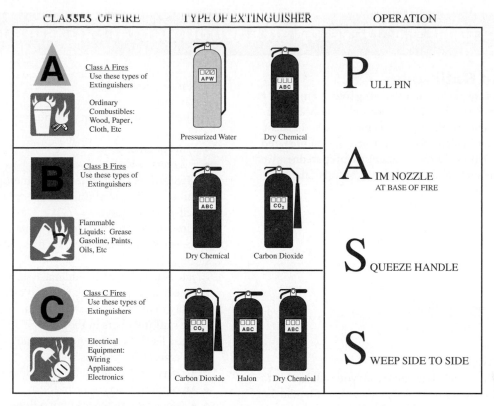

Figure 15-18 ◆ PASS method of firefighting: pull the pin, aim at the base of the fire, squeeze the trigger, and sweep from side to side.

Source: The University of Texas Health Science Center at Houston Environmental Health and Safety Department.

During a fire, the medical assistant should be aware that if a person's clothes are on fire, that person should stop, drop, and roll until the fire is extinguished. Running makes the fire burn faster.

In order to escape a fire, the medical assistant should check closed doors for heat before opening. This is done by using the back of the hand to feel the top of the door, the doorknob, and the crack between the door and the door frame before opening the door. If the door is hot, it should not be opened and another route of escape should be sought. If the door is cool, it should be opened slowly.

When escaping a fire, the medical assistant should crawl low under any smoke on the way to the exit and close doors as they are passed through to delay the spread of fire. Once out of the building, the medical assistant should not attempt to reenter until or unless the fire department declares that action to be safe.

Floods

FEMA declares floods to be the most common hazard in the United States. Some floods can develop over days of rainy weather, others may be in the form of flash floods and may come on very quickly. The MA should be aware of the flood dangers that exist in his or her local area.

During a flood, the medical assistant should listen to the radio for information. In the event of a flash flood, the medical assistant should move to higher ground. If there is time before evacuating, the medical assistant should be sure to disconnect any electrical equipment and shut off utilities at their main valve.

When evacuating, the medical assistant should be careful not to walk through moving water. Just six inches of moving water can make a person fall.

Hurricane

Hurricanes can strike with little warning, though most will allow for some advance warning, giving the medical office staff time to prepare. If the office is in the path of the hurricane, the windows may need to be secured. This can be done using plywood. Trees and shrubs around the office should be well trimmed.

If the medical office is to be evacuated before a hurricane, the medical assistant should listen to the radio or television for information provided by local emergency management personnel.

During the hurricane, the medical assistant should listen to the radio or television for information and prepare for high winds and possible flooding.

Terrorism

In the event of a terrorist attack, the medical assistant should be aware of the steps to take in an emergency.

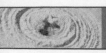

PROCEDURE 15-8 Develop an Environmental Exposure Plan

Theory and Rationale

Medical assistants are playing an increasing role in emergency preparedness. Emergencies include not only medical emergencies, but also natural disasters and man-made disasters. The most important rule to follow is to always be prepared for any situation that may arise. By adequate preparedness we not only help ourselves and our patients, but also the community that surrounds us.

Materials

- Pen
- Paper
- Computer
- Copy machine
- Various emergency supplies
- Waterproof containers

Competency

(**Condition**) With the necessary materials you will be able to (**Task**) develop an environmental exposure plan (**Standards**) with correct items in the time designated by the instructor.

1. Create an emergency kit that can be used by your office in the event of an environmental emergency. Supplies may include:
   - Flashlights
   - Batteries
   - Bottles of water
   - Nonperishable food
   - Bandages
   - Alcohol and hydrogen peroxide
   - Blankets
   - Vinyl or latex gloves
   - Tweezers, scissors
   - Medication—ibuprofen, acetimetophen, antihistamines, antibiotic ointment, tetanus vaccines, etc.
   - Self-powered radio
2. Enclose the kit in a waterproof container.
3. Place the kit in a safe area, such as a medicine closet or storage closet.
4. Create evacuation plans and make sure that every room in the medical office shows a detailed exit route.
5. Create a delineation chart that outlines responsibilities of office staff members in the event of an emergency.
6. Create a list of "safety zones" that can be used in the event of an emergency. For instance:
   - A safety zone in the event of a tornado
   - An outdoor safety zone in the event of a fire
   - A safety zone in the event of a flood
7. Make photocopies of the safety zone list, evacuation plan, and delineation chart for everyone in the office. Laminate and hang copies in the employee break room.
8. Train all office staff on the environmental exposure plan within 10 days of hire.

Explosions

In the event of a bomb threat, the medical assistant should try to obtain as much information from the caller as possible:

- When is the bomb going to explode?
- Where is the bomb right now?
- What does it look like?
- What kind of bomb is it?
- What will cause it to explode?

This information should be immediately provided to the police and their directions should be followed.

If an explosion has occurred, the medical assistant should respond by following the steps as if an earthquake and/or fire has happened.

Biological Threats

There are four methods of delivery of a biological agent:

1. Aerosols—agents are dispersed into the air, forming a mist that may drift for miles.
2. Animals—some diseases are spread by insects or animals.
3. Food and water contamination—some agents are placed in the food or water supply.
4. Person-to-person—some spread of agents is possible via direct contact between people.

In order to prepare for a biological attack, the medical facility may have a high efficiency particulate air (**HEPA**) filter installed.

In the event of a biological attack, the medical assistant should be prepared to move away quickly, wash with soap and water, contact authorities, listen to the radio for instructions, and remove and bag clothing if contaminated.

Nuclear Blast

In the event of a nuclear attack, the medical assistant should take cover as quickly as possible, below ground if the building has a basement. The medical assistant should remain in a safe location, listening to the radio for instructions. The medical assistant should not look at the flash or fireball, lie flat on the ground with the head covered, and seek shelter as quickly as possible.

Mock-Environmental Exposures

Medical assistants can play a vital role in the event of an environmental emergency. It is helpful to be prepared for such events, understanding how to help victims and provide assistance to other healthcare providers.

Organizations within the community, colleges, and hospitals may offer mock-environmental exposure events. These events provide real-life scenarios and situations that may arise during times of disaster. Scenarios of mock-environmental events may include a tornado site with injured victims, an exposure to a biological chemical, or treating injured victims of flash floods or hurricanes. The role of the medical assistant will vary in every situation; however, overall, MAs may be able to provide assistance by:

- Aiding in evacuation plans
- Triaging patients to determine which patients require immediate attention
- Assisting in first-aid response for wounded individuals
- Administering tetanus and other vaccines under the direction of a physician
- Facilitating order and organization in the midst of chaos
- Implementing and following through on an environmental safety plan

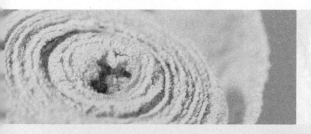

REVIEW

Chapter Summary

- Medical assistants have distinct and vital roles in medical emergencies.
- A number of supplies and equipment help support life-saving objectives in emergency situations.
- When an emergency arises, preparedness, training, and organization can mean the difference between measured, effective response and chaos.
- To ensure appropriate responses, members of the health care team should call emergency services to the medical office as needed.
- Rescue breathing and cardiopulmonary resuscitation (CPR) are just two means medical staff have to address emergency situations.
- A crash cart holds a number of supplies and equipment needed in emergencies.

- An automated external defibrillator is used to treat patients with no pulse.
- Medical assistants should be trained to stop bleeding, as well as take all comfort measures for patients in varied types of emergencies.
- The medical assistant should be knowledgeable in the area of emergency preparedness, and understand how to respond in the event of a man-made disaster or a natural disaster.
- Mock environmental exposure events may be offered within the community, at colleges and hospitals. These events provide real-life scenarios and situations that may arise during times of disaster.

Chapter Review

Multiple Choice

1. Which of the following items would be found on a crash cart?
   a. Steristrips
   b. Ambu bag
   c. Blood pressure cuff
   d. All of the above

2. The American Association of Medical Assistants (AAMA) requires certified medical assistants to renew their first aid and CPR training:
   a. Yearly
   b. Biyearly
   c. Every 3 years
   d. Every 5 years

3. Which of the following situations could create an accident in the medical office?
   a. Toys on the floor in the reception room
   b. Medications left unattended
   c. Water spilled on the restroom floor
   d. All of the above

4. Which of the following telephone numbers should the medical assistant have available in the event of an emergency?
   a. Local police department
   b. Local fire department
   c. Poison Control
   d. All of the above

Chapter Review (continued)

True/False

T F 1. A patient with a nosebleed should be asked to sit, lean forward, and pinch the nose.

T F 2. One of the responsibilities of the administrative medical assistant in an office emergency is to direct patients and family members as needed.

T F 3. When emergency personnel services must be summoned to the medical office, physicians should call because they have the greatest knowledge of the situations.

T F 4. When administering oxygen to a patient, the medical assistant will always use a nasal cannula.

T F 5. Standard precautions are used to prevent spread of infection.

T F 6. Patients who are choking and have blocked airways can still speak.

T F 7. An automated external defibrillator will not shock a patient who does not need to be shocked.

Short Answer

1. To stop bleeding, the medical assistant should apply _____ to the wound.

2. Describe the purpose of a CPR mouth barrier.

3. Describe the comfort measures that should be taken with a patient who has suffered a fracture.

4. What steps would make a medical office safe for small children?

5. Why is knowing the cause of a burn important?

6. What are two reasons a patient might be in shock?

7. What are two reasons a patient might faint?

8. How does adult choking treatment differ from child choking treatment?

9. What is the proper treatment of a patient who is in shock?

Research

1. Using the Internet as a resource, look up information on handling medical emergencies in the healthcare setting. What information do you find?

2. Call your local medical assisting chapter. Ask them if they offer any continuing education classes that touch on the topic of handling medical emergencies. What kind of classes do they suggest?

3. Speak with one of your instructors in the medical assisting program you are attending. Ask the instructor what kind of reading material he or she would recommend on the subject of handling medical emergencies in the medical office.

Externship Application Experience

Willie Harrison has brought his 2-year-old daughter, Sonya, to his weekly blood draw. While Willie and his daughter are waiting in the medical office, Sonya finds an object on the floor and places it in her mouth. Seconds later, Willie begins shouting that his daughter is choking. What should the medical assistant do?

Resource Guide

American Heart Association
7272 Greenville Avenue
Dallas, TX 75231
Phone: (800) 242-8721
http://www.americanheart.org/

American Red Cross
www.redcross.org

Federal Emergency Management Agency (FEMA)
500 C Street SW
Washington, DC 20472
Disaster Assistance: (800) 621-FEMA
www.fema.gov

National Highway Traffic Safety Administration
1-888-327-4236

U.S. Department of Transportation (USDOT)
400 7th St., SW
Washington, DC 20590
www.dot.gov

U.S. National Library of Medicine
8600 Rockville Pike
Bethesda, MD 20894
http://www.nlm.nih.gov/medlineplus

MedMedia

http://www.MyMAKit.com

More on this chapter, including interactive resources, can be found on the Student CD-ROM accompanying this textbook and on http://www.MyMAKit.com.

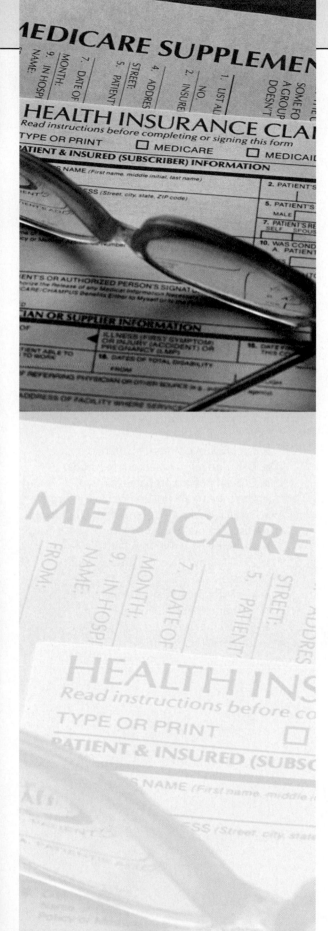

SECTION IV

Practice Finances and Management of the Medical Office

My name is Amy Walter and I love my job as a medical assistant. I get to help people every day. My days consist of taking vitals, giving shots, scheduling appointments, assisting the doctor, making multiple phone calls, and sending faxes—sometimes all at once! It is a fast-paced, but rewarding job. Every day there is a new challenge that I must face. Patients come to me for help, and I do everything in my power to get them the help that they need.

I feel so lucky to be working in a large family practice with an amazing doctor. The doctor–medical assistant relationship is so important for excellent patient care. It is imperative for the medical assistant to have an open line of communication with doctors and other medical office staff. The most valuable thing I have learned working as a medical assistant is that it is okay to say "I don't know." Individuals will become better providers if they are able to admit that they don't know everything. It is okay to ask questions and look things up.

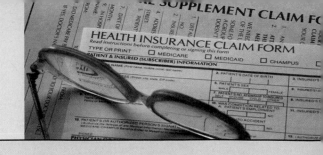

CHAPTER 16

Insurance Billing and Authorizations

Case Study

Martin Zamora is a patient at Woodway Health Care. Martin has recently gotten married and his new wife has health coverage through her employer. Martin says he believes his wife's coverage is better than what he has through his own employer, and he wants her policy billed for his care.

Objectives

After completing this chapter, you should be able to:

- Define and spell the key terminology in this chapter.
- Define the medical assistant's role in insurance claim processing.
- Describe the history of health insurance.
- Define health insurance terminology.
- Describe private health insurance and the various sources of coverage.
- Describe the types of managed care plans.
- Describe the various types of coverage available.
- Explain government insurance.
- Describe reimbursement methods.
- Explain how to prepare claims.
- Describe health insurance claims forms.
- Explain how to work with fee schedules.
- Discuss how to post payments.
- Describe how to trace claims.
- Explain how to reconcile payments and rejections.
- Describe the role of the office of the insurance commissioner.
- Explain health insurance costs in the future.

MedMedia
http://www.MyMAKit.com

Additional interactive resources and activities for this chapter can be found on http://www.MyMAKit.com. For a video, tips, audio glossary, legal and ethical scenarios, on-the-job scenarios, quizzes, and games related to the content of this chapter, please access the accompanying CD-ROM in this book.

Video: *Getting Precertification*
Legal and Ethical Scenario: *Insurance Billing and Authorizations*
On the Job Scenario: *Insurance Billing and Authorizations*
Tips
Multiple Choice Quiz
Audio Glossary
HIPAA Quiz
Games: Spelling Bee, Crossword, and Strikeout

➕ MEDICAL ASSISTING STANDARDS

CAAHEP ENTRY-LEVEL STANDARDS	ABHES ENTRY-LEVEL COMPETENCIES
▪ Identify types of insurance plans (cognitive) ▪ Identify models of managed care (cognitive) ▪ Discuss workers' compensation as it applies to patients (cognitive) ▪ Describe procedures for implementing both managed care and insurance plans (cognitive) ▪ Discuss utilization review principles (cognitive) ▪ Discuss referral process for patients in a managed-care program (cognitive) ▪ Describe how guidelines are used in processing an insurance claim (cognitive) ▪ Compare processes for filing insurance claims both manually and electronically (cognitive) ▪ Describe guidelines for third-party claims (cognitive) ▪ Discuss types of physician fee schedules (cognitive) ▪ Describe the concept of RBRVS (cognitive) ▪ Define Diagnosis-Related Groups (DRGs) (cognitive) ▪ Describe liability, professional, personal injury, and third-party insurance (cognitive) ▪ Apply both managed care policies and procedures (psychomotor) ▪ Apply third-party guidelines (psychomotor) ▪ Complete insurance claim forms (psychomotor) ▪ Obtain precertification, including documentation (psychomotor) ▪ Obtain preauthorization, including documentation (psychomotor) ▪ Verify eligibility for managed care services (psychomotor) ▪ Incorporate the Patients' Bill of Rights into personal practice and medical office policies and procedures (psychomotor) ▪ Respond to issues of confidentiality (psychomotor) ▪ Demonstrate assertive communication with managed-care and/or insurance providers (affective) ▪ Demonstrate sensitivity in communicating with both providers and patients (affective) ▪ Communicate in language the patient can understand regarding managed care and insurance plans (affective)	▪ Maintain confidentiality at all times ▪ Use appropriate guidelines when releasing records or information ▪ Be cognizant of ethical boundaries ▪ Monitor legislation related to current healthcare issues and practices ▪ Apply computer concepts for office procedures ▪ Use manual and computerized bookkeeping systems ▪ Serve as a liaison between physician and others ▪ Perform billing and collection procedures ▪ Exercise efficient time management ▪ Receive, organize, prioritize, and transmit information expediently ▪ Analyze and use current third-party guidelines for reimbursement ▪ Perform billing and collection procedures ▪ Complete insurance claim forms ▪ Implement current procedural terminology and ICD-9 coding ▪ Use physician fee schedule

Key Terminology

abstract—the process of locating data in multiple source documents and accurately transferring it to a form

accept assignment—physician agrees to accept the amount approved by the insurance company as payment in full for a given service

advance beneficiary notice—a form patients sign agreeing to pay for covered Medicare services that may be denied due to medical necessity or frequency

allowed amount—the dollar amount for a service that an insurance company considers acceptable and uses to determine benefit payments; also called *approved amount*

ancillary coverage—insurance coverage for services provided by other than a physician or hospital, such as dental, vision, or chiropractic care

appeal—process of asking for a review of a denied service or claim

approved amount—see *allowed amount*

assignment of benefits—request made by a patient to allow the insurance carrier to pay the health care professional directly rather than issuing monies to the patient

balance billing—billing a patient for the dollar difference between the provider's charge and the insurance approved amount; usually not permitted for participating providers

beneficiary—person who is eligible to receive benefits/services under an insurance policy

birthday rule—according to this rule, the parent with the birthday earlier in the year is the primary carrier for the children; the parent with the later birthday is the secondary carrier

bundling—combining multiple services under a single all inclusive CPT code and one charge

capitation plans—health care plans in which providers are paid set fees per month per member patients

caretaker—person or entity responsible for determining when and if a patient needs specific types of health care; also called gatekeeper or primary care provider (PCP)

carve outs—services that are reimbursed in addition to the base rate for the patient

catastrophic—large and usually unforeseen

Key Terminology *(continued)*

categorically needy—Medicaid eligible patients who quality for cash assistance as well as medical services

certificate of coverage—a letter from the insurance company that provides proof of type and timeframe of coverage when a patient terminates a health insurance policy

charge slip—document on which the physician indicates procedure and diagnosis codes; also called a routing slip, or *see* an encounter form

clean claim—insurance claim with no data errors

coinsurance—percentage of medical charges patients are responsible for according to their insurance plan contracts

commercial insurance—see *private insurance*

consumer-directed health care plans—health insurance plans that place patients in charge of how their health care dollars are spent

conversion factor—a constant dollar value multiplied by the relative value unit to determine the price of individual services

coordination of benefits—the process of determining which insurance policy should be billed first, second, or third when a patient is covered by multiple policies

copayment—set dollar fee per visit or service that patients are responsible for according to their insurance plan contracts

covered—services potentially eligible for reimbursement

deductible—monetary amount patients must pay to the provider for health care services before their health insurance benefits begin to pay

denied—a claim processed by an insurer and determined not eligible for payment

dependent—a family member or other individual who qualifies for coverage on the insured's policy; also called *beneficiary*. See also *insured; policyholder*

disability insurance—insurance that covers lost wages and certain other benefits due to a disability that prevents the individual from working

e-billing—process of sending health insurance claims electronically

elective procedure—procedure that will benefit the patient but does not need to be scheduled immediately

eligibility—the process to determine if a patient is qualified to receive coverage/paid benefits according to the insurance policy guidelines

encounter form—document on which the physician indicates procedure and diagnosis codes; also called a routing slip or charge slip

end-stage renal disease—total or nearly complete failure of the kidneys

exclusions—procedures or services not covered under an insurance plan

exclusive provider organization—a managed care contract with a smaller network of providers under which the employer agrees to not use any other networks in return for favorable pricing

explanation of benefits—a statement that accompanies payment from the insurance company which summarizes how the payment for each billed service was calculated and gives reasons for any items not paid

fee-for-service—process in which insurance companies pay providers fees for each service provided to covered patients

fee schedule—list of the approved fees insurance carriers agree to pay to participating providers who agree to contract with the carriers; also refers to the standard set of fees the provider charges to all insurers

flexible spending account—account into which employees place pretax earnings for projected medical expenses; also called *health care reimbursement account*

form locators—the boxes to be completed on the CMS-1500 claim form.

formulary—tiered list of drugs covered by an insurance company

gatekeeper—see *caretaker*

generic drugs—low-cost medications that duplicate their name-brand counterparts in active ingredient and effect

geographic adjustment factor (GAF)—a numeric multiplier used by Medicare to adjust fees for the varying costs of practicing medicine in different areas of the country

group health insurance—a commercial insurance policy with rates based on a group of people, usually offered by an employer

health care reimbursement account—see *flexible spending account*

health maintenance organization—a group of physicians or medical centers that provides comprehensive service to members under a capitated payment plan; members' care is covered only when using these designated providers

health savings account—tax-free savings accounts used for medical expenses in conjunction with a high-deductible health plan

hospice—facility or service for patients who are diagnosed with terminal illnesses and are expected to have 6 or fewer months to live

hospital services—patient care provided by a licensed acute-care hospital

indemnity—see *fee-for-service*

individual insurance—a commercial insurance policy with rates based on individual health criteria

individual practice association—HMOs that are the most decentralized and involve contracting with individual physicians to create a healthcare delivery system.

inpatient—a person who is admitted to the hospital for a minimum of 24 hours

insured—person who holds or owns an insurance policy; same as the member or the policyholder

liability insurance—type of insurance that covers injuries that occur on, in, or because of the insured's property

lifetime maximum benefit—monetary amount allowed by an insurance carrier for a covered member's covered expenses over the member's lifetime

limiting charge—the maximum amount a Medicare non-PAR provider may bill the patient on an unassigned claim; 115% of the non-PAR fee schedule

long term disability insurance—insurance that covers lost wages and certain other benefits due to a disability that prevents the individual from working, usually for more than one year

managed care—a system of healthcare delivery focused on reducing costs by transferring risk to the provider and may limit the type and frequency of care members may receive

Medicaid—a joint federal and state program that helps with medical costs for some people with low incomes and limited resources

medical necessity—criteria establishing when a service is appropriate

medical savings account—tax-free savings account for small employers and self-employed; used for medical expenses in conjunction with a high-deductible health plan

medically needy—Medicaid-eligible patients who are eligible for medical services, but not cash assistance

Medicare—federal program that covers medical expenses for those aged 65 and over, those with end-stage renal disease, and those with long-term disabilities

member—the person who owns the insurance policy

negotiated fee schedule—a common reimbursement method in managed care whereby the MCO develops a list of fees for providers that they agree to accept in the participating provider contract. Fees may be determined based on a percentage of the provider's usual fee or arrived at through negotiation.

non-covered—services not eligible for reimbursement under any circumstance

nonparticipating provider—health care provider who has not contracted with a particular health insurance carrier

Key Terminology *(continued)*

outliers—exceptional circumstances that cost far more or less than the average

outpatient—a person who receives medical care at a hospital or other medical facility but who is not admitted for more than 24 hours

participating provider—health care provider who has contracted with a particular health insurance carrier

past timely filing limits—time beyond which an insurance carrier will accept an insurance claim

payor number—unique identifying number assigned to each insurance carrier for the purpose of directing electronic claims

per case—*per case* payment method used for hospitals; under this method, the hospital receives a pre-established amount per patient for the entire stay, based on the patient's diagnosis, regardless of how long they are in or what services are provided

per diem—*per day* payment method whereby the facility is paid a flat amount per day the patient remains, regardless of what services are provided

physician services—patient care provided by a licensed physician

point of service—an insurance offering in which a patient has access to multiple plans, such as an HMO, PPO, and indemnity, and may choose to use any of them for any given service

policyholder—person who holds or owns an insurance policy; same as the member or the insured

preauthorization—approval for treatment or service obtained from an insurance company before the care is provided

precertification—see *preauthorization*

pre-existing condition—condition for which a patient received treatment in a certain period before beginning coverage with a new insurance plan

preferred provider organization—organization that contracts with independent providers to perform services for members at discounted rates

premium—dollar amount paid to the insurance company to have coverage in force; usually paid monthly; employers may pay part or all of the premium as an employee benefit

preventive care—health care designed to keep a person healthy

private insurance—insurance not provided by the government but by an independent not-for-profit or for-profit company; also called *commercial insurance*

rejected—a claim that is returned to the provider without processing due to a technical error

relative value unit—unit of measure assigned to medical services based on the resources required to provide it; includes work, practice expense, and liability insurance

resource-based relative value scale—the methodology Medicare uses to establish physician fees, based on the relative value unit, the geographic adjustment factor, and the conversion factor

respite care—temporary care provided by an outside party to relieve the usual caregiver

self-insurance—type of insurance where rather than purchasing a commercial insurance policy, an employer sets aside a large reserve fund to directly reimburse employees for medical expenses

skilled nursing facility—a licensed facility which primarily provides inpatient, skilled nursing care to patients who require medical, nursing, or rehabilitative services but does not provide the level of care or treatment available in a hospital

sliding fee scale—a provider's fee schedule that charges varying fees for a service based on a patient's financial ability to pay

staff model HMO—employs salaried physicians who treat members in facilities owned and operated by the HMO

stop loss—the maximum amount the patient must pay out-of-pocket for copayments and coinsurance

subscriber—person who holds or owns an insurance policy; same as the member, or *see* the insured

superbill—document on which the physician indicates procedure and diagnosis codes; also called a routing slip or an encounter form

third-party administrator—a company that processes paperwork for claims for a self-insured employer

TRICARE—health insurance administered by the U.S. Department of Defense for active duty military personnel, retired service personnel, and their eligible dependents; formerly known as Civilian Health and Medical Program (CHAMPUS)

unbundling—billing multiple services with separate CPT codes and separate charges that should be combined under a single CPT code and one charge

usual, customary, and reasonable (UCR) fee—a fee determined by third-party payers to reimburse providers based on the provider's normal fee, the range of fees charged by providers of the same specialty in the same geographic area, and other factors to determine appropriate fees in unusual situations

waiting period—period after a new health insurance plan begins during which certain services are not covered

waiver—see *advance beneficiary notice*

worker's compensation—insurance coverage for job-related illness or injury provided by employers

Abbreviations

ABN—advance beneficiary notice

ADA—American Dental Association

CDHP—Consumer Directed Health Plan

CF—conversion factor

CHAMPUS—Civilian Health and Medical Program for the Uniformed Services

CHAMPVA—Civilian Health and Medical Program of the Veterans Administration

CMS—Centers for Medicare and Medicaid Services

COB—coordination of benefits

COBRA—Consolidated Omnibus Budget Reconciliation Act

CPT—Current Procedural Terminology

CSRS—civil service

DEERS—defense enrollment eligibility reporting system

DME—durable medical equipment

EMC—electronic media claims

EOB—explanation of benefits

EPO—exclusive provider organization

ESRD—end-stage renal disease

FERS—Federal employee retirement system

FL—form locator

FSA—flexible spending account

GAF—geographic adjustment factor

HCFA—Health Care Financing Administration

HCRA—health care reimbursement account

HIPAA—Health Insurance Portability and Accountability Act

HMO—health maintenance organization

HSA—Health Savings Account

Abbreviations *(continued)*

ICD-9-CM—*International Classification of Diseases*, 9th ed., *Clinical Modification*

IPA—individual practice association

IRS—Internal Revenue Service

LC—limiting charge (Medicare)

MAC—Medicare administrative contractor

MCO—managed care organization

MFS—Medicare fee schedule

MSA—medical savings account

MSP—Medicare as secondary payor

NON-PAR—non-participating physician (Medicare)

NPI—national provider identifier

OCR—optical character recognition

OHI—other health insurance (Medicare)

PAR—participating physician (Medicare)

PCP—primary care provider

PIP—personal injury protection

POS—point of service

PPO—preferred provider organization

RBRVS—resource-based relative value scale

RVU—relative value unit

SCHIP—State Children's Health Insurance Program

SSDI—social security disability insurance

SSI—supplemental security income

TEFRA—Tax Equity and Fiscal Responsibility Act

TPA—third party administrator

TPL—third-party liability

UCR—usual, customary, and reasonable

UPIN—unique provider identification number

✓ COMPETENCY SKILLS PERFORMANCE

1. Calculate deductible, coinsurance, and allowable amounts.
2. Verify a patient's insurance eligibility.
3. Obtain a managed care referral.
4. Obtain authorization from an insurance company.
5. Abstract data to complete a paper CMS-1500 form.
6. Complete a computerized insurance claim form.
7. Handle a denied insurance claim.

Introduction

Processing insurance claims accurately is vital to the success of any medical practice. Just as basic knowledge of medical terminology is the first step to medical assisting success, an understanding of basic insurance terminology is vital to those responsible for processing claims.

Medical assistants must be able to answer patients' questions regarding how managed care works and how owed amounts are determined for any given procedure. Medical assistants must also be able to verify patients' insurance coverage and explain that coverage to the patients. In addition, MAs must know how to process health insurance claims accurately, follow up on past-due claims, and pursue accounts collection.

Developing skills in this area will enable the MA to be a patient advocate, helping patients obtain the benefits they are eligible for and helping them understand the reasons when a cost is not covered. Just as in other areas of medical assisting, the medical assistant's involvement in the insurance billing area will depend on the type of practice. In a large physician's office, there often is a separate department that handles most of the insurance matters. In a smaller office, the medical assistant may have more responsibilities in this area. Regardless of the type or size of office, in every situation the medical assistant is a vital team player in helping patients access their insurance benefits.

The History of Health Insurance

Health insurance in the United States began in the mid-1800s, when it was used to replace the income of people injured in accidents or ill from certain diseases. The first group policy giving comprehensive benefits was offered by Massachusetts Health Insurance of Boston in 1847. Insurance companies issued the first individual disability and illness policies around 1890. Hospital insurance coverage began in 1929, when a group of schoolteachers in Texas formed a contract with a local hospital to guarantee up to 21 days of hospital care for a premium of $6 per year. This plan became quite popular, and other groups of employers joined the plan, which eventually became known as the Blue Cross Plan.

During World War II, when wages froze, employers began offering their employees **group health insurance** as a benefit. Group health insurance plans cover entire groups of individuals, usually through employers or other large associations or defined groups. These early plans were designed to protect employees from the high costs of hospitalization and eventually evolved into the health care plans common today.

Employee benefit plans became popular in the 1940s and 1950s. The unions that represented large groups of workers bargained for better benefit packages, including tax-free, employer-sponsored health insurance.

During the 1950s and 1960s government programs began to cover health care costs. Social security coverage included disability benefits for the first time in 1954 and the government created the Medicare and Medicaid programs in 1965. By the end of 1995, individuals and companies paid for about one-half of the health care received in the United States, with the government paying for the other half.

The 1980s and 1990s saw a rapid rise in the cost of health care. During this time the majority of employer-sponsored group insurance plans moved to less expensive managed care plans. This move had been facilitated by the federal HMO Act of 1973, which allowed use of federal funds and policy to promote health maintenance organizations (HMO), and the Tax Equity and Fiscal Responsibility Act (TEFRA) in 1982, which made it easier and more attractive for HMOs to contract with the Medicare program. By the mid-1990s, most Americans who had health insurance were enrolled in managed care plans.

Patient Education

Although most insurance plans began as safety mechanisms in the event of **catastrophic** health events, most plans today cover **preventive care.** Catastrophic health events are defined as chronic illnesses or serious injuries that require expensive, specialized, or long-term care. An example is a person diagnosed with cancer or a person who needs several surgeries after a serious accident. Preventive care is care a patient receives to stay well. Examples include well-child checks and yearly mammograms or physicals.

Health Insurance Today

Today, Americans obtain health insurance from a variety of sources. Medical assistants need to be knowledgeable about the rules and requirements of each. These will be discussed in detail later in the chapter.

About half of insured Americans have health insurance through a private or commercial insurance company. Usually this is through a group health insurance policy sponsored by an employer. Some employers **self-insure**, paying directly for employees' medical bills. Individuals who do not have employer-sponsored health insurance may purchase an **individual health insurance** policy. **Liability insurance**, such as automobile and homeowner insurance, provides for medical expenses related to certain accidents.

Most Americans who do not have private insurance receive health insurance benefits from the state or federal government. Government programs include **Medicare**, a federal program for persons over age 65, the disabled, and **end-stage renal disease** (**ESRD**) patients; **Medicaid**, a federal/state program primarily for low income people; **TRICARE**, for active duty and retired service personnel and their families; and **CHAMPVA** for veterans with service-related disabilities. **Workers' compensation** provides coverage for employees for job-related injuries or illnesses.

Despite the many options available for health insurance, it is estimated that 45 to 50 million Americans have no health insurance coverage. Often this is because individuals do not have or do not qualify for employer-based coverage, do not qualify for federal programs, and cannot afford individual policies. For these patients, many offices establish a **sliding fee scale** that charges fees based on a patient's financial ability to pay. Some cities also have free or low-cost clinics established and run by volunteers or not-for-profit agencies.

In addition to determining the source of patients' insurance, medical assistants need to determine what type of coverage they have. Insurance may cover **hospital services**, **physician services**, **preventive** care, **catastrophic** care, **long term care**, **ancillary services** such as prescription drug, vision, dental, chiropractic, and special risks such as cancer. With each type of coverage and each source of coverage, medical assistants need to identify how patients' insurance relates to the specific services being provided in a specific situation. Research, attention to detail, careful communication and patient advocacy are skills that successful medical assistants use in the insurance arena.

Health Insurance Terminology

Just as medical assistants need to understand medical terminology to provide physical care for patients, a knowledge of insurance terminology is critical to helping patients utilize their health insurance. In many situations, there are multiple terms that essentially have the same meanings. In other situations, terms that seem similar to the layperson have different and specific meanings in the world of health insurance. Patients are often unfamiliar with their insurance benefits and may not understand the terms they hear. Medical assistants who understand insurance terms can advocate for patients and communicate in ways that patients understand.

Members and Their Families

Health insurance, also called medical insurance, is a contract between an insurance carrier and the person who owns the insurance policy, known as the **member**, **subscriber**, **insured**, or **policyholder**. For those who receive insurance through their employers, the member is the employee. For those who buy individual policies, the member is the person who purchased the plan. For those covered by government policies, the term **beneficiary** is often used and refers to the individual who qualifies for the program.

Many commercial policies allow members to include family members on the plan. Family members are called **dependents** and may include a spouse, children, unmarried domestic partners, and stepchildren. Inclusion of family members is not automatic and it is possible for some, but not all, family members to be covered. The member must obtain forms from the employer or the insurance company to specifically designate dependents' coverage. The medical assistant will need to ask the patient, and possibly call the insurance company, to determine who is eligible for benefits. It is also important to know exactly how each dependent is legally related to the member.

Premiums

In order to obtain a commercial health insurance policy, the policyholder pays a **premium** to the insurance carrier. The premium is usually paid in monthly installments for the next month's coverage. In group coverage, the employer often pays the majority of the premium and employees authorize the remainder to be deducted from paychecks. If dependent coverage is selected, the premium is higher. Some government plans require a premium as well.

Fee Schedules and Approved Amounts

Providers establish a **fee schedule** which lists their charge for each service they provide. This is normally organized by type of service and CPT code. See Figure 16-1 ◆. Providers may set their charges in any manner they desire; however, in most states

New Patient Examinations		
Office Visit, Level 1	99201	$ 55.00
Office Visit, Level 2	99202	$110.00
Office Visit, Level 3	99203	$154.00
Office Visit, Level 4	99204	$226.00
Office Visit, Level 5	99205	$299.00
Established Patient Examinations		
Office Visit, Level 1	99211	$ 45.00
Office Visit, Level 2	99212	$ 60.00
Office Visit, Level 3	99213	$ 80.00
Office Visit, Level 4	99214	$123.00
Office Visit, Level 5	99215	$199.00

Figure 16-1 ◆ Sample fee schedule.

they are required to charge the same fee to every patient and every insurance company. They cannot discuss their fees with other providers and use that information to set prices, a practice known as price fixing. The charge on the fee schedule is known as the providers usual charge.

Insurance companies are not required to pay providers' usual charges. Insurers can use any method they desire to establish a payment level. Often they calculate what they determine to be an average or customary price among providers of the same specialty and in the same geographic area. This is called the **approved** or **allowed amount**. When a provider's actual charge is less than the allowed amount, the insurer will pay the actual charge. Providers cannot increase their charge for a given service to selected insurance companies in order to receive higher payment. When providers' charges are more than the insurance allowable, the insurance pays the allowed amount. This method of determining insurance payments is called **usual, customary and reasonable (UCR).** When calculating benefits and amounts owed, the first step is to identify the allowed charge.

Deductibles

Few health insurance plans cover 100% of the care patients receive, so patients will experience several different kinds of out-of-pocket expenses. Before the insurance plan pays any benefits, patients may have a **deductible** to meet. The deductible is a monetary amount patients must pay to the provider for health care services before health insurance benefits begin to pay. Deductible amounts can be as low as $100 or as high as $10,000. Plans with low deductibles tend to have higher premiums than plans with high deductibles. Some government plans also have deductibles. When calculating benefits and amounts owed, the second step is to subtract the deductible from the allowed charge. See Figure 16-2 ◆.

In some policies, the deductible will not be required for all services. A preventive care visit may not require a deductible, whereas a sick visit will. This is to encourage patients to seek preventive care. When patients include family members on the policy, there is usually an individual deductible and a family deductible. The individual deductible is the maximum deductible that any given family member must pay; the family deductible is the maximum deductible for all family members combined.

For example, John Jacobs is the policyholder and carries his wife, Jeanne, and his two children, Jana and James, on the policy. The individual deductible is $100 and the family deductible is $300. Jeanne receives medical care for a cost of $150; she pays her deductible of $100 and insurance benefits will apply to the remaining $50. A short time later, Jana becomes ill and sees the doctor for a charge of $50. The entire $50 will be applied to her deductible and must be paid out-of-pocket. Now the family has accumulated $150 towards the family deductible. Next, John receives care for $200. He has not met his individual deductible and the family deductible has not been met yet. He will pay $100 out-of-pocket for his individual deductible and insurance benefits will apply to the remaining $100 of his bill. $250 of the family deductible has now been met. Unfortu-

> **Scenario 1:** Martina Kahlo has health insurance through her employer's plan. She has a $100 yearly deductible, and then she is covered at 100 percent. Martina sees Dr. Jacobson for an office call that includes lab work. The cost of the office call is $128. How much does Martina owe for her visit?
>
> **$128 charge for medical services.**
>
> **$100 for Martina's annual deductible**
>
> **Martina must pay her $100 deductible. The insurance company will pay the $28 balance.**
>
> **Scenario 2:** Jorge Garcia has an individual health insurance plan. He has a $1,000 yearly deductible, and then he is covered at 80 percent. Jorge sees Dr. Jacobson for an office call that includes lab work and two X-rays. The cost of the office call is $217. How much does Jorge owe for his visit?
>
> **$217 charge for medical services**
>
> **$1,000 for Jorge's annual deductible**
>
> **Insurance company will pay $0 because Jorge has not met his $1,000 annual deductible. Jorge must pay the $217 charge.**

Figure 16-2 ◆ Calculating a patient's insurance deductible.

nately, James becomes ill and sees the doctor for a $100 visit. Even though he has not met his individual deductible, only $50 is owed on the family deductible, so $50 is paid out-of-pocket for James and insurance benefits apply to the remaining $50. Now that the $300 family deductible has been met, no family member will be required to pay a deductible for the remainder of the year, even if the individual deductible for that dependent has not been met. The family deductible presents a savings for families of more than three members.

Copayments and Coinsurance

After the deductible is met, most patients still have out-of-pocket expenses they are responsible for. **Copayments** are set dollar amounts that patients pay at the time of service, such as $5 or $10 per visit. **Coinsurance** is a set percentage of charges that patients pay. An 80/20 coinsurance plan means that the insurance company pays 80% of approved charges and the patient pays 20%. A 70/30 plan means that the insurance company pays 70% of approved charges and the patient pays 30%. Different types of visits or different types of providers may have different copayment or coinsurance amounts. For example, preventive care may have no copayment or coinsurance while sick care does. A specialist visit may require a higher copayment or coinsurance than a primary care visit. The specific rules are set by the insurance company and clearly spelled out in the patient's policy. Most government programs require a copayment or coinsurance.

When calculating benefits and amounts owed, after the deductible is subtracted from the allowed amount, coinsurance is calculated by multiplying the remaining balance times the coinsurance percentage. Then, subtract the copayment or coinsurance amount from the remaining balance.

When providers have a **participating** or **preferred** provider contract with the insurance company, they agree to accept the insurance allowed amount as payment in full and cannot bill patients the difference between their actual charge and the allowed amount. However, when the provider is not participating or contracted with an insurance company, the patient is responsible for the entire balance not covered by insurance. This is called **balance billing**. The insurance company calculates deductibles, coinsurance, and copayments based on the allowed amounts, which may be less than the provider's actual charge. Figure 16-3 ◆ shows how copayments and coinsurance amounts are calculated.

Stop Loss and Lifetime Maximum

Many insurance policies have **stop loss** and **lifetime maximum** benefits clauses. A stop loss is the maximum amount the patient must pay out-of-pocket for copayments and coinsurance. After this amount is reached in a year, the insurance pays 100% of the remaining expenses. The stop loss amount starts over the next year. Lifetime maximum benefit is the maximum amount the insurance company will pay for individual members over the course of the patient's life. A common lifetime maximum benefit is $1 million, but it could be as low as $100,000 in a very inexpensive policy. Sometimes patients will select a low cost policy and not be aware of provisions such as the lifetime maximum. While $1 million or even $100,000 may sound like a lot of money, medical expenses can accumulate very quickly with a serious illness such as cancer or an organ transplant.

> **Scenario 1:** Dr. Jones charges $75 for an office call. Mary Smith is insured with Premera Blue Cross Insurance and has a 20 percent coinsurance obligation. Dr. Jones is a preferred provider with Premera Blue Cross and has agreed to accept $64.25 as payment in full for his office call. Mary owes 20 percent of the $64.25 fee ($12.85).
>
> **Scenario 2:** Dr. Barro charges $70 for an office call. Molly Manchero is insured with Regence Blue Shield Insurance and has a $10 copayment obligation. Dr. Barro is a preferred provider with Regence Blue Shield and has agreed to accept $62.50 as payment in full for his office call. Molly owes $10 of the $62.50 fee.

Figure 16-3 ◆ Calculating copayments and coinsurance.

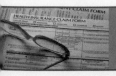

PROCEDURE 16-1 Calculate Deductible, Coinsurance, and Allowable Amounts

Theory and Rationale

The medical assistant will frequently explain to patients how their deductible, coinsurance, and allowable amounts are calculated. Attention to detail is very important as misquoted figures can be cause for patients to become dissatisfied with the medical staff.

Materials

- Pen
- Paper
- Insurance verification form
- Patient's insurance identification card

Competency

(**Conditions**) With the necessary materials, you will be able to (**Task**) calculate deductible, coinsurance, and allowable amounts (**Standards**) correctly within the time limit set by the instructor.

1. After the patient's insurance coverage has been verified, locate the information on the verification form regarding any deductible and coinsurance amount.
2. Inform the patient of the deductible amount that will need to be paid at the beginning of the calendar or fiscal year.
3. Explain to the patient that the amount charged for any particular procedure in the medical office will likely be reduced to a lower amount (called the allowed amount) when processed by the insurance carrier.
4. Imagine the patient has a $100 yearly deductible and a 10% copayment. The patient has had an examination, with a charge of $95.00, an X-ray with a charge of $75.00, and laboratory work with a charge of $102.00.
5. Imagine the insurance carrier in this situation allows $72.00 for the examination, $51.00 for the X-ray, and $80.00 for the laboratory work.
6. Calculate the patient's amount owing by adding the allowed figures to come to a total of allowed charges.
7. Subtract the $100.00 deductible from the total of the allowed charges.
8. Multiply 20% by the remaining allowed amount to determine the patient's coinsurance.
9. Add the $100.00 deductible to the 20% coinsurance amount to determine the amount the patient will need to pay out of pocket for the visit.
10. Explain the figures to the patient and collect the fees.

Waiting Period, Exclusions, and Pre-Existing Conditions

In addition to out-of-pocket expenses, many health insurance plans have **waiting periods** and **exclusions** that limit what the insurance plan needs to pay in benefits. A waiting period is a set period of time that must pass before a member's **pre-existing condition** is covered. A pre-existing condition is any condition a patient was diagnosed with or treated for, including receiving prescription medications, before beginning coverage with a new insurance plan.

HIPAA Compliance

Although waiting periods for pre-existing condition coverage vary from one insurance plan to another, a pre-existing condition is covered without a waiting period when the patient has been insured the 24 months before joining the new plan. Therefore, if patients remain insured for 24 or more months, they can change jobs and retain pre-existing condition coverage without added waiting periods even when they have chronic illnesses. Patients should obtain a **certificate of coverage** from the previous insurance plan. This letter documents the nature and length of coverage with the plan. Patients submit it to the new plan to establish proof of continuous coverage. If patients have had more than one insurance plan during the previous 24 months, certificates of coverage from each plan should be submitted. Even when patients have not been insured the 24 months before joining new insurance plans, Health Insurance Portability and Accountability Act (HIPAA) legislation restricts insurance companies from requiring patients to wait any longer than 12 months from the dates their new insurance coverage began.

Any uncovered services or diagnoses are called **exclusions.** Some plans exclude such things as routine eye exams and hearing tests. Others exclude any service related to an uncovered or excluded diagnosis. For instance, if a patient's insurance plan does not cover services related to a "hearing loss" diagnosis, that patient would have no coverage for hearing tests. If, however, that same patient presented with complaints of multiple ear infections, hearing tests with a diagnosis of "ear infection" may be covered.

Private Health Insurance

An overview of the health insurance industry and a basic understanding of key insurance terms has been presented. Next is a discussion of private and commercial insurance. A number of national commercial insurance carriers, including Blue

Cross/Blue Shield, Aetna, and Cigna, offer health insurance coverage. Some national carriers offer both managed care and preferred provider policies; most offer policies that can be purchased secondary to Medicare, which is described in the following section. Policies through national commercial carriers might be purchased by employers for a group of employees or by individuals who lack health insurance through their places of employment. Coverage amounts and premiums vary according to policy type.

Sources of Coverage

The most common sources of private health insurance are group insurance through an employer or other organization, a self-insured plan through an employer or labor union, COBRA continuation of group coverage, and individual insurance.

Group Insurance

Group insurance is a policy offered to groups of people where the risk or cost of insurance is spread across everyone equally for a given level of coverage. It is usually the least expensive type of insurance because statistics show that a few people in a group will use a large amount of services, but many people in the group will use few if any services. Everyone pays the same rate for protection, so the high costs of a few members are shared equally by everyone in the group. The most common group is the employees of a company. However, various professional organizations also offer group coverage. Group insurance is the most common source of private insurance in the United States.

Employers initiate negotiations with an insurance company to cover their employees. Employers determine how large their financial budget is for employee health insurance premiums and how much they want employees to contribute towards the premium. The insurance company then presents a list of benefits available for that price. The more that can be paid in premiums, the more benefits will be available. Employers will select the insurance company and the benefit package that best meets the budget and the employees' anticipated needs.

It is common for an employer to allow employees to select among a variety of benefit packages from the chosen insurance company. The employer designates the amount the company will pay per month towards the premium, which is usually constant among all packages. Employees are able to select the package that best meets their needs for medical care and premium cost. Packages with high deductibles and copayments or coinsurance will cost less than packages with low deductibles and out-of-pocket expenses. Employees may have the option to add dependents for an additional premium. Some employers pay part of the dependents' premiums and others require the employee to pay the full amount. Because most companies offer a variety of health insurance options for employees, two patients with the same employer and the same insurance company may have different benefits. Figure 16-4 ◆ gives such a sample scenario. To avoid giving out incorrect information, it is important for medical assistants to determine the specific benefits available to each patient. Often this information is available online through the insurer's secured Web site or by calling the insurance company.

Two patients, Sara and George, present Premera Blue Cross insurance identification cards. ABC Marketing, a large employer that provides its employees an extensive insurance plan, employs Sara. Lone Star Plumbing, a small employer that has purchased a plan with minimal employee coverage, employs George. Although they present similar insurance cards, Sara and George have vastly different coverage.

Figure 16-4 ◆ Same insurance company, different benefits.

—Critical Thinking Question 16-1—
How should the medical assistant explain to Martin that his wife will need to add him to her policy if she has not yet done so?

Employer-based coverage typically begins with the next calendar month following 30 days of employment, but this timeframe can vary. It is important to determine when coverage begins for a patient who has recently changed jobs. It is also important to determine when coverage ends for a patient leaving a job. Coverage may end the last day of employment, the end of the month, or the end of the following month.

Self-Insured Plan

For patients, health insurance through a self-insured plan is very similar to group insurance. In fact, employees may not even recognize the difference. An employer or labor union who self-insures does not purchase a policy through a commercial insurance company. Instead, they set aside a large pool of money, or reserve, and use that fund to reimburse employees for their health care expenses. Sometimes they will contract with a **third party administrator (TPA)**, an outside company that processes the paperwork for claims, but any payments come from the employer's or labor union's funds, not an insurance company.

—Critical Thinking Question 16-2—
Is it advisable to call the insurance carrier of Martin's wife to check on benefits and spousal eligibility? Why or why not?

COBRA Coverage

When employees have been covered under group insurance and leave employment, they may have the opportunity to continue the group coverage at their own expense. The premium is the same as that for the group, but because often the employer has been paying a large portion of the employees' premium, patients may be surprised at the cost of the premium. Nonetheless, the premium is usually less, and the benefits better, than an individual policy. This option allows employees to keep insurance in force until they obtain new insurance coverage.

The federal Consolidated Omnibus Reconciliation Act (**COBRA**) requires employers to extend health insurance coverage at group rates, usually for up to 18 months, to any employee who is laid off, quits, or is fired, except under certain circumstances (Figure 16-5 ◆).

COBRA coverage is available to employees who work for employers with 20 or more employees. Both full- and part-time employees are counted to determine whether a plan is subject to COBRA. A qualified beneficiary is typically an individual who was covered by the employer's group health insurance plan on the day before a qualifying event. This beneficiary can be the employee, the employee's spouse, and the retired employee's dependent children or any child born to or placed for adoption with a covered employee during the period of COBRA coverage.

In order to be qualified for COBRA coverage, the qualified beneficiary must have experienced a qualifying event. Qualifying events for employees include:

- The voluntary or involuntary termination of employment for reasons other than gross misconduct
- Reduction in the number of hours of employment resulting in the termination of health insurance coverage

Qualifying events for spouses include:

- The covered employee's becoming entitled to Medicare coverage
- Divorce or legal separation of the covered employee
- Death of the covered employee

Qualifying events for dependent children include:

- Loss of dependent child status under the plan rules
- Voluntary or involuntary termination of the covered employee's employment for any reason other than gross misconduct
- Reduction in the hours worked by the covered employee resulting in the termination of health insurance coverage

Keys to Success
PROVIDING COVERAGE INFORMATION TO PATIENTS

Most patients are only vaguely aware of their insurance plan coverage. Therefore, be sure to check with patients' insurance companies before providing patients expensive treatment and to relay coverage information to patients. Remember that insurance companies only give reviews of patients' benefits. They do not guarantee actual benefit when claims are received. Make sure patients understand that you are only relaying information from their insurance carriers. Direct any questions the patient may have about coverage to those carriers.

- Covered employee's becoming entitled to Medicare
- Divorce or legal separation of the covered employee
- Death of the covered employee

In order to be eligible for COBRA coverage, a qualified beneficiary must notify the employer's plan administrator of a qualifying event within 60 days after divorce or legal separation or a child's ceasing to be a dependent under plan rules. Employers must notify the plan administrator of a qualifying event within 30 days after an employee's death, termination, reduced hours of employment, or entitlement to Medicare.

Individual Health Insurance Policies

Another type of insurance plan is the individual plan or policy, which individuals buy directly through insurance carriers. These plans are often the most expensive, because group rates are unavailable.

The benefits are often not as good as group policies, resulting in higher deductibles and other out-of-pocket expenses. The minimum level of benefit package for individual insurance policies is regulated by each state and in some states, only a few companies offer individual policies due to restrictive requirements. Employees who have been on a COBRA plan can convert to an individual policy with the same insurance company when the COBRA benefits expire, but the group rates and benefits will no longer apply.

Types of Plans

Since the passage of the HMO ACT of 1973 and the Tax Equity and Fiscal Responsibility Act (**TEFRA**), the insurance industry has introduced health insurance plans that allow patients a variety of ways to access providers and share in the cost of care. These various plans also differ in how insurance companies pay providers.

Fee-for-Service Plans

Back in the 1980s, **fee-for-service**, also known as **indemnity**, plans were the norm. Rare today, and typically among the most expensive offerings, fee-for-service plans allow patients to seek

Congress passed COBRA health benefit provisions in 1986 to provide certain former employees, retirees, spouses, former spouses, and dependent children the right to temporarily continue health coverage at group rates. To be eligible for COBRA coverage, employees must have been enrolled in their employers' health plans when they worked and those health plans must continue to be in effect for active employees.

Figure 16-5 ◆ COBRA overview.

care with any covered health care providers, for any covered services. Neither the list of physicians patients may see, nor the fee schedules are prearranged. These plans are private health insurance plans that reimburse health care providers on the basis of a fee for each health service provided to the covered person. Fee-for-service plans typically include a yearly deductible, after which the insurance company will pay at a certain coinsurance rate. Most commonly the coinsurance rate is 70/30 or 80/20 percent, with the insurance company paying the higher percentage and the member paying the lower.

Fee-for-service plans are among the most expensive because they do not contain managed care or cost-control measures. The type of person who generally opts for the fee-for-service plan is an individual with a serious medical condition who needs frequent treatment, and those who can afford the plan and want to have complete freedom of choice to see the provider of their choice whenever they wish.

Managed Care Plans

Today, most patients are covered by **managed care.** Managed care plans control the costs associated with plan purchase by controlling the amounts they reimburse health care providers. Managed care organizations (**MCOs**) contract with health care providers to provide care for a certain group of patients. Those providers, called **participating providers,** sign a contract with the MCO that stipulates discounted reimbursement rates, billing guidelines, and other rules. A provider will usually have contracts with several different MCOs. The MCO then contracts with insurance companies to offer lower reimbursement rates through its network of participating providers. The MCO will list the provider's name in a directory given to patients. Patients will have lower out-of-pocket expenses if they use a participating provider.

Providers who do not contract with a specific MCO are called **nonparticipating providers.** Some MCOs cover patients who see nonparticipating providers, but usually at the patients' higher out-of-pocket expense. Other MCOs offer no coverage if the insured sees a nonparticipating provider. Therefore, it is important for medical assistants to let patients know whether providers participate with the patients' health plans. A provider may be participating with some patients' MCOs and nonparticipating with others. Most offices ask about health care coverage the first time patients call. When in doubt, assistants should ask patients for their insurance information and then call or research the insurance companies online.

Managed care plans are divided into four basic types: Health Maintenance Organizations (**HMOs**), Preferred Provider Organizations (**PPOs**), Exclusive Provider Organizations (EPOs), and Point of Service (**POS**) Plans.

Table 16-1 summarizes the various types of MCOs and their characteristics.

In Practice

Georgia Collins calls the medical office to schedule an appointment as a new patient. When the medical assistant asks her about her insurance coverage, she says she is unsure of her insurance company's name and cannot locate her insurance card. How should the medical assistant respond? Is insurance information needed before patients seek care? Why or why not? If Georgia becomes angry, how should the medical assistant react?

Preferred Provider Organizations

The **preferred provider organization** (PPO) contracts with physicians and facilities to perform services for PPO members at specified rates. These rates, or fees, are contractually adjusted so that the PPO member is charged less than nonmembers. The PPO gives subscribers a list of PPO member-providers from which subscribers can receive health care at PPO rates. If a patient chooses to receive treatment from a provider who is not in the PPO network, the patient has to pay any difference between the PPO's rate and the outside provider's rate. PPOs generally require preauthorization for major medical services.

Each physician in a practice may be a member of more than one PPO, and all the doctors in the practice may not necessarily belong to the same PPO. Some of the main features of PPOs include the following:

- PPOs are similar to HMOs in that they enter into contractual arrangements with healthcare providers (e.g., physicians, hospitals, and other healthcare professionals) and together form a provider network.
- Unlike an HMO, members don't have a PCP (gatekeeper) nor do they have to use an in-network provider for their care. However, PPOs offer members higher benefits as financial incentives to use network providers. The incentives may include lower deductibles, lower copayments, and higher reimbursements. For example, if the subscriber sees an in-network family physician for a routine visit, she may only have a small copayment or deductible. If she sees a non-network family physician for a routine visit, she may have to pay as much as 50% of the total bill.
- PPO members typically do not have to get a referral to see a specialist. However, there is a financial incentive to use a specialist who is a member of a PPO's provider network.
- PPOs are less restrictive than HMOs in the choice of healthcare provider. However, they tend to require greater out-of-pocket payments from their members.*

?—Critical Thinking Question 16-3—

Assume the medical assistant determined that Martin's wife's insurance plan was not one of the physician's preferred plans. What should the medical assistant say to Martin?

*Source: Vines, Deborah, Braceland, Ann, Rollins, Elizabeth, and Miller, Susan. *Comprehensive Health Insurance: Billing, Coding, and Reimbursement.* © 2008, pp. 29–30. Reprinted by permission of Pearson Education, Inc. Upper Saddle River, NJ.

TABLE 16-1 VARIOUS TYPES OF MCOs AND THEIR CHARACTERISTICS

HMO	PPO	POS	EPO
■ State licensed ■ Most stringent guidelines ■ Limited network of providers ■ Members assigned to PCPs ■ Members must use network except in emergencies or pay a penalty ■ Usually there is a financial reward to providers for managing the cost of care	■ Limited network of providers but larger than HMO ■ Members may be assigned to PCPs but restrictions on accessing other physicians not as tight as in HMO ■ Financial penalty for accessing non-network providers less severe than in an HMO ■ Usually there is no reward to providers for managing the cost of care	■ Hybrid of HMO and PPO networks ■ Members may choose from a primary or secondary network ■ Primary network is HMO-like ■ Secondary network is often a PPO network ■ Out-of-pocket expenses are lower within the primary network and higher when using the secondary network ■ Members have more choices with less expense than with a PPO	■ Doesn't have an HMO license ■ Members are eligible for benefits only when they use network providers ■ Financial penalties for members leaving the network are similar to those of HMO ■ Priced lower than a PPO but higher than an HMO
IPA Model HMO	**Staff Model HMO**	**Network Model HMO**	**Group Model HMO**
■ An association formed by physicians with separately owned practices (solo or small group) ■ HMO may contract with physicians separately or through the IPA	■ HMO hires the physicians and pays them salaries ■ HMO owns the network ■ HMO owns the clinic sites and health centers	■ HMO uses two or more group practices or a group practice plus a combination of staff physicians and contracted independent physicians to form a network of providers ■ Allow members to choose their providers	■ HMO contracts with multi-specialty groups ■ May be open-panel or closed-panel

Source: Vines, Comprehensive Health Insurance: Billing, Coding, and Reimbursement, *p. 34.*

Health Maintenance Organizations

Health maintenance organizations (HMOs) are managed care plans that cover members only when those members seek care from a list of health care providers and suppliers who have contracted with the HMO. When members wish to seek care from providers not on the list, they must pay for the care. Most HMOs require patients to choose primary care providers (PCPs) who belong to the network of covered providers. The primary care provider serves as the **caretaker** or **gatekeeper,** the person who arranges any specialist services or hospitalizations.

The plans have various rules for copayment, coinsurance, and deductible amounts. The subscriber to an HMO plan is able to obtain health care on a regular basis with unlimited medical attention. Thus, HMOs encourage subscribers to take advantage of preventive healthcare services in an attempt to make healthcare coverage more cost efficient. HMOs do tend to cover more preventive procedures such as annual physicals, prostate cancer testing, and mammography.

■ A distinctive feature of an HMO is that the subscriber chooses a primary care physician. The PCP arranges, provides, coordinates, and authorizes all aspects of a member's health care. PCPs are usually family doctors, internal medicine doctors, general practitioners, or OB/GYNs.

■ An HMO enters into contractual arrangements with healthcare providers (e.g., physicians, hospitals, and other healthcare professionals) and together form a provider network.

■ Members are required to see only providers within this network if they are to have their health care paid for by the HMO. If the member receives care from a provider who isn't in the network, the HMO will not pay for care unless it was preauthorized by the HMO or deemed an emergency.

■ Members can only see a specialist (e.g., cardiologist, dermatologist, rheumatologist) if they are referred and the PCP authorizes the service. The referral must be approved by the HMO. If the member sees a specialist without a referral, the HMO will not pay for the service.

■ HMOs are the most restrictive type of health plan because of the restrictions the members have in selecting a healthcare provider. However, HMOs typically provide members with a greater range of health benefits for the lowest out-of-pocket expenses, such as either no or a very low copayment and deductible.

The four main types of HMOs, discussed next, vary in the way they link providers in order to create a healthcare delivery system.

Group Model HMO   A group model HMO is an organization that contracts with a multispecialty physicians' group to provide physician services to an enrolled group. Physicians are employees of the group practice and generally are limited to providing care only to the HMO's members.

Individual Practice Association HMO   **Individual practice association (IPA)** HMOs are the most decentralized and involve contracting with individual physicians to create a healthcare delivery system. The HMO contracts with community hospitals and providers of services such as laboratories and diagnostics. Pharmacy services are provided through a contracted network of independent and chain community pharmacies and mail order service.

Network Model HMO   Network HMOs contract with more than one community-based multispecialty group to provide wider geographical coverage. The group practices under contract with one HMO vary from large to small, from primary care to multispecialty practice.

Staff Model HMO   The **staff model HMOs** employ salaried physicians who treat members in facilities owned and operated by the HMO. Most services, including diagnostic, laboratory, and pharmacy services, are provided on-site. A team of health professionals delivers the care.*

Exclusive Provider Organizations

Exclusive provider organizations (EPOs) are types of managed care plans that cover members who seek care from health care providers in a small network. In these plans, groups of health care providers often form their own networks and then contract with employers to provide exclusive care to their employees. EPOs often have hospitals in their networks, and physicians contracted with these networks must perform their hospital services in the contracted hospitals. Just like with an HMO, members who wish to seek care outside the exclusive network must fund the care.

An EPO is referred to as *exclusive* because employers agree not to contract with any other plan. Members are eligible for benefits only when they use the services of the network of providers with certain exceptions for emergency or out-of-area services. If a patient decides to seek care outside the network, generally he is not reimbursed for the cost of treatment. Technically many HMOs can be considered EPOs except that EPOs are regulated under insurance statutes rather than federal and state HMO regulations. As a result, the EPO is priced lower than a PPO to the employer, but an EPO's premiums are usually more expensive than an HMO's premiums.

Point-of-Service (POS) Options

Because many patients do not wish to accept services from only their HMO providers, some HMO plans add a **point-of-service** option. Patients who choose this option do not have to use only the HMO's physicians. However, if they choose to see physicians outside the network, they must pay increased deductibles and coinsurance. This option makes the HMO more like a PPO, in terms of choices available to the patients.

- The reason it is called a *point-of-service* option is because members choose which option—HMO or PPO—they will use each time they seek health care.
- Like an HMO and a PPO, a POS plan has a contracted provider network.
- POS plans encourage, but do not require, members to choose a primary care physician. As in a traditional HMO, the PCP acts as a "gatekeeper" when making referrals. Members who choose not to use their PCPs for referrals (but still seek care from an in-network provider) still receive benefits but will pay higher copays and/or deductibles than members who use their PCPs.
- POS members also may opt to visit an out-of-network provider at their discretion. If that happens, the member's copayments, coinsurance, and deductibles will be substantially higher.†

A triple option plan is a type of POS that offers patients a choice between an HMO, a PPO, and a traditional indemnity plan. For example, they may choose to use the HMO or PPO, where their out-of-pocket costs are lower for routine checkups, but may have an out-of-network specialist they have seen for many years for a particular medical problem, and choose to pay a higher out-of-pocket cost to continue to see that specialist under the traditional indemnity plan. A POS offers patients the greatest amount of control over both their providers and their out-of-pocket costs.

Consumer-Directed Health Care Plans

The newest type of insurance plan, which is becoming increasingly popular in response to rising health care costs, is the **consumer-directed health care plan.** These plans place consumers in charge of how their health care dollars are spent, rendering those consumers more likely to ask questions about, or research the need for, their health-related services. Just as with traditional employer-paid plans, employers who support

*Source: Vines, Deborah, Braceland, Ann, Rollins, Elizabeth, and Miller, Susan. *Comprehensive Health Insurance: Billing, Coding, and Reimbursement.* © 2008, pp. 28–29. Reprinted by permission of Pearson Education, Inc. Upper Saddle River, NJ.

†Source: Vines, Deborah, Braceland, Ann, Rollins, Elizabeth, and Miller, Susan. *Comprehensive Health Insurance: Billing, Coding, and Reimbursement.* © 2008. pp. 30–31. Reprinted by permission of Pearson Education, Inc. Upper Saddle River, NJ.

consumer-directed health care plans retain a certain amount of money from employees' paychecks to fund health care premiums. Generally, a consumer-driven health plan includes a three-tier structure of payment for health care: a tax-exempt health savings account or medical savings account that an individual uses to pay for health expenses up to a certain amount, a high-deductible health insurance policy that pays for expenses over the deductible, and a gap between those two in which the individual pays any healthcare expenses out of their own pocket. These out-of-pocket expenses may be eligible for reimbursement through a flexible spending account. Accounts are administered by insurance companies, which process claims and issue payments. Employees receive lists of covered services, just as with traditional plans.

From the medical provider's point of view, consumer-directed health care plans work much the same as traditional health insurance plans in that the physician's office sends bills directly to health care plans and is reimbursed by health care plans. Patients pay any portion not covered by the health care plan.

Blue Cross/Blue Shield Plans

Patients may have Blue Cross (BC) and Blue Shield (BS) plans through group health coverage or individual insurance. According to the BCBS Association (BCBSA), nearly one-third of Americans are covered by some type of BCBS plan (www .bcbsa.com). BC began at Baylor University Hospital in Texas to provide teachers with prepaid hospitalization benefits. BS was begun in Palo Alto, California, in 1939 as a response to an AMA resolution encouraging physicians to cooperate with prepaid health plans. Historically BC plans provided hospital service benefits and BS plans provided physician service benefits. Each BC and BS plan was an independent not-for-profit health plan, with one or more plans in most states across the country. The national associations merged in 1977 to form BCBSA, with 450 member plans. Today the national association is for-profit and many of the local plans have either gone for-profit or have been purchased by for-profit insurance companies.

Patients may have a BC plan, a BS plan, or a combination BCBS plan depending on the geographic area. It is important to remember that each BCBS plan is separate and unique in terms of benefits, cost sharing, and other requirements, just as private commercial insurance companies are unique from each other.

BCBS coverage includes fee-for-service traditional coverage, managed care plans, a federal employee program (FEP), Medicare supplemental plans and healthcare anywhere plans. The type of coverage is indicated on the member ID card. Members with a PPO plan have cards that contain the letters "PPO" in the upper right hand corner. FEP member cards display a logo of an outline of the USA map and the words "federal employee program" and "government-wide service benefit plan." The healthcare anywhere coverage, also called BlueCard, contains a logo of a suitcase. This coverage enables members traveling in the service area of another BCBS plan to utilize local preferred providers and receive benefits under their home plan. Most BCBS member ID numbers begin with three letters that are a code indicating the member's home plan. It is essential to include these letters when reporting the member ID number on a claim. Figure 16-6 ◆ shows a sample BCBS member ID card.

Each BCBS processes its own claims, so medical assistants need to verify the correct filing address. In the past, most local BCBS plans would forward claims to the correct home plan, but that practice has become less common in recent years as many plans have joined commercial for-profit companies.

Other Related Benefits

Legislation has created the opportunity for several types of tax-advantaged financial accounts in which patients can set aside some of their income to help cover health care expenses not paid by insurance. Employers are able to contribute to some of these funds. Patients submit their own expenses for reimbursement to these funds, so medical assistants are not directly

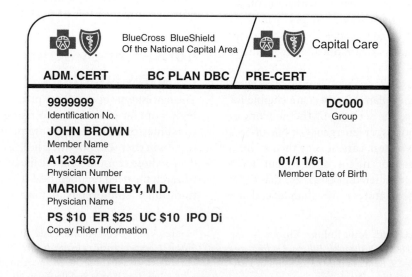

Figure 16-6 ◆ Sample BCBS member ID card.

involved in the billing. But, it is important to be aware of them in case patients have questions or need receipts or other documentation from the provider to submit to these plans.

Health Savings Accounts

Health savings accounts (HSAs) are personal savings accounts that can be used along with a high-deductible health plan to help pay for unreimbursed medical expenses. These accounts offer certain tax advantages to the individual in that the employee places pretax dollars into the savings accounts. Contributions to HSAs can be made by employers and/or individuals. Annual contributions are limited, as are out-of-pocket maximums, though persons aged 55 and over can make additional contributions. HSAs are portable from one job to another.

Medical Savings Accounts

The Health Insurance Portability and Accountability Act of 1996 (HIPAA) permits eligible individuals to establish a **medical savings account (MSA)**. These accounts may be used to pay for medical expenses along with a high-deductible health insurance plan. In order to be eligible for a medical savings account an individual must be employed by a small employer that provides a high-deductible health insurance plan or be self-employed and covered by a high-deductible health insurance plan. Contributions may be made by the individual and/or the employer, but not both in the same year.

Flexible Spending Accounts

Flexible spending accounts (**FSA**), also called healthcare reimbursement accounts (**HCRA**), allow individuals to set aside a portion of their pretaxed wages to pay for certain out-of-pocket health care expenses. Money from flexible spending accounts can be used to pay for expenses not covered by health insurance such as:

- Deductibles and copays
- Prescription drugs and medical supplies
- Dental services, dentures and orthodontics
- Eyeglasses, contacts, solutions and eye surgery
- Chiropractic services
- Psychiatric care and psychologist's fees
- Smoking cessation programs

Money set aside in flexible spending accounts in any given year must be spent by a certain date, typically March 15th of the following year or the money is forfeited. Figure 16-7 ◆ explains how a flexible spending account works.

Third Party Liability

When patients are involved in a non–work-related accident, there may be third party liability (**TPL**) insurance that covers medical bills. Most businesses, home owners, and vehicle owners have liability insurance to cover injuries that occur on their properties or in vehicle accidents. For example, when patients are injured in an automobile accident, the automobile owner's auto liability insurance typically covers the patients' medical expenses.

Chris Tamparo works for an employer that offers to put Chris's pretax earnings into a flex spending account for Chris' health care expenses. Chris has a health insurance plan through his employer that has a $500 deductible and then coverage for 80 percent of his care.

Chris visits his physician for an office call and lab work. The cost for the visit is $145. During the office call, Chris gets a prescription that costs $43. Chris's health insurance policy lacks a prescription drug benefit.

Cost of physician visit and lab work: $145
Cost of prescription medication: $ 43
Total $188

Chris has a $500 annual deductible, so his insurance plan will pay $0 of the physician visit. Because Chris lacks prescription drug coverage, his insurance plan will pay $0 of the prescription cost. Chris pays the full $188 and gives the receipts to his employer. The employer reimburses Chris $188 out of Chris' flex spending account.

Figure 16-7 ◆ Flex spending or health care savings accounts.

State laws vary regarding how automobile insurance is handled, but many states have no-fault coverage. Under no-fault coverage, the injured person's own auto insurance pays the medical bills, even if someone else was at-fault. This is paid under the personal injury protection (PIP) of the injured person's policy. Their auto insurance company then works with the at-fault party's company to recover the expenses. If the injured person does not have PIP coverage, or expenses exceed the limit, then the at-fault party's insurance is billed. If the injured party files a lawsuit against the at-fault party, then medical bills may be sent to the patient's attorney. In these cases, the provider may need to wait until the case is settled to receive payment, which can take several years. Providers should ask their own attorney to file a lien with the patient's attorney, which establishes the provider's legal right be paid upon settlement.

If payment from a TPL company is delayed more than a specified number of days, such as 45 or 60 days, some insurers will *pay and pursue.* This means they will accept claims for services related to the injuries, pay them, then pursue the TPL insurance for reimbursement. If the provider or patient receives payment or a settlement from the TPL, they need to reimburse the plan that originally paid the bills. When patients' bills exceed the amount covered by the TPL, private and government plans can be billed for the denied expenses.

Patients often are responsible for a deductible and sometimes copayments or coinsurance on a TPL policy. Insurers often have a maximum approved charge that they will pay.

Usually balance billing is permitted because providers are not contracted with TPL insurers.

When injured patients are already established in the practice, a new medical record and a new financial account should be created specifically for treatment related to the accident. This helps clarify what services are accident-related and what services are part of patients ongoing health care. It also makes it easier to provide copies of accident-relevant records which will be required by the insurers. When registering patients involved in an accident, medical assistants should gather as much information as possible regarding the accident, the patient's automobile coverage if an auto accident, the at-fault party's name and insurance information, as well as the patient's private health insurance or Medicare coverage. While this information can be confusing to collect and organize, thoroughness up front will make it easier to bill and collect for services later.

Types of Coverage

Regardless of patients' source of coverage or the type of plan they have, many alternatives exist as to the type of coverage included in a plan. Type of coverage refers to the specific services covered under the plan. Each insurance policy is tailored to include the benefits most desired and most affordable for each group or individual. Understanding some of the most common alternatives for coverage types will enable medical assistants to clarify for patients what can be expected from their policies (Vines, p. 35).

Hospital

Hospital coverage provides protection against the costs of hospital care. It generally provides a room allowance (a stated amount per day for a semiprivate room) with a maximum number of days per year. Special provisions are made for operating room charges, X-rays, laboratory work, drugs, and other medically necessary items while the insured person is an **inpatient.** An inpatient is a person who is admitted to the hospital for a minimum of 24 hours.

Medical

Medical coverage provides benefits for **outpatient** medical care including physicians' fees for hospital visits and nonsurgical procedures. The term *medical* refers to physicians' costs. Special provisions are made for diagnostic services such as laboratory, X-ray, and pathology costs. An outpatient is a person who receives medical care at a hospital or other medical facility but who is not admitted for more than 24 hours.

Surgical

Surgical coverage provides protection for the cost of a physician's fee for surgery, whether it is performed in a hospital, in a doctor's office, or elsewhere, such as a surgical center. Charges for anesthesia generally are covered by surgical insurance.

Outpatient

Outpatient coverage usually provides protection for emergency department visits and other outpatient divisions in a hospital or medical facility such as X-ray, pathology, and psychological services.

Major Medical

Major medical insurance offers protection for large medical expenses established by a regular health insurance policy. There is usually an added cost for this type of insurance coverage.*

Home Health Care

Home health coverage provides benefits for services received by a homebound patient including nursing care, physical, speech and occupational therapy, personal caregivers, and other related needs. It is much less expensive to provide these services at home than in a facility, so many policies provide high levels of coverage for these services when prescribed by a physician.

Catastrophic Health Insurance

Catastrophic insurance provides protection only for the most expensive medical needs and are only suitable for individuals with the financial means to handle routine illnesses and hospitalizations. It is among the least expensive forms of health insurance because deductibles are generally large and there may be caps on the amount the policy will pay.

Specialized Policies

Patients can also purchase separate specialized policies to provide protection for unique situations. Special risk insurance provides protection against specific illnesses, such as cancer, or against certain types of high-risk accidents that may be excluded from traditional policies, such as sky diving or mountain climbing.

Long-term care insurance covers custodial services such as assistance with personal and household chores either at home or in a facility. The degree of care is based on the condition and requirements of the patients. Long-term care insurance is best purchased many years before a person anticipates needing it, because the annual premium increases with age and health status decline. Many financial advisers recommend that people consider purchasing long-term care policies in their early 50s.

Ancillary Coverage

Ancillary coverage is insurance for services provided by other than a physician or hospital, such as prescription drugs, vision, dental, and alternative care. These are often packaged in with the main policy, but are actually provided by other insurance companies and other MCOs. Usually patients have separate

*Source: Vines, Deborah, Braceland, Ann, Rollins, Elizabeth, and Miller, Susan. *Comprehensive Health Insurance: Billing, Coding, and Reimbursment.* © 2008. Reprinted by permission of Pearson Education, Inc. Upper Saddle River, NJ.

deductibles and copayments/coinsurance for ancillary coverage. Out-of-pocket costs from these plans may not count toward the overall stop lost provision.

Prescription Drug Coverage

Most insurance plans today have some form of prescription drug coverage. Prescription medications are often very expensive, and name brands are often far more costly than their generic counterparts. On behalf of pharmaceutical companies, pharmaceutical representatives visit medical offices to showcase the latest drugs on the market. As a marketing tactic, representatives often leave free samples for physicians to dispense. Through free samples on a short-term basis, physicians can provide needed medications to patients with financial issues or insurance companies that do not offer coverage. Physicians may also use free samples as trials before writing prescriptions.

Plans typically have a **formulary**, a list of drugs they will cover. Usually the formulary is subdivided into two or more tiers with each tier having a different level of coverage (Figure 16-8 ◆). For example, tier 1 may include most **generic drugs** and perhaps a few brand name drugs that have no generic equivalent. Patients might have a small copayment, perhaps only a few dollars, for tier 1 drugs. Tier 2 may include preferred brand name drugs, ones for which there is no generic equivalent. Patients would have a slightly higher copayment for these drugs. Tier 3 may include brand name drugs that have generic equivalents or similar brand name drugs at a lower cost. Patients would have the highest out-of-pocket expense for these drugs, perhaps as high as 50% coinsurance. There may be some drugs that are not on the formulary at all. Patients need to present evidence of medical necessity in order to receive coverage for non-formulary drugs. Medical assistants can advocate for patients if their plan will not cover a specific drug the provider

prescribed. They can help identify potentially similar medications from the formulary or from a lower tier of the formulary that the provider could evaluate and consider prescribing for the patient. This could create a financial savings to the patient while maintaining safe and high-quality care.

Most drug plans are administered separately from the main insurance plan. Patients usually have a separate deductible and different copayments or coinsurance amounts than their core health insurance plan. This can be confusing to patients who think they have met the medical deductible, only to find out they owe a drug deductible as well.

Some drug plans provide a mail order option for maintenance medications, which are medications patients take on a long-term basis to treat a chronic condition such as high cholesterol, arthritis, or heart conditions. The mail order plan may allow patients to order three months of medication for two copayments. This saves the patient four copayments per year for each medication ordered in this manner. In order to fill prescriptions in this manner, the mail order pharmacy will require that the prescription be written to dispense 90 days of medication at a time, with three refills for the remainder of the year. Medical assistants may need to make the prescriber aware of this requirement so the script can be written in the appropriate format.

Vision

Vision benefits include examinations and corrective hardware. Usually patients can receive these services from an ophthalmologist or a licensed optometrist (D.O.). An ophthalmologist is a medical doctor who specializes in examining, diagnosing, and treating eyes and eye diseases. An optometrist is an eye care professional who is a PCP for most vision and ocular healthcare concerns.

Examinations may be allowed annually or bi-annually. Contact lens wearers have a vision examination followed by a contact lens fitting/examination. If contact lenses are not medically necessary, the cost of the contact lens exam may not be covered.

Corrective hardware includes lenses, frames, and contact lenses. Hardware usually has a maximum dollar amount approved annually. Contact lenses needed after cataract surgery are usually covered under the patient's medical benefit, not the vision benefit.

Dental

Dental services are provided by a licensed dentist (D.D.S or D.M.D.) or denturist, as well as a registered hygienist operating under a licensed dentist. Benefits may include diagnostic/preventive, basic, major, and orthodontia. Diagnostic/preventive services typically include examinations, cleaning, X-rays, space maintainers, and fluoride treatments. Basic may include amalgam fillings, simple and surgical extractions, endodontics, root canal, and treatment of periodontal disease. Major service covers crown, bridges, partials, and dentures. Orthodontia includes initial banding fees as well as monthly maintenance fees. Certain high-cost services such as dentures and orthodontia may require a significant waiting period before being eligible for

Tier 1
Penicillin G Sodium
Penicillin V Potassium
Trimox

Tier 2
Avelox (Tablet)
Timentin

Tier 3
Avelox (Solution)
Penicillin G Procaine
Piperacillin Sodium
Zosyn

Figure 16-8 ◆ Sample tiered drug formulary for antibiotics.

coverage. Dental services directly related to medical conditions can often be billed to medical rather than dental insurance. An example of this would be tooth decay as a result of radiation therapy for a bone tumor in the jaw.

Alternative Care

Alternative care, also called complementary care, includes services such as chiropractic, massage therapy, and acupuncture. A chiropractor (D.C.) diagnoses and treats back problems by manually manipulating the bones in the spine to ease pain and restore mobility. "Chiropractors are . . . also trained to recommend therapeutic and rehabilitative exercises, as well as to provide nutritional, dietary, and lifestyle counseling. Chiropractic care is used most often to treat neuromusculoskeletal complaints, including but not limited to back pain, neck pain, pain in the joints of the arms or legs, and headaches" (American Chiropractic Association). Depending on the state and the insurance company, chiropractic coverage may or may not require a referral from a medical doctor.

Massage therapy is "a profession in which the practitioner applies manual techniques, and may apply adjunctive therapies, with the intention of positively affecting the health and well-being of the client" (American Massage Therapy Association). Massage therapy improves functioning of the circulatory, lymphatic, muscular, skeletal, and nervous systems and may improve the rate at which the body recovers from injury and illness. It is often used in treating musculoskeletal conditions and injuries. Training and licensing requirements for massage therapists vary from state to state. Insurance coverage for services of a massage therapist usually requires a prescription from a chiropractor or medical doctor.

Acupuncture is part of traditional Chinese medicine. Acupuncture is the stimulation of specific points on the body by a variety of techniques, including the insertion of thin metal needles though the skin. It aims to restore and maintain health through the stimulation of specific points on the body. The service is provided by a licensed acupuncturist (L.Ac.).

Some plans require a referral or authorization from the PCP in order for a patient to receive benefits for alternative care services. Medical assistants may need to facilitate such requests for referrals. Other plans will allow the patient to self-refer, meaning the patient receives these services without a referral or authorization. Typically, chiropractic, massage therapy, and acupuncture visits are limited in terms of how often the patient may receive them and the number of visits in a year. Anything above this cap may need a PCP referral or may not be covered at all. It is important for medical assistants to help patients understand how their policies are structured in this area.

Government Insurance

The United States government provides health insurance through a number of different programs for designated groups of people, such as the elderly, disabled, military personnel and retirees, and injured workers. Each of these programs has its own eligibility requirements and benefit structure. An overview of these programs follows.

Medicare Coverage

Medicare established in 1965, is a federal program that provides health insurance for approximately 43 million Americans, including people aged 65 and older, patients who have been disabled for more than 24 months, and patients with end-stage renal disease (ERSD).

The program is administered by the Centers for Medicare and Medicaid Services (**CMS**) formerly known as the Health Care Financing Administration (**HCFA**). CMS contracts with private companies called Medicare Administrative Contractors (**MAC**) to educate and work with providers, process claims, and other functions. (Prior to 2008, the administrators for Part A were called carriers and the administrators for Part B were called carriers.)

One of CMS's obligations is to keep providers informed about proper Medicare billing. To this end, there is vast array of information available to providers free of charge on the CMS Web site, www.cms.gov. A section called MedLearn provides free online training on many Medicare topics, free newsletters, articles, and other informative products.

The MACs also disseminate free billing information relevant to that particular region. Providers can sign up for e-mail alerts and announcements from the MAC to be sure they remain up to date. The MACs for each region are listed on the CMS Web site. Medical assistants involved in Medicare billing should learn how to access and use this vital information. Just as in many other areas of law, ignorance of Medicare rules is not an acceptable response.

Medicare claims should be submitted within 365 days of date of service. Those submitted later than this will be subject to a 10% penalty, unless the provider can prove that late submission was due to factors beyond their control, such as obtaining information from the MAC. The final submission deadline for claims to be considered at all is determined by a unique timetable based on the Medicare fiscal year. To simplify, services provided from January 1 through September 30 should be billed by the end of the next calendar year. Services provided between October 1 and December 31 have until the end of two calendar years to be billed. Figure 16-9 ◆ illustrates the schedule.

This means that providers have 13 to 27 months to bill for services, depending on the date the service was provided. This is longer than many private carriers allow and longer than many providers think they have. Medical assistants should not assume that a Medicare bill more than a year old is too old to submit, even though it will usually be penalized 10%. The MA should keep a chart like that in Figure 16-9 handy for quick reference to determine what deadlines exist.

The Medicare program has major component parts called Part A (hospital insurance), Part B (provider coverage), Part C (Medicare Advantage), and Part D (prescription drug).

The National Provider Identifier (NPI)

A national provider identifier (**NPI**), a unique, ten-digit number assigned to health care providers by the CMS, replaces the unique provider identification number (**UPIN**) CMS formerly assigned. NPI use was mandated as part of HIPAA administrative simplifications language. As of May 2007, all health care providers must use NPIs on patient billing forms.

Service provided (date)	Should be billed by (date)
10/1/07–9/30/08	12/31/09
10/1/08–9/30/09	12/31/10
10/1/09–9/30/10	12/31/11
10/1/10–9/30/11	12/31/12

Figure 16-9 ◆ Medicare submission deadlines.

NPI numbers must be used by all covered entities. A covered entity is any provider who submits claims to Medicare. Specialists who receive referrals from other physicians must place not only their own NPI number on the CMS-1500 claim form, they must also include the referring physician's name and NPI number. Not only does each individual provider have an NPI, but the facility or medical group that bills for individual providers will have a facility or group NPI. Both the rendering provider NPI and group NPI will be entered on the CMS-1500 in specific locations.

All members receive Medicare identification cards that list their names, identification numbers, plans (Part A, Part B, or both), and effective dates (Figure 16-10 ◆).

Medicare Part A

Part A Medicare coverage is hospital insurance that covers most care for patients who have been hospitalized (for up to 90 days in a given period of time), patients in **skilled nursing facilities** (facilities for long-term care or other care facilities where patients must be monitored by nursing staff regularly) for given periods, patients who receive medical care at home, patients with life-limiting illnesses requiring **hospice** care (comfort care provided to patients who have 6 or fewer months to live), patients who require psychiatric treatment for given periods, and patients who require **respite** care (care provided in a skilled nursing facility on a short-term basis for patients normally treated at home). Citizens who receive Social Security benefits are automatically enrolled in Medicare Part A benefits with no premiums. There are deductibles and coinsurance for most services in Part A.

Medicare Part B

Part B Medicare coverage covers such services as physician care, therapy, and laboratory testing. Because Part B is voluntary, members must pay income-based premiums to enroll, which is a requirement as of January 1, 2007. In 2008, the standard

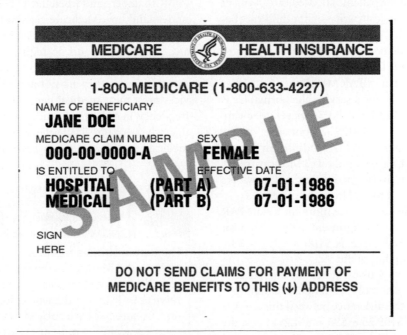

Figure 16-10 ◆ A Medicare ID card.

monthly premium was $96.40 though this premium fluctuates depending upon the Medicare recipient's income level. Patients also have out-of-pocket expenses under Part B. There is an annual deductible ($128 in 2008) which increases each year and 20% coinsurance on most services.

Physicians must choose if they will participate with Medicare. A participating provider, also called PAR, must accept the Medicare fee schedule (MFS) amounts as payment in full for their services. If the MFS is higher than the physician's normal fee for a service, the normal fee is the maximum amount that can be billed. They need to bill Medicare for all services, even those known to not be covered by Medicare. They also **accept assignment** on all claims, which means they accept the MFS amounts and the payment is sent to the provider. Approximately 95% of all physicians are PAR.

For example, consider an office visit with a physician charge of $118 and an assumed rate of $100 on the MFS. The PAR physician receives $100 × 80% = $80 from Medicare and must collect $100 × 20% = $20 coinsurance from the patient. The Medicare payment is sent to the physician. The physician writes off the difference between the MFS and the normal charge: $118 − $100 = $18.

Nonparticipating physicians (non-PAR) also need to bill Medicare for all services, including those not covered. However, they can decide to accept assignment on a case-by-case basis. If they accept assignment, they agree to accept the non-PAR MFS as payment in full. The non-PAR MFS is 5% less than the PAR MFS, so non-PAR physicians are paid less than PAR physicians on assigned claims. Medicare sends the payment to the non-PAR physician on assigned claims. Approximately 5% of all providers are non-PAR.

For example, consider the example above for a non-PAR physician who accepts assignment. The office visit charge is $118. The non-PAR MFS is $100 × 95% = $95. The non-PAR physician receives $95 × 80% = $76 from Medicare and must collect $95 × 20% = $19 coinsurance from the patient. The Medicare payment is sent to the physician. The physician writes off the difference between the MFS and the normal charge: $118 − $95 = $23.

If non-PAR providers do not accept assignment, they must accept the **limiting charge (LC)** as payment in full. The LC amount is 15% higher than the non-PAR MFS. If the LC is higher than the physician's normal fee for a service, the normal fee is the maximum amount that can be billed. However, Medicare will reimburse 80% of the non-PAR MFS amount only. Patients pay 20% coinsurance of the non-PAR MFS and also pay the additional 15% difference that makes up the LC. Medicare sends payment to the patient on non-assigned claims and providers must collect the full amount of the LC from the patient.

Consider the example above once more for a non-PAR physician who does not accept assignment. The office visit charge is $118. The non-PAR MFS is $100 × 95% = $95. Medicare sends its portion to the patient $95 × 80% = $76. The patient has out-of-pocket responsibility for the coinsurance $95 × 20% = $19. The LC is $95 × 115% = $109.25, and the patient is also responsible for the difference between this and the Medicare approved charge $109.25 − $95 = $14.25. Thus, the patient's total responsibility is $19 + $14.25 = $33.25. The total amount of $109.25 must be collected from the patient. The physician writes off the difference between the LC and the normal charge $118 − $109.25 = $8.75.

On nonassigned claims, non-PAR physicians can be paid at higher rates than PAR physicians, but the higher amount is the responsibility of the patient, not Medicare. In addition, the provider must devote more time and effort to collections because the entire amount must be obtained from the patient.

Physicians, dentists, podiatrists, and selected non-physician providers may also choose to opt out of Medicare completely and enter into private contracts with patients. They do not bill Medicare for any services and collect their entire fee from the patient. There is no limit on what physicians can charge. Patients bill Medicare themselves and receive reimbursement. Physicians who opt out must opt out for all patients and cannot re-enroll for two years. Less than 1% of providers choose to opt out. Some non-physician providers such as chiropractors cannot opt out and are required to bill Medicare for all patients.

One very important aspect to billing Medicare is a form called the **Advance Beneficiary Notice (ABN)** or **waiver** (Figure 16-11 ◆). The ABN must be signed by patients before receiving covered services that may be denied payment by Medicare. If during the encounter, physicians recommend services that may be denied, patients need to be informed and given the opportunity to accept or decline the service, knowing they will be obligated to pay if Medicare does deny it. If patients do not understand that Medicare could deny the service, they are not obligated to pay for and cannot be billed for it. Medical assistants are vital to facilitating this because they are the link between the medical care and the billing rules. Medical assistants need to review the ABN with the patient and obtain a signature before the service is provided. The ABN notifies patients that the service may not be paid by Medicare and patients agree to be responsible for payment. Medicare does not allow the ABN to be completed after the service is provided.

To understand when the ABN is needed, it is important to understand how Medicare classifies its services. **Non-covered** services are those that are not eligible for reimbursement under any circumstance and do require an ABN to be completed. **Covered** services are those potentially eligible for reimbursement; however, they are not automatically paid. Covered services must meet **medical necessity** and other criteria, such as frequency, in order to be paid. Medical necessity refers to more than whether a physician believes the service is needed. Medicare medical necessity means services or supplies that are proper and

Keys to Success
EXPLAINING MEDICARE COVERAGE

The administrative medical assistant should clearly explain to the Medicare-covered patient any services and costs that may not be paid by Medicare. Medicare requires services be listed on the waiver form that the patient must sign. Be sure to give a copy of the form to the patient, and keep a copy in the patient's permanent file.

(A) Notifier(s):
(B) Patient Name: _____   **(C)** Identification Number: _____

ADVANCE BENEFICIARY NOTICE OF NONCOVERAGE (ABN)

NOTE: If Medicare doesn't pay for **(D)**_____ below, you may have to pay.

Medicare does not pay for everything, even some care that you or your health care provider have good reason to think you need. We expect Medicare may not pay for the **(D)**_____ below.

(D)_____	**(E) Reason Medicare May Not Pay:**	**(F) Estimated Cost:**

WHAT YOU NEED TO DO NOW:

- Read this notice, so you can make an informed decision about your care.
- Ask us any questions that you may have after you finish reading.
- Choose an option below about whether to receive the **(D)**_____ listed above.
  Note: If you choose Option 1 or 2, we may help you to use any other insurance that you might have, but Medicare cannot require us to do this.

(G) OPTIONS: **Check only one box. We cannot choose a box for you.**

❏ **OPTION 1.** I want the **(D)**_____ listed above. You may ask to be paid now, but I also want Medicare billed for an official decision on payment, which is sent to me on a Medicare Summary Notice (MSN). I understand that if Medicare doesn't pay, I am responsible for payment, but **I can appeal to Medicare** by following the directions on the MSN. If Medicare does pay, you will refund any payments I made to you, less co-pays or deductibles.

❏ **OPTION 2.** I want the **(D)**_____ listed above, but do not bill Medicare. You may ask to be paid now as I am responsible for payment. **I cannot appeal if Medicare is not billed**.

❏ **OPTION 3.** I don't want the **(D)**_____ listed above. I understand with this choice I am **not** responsible for payment, and **I cannot appeal to see if Medicare would pay**.

(H) Additional Information:

This notice gives our opinion, not an official Medicare decision. If you have other questions on this notice or Medicare billing, call **1-800-MEDICARE** (1-800-633-4227/**TTY**: 1-877-486-2048).

Signing below means that you have received and understand this notice. You also receive a copy.

(I) Signature:	**(J)** Date:

Form CMS-R-131 (03/08)   Form Approved OMB No. 0938-0566

Figure 16-11 ◆ Advance Beneficiary Notice Form (ABN).

needed for the diagnosis or treatment of the patient's medical condition are provided for the diagnosis, direct care, and treatment of the medical condition, meet the standards of good medical practice in the local area, and are not mainly for the convenience of the patient or provider. If they do not meet these criteria, services may be denied. It is providers' responsibility to become familiar with what covered services may be denied under what circumstances, based on their specialty. Medicare does not allow blanket ABNs, which is the practice of having all Medicare patients sign ABNs for any service provided. The ABN must be specific to the patient's particular circumstance.

For example, Medicare limits how often B-12 injections are given, depending on the diagnosis. In a particular situation the physician may recommend more than the stipulated number of injections, believing the patient will receive the most benefit. The medical assistant would ask the patient to sign the ABN and agree to pay for the additional injection if Medicare denies payment.

Medicare has very specific rules about what services can be billed together. For example, Medicare will not pay for an office visit and an injection on the same day, unless the office visit was clearly a distinct service, such as a physical examination. Many surgical procedures are **bundled**, meaning that multiple procedures are covered with one charge. For example, a surgeon who performs an abdominal hysterectomy with oopherectomy and salpingectomy must bill one charge only, which includes all three procedures. To bill this as three separate services would be called **unbundling**, which is considered fraud. This will be discussed further in ∞ Chapter 19, Procedural Coding.

Medicare Part C: Advantage Plan

Medicare Part C is managed care, known as Medicare Advantage plans. Formerly known as Medicare + Choice, these plans are offered by private insurance companies and replace Parts A, B, and D. The benefit to the patient is potentially more comprehensive care at the same or lower cost than Medicare. The disadvantage, as with any managed care plan, is that the choice of providers is limited. Patients keep their Medicare identification card and receive an additional card from the Advantage plan. Because patients may not understand the difference between the two cards, it is a good practice for medical assistants to ask patients if they belong to an Advantage plan or have another identification card. When billing, the Medicare Advantage plan is billed, not Medicare. When patients have secondary coverage, medical assistants bill the secondary plans after the Medicare Advantage plan has made a payment or decision.

Medicare Part D

As of January 2006, the newest Medicare coverage plan is Part D, the prescription drug plan. Members covered by Medicare may opt to purchase Part D coverage, which covers both name-brand and generic prescription drugs at participating pharmacies. The Part D plans are provided by private companies. Not all drugs are covered under every plan, so patients need to determine which plans cover their most common or most ex-

pensive medications. Medical assistants can assist patients by providing them with complete medication lists. The Medicare Web site for patients, www.medicare.gov, has a prescription drug plan finder tool to assist patients to evaluate their options. Medicare Part D has an annual deductible, copayments or coinsurance, and a maximum benefit level, and a stop loss for patients who have out-of-pocket costs over a certain level. The deductible and stop loss levels are updated annually.

Medicare Part D enrollees have several mail-in pharmacy options from companies that typically offer low out-of-pocket expenses. Enrollees should view this option cautiously, however. It may be less than ideal for patients on short-term medications, like antibiotics, because delivery may take a week or more.

Medigap Plans

Medigap or Medicare Supplemental Plans are insurance plans offered by private companies to reimburse patients for the out-of-pocket expenses they incur with Medicare. CMS regulates what benefits can be offered by these plans and which companies can offer them. Not all Medigap plans cover the same expenses. The basic benefit is coverage of patients' coinsurance, but some also offer coverage of deductibles for Parts A and B, skilled nursing facility coinsurance, foreign travel, and other specific expenses. Medigap is billed after Medicare has determined its portion of the payment. Most Medigap plans have an agreement with CMS so that the MACs will electronically send the claims information to the Medigap carrier, relieving the provider of the need to directly bill the Medigap policy. Medical assistants should ask patients if they have a Medigap policy so that information can be included on the billing to Medicare.

Medicare and Other Health Insurance (OHI)

Patients may have other health insurance (OHI) in addition to Medicare. CMS requires providers to be very vigilant in determining when Medicare is obligated to pay first and when they are the secondary payer. These are known as Medicare Secondary Payer (MSP) rules. When Medicare is the secondary payer they pay a lower portion of the bill than when they are primary. Medicare provides a detailed questionnaire on the CMS Web site that medical assistants should review with patients to determine MSP. In general, Medicare is primary to Medicaid and secondary to most other insurance, including workers' compensation, liability, TRICARE, or when covered by a spouse's group health policy. Medicare is usually secondary when patients over age 65 are still working and covered by an employer's group heath plan. There are exceptions to this, which the MSP questionnaire will aid in determining.

Providers Participating in Medicare

Medicare must accredit any health care providers who wish to participate in its program in a process very similar to the application process of any managed care plan. Because most health insurance plans follow Medicare's lead when it comes to accreditation and fee schedules, it is crucial for medical assistants or office managers to stay up to date by consulting Medicare's published guidelines or Web site.

As of July 2005, Medicare requires all medical offices to file medical claims electronically, or via **e-billing**. Some clinics may be allowed to continue to bill claims on paper. Those clinics must have no more than 10 full time employees, or the equivalent of 10 full-time employees, such as 20 part-time employees whose combined working hours total that of 10 full-time employees.

Medicare prefers to use electronic funds transfer for payment to physicians and medical facilities. This is set up by filling out an Authorization Agreement for Electronic Funds Transfer form. This form is returned to Medicare along with a copy of a voided check or deposit ticket. After receipt of this information, Medicare will begin directly depositing funds into the physician or facility's account within 3 weeks.

Medicare maintains a provider directory of participating providers nationwide. A search for a provider can be performed by state or specialty. This list contains the provider's name, specialty, education, residency, gender, foreign languages spoken by the physician, hospital affiliation, and practice location.

Medicare provides a variety of in-person as well as online workshops for providers to learn more about topics such as payment notices and reimbursements, the appeals process, using the Medicare Web site, and updates on changes that apply to physicians or medical facilities.

Medicaid

Medicaid coverage is a health benefit program for low-income patients. Like Medicare, Medicaid is run by **CMS,** although each state dictates the amount and type of services Medicaid covers. The federal government provides funds to every state, and every state adds its own funds to cover qualified enrollees. As of 2001, the last year for which Medicaid has compiled extensive data, more than 46 million persons received healthcare services through the Medicaid program. Because every state runs its own Medicaid program, identification cards or coupons differ (Figure 16-12 ◆).

Because Medicaid reimbursement is extremely low in most states, most health care providers cannot afford to treat a large number of Medicaid patients. The low reimbursement rate has caused many health care providers to stop accepting Medicaid patients altogether, or to stringently limit the number of patients. As a result, Medicaid-covered patients may wait longer for care or travel to find accepting providers.

If they wish to accept Medicaid patients, health care providers must apply to become Medicaid accredited in their state. As part of this process, which is very similar to any other managed care application process, Medicaid provides physicians fee schedules of covered expenses.

Medicaid programs offer coverage on a month-to-month basis in most states, which means that Medicaid may not cover a patient one month just because Medicaid covered the patient in a previous month. It is vital for medical assistants to know the Medicaid rules and regulations in their state as those rules and regulations apply to their practice types and to ask Medicaid patients for proof of coverage in the plan.

Low-income elderly or disabled patients often have both Medicare and Medicaid coverage. Medicare is always primary in these cases, and Medicaid is secondary. Often, Medicare's reimbursement rate is higher than what Medicaid will allow, resulting in no Medicaid payment. The CMS estimates that there are approximately 6.5 million persons receiving benefits from both Medicare and Medicaid. When physicians **accept assignment** from both Medicare and Medicaid, or participate in both programs, those physicians must accept what the two agencies together pay as payment in full for covered services. In these cases, billing patients for any portion of covered services is illegal. To do so can result in fines and/or removal from the Medicare and/or Medicaid programs as a participating provider.

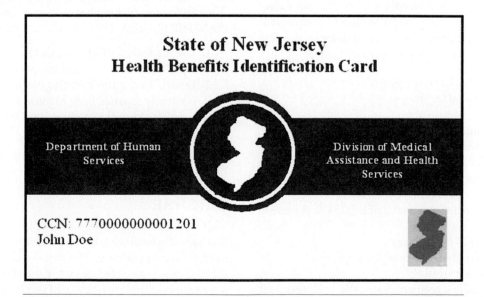

Figure 16-12 ◆ Medicaid coupon from New Jersey.

It is important to note that Medicaid coverage is not simply based upon a person's income level. An individual may be considered low income yet not qualify for Medicaid benefits within their state. Medicaid coverage is based upon a list of qualifications, including the person's age, whether the patient is pregnant, disabled, or blind, whether or not the person is a U.S. citizen or a lawfully admitted immigrant, as well as income level. Medicaid also includes special rules for persons who live in nursing homes or disabled children who live at home.

Medicaid eligible patients may qualify under different sets of criteria for different programs. One major distinction is between the **categorically needy (CN)** and **medically needy (MN)**. CN patients qualify for cash assistance as well as medical services. MN patients generally have a higher income than CN patients and are eligible for medical services but not cash assistance. In addition, they may be eligible for fewer medical services than CN patients. Medical assistants need to verify which specific services and programs covered patients are eligible for. For example, some patients will be eligible for certain children's programs that cover a subset of specific services.

Medicaid is always the "payer of last resort," meaning that all other insurances should be billed before Medicaid. If the payment from the other insurance is higher than Medicaid's approved rate, Medicaid will pay nothing.

Medicaid has introduced cost-sharing in recent years which means that some patients may be responsible for copayments, deductibles, or premiums based on income level, family size, and other factors. If working for Medicaid providers, medical assistants should become familiar with their state's Medicaid identification card and eligibility verification system, as these tools provide much information about patients' coverage, eligibility, and financial responsibility.

Covered Medicaid Services

Though each state determines who will be covered by Medicaid, what type of services will be covered, and the reimbursement provided for the covered services, the federal government requires certain basic services be provided in order for the state to qualify for federal funding. These services include:

- Inpatient hospital services
- Outpatient hospital services
- Prenatal care
- Vaccines for children
- Physician services
- Nursing facility services for persons aged 21 or older
- Family planning services and supplies
- Rural health clinic services
- Home health care for persons eligible for skilled-nursing services
- Laboratory and X-ray services
- Pediatric and family nurse practitioner services
- Nurse-midwife services
- Early and periodic screening, diagnostic, and treatment services for children under age 21

The federal government also lists certain optional services for which states will receive matching funds for providing. These include:

- Diagnostic services
- Clinic services
- Intermediate care facilities for the mentally retarded
- Prescribed drugs and prosthetic devices
- Optometrist services and eyeglasses
- Nursing facility services for children under age 21
- Transportation services
- Rehabilitation and physical therapy services
- Home and community-based care to certain persons with chronic impairments

Along with the Medicaid program, the federal government also reimburses states for 100 percent of all costs associated with providing health care in facilities of the Indian Health Service. This program is responsible for providing health services to native Americans and Alaskan natives. The federal government also provides financial assistance to the 12 states that provide the highest number of emergency services to undocumented aliens.

State Children's Health Insurance Program (SCHIP)

In 1997, as part of the Balanced Budget Act, Congress created the State Children's Health Insurance Program (**SCHIP**). This program was created to cover children who did not have another form of health insurance coverage. Similar to basic Medicaid, SCHIP was designed to function as a federal/state joint program. Children within families who earned too much income to qualify for Medicaid, but not enough income to purchase other health insurance, are to be covered by the SCHIP program.

Beginning in October 1997, the federal government provided $24 billion in funds over 5 years to help states expand healthcare coverage to the estimated 5 million uninsured children who fall into the category targeted by SCHIP. There are three options states can choose from in order to comply with the SCHIP program. These choices are the following:

1. Use the federal SCHIP funds to expand Medicaid eligibility to children who did not previously qualify
2. Design a separate children's health insurance fund that is entirely separate from Medicaid
3. Combine both the Medicaid and the separate children's health insurance fund

Every state had an approved SCHIP program in place by October 1999.

TRICARE

TRICARE, formerly called CHAMPUS, is a federal program that provides healthcare benefits to families of current and retired military personnel. The active duty service member is called a *sponsor* and eligible family members are called *beneficiaries*. To be eligible for TRICARE, sponsors and beneficiaries must be enrolled in the Defense Enrollment Eligibility Reporting System (**DEERS**). TRICARE offers three benefit types: (1) TRICARE Standard, a fee-for-service plan; (2) TRICARE Extra, a PPO; and (3) TRICARE Prime, an HMO. Active duty families on TRICARE Standard and TRICARE Extra and most retirees will usually owe copayments and deductibles. Medical assistants should be alert to the fact that TRICARE's deductible year begins October 1, not January 1 as is common with many insurance plans. All TRICARE enrollees are automatically enrolled in TRICARE Standard and TRICARE Extra. TRICARE Prime is an optional plan which enrollees must specifically enroll in. Some patients have TRICARE for Life, a plan that acts as secondary insurance coverage for patients over age 65. For primary insurance, these patients have Medicare. TRICARE requires preauthorization for medical services, and patients must use in-network providers.

TRICARE requires participating providers to submit claims within 60 days of the date care was provided. Non-network providers have up to one year from the date the care was provided to submit claims.

CHAMPVA

The Civilian Health and Medical Program of the Veterans Administration (**CHAMPVA**) is a federal program that covers the health care expenses of the families of veterans with total, permanent, service-related, covered disabilities and the spouses and dependent children of veterans who died in the line of duty. Patients with CHAMPVA coverage may use any civilian health care provider, without preauthorization.

If a patient has other coverage besides CHAMPVA, the other coverage should be billed first. By law, CHAMPVA is always the secondary payer, except to Medicaid, State Victims of Crime Compensation, and supplemental CHAMPVA policies. Once the primary insurance carrier has made payment, a CMS-1500 claim form is sent to CHAMPVA along with a copy of the primary carrier's explanation of benefits.

CHAMPVA requires pre-authorization in the following areas only:

- Organ and bone marrow transplants
- Hospice care
- Dental care
- Durable medical equipment (**DME**) worth more than $300
- Most mental health or substance abuse services

Worker's Compensation Insurance

Worker's compensation insurance covers employees injured in the workplace or suffering from a workplace-related illness. Occupational injuries are those that occur during the course of employment, but do not have to be on company property or while performing work duties. Accidents that occur off-site, such as while driving on company business, at a remote work site, or during a paid break are covered. Occupational illnesses are conditions that arise from short- or long-term exposure to

a workplace hazard or condition, such as dust, chemical allergens, radiation, repetitive motion, and loud noises. The challenge with occupational illnesses is identifying, diagnosing and reporting them, as some such as repetitive stress injuries (RSI), hearing loss, and various respiratory disorders may take years to manifest themselves.

All employers must offer workers' compensation insurance, although laws vary from state to state. Insurance may be obtained from a state-managed fund, private insurers, or employer self-insurance. Some states do not allow private insurers to offer workers' compensation policies, so coverage must be obtained from the state or through self-insurance. Federal laws cover workers in Washington, D.C, coal miners, federal employees, and maritime workers.

A workers' compensation claim is initiated by filing the First Report of Illness or Injury. State laws vary widely on the time frame required for filing and the responsible party. In some states, the employer may be required to file this report and in other states the first provider who treats the injured worker is responsible. Medical assistants need to be familiar with how the filing process works in their state.

Benefits to the injured worker include coverage of the cost of medical care related to the illness or injury, wages for time lost from work due to illness or injury, death benefits for survivors when the accident is the cause of the worker's death, and rehabilitation or retraining benefits that enable the worker to return to work or learn a different line of work if necessary.

A non-disability (ND) claim means the worker was injured and treated by a physician, but no time was lost from work. In a ND claim, no lost wages are paid. Temporary disability (TD) means that the worker is able to return to previous or modified work at a later time. Permanent disability (PD) means that no further improvement is expected and the worker is unable to return to work.

Healthcare providers must enroll with their states' worker's compensation programs before accepting worker's compensation cases. Providers receive identification numbers for billing purposes. Worker's compensation programs reimburse physicians based on an established schedule. If physician charges are higher than the reimbursement amount, patients cannot be balance billed. In some states, worker's compensation operates under a managed care model.

To ensure the program runs properly, healthcare providers must keep good records on worker's compensation cases. This includes verifying patients' injuries with employers and contacting insurance companies to obtain claim numbers and verify the date of injury on file. Medical assistants must know their state laws for worker's compensation coverage should patients need preauthorization before care.

Patients in worker's compensation cases should have new files created so the medical office can separate that documentation from patients' other records, and thereby keep reporting and claim filing accurate. Most states' labor departments provide free physician reporting forms and claim information for injured workers.

HIPAA Compliance

Medical providers often receive requests for copies of medical records for patients who have been injured on the job or elsewhere. To practice within HIPAA guidelines for information release, be sure to look closely to determine the exact information being requested. For example, a requesting agency may ask for medical records pertaining to injury care only. A separate file for injury claims makes it easier to determine the information that is to be copied and sent. Also, be sure you have a signed release from the patient or a court order before releasing any information to a third party.

Disability Insurance

Disability insurance reimburses a patient for lost wages due to a non–work-related disability that prevents the individual from working. Benefits are based on a percentage of employees' wages, often 66%, because benefits are not subject to income tax. Lost wages due to a work-related disability are covered by worker's compensation insurance; lost wages due to a disability related to an automobile or other liability accident are covered by liability insurance.

With only a few exceptions, disability insurance does not pay for medical treatment; therefore, medical assistants will not often be billing a disability plan for medical services. However, medical assistants may need to assist patients who are applying for disability coverage or benefits by providing information from the medical record regarding a patient's past health history or current disability. Even though patients have disability insurance, they may not have medical coverage because they are not employed and cannot afford or are not eligible for individual health insurance policies.

Types of Disability Insurance

Disability insurance is offered by federal, state, and private sources. Federal disability policies include Social Security Disability Insurance (**SSDI**) for workers who are permanently disabled, but not from a job-related incident; and Supplemental Security Income (**SSI**) for low-income disabled persons without a qualifying work history; Veteran's Disability Compensation for veterans whose injuries or diseases are the result of active duty service; Veteran's Disability Pension Benefits for wartime veterans with limited income and who are no longer able to work; Civil Service (**CSRS**) and Federal Employees Retirement System (**FERS**) disability for federal and civil service employees who become disabled. Veterans benefits include certain medical services, which medical assistants will submit bills for and for which the insurance payment must be accepted as payment in full. Five states (California, Hawaii, New Jersey, New York, and Rhode Island) and Puerto Rico provide disability insurance. State policies tend to provide short-term coverage which begins about a week after disability and extends from six to 12 months. Private policies may be obtained through employers or purchased individually. Usually a waiting period after the disability begins is required before benefits are paid. A

longer waiting period will result in a lower premium. An employer-sponsored policy will be terminated when employment ends. The advantage of an individual policy is that employees keep it when changing employers, and it can be renewed without regard to health status.

Definition of Disability

No standard definition of a disability exists; rather, the conditions of a disability are defined by each individual plan. The Social Security definition of a disability is the strictest and own-occupation disability offered by some private companies is the most liberal. Under the Social Security definition, patients are considered disabled if they cannot do work that they did before, they cannot adjust to other work because of their medical condition(s), and their disability has lasted or is expected to last for at least one year or to result in death. Social security pays no benefits for temporary or partial disability. This definition applies to both SSI and SSDI.

Own-occupation disability means that, because of sickness or injury, patients are not able to perform the substantial duties of their occupation which they were performing at the time of disability. Patients may be considered totally disabled even if they are at work in some other capacity so long as they are not able to work in their occupation. Of course, a private own-occupation disability policy will be more expensive to purchase than one with a more strict definition, similar to the one used by Social Security. Patients may be tempted to purchase the least expensive policy only to be disappointed when they find the definition of disability is so strict that it is difficult to meet eligibility requirements.

SSDI and SSI

To establish disability under SSDI or SSI, individuals complete the required forms, usually with the help of a social worker, and go through a determination process. Patients' personal physicians do not make a determination regarding whether a patient is disabled or not; this is determined by the insurance plan based on medical information in the patient's record. An appeals process is also available for patients who disagree with the determination of disability.

To be eligible for SSDI, workers must meet Social Security eligibility standards in terms of number of quarters worked and the amount of wages earned per quarter. Eligible workers include disabled workers under the age of 65 and their families; individuals who become disabled before age 22 if a parent who is covered under Social Security retires, becomes disabled, or dies; certain disabled widows, widowers, or divorced spouses; and blind workers meeting specific vision criteria. After 24 months of disability payments, disabled individuals become eligible for Medicare, which will cover many of the medical expenses.

SSI was created for disabled individuals with low incomes not meeting the work and wage criteria for SSDI. Eligible persons include disabled individuals under the age of 65 with very limited income and resources; disabled children under the age of 18; and blind adults and children meeting specific vision criteria. Many SSI recipients also qualify for Medicaid and as such, some of their medical expenses may be covered.

The Medical Assistant's Role with Disability Insurance

Medical assistants should be familiar with the various ways physicians may be involved with the disability determination process, for both government and private insurers. Physicians may be treating disability applicants and need to provide medical records or testimony regarding patients' functioning. Information provided may include facts such as the date the disability occurred, a description of how the disability occurred, description of how the disability prevents the patient from working, examination and test results that document the extent of disability, and the level and timeframe of expected recovery. The wording of information provided by physicians can affect the determination, based on the disability definition being used by the insurer. Physicians may also work as paid consultative examiners who provide an outside medical or psychological examination of applicants. In this case, patients who are disability applicants and not part of the physician's established patient base may come to the office. Physicians also may be paid medical review officers who review claims from a medical perspective for the insurer. Part of the physician's regular schedule may be set aside for this activity.

Reimbursement Methods

Insurance companies reimburse providers using a variety of methods, so it is important for medical assistants to understand how this impacts the practice. The most traditional reimbursement method is a usual, customary, and reasonable (UCR) fee schedule maintained by each insurance company. The insurer establishes an acceptable "customary" fee based on the range of what other providers of the same specialty in the same geographic area charge. The insurer will pay either this amount or the provider's normal fee ("usual"), whichever is less. In unusual circumstances, they will negotiate a specific "reasonable" for a given bill. The insurer is not required to publicize what their UCR fees are, but the practice learns by experience the amount each company approves.

A common reimbursement method in managed care is a **negotiated fee schedule**. The MCO develops of list of fees for providers that they agree to accept in the participating provider contract. Fees may be determined based on a percentage of the provider's usual fee (for example, 80%) or may be arrived at through negotiation.

Capitation is most often used by HMOs. *Capitation* means *per head*. Under a capitation plan, the insurer pays providers a flat amount per member per month, regardless of what services the patient uses. If they come in many times, or not at all, the provider receives the same payment. The objective of capitation is to put the responsibility and risk on the provider to manage the patient's care in a cost effective yet medically appropriate manner.

For inpatient care a **per diem** or *per day* payment method may be used. The facility is paid a flat amount per day the patient remains, regardless of what services are provided. This method places much cost management on the facility to provide the services that are medically appropriate because they will not be paid more for unnecessary services. The risk is partially shared with the insurer, who pays more for a longer stay than a shorter one. However, there may be a maximum number days that will be paid for any given condition.

Per case payment is also used for hospitals. Under this method, the hospital receives a pre-established amount per patient for the entire stay, based on the patient's diagnosis, regardless of how long they are in or what services are provided. When Medicare uses this form of reimbursement, it is called Diagnosis Related Groups (DRG) because patients with similar conditions and care requirements are classified or grouped together and all are eligible for the same amount of reimbursement.

In capitation, per diem, and per case reimbursement methods, it is not uncommon for additional payment to be made for **outliers**, or exceptional circumstances that cost far more or far less than the average. Most contracts also include **carve outs**, services that are reimbursed in addition to the base rate for the patient. The details of each MCO contract are different; there are no general rules. The medical assistant needs to become familiar with the details of each contract the provider has to be sure the billing and payment are appropriate.

Processing Claims

The first step to properly reimbursing insurance claims is obtaining accurate information. Many medical offices ask patients for their health insurance information over the phone, before their first visits. Other offices simply ask patients for their insurance type over the phone and then ask those patients to bring their insurance card to their visit.

Patient Registration

Each new patient in the medical office should complete a registration form (Figure 16-13 ◆) that is verified at each visit and updated annually. Before releasing private patient information to insurance carriers, medical assistants must obtain signed authorization from patients. To do otherwise is to violate HIPAA regulations for patient confidentiality. Insurance claim forms give patients' names, addresses, birth dates, diagnoses, and types of treatment, all highly protected patient information.

Keys to Success
MEDICAL CLAIMS FOR INJURIES

Any patient who has a medical claim for an injury, whether through workmen's compensation or other liability insurance, will have a claim number and a claims manager or department to handle the claim. At the beginning of the patient's care in the medical office, locate the name and phone number of the claims manager. Readily available contact information will allow the office easily to contact the claims manager in the event the physician orders tests or procedures that require preauthorization.

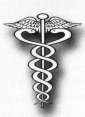

Victory Medical Center
4100 SW Highway 6
Victorville, WA 12345
(509) 555-9832

Patient Name: _____
          Last Name   First Name   Middle Initial

Address: _____
         Street   City   State   Zip

Home Phone: _____ Work Phone:_____

Mobile Phone: _____ Birthdate:_____

Social Security Number: _____ Age:_____

Sex: _____ Marital Status: S M D W Children: _____

How do you prefer to be addressed? _____

Spouse's Name:_____

Primary Care Physician: _____ Phone No:_____

Name of Person Responsible for Bill: _____

Relationship to Patient: _____ Phone No: _____

Address of Person Responsible for Bill: _____

Patient's Employer: _____ Phone No: _____

Occupation: _____

Spouse's Employer: _____ Phone No:_____

Occupation: _____

INSURANCE INFORMATION

Primary Insurance: _____ Policy No: _____

Name of Policyholder: _____ Birthdate: _____

SS#: _____ Relationship to Insured: _____

Secondary Insurance: _____ Policy No: _____

Name of Policyholder: _____ Birthdate: _____

If Injured: Date:_____ Place: _____

Claim Number: _____ Nature or Cause of Injury: _____

Employer at Time of Injury: _____ Phone No: _____

EMERGENCY INFORMATION

In case of emergency, local friend or relative to be notified (not living at same address)

Name:_____ Relationship to Patient: _____

Address: _____ Phone No: _____

I hereby authorize the healthcare professionals in this clinic to diagnose and treat my condition. I clearly understand and agree that all services rendered me are charged directly to me and that I am personally responsible for payment. I agree that I am responsible for all bills incurred at this clinic. I hereby authorize assignment of my insurance rights and benefits directly to the provider for services rendered. I also authorize the healthcare professionals to discuss my care with other health care providers who I am currently treating with.

_____   _____
Patient's Signature   Date   Parent or Guardian Signature   Date

Figure 16-13 ◆ Sample new patient registration form.

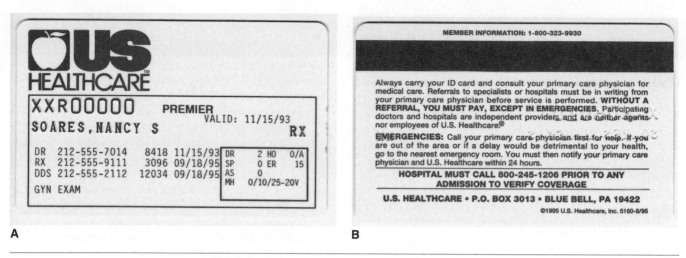

Figure 16-14 ◆ (a) The front of an insurance identification card; (b) the back of an insurance identification card.

After obtaining pertinent patient information, medical assistants must identify the name and birth date of the insured. When the patient is the spouse or child of the insured, the medical assistant must ask the patient for the additional information. The assistant will need to know if the patient is covered by more than one plan. If so, the assistant will then have to determine which plan is primary and which is secondary.

Either way, medical assistants must photocopy both sides of patients' insurance identification cards when patients arrive for their first visits. The front of cards typically carry the names and identification numbers of the insured or members. Each patient is uniquely identified by a member identification number assigned by the insurance company. Patients have a different number with each separate insurance plan they may have. HIPAA originally made provision for a unique patient identification number that would be the same for all insurance companies, but concerns about privacy and identity theft have put this on hold indefinitely.

In today's world of identify theft, most insurance plans no longer use Social Security numbers for identification. Instead, many identification numbers now have alphabetic prefixes followed by numbers. Some have alphabetic characters only. Plans may have their own group or plan numbers, as well. A **payor number,** a number that identifies an insurance company, allows medical offices to submit claims electronically. The back of the card typically has the claims mailing addresses (Figure 16-14 ◆). Insurance telephone numbers appear on the front or back of cards. Typically, one number is for "customer or member service" and another is for "providers." Medical assistants call the latter for information on patients' coverage or claims.

Verification of Benefits

After obtaining insurance information from patients, medical assistants should verify coverage with the insurance company. By doing this, medical assistants ensure they have the most current and accurate information possible. However, even verifying benefits with the insurance company is not a guarantee of payment because there may have been recent changes in the patient's status, such as adding or dropping coverage, that have not been input into the computer system at the time of verifi-

cation. The most common way to verify benefits is to make a phone call to the insurance company. Some companies have a separate phone number for verification. The process may be completely automated or may include personally speaking with a representative. Many companies also offer the option of verifying benefits online through a secure Web site. It is worthwhile to make arrangements for online verification with providers' largest insurance carriers because it is usually faster and more convenient for medical assistants.

Determining Coordination of Benefits

Patients may be covered by more than one insurance plan. Most often this is because spouses each have a group health plan and each has purchased coverage for the other. Also, both spouses may elect to cover their children under both policies. Insurance companies, in cooperation with state insurance commissioners, have established specific rules that determine which coverage is billed first, called primary, and which is billed second, called the secondary policy. This process is called **coordination of benefits (COB)**. Patients do not have the option of specifying which insurance should be primary or secondary.

When spouses or partners are covered by each other's policy, the patient's own policy is always primary for them, and the spouse's or partner's policy is secondary. Likewise, when spouses are patients, their own policy is primary. Medical assistants should not assume that spouses are covered by each other's policy because such coverage is entirely their choice, based on their insurance needs and costs associated with covering other family members. It is possible, for example, for the husband's insurance to cover himself and his wife, but the wife's insurance may cover only her. In this case, the husband would have only one insurance, his own. The wife would have two policies; hers would be primary and her husband's would be secondary.

When both parents carry coverage for the children, most health insurance plans decide which insurance plan is primary and which is secondary based on the **birthday rule** (Figure 16-15 ◆). According to this rule, the parent with the birthday earlier in the year is the primary carrier for the children; the parent with the later birthday is the secondary carrier for the children.

PROCEDURE 16-2 Verify a Patient's Insurance Eligibility

Theory and Rationale

Many patients who seek medical care are covered by some form of medical insurance. Verifying a patient's eligibility is an important part of the medical assistant's job. Verifying benefits with the insurance company ensures that the medical assistant has the most current and accurate information possible.

Materials

- Insurance identification card
- Patient's registraton form
- Telephone
- Paper
- Pen

Competency

(**Conditions**) With the necessary materials, you will be able to (**Task**) verify a patient's insurance eligibility (**Standards**) correctly within the time limit set by the instructor.

1. Looking at the patient's registration form, locate the patient's birthdate and the patient's relationship to the insured.

2. Looking at the patient's insurance identification card, locate the name of the insured, the insured's member identification number, and the telephone number of the insurance company.
3. Call the insurance company at the provider customer service telephone number listed on the insurance identification card.
4. When the customer service representative answers the call, write down the name of the customer service representative, and the date and time of the call.
5. Verify spelling of policyholder's name and birthdate.
6. Verify patient's name and birthdate.
7. Verify coverage for type of service to be rendered, including frequency or number of visits.
8. Verify when preauthorization is needed.
9. Verify patient's financial responsibility for deductible, co-payment, or coinsurance amounts.
10. Verify coordination of benefits rules if more than one policy covers the patient.
11. Verify provider's participating or non-partipating status.
12. Verify the address where insurance claims are to be mailed or the payer number needed for electronic billing.

Mary and Josiah Banks have a son, Ian. Mary has an insurance policy through Aetna U.S. Health Care that provides family coverage. Josiah has an insurance policy through Premera Blue Cross that also provides family coverage. Mary's birthday is January 10, 1977, and Josiah's birthday is April 15, 1968. According to the birthday rule, the primary and secondary coverage for this family would be as follows:

	Primary Coverage	Secondary Coverage
Mary	Aetna U.S. Healthcare	Premera Blue Cross
Josiah	Premera Blue Cross	Aetna U.S. Healthcare
Ian	Aetna U.S. Healthcare	Premera Blue Cross

Because Mary's birthday falls earlier in the year than Josiah's, her policy is primary for her and Ian. Because Josiah's birthday falls later, his plan is secondary for Ian. Policyholders are primary on their own policies, so Josiah's primary carrier is his own policy through Premera Blue Cross.

Figure 16-15 ◆ Using the birthday rule.

The birthday rule relies only on the month and day of the parent's birthday. The year is not used. The insurance commissioners of most states have agreed to use the birthday rule. If a state does not use the birthday rule, the COB rules of plan in the non-birthday rule state apply. Medical assistants need to ask about this when verifying benefits.

Complicated issues can arise with child patients covered by three companies, perhaps through both biological parents and one stepparent. In these cases, typically the custodial parent's plan is primary, the spouse of the custodial parent's plan is secondary, and the noncustodial parent's plan is tertiary. The easiest way to get patients' claims paid on time is to ask the insurance carriers to identify the order in which to bill.

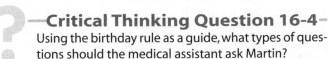

?—Critical Thinking Question 16-4

Using the birthday rule as a guide, what types of questions should the medical assistant ask Martin?

Preparing Referrals, Authorizations, and Precertifications

Before scheduling any nonemergency procedures or costly tests, medical assistants should call insurance carriers to both verify patients' eligibility for those services and to complete any needed **preauthorizations.** Preauthorization, sometimes called **precertification,** is the process of calling the patient's insur-

Keys to Success
DOCUMENTING THE PATIENT FILE

Any service billed by the medical office must be documented in the patient's file. Billing for services that have not been documented is considered fraud and is illegal. Therefore, it is crucial that all billed-for services and diagnoses are documented as patient complaints or services performed by members of the health care team.

ance carrier to obtain permission for patients to receive prescribed procedures. Depending on the insurance plan, some managed care companies require referrals from patients' primary care providers for specialized care. In these cases, medical assistants may need to call patients' primary care providers to coordinate the patients' referrals. Any time assistants receive preauthorization or precertification numbers for patients, they should include those numbers on the CMS-1500 insurance billing form as well as make note of them in the patient's file.

When patients require specialist care, managed care plans may require referrals from patients' **PCPs.** Medical assistants who work for PCPs may be asked to arrange those specialist referrals, which entails verifying that specialists are covered under patients' managed care plans. To accomplish this task, assistants can either phone insurance carriers' customer service departments or look online. Medical assistants in specialist offices must ensure that patients' PCPs have arranged referrals before those patients visit the specialists' offices.

Many HMOs penalize physicians who fail to obtain authorization before rendering service. Many times, insurance carriers will deny claims that were not properly preauthorized. In managed care, physicians are then restricted from billing patients for denied services. In effect, the physicians perform the procedures for free. With penalties this severe, it is imperative that health care providers verify the need for referrals, authorizations, or precertifications before providing service.

Documenting Insurance Company Calls

While comprehensive, in-depth knowledge of all insurance plans is unrealistic, administrative medical assistants should know where to find answers and information. Many insurance companies provide coverage information on line. Insurance companies' Web site addresses typically appear on patients' identification cards. These resources are recommended for general information, not procedure authorization. When assistants have questions about patients' insurance coverage, the provider customer service departments of the patients' insurance carrier is the best place to call.

Medical assistants should document any calls made to an insurance carrier, including date and time, number used, party on the phone, and information obtained. Such data becomes part of patients' permanent financial record and can be refer-

enced should there ever be a discrepancy between what the medical assistant was told by the insurance carrier and how the insurance carrier processed the claim.

Health Insurance Claim Forms

Before the 1990s, health insurance carriers required health care providers to use unique forms to bill for patient services. Patients were required to obtain these forms from their employers or insurance carriers. Health care providers would attach **superbills,** also called **charge slips** or **encounter forms,** which are preprinted lists of procedures and diagnosis codes commonly used in the office. Providers would circle the services they provided, along with the applicable diagnoses; attach the superbill to the unique insurance claim form; and mail the form to the appropriate insurance carrier for reimbursement.

The CMS-1500 Claim Form

To help standardize the insurance billing industry, the former HCFA (now CMS), created a uniform billing form to be used by physicians and other professional providers. This form, now called the CMS-1500, is used today by all health insurance carriers, including Medicare, Medicaid, and workmen's compensation carriers, to complete paper billed claims (Figure 16-16 ◆). Dental claims are sent via the American Dental Association (**ADA**) standard form. The ADA form and the CMS-1500 are the only two insurance claim forms medical assistants use to submit paper claims today.

The boxes to be completed on the CMS-1500 form are referred to as **form locators** (FL). The form is divided into two major sections: Patient and Insured Information (FL 1–13) and Physician or Supplier Information (FL 14–33). The top right margin is the Carrier's Area and is used to print the insurance company's address on the form.

Specific guidelines exist for completing a CMS-1500 claim form. TRICARE, CHAMPVA, Medicare, Medicaid, and workers' compensation carriers have their own rules. Private insurance companies also have their own variations. Because guidelines vary at the state and local levels for completing the CMS-1500, the medical assistant should check with his local intermediaries or private carriers. For Blue Cross Blue Shield claims, the medial assistant should refer to the provider manual for their state's Blue Cross Blue Shield plans for guidelines for completing the CMS-1500 claim form.

When completing the form, medical assistants will be **abstracting** data, or using several source documents to find the required information. It is the medical assistant's responsibility to locate all needed data on established documents and accurately transfer it to the CMS-1500 form. The patient registration form provides information about the patient's and insured's name, address, birthdate, and related data. The insurance card provides information on the insurance policy, identification and group numbers, mailing address for claims, as well as basic coverage and cost information. The clinic's encounter form will provide the date of service, services rendered, and treating

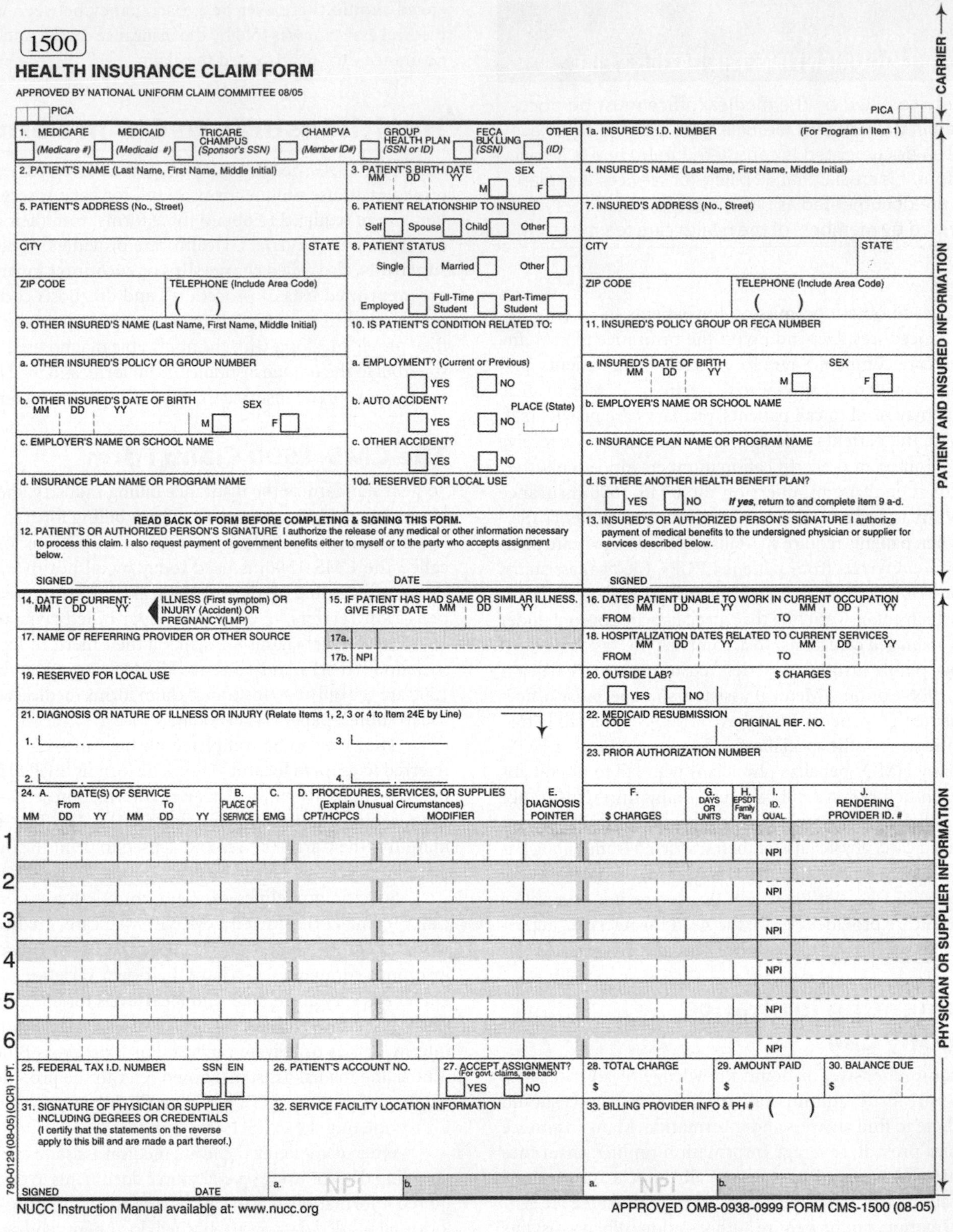

Figure 16-16 ◆ CMS-1500 claim form.

provider. The encounter form may contain fees or the medical assistant may need to refer to the clinic's fee schedule for charges. The encounter form or patient registration form may contain the clinic's address, tax identification number, and NPI numbers, or the medical assistant may need to refer to other office records for this information. Table 16-2 provides general guidelines for completing the form and identifies the most common source documents needed for each form locator. Accuracy in identifying and transferring the data is paramount; a single transposition in a critical field such as name, identification number, birthdate, or CPT code could cause the claim to be rejected. A few extra minutes spent proofreading data will prevent the need to rework claims later.

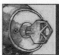

Keys to Success
PATIENT ACCOUNT NUMBERS

Including the medical office's patient account number on the CMS-1500 claim form helps identify the patient when payment is made. Most insurance companies list offices' patient account numbers on the explanation of benefits, making patient accounts easier to find and payments easier to post in computer systems.

TABLE 16-2 INSTRUCTIONS FOR COMPLETING THE CMS-1500 CLAIM FORM

FL Number, Name, and Use (R = required; C = conditional depending on claim)	Source Document
Carrier area (top right hand margin) Enter the insurance plan's mailing address for claims from this policy. Be sure to verify. Some insurance companies have different addresses and different PO boxes for different types of plans, such as group, individual, or government.	Insurance ID card
Fl 1–FL 13: PATIENT AND INSURED INFORMATION	
FL 1: Type of Insurance (R) FL 1 identifies what type of insurance the patient carries. The form lists five government plans: Medicare, Medicaid, TRICARE/CHAMPUS, CHAMPVA, and FECA/Black Lung. There are two other options: Group Health Plan and Other. These are utilized based on what type of plan the insured is enrolled in. BCBS is usually marked Other.	Insurance ID card
FL 1a: Insured's ID Number (R) FL 1a asks for the insured's insurance ID number as reflected on the insurance card. The insured could be the patient or it could be someone else such as spouse, mother, or father.	Insurance ID card
FL 2: Patient's Name (R) In FL 2, enter the name of the patient who received services. This information is input last name, first name, and middle name or initial. The spelling should match the insurance card exactly. If the name on the card is misspelled, then the name in the computer should be misspelled until the patient provides a new card with the correct spelling.	Patient registration form Encounter form
FL 3: Patient's Date of Birth/Sex (R) In FL 3, enter the patient's date of birth and sex/gender. The date of birth is entered using the eight-digit format: MMDDCCYY. Enter an X in the correct box for male or female. Do not try to guess the gender based on the patient's name.	Patient registration form Encounter form
FL 4: Insured's Name (R) FL 4 asks for the name of the person who is the insured. This may or may not be the patient. If the patient is the insured, the word "SAME" should be entered. The insured's name should be entered last name, first name, middle name or initial.	Insurance ID card
FL 5: Patient's Address (R) Enter the patient's home address and telephone number in FL 5. This information is taken from the patient information form when the patient registers in the office. The address should include the street name and number, city, state (two-letter abbreviation), and zip code. Do not use commas, periods, or other punctuation in the address. Do not use the # sign for apartment numbers. When entering a nine-digit zip code, include the hyphen. Do not use a hyphen or space as a separator within the telephone number.	Patient registration form
FL 6: Patient's Relationship to the Insured (R) Once FL 4 has been completed, in FL 6 enter an X in the correct box to indicate the patient's relationship to the insured. Options include Self, Spouse, Child, or Other. If the patient is the insured person, the "Self" entry is marked here. Only one box can be marked.	Patient registration form
FL 7: Insured's Address (R) In FL 7, enter the insured's address. If the insured person is not the patient (see FL 4), then this field should be completed. This information should include the street name and number, city, state (two-letter abbreviation), zip code, and phone number. If the patient is the insured, leave this FL blank.	Patient registration form

continued

TABLE 16-2 INSTRUCTIONS FOR COMPLETING THE CMS-1500 CLAIM FORM (CONTINUED)

FL Number, Name, and Use (R = required; C = conditional depending on claim)	Source Document
FL 8: Patient Status (R) Indicate the patient's status in FL 8: Single, Married, or Other. It also requires the patient's employment status: Employed, Full-Time Student, or Part-Time Student. Enter an X in the box for the patient's marital status and for the employment or student status. Only one box on each line can be marked. Divorced and widowed should be marked as Single. Full-Time Student indicates that the patient is registered as a full-time student as defined by the postsecondary school or university. Do not mark this box for students in elementary or high school. This information is important for determination of liability and coordination of benefits.	Patient registration form
FL 9: Other Insured's Name (C) If FL 11d is marked YES, complete form locators 9 and 9a–d; otherwise, leave them blank. FL 9 indicates that there is a holder of another policy that may cover the patient. When there is additional group health coverage, enter the other insured's full last name, first name, and middle initial of the enrollee in another health plan if it is different from that shown in FL 2. If there is no secondary policy, FL 9 is left blank.	Insurance ID card
FL 9a: Other Insured's Policy or Group Number (C) Enter the policy number or group number of the secondary insurance policy in FL 9a. The number should be entered exactly as it appears on the insurance card.	Insurance ID card
FL 9b: Other Insured's Date of Birth/Sex (C) FL 9b requires the date of birth of the insured of the secondary policy. The date of birth should be entered in the eight-digit format: MMDDCCYY. Choose either male or female accordingly.	Insurance ID card Patient registration form
FL 9c: Employer's Name or School Name (C) Enter the name of the insured's employer or school in FL 9c.	Patient registration form Insurance ID card
FL 9d: Insurance Plan Name or Program Name (C) FL 9d asks for the name of the secondary insurance plan. This information is taken directly from the secondary insurance card. Enter the name exactly as it appears on the card.	Insurance ID card
FL 10a–c: Is Patient's Condition Related To? (R) FL 10 identifies whether the patient's visit was related to an employment accident, auto accident, or other accident. This FL is used when filing workers' compensation claims, auto accident claims, or claims for other types of injuries. If the patient's visit does not pertain to an accident of any kind, the default answer will be NO. Enter an X in the correct box. If this box is not marked, or marked incorrectly, the claim could be delayed.	Encounter form Medical record
FL 10d: Reserved for Local Use (C) Different insurance carriers for different reasons use FL 10d. One example of use would be a specific insurance carrier requiring the word "Attachment" to be placed here in the event that there are paper attachments with the claim. This box is completed with the Medicaid ID number on Medi-Medi claims.	
FL 11: Insured's Policy Group or FECA Number (C) If FL 4 is completed, then FL 11 should be completed. FL 11 identifies the insured's policy group number listed on the insurance card. This number should be entered exactly as it appears on the insurance card. A FECA number (nine-digit alphanumeric identifier) is listed here when employees of the federal government are filing workers' compensation claims.	Insurance ID card
FL 11a: Insured's Date of Birth/Sex (C) In FL 11a, list the date of birth of the insured. The date of birth should be listed in the eight-digit format: MMDDCCYY. If the patient and the insured are the same person, this space can be left blank. Mark an X in either male or female accordingly. If gender is unknown, leave blank.	Insurance ID card Patient registration form
FL 11b: Employer's Name or School Name (C) In FL 11b, list the insured's place of employment or school that is attended, if a full time university student as marked in FL 8. If the patient/insured is unemployed, leave blank.	Insurance ID card Patient registration form
FL 11c: Insurance Plan Name or Program Name (C) FL 11c identifies the insurance plan name. The information should be taken directly from the insurance card and spelled exactly as it appears on the card.	Insurance ID card
FL 11d: Is There Another Health Benefit Plan? (R) In FL 11d, indicate whether there is another health benefit plan. If there is another plan, YES is marked with an X and the information is entered into form locators 9a–d. If there is no additional insurance plan, NO is marked.	Patient registration form

TABLE 16-2 INSTRUCTIONS FOR COMPLETING THE CMS-1500 CLAIM FORM (CONTINUED)

FL Number, Name, and Use (R = required; C = conditional depending on claim)	Source Document
FL 12: Patient's or Authorized Person's Signature (R) FL 12 is where the patient or guarantor signs, allowing the release of any medical information to the insurance company for billing purposes. This release is only valid for billing information. Any other request for records will require a formal release of information form to be signed by the patient or guarantor. This signature is good for 1 year from the date it is signed and should be updated annually. When submitting claims the words "Signature on File" or "SOF" may be printed here in place of a signature. The actual patient signature will be on file in the patient's chart. If the patient signs the form, enter the date in the six-digit format (MM/DD/YY) or eight-digit format (MM/DD/CCYY). If "Signature on File" or "SOF" is entered, do not enter a date. If there is no signature on file, leave blank or enter "No Signature on File."	Patient registration form
FL 13: Insured's or Authorized Person's Signature (C) FL 13 is where the patient or insured signs, authorizing the insurance company to reimburse the physician or supplier directly. As just stated, the words "Signature on File" or "SOF" may be printed here in place of a written signature when filing claims. If the patient signs the form, enter the date in the six-digit format (MM/DD/YY) or eight-digit format (MM/DD/CCYY). If "Signature on File" or "SOF" is entered, do not enter a date. If there is no signature on file, leave blank or enter "No Signature on File." Not required for government claims such as Medicare, Medicaid, Workers' Compensation.	Patient registration form
Fl 14–FL 33 PHYSICIAN OR SUPPLIER INFORMATION	
FL 14: Date of Current: Illness, Injury, Pregnancy (C) Indicate the first date of the current illness, injury, or pregnancy in FL 14. The date should be entered in the six-digit (MM/DD/YY) or eight-digit format (MM/DD/CCYY). For a pregnancy, the first day of the woman's last menstrual period (LMP) is used. If this information is not known, leave blank.	Encounter form Medical record
FL 15: If Patient Has Had Same or Similar Illness (C) In FL 15, enter the first date of treatment for the same or similar illness in the past. The date should be entered in the six-digit (MM/DD/YY) or eight-digit format (MM/DD/CCYY). If the information is not known, leave blank.	Encounter form Medical record
FL 16: Dates Patient Unable to Work in Current Occupation (C) In FL 16, list the dates the patient is unable to work due to his illness or injury. These dates will be required when filing workers' compensation or disability claims. The dates should be entered in the six-digit (MM/DD/YY) or eight-digit format (MM/DD/CCYY). If the information is not required, leave blank.	Encounter form Medical record
FL 17: Name of Referring Physician or Other Source (C) FL 17 requests the name of the physician referring the patient. Some insurance companies, such as health maintenance organizations (HMOs) or exclusive provider organizations (EPOs), require this information to be on a claim. The information entered should include the physician's last name, first name, and credentials. If multiple providers are involved, enter one provider using the following priority order: 1. Referring provider 2. Ordering provider 3. Supervising provider. If there is no referring physician, leave blank.	Encounter form Referral form
FL 17a: ID Number of Referring Physician (C) The insurance plan's ID number of the referring, ordering, or supervising provider is reported in FL 17a, if required by the plan. Since the implementation of the NPI, this field is rarely used.	Referral form
FL 17b: NPI Number (C) Enter the NPI number of the referring, ordering, or supervising provider in FL 17b.	Referral form
FL 19: Reserved for Local Use (C) FL 19 is used for miscellaneous information that may be required by the insurance policy.	
FL 20: Outside Lab (C) FL 20 is used only if lab tests appear in section 24. A YES answer indicates that an entity other than the entity billing for the service performed the purchased services. If YES is chosen, enter the purchased price under Charges and complete FL 32. If the lab tests were performed by the provider's office mark NO. If no lab tests were ordered, leave this FL blank.	Encounter form Medical record

continued

TABLE 16-2 INSTRUCTIONS FOR COMPLETING THE CMS-1500 CLAIM FORM (CONTINUED)

FL Number, Name, and Use (R = required; C = conditional depending on claim)	Source Document
FL 21: Diagnosis or Nature of Illness or Injury (R) In FL 21, the ICD-9 codes for the diagnoses applied to this claim are entered. At least one code must be entered and up to four codes can be used on a claim. They are placed in order of precedence, line 1 being the primary diagnosis, and so forth. No diagnosis descriptions are used on a claim form. The ICD-9 codes should be checked for medical necessity to make sure they are used appropriately with the CPT codes used in FL 24D. Relate lines 1, 2, 3, and 4 to the lines of service in 24E by line number.	Encounter form Medical record
FL 22: Medicaid Resubmission Code (C) If required, FL 22 is where the Medicaid resubmission code used for Medicaid claims is entered. List the original reference number and the code for resubmitted claims.	Medicaid EOB Phone call to insurance company
FL 23: Prior Authorization Number (C) Some insurance plans, such as those of HMOs and PPOs, require a prior authorization number. If required, when preauthorization is obtained from an insurance company for services, the number assigned is input in FL 23. Also, HMO required referral numbers are input in this form locator. If prior authorization is required and is omitted, the claim will be denied. If no prior authorization is required, leave blank.	Referral form
Section 24 The six service lines in Section 24 were divided horizontally to accommodate submission of supplemental information to support the billed service, such as anesthesia and drug information.	
FL 24A: Dates of Service (R) In FL 24A, enter the dates of service for the services provided. Depending on the insurance carrier, these columns are filled in using different formats. Some require both the To and From dates to be listed in six-digit format (MM/DD/YY). Some require just the From date to be listed or just the To date. If the same procedure was provided multiple times on a single date, the specific date is entered once and the number of procedures is listed in FL 24G.	Encounter form Medical record
FL 24B: Place of Service (R) Place of service in FL 24B is a mandatory field to be completed because it describes the place where the procedure or service was performed. This place could be many places, such as the physician's office, hospital, emergency department, skilled nursing facility, or even the patient's home. A code is used (see following list) to indicate the place of service. Note that the CMS has stated that the place of service must also be fully written out in FL 32. Consider this example: The patient was an inpatient (hospital) and the physician saw the patient in the hospital for an evaluation and management service. Therefore, the code 21 (see following list) would be entered in FL 24B and the name and address of the hospital entered in FL 32: Common place of service codes include the following: 11. Physician's office 20. Urgent care facility 21. Inpatient hospital 22. Outpatient hospital 23. Hospital emergency department 31. Skilled nursing facility	Encounter form Medical record
FL 24C: EMG (Emergency) (C) FL 24C is used only with Medicaid to indicate whether the service was provided on an emergency basis. This FL should be marked with a Y for YES or left blank for NO. The definition of an emergency can be defined differently by each payer.	Encounter form Medical record
FL 24D: Procedures, Services, or Supplies (R) In FL 24D, enter the CPT or HCPCS codes used to identify the procedures, services, or supplies provided. Modifiers are also listed in FL 24D. If more than three modifiers are used, list 99 here and enter the modifiers in FL 19.	Encounter form Medical record
FL 24E: Diagnosis Pointer (R) FL 24E indicates the line number (1, 2, 3, and 4) of the diagnosis code listed in FL 21 as it relates to each service or procedure. If more than one diagnosis is attached to a single procedure or service, list the primary diagnosis first. Leave a space between each number. It is critical to be sure that each CPT code has a corresponding diagnosis code to justify the need. Some insurances, such as Medicare, require only one diagnosis reference number per service.	Encounter form Medical record

TABLE 16-2 INSTRUCTIONS FOR COMPLETING THE CMS-1500 CLAIM FORM (CONTINUED)

FL Number, Name, and Use (R = required; C = conditional depending on claim)	Source Document
FL 24F: Charges (R) FL 24F lists the charges that are assigned to each CPT or HCPCS code listed. The amount should be entered without a decimal point or dollar sign. If multiple units are entered in FL 24G, the charges should reflect the total charge for amount of the procedure times the number of units. It is not a per unit charge. The charge entered should be the provider's established fee schedule, not the discounted or contracted rate. Medicare claims should contain the Medicare fee schedule charge.	Encounter form Physician fee schedule
FL 24G: Days or Units (R) Enter the number of units per procedure or service provided to a patient in FL 24G. If multiple units are entered in 24G, the charges should reflect the amount of the procedure multiplied by the number of units. When required by payers to provide supplemental information such as the National Drug Code (NDC) units in addition to the HCPCS units, enter the applicable NDC units' qualifier and related units in the shaded line. The following qualifiers are to be used when reporting NDC units: F2 International Unit ML Milliliter GR Gram UN Unit.	Encounter form Medical record
FL 24H: EPSDT Family Plan (C) FL 24H is used on Medicaid claims only, to identify whether the patient is receiving her services through Medicaid's Early and Periodic Screening, Diagnosis, and Treatment (EPSDT) program. Enter "Y" for YES or "N" for NO or follow state-specific guidelines.	Insurance (Medicaid) ID card
FL 24I: ID Qualifier (C) If the insurance plan requires use of a plan specific provider ID number for the provider who delivered the service, enter the code for type of plan. Otherwise, leave blank.	Office records
FL 24J: Rendering Provider (R) The provider rendering the service is reported in FL 24J. Enter the NPI number in the unshaded area of the field. If the insurance plan also requires use of a plan specific provider ID number for the provider who delivered the service, enter the ID number in the shaded portion. Otherwise, leave the shaded portion blank.	Encounter form Medical record
FL 25: Federal Tax I.D. Number (R) List in FL 25 the physician's federal tax I.D. number or the employer identification number (EIN) of the billing entity. Do not enter hyphens with numbers. The appropriate box (SSN or EIN) should be marked with an X.	Encounter form Office records
FL 26: Patient's Account Number (C) In FL 26, enter the patient's account number assigned by the medical office. The computer system used in the office will generate the number and it should be entered on the claim. This in turn will allow for the account number to appear on the Explanation of Benefits (EOB) form, which makes it easier to locate the correct patient to post insurance payments.	Encounter form Medical record
FL 27: Accept Assignment? (C) FL 27 is used with Medicare claims to indicate whether or not the physician accepts assignment on this claim. PAR physicians will always mark YES. Non-PAR physicians must select YES or NO on each claim.	Encounter form Office records
FL 28: Total Charge (R) FL 28 lists the total charges, added together from those listed in FL 24F. The charges should be checked for accuracy to ensure proper reimbursement. Do not use decimal points or dollar signs in this entry.	Calculator
FL 29: Amount Paid FL 29 indicates the amount paid by primary insurance on this claim. This amount is added after the primary EOB is received and payment is posted. A secondary claim is printed to be sent to the secondary insurance carrier along with a copy of the primary insurance carrier's EOB. Do not use decimal points or dollar signs in this entry. Do not enter any patient payments unless instructed to do so by the insurance plan. Some managed care plans require copayments to be reported here.	Encounter form
FL 30: Balance Due (C) FL 30 is used to record the difference between the amounts in FL 28 and 29. If FL 29 is blank, leave FL 30 blank also. This amount is the balance due for the claim being submitted. When a claim is submitted electronically this locator or "balance due" does not appear. Do not use decimal points or dollar signs in this entry.	Calculator
FL 31: Signature of Physician or Supplier Including Degrees or Credentials (R) FL 31 identifies the name of the physician or supplier who has provided the services to the patient along with professional credentials (M.D., PA-C, or NP). If a paper claim is submitted, the physician or supplier's name must be typed/printed. "Signature on File" or "SOF" is not acceptable in this FL. Enter a six-digit date (MM/DD/YY), eight-digit date (MM/DD/CCYY), or alphanumeric date. A signature stamp may be used instead of a written signature. The stamp must leave a clear, nonsmeared image on the claim.	Typed Signature stamp

continued

TABLE 16-2 INSTRUCTIONS FOR COMPLETING THE CMS-1500 CLAIM FORM (CONTINUED)

FL Number, Name, and Use (R = required; C = conditional depending on claim)	Source Document
FL 32: Name and Address of Facility Where Services Were Rendered (C) FL 32 identifies the name of the facility where services were provided. Enter the name, address, zip code, and NPI number. When more than one supplier is used, a separate CMS-1500 form should be used for each supplier.	Encounter form Medical record
FL 32a: NPI Number (C) Enter the NPI number of the service facility location in FL 32a.	Encounter form Office records
FL 32b: Other ID Number (C) If required by the insurance plan, enter the plan specific ID number here.	Encounter form Office records
FL 33: Billing Provider Information and Phone Number (R) Enter the provider's or supplier's billing name, address, zip code, and phone number in FL 33. The phone number is to be entered in the area to the right of the field title. Enter the name and address information in the following format: First line: Name Second line: Address Third line: City, state, and zip code.	Encounter form Office records
FL 33a: NPI Number (R) Enter the NPI number of the billing provider in FL 33a.	Encounter form Office records
FL 33b: Other ID Number (C) If required by the insurance plan, enter the plan specific ID number here.	Encounter form Office records

Source: Adapted from Vines, Deborah, Braceland, Ann, Rollins, Elizabeth, and Miller, Susan. Comprehensive Health Insurance: Billing, Coding, and Reimbursement. © 2008, pp. 223–232. Reprinted by permission of Pearson Education, Inc. Upper Saddle River, NJ.

Optical Character Recognition

The CMS-1500 is printed in red ink so that it is recognizable by OCR scanners. Optical character recognition (OCR) devices (scanners) are being used frequently across the nation for processing paper insurance claims because of their speed and efficiency.

A scanner can transfer printed or typed text and bar codes to the insurance company's computer memory. Scanners read at such a fast speed that they reduce the cost of data entry and decrease the processing time. More control is gained over data input by using OCR. It improves accuracy, thus reducing coding errors because the claim is entered exactly as coded by the medical assistant.

The CMS-1500 form was developed so insurance carriers could process claims efficiently by OCR. Keying a form for OCR scanning requires different techniques than preparing one for standard claims submission. Because the majority of insurance carriers accept the OCR format, it is suggested that it be routinely used. Successful OCR begins with the proper submission of claims data. Printed characters must conform to the preprogrammed specifications relative to character size and alignment on the CMS-1500 form. Only the current CMS-1500 form with red dropout ink is acceptable for OCR. These characteristics cannot be copied; therefore, original forms are necessary. OCR guidelines include:

■ Use original approved forms only.
■ Use all capital letters.
■ Use a standard mono-spaced serif font (one that has little lines on the ends of the letters such as Courier).
■ Do not use any punctuation such as . , / # -.

■ Keep all text within the boundaries of the red box for each FL.
■ Use eight digit dates for birthdates. Other dates can be either six or eight digits, but should be consistent.
■ Do not erase, strike out, overtype, or white out. If you make a mistake, start over.
■ Do not use highlighters or pen to make any extra markings on the form.
■ Do not tape or staple anything to the form.*

Using diagnostic coding (**ICD-9-CM**) ∞ (Chapter 17) and procedural (CPT) coding ∞ (Chapter 18), medical assistants can file accurate CMS-1500 health insurance claim forms. Most medical offices have software that creates these forms, but medical assistants must input proper, comprehensive information to obtain accurate results. For example, assistants enter an insurance company's address in the blank portion in the upper right of the form. When preparing to send printed documents, assistants should fold the CMS-1500 such that address information shows through a window envelope (Figure 16-17 ◆).

HIPAA Compliance

Once completed, CMS-1500 claim forms contain confidential patient information. As a result, these forms must be protected from view by anyone who is unauthorized to see patient

*Source: Adapted from Vines, Deborah, Braceland, Ann, Rollins, Elizabeth, and Miller, Susan. *Comprehensive Health Insurance: Billing, Coding, and Reimbursement.* © 2008, p. 35. Reprinted by permission of Pearson Education, Inc. Upper Saddle River, NJ.

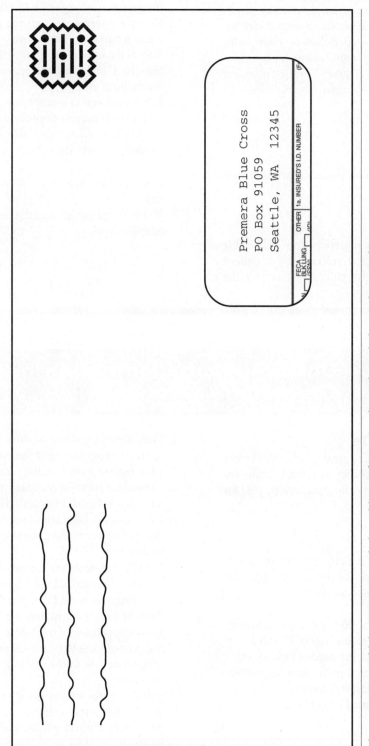

Figure 16-17 ◆ Fold the CMS-1500 such that address information shows through the window envelope.

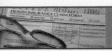

PROCEDURE 16-3 Obtain a Managed Care Referral

Theory and Rationale

Medical assistants in primary care or family practice physicians' offices are often required to obtain managed care referrals for patients who need to see specialists or other health care providers. Whenever needed, medical assistants in specialists' office should ensure that managed care referrals are obtained for patients covered by managed care policies.

Materials

- Telephone
- Patient's medical chart
- Name and telephone number of patient's primary care provider

Competency

(**Conditions**) With the necessary materials, you will be able to (**Task**) obtain a managed care referral for a patient (**Standards**) correctly within the time limit set by the instructor.

1. Call the patient's primary care provider's office, and ask for the person in charge of referrals.
2. Give the referral assistant the patient's information, including name and birth date.
3. Inform the referral assistant of the need for a referral to the physician, including the reason for the patient's visit in the medical office.
4. Ask the referral assistant if any information from the patient's file is needed to process the referral.
5. Ask the referral assistant when to expect the referral. If needed, provide the office fax number for information transmittal.
6. Document in the patient's file the content of the telephone call.
7. Notify the physician and the patient of the content of the telephone call.

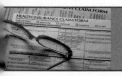

PROCEDURE 16-4 Obtain Authorization from an Insurance Company for a Procedure

Theory and Rationale

Most insurance companies require preauthorization before physicians perform any nonemergency services. Without insurance carrier authorization, physicians may not be paid for their services.

Materials

- Patient insurance information (i.e., ID number, birth date of the insured, name and telephone number for provider customer service at the insurance company)
- Paper and pen
- Description of the procedure the doctor has prescribed, including Current Procedural Terminology (**CPT**) code
- Patient's diagnosis pertaining to the needed procedure
- Location where procedure is to be performed (e.g., office, outpatient surgery, inpatient hospitalization)
- Date by which the procedure must be performed

Competency

(**Conditions**) With the necessary materials, you will be able to (**Task**) obtain an authorization from an insurance carrier for a procedure (**Standards**) correctly within the time limit set by the instructor.

1. Write down the date and time of the call, the name of the insurance company, and the name of the insurance company representative on the phone.
2. Give the insurance company representative your name and your office's/physician's name.
3. Give the insurance company representative the name of the patient, the name of the insured, and the insured's ID number.
4. Let the representative know what the procedure is your doctor has prescribed for the patient and the date by which the procedure must be performed.
5. Provide the representative any other requested information (e.g., procedure code, diagnosis code, and place where the procedure is to be performed).
6. Write down the authorization number the representative provides.
7. Ask the representative if any supporting documentation (e.g., chart notes, operative report, laboratory report, or pathology report) will be needed with the CMS-1500 billing form. If so, write down the required documentation.
8. Keep all preceding information in the patient's file for reference in case the claim is not paid by the insurance carrier.

information. Keep these forms in a secure area, never in a non-secure area even when in envelopes. When errors are made on CMS-1500 claim forms and new ones must be printed, shred the forms with errors to protect patient privacy.

The CMS-1500 form accommodates only four diagnostic codes, which should appear in order of importance. The first code is always for the patient's chief complaint. Box 24E on the CMS-1500 form links each service on the form to the appropriate diagnosis code in Box 21. Table 16-2 provides further instructions for correct CMS-1500 form completion (Figure 16-18 ◆).

Filing Timelines

Most insurance carriers accept claims up to 1 year from the date of service, although some have much shorter timelines, such as 90 days. After filing timelines pass, claims are considered **past timely filing limits** and will likely be rejected. With most managed care plans, claims rejected due to timely filing limits cannot be billed to the patient. To avoid rejection, it is best to submit claims soon after service is rendered.

Billing Insurance Companies Electronically

Electronic claims, also called electronic media claims or EMCs, are submitted to the insurance carrier via a central processing unit (CPU), tape diskette, direct data entry, direct wire, telephone line via modem, or personal computer. Electronic claims are never printed on paper. When claims are sent electronically to the insurance carriers for processing, an electronic signature is used to verify that the information received is true and correct. Medicare requires electronic transmission of claims for providers with 10 or more employees or facilities with 25 or more employees. Paper claims will not be processed for these submitters.

Electronic claims have a number of advantages:

- Administrative costs are lower because fewer personnel hours are needed to prepare forms, and supply and postage costs are lower.
- Fewer claims are rejected because technical errors are detected and corrected before the claim arrives at the payer.
- Processing is faster with fewer errors. An electronic claim is received by the payer in minutes. The payer does not have to perform data entry, so there is less opportunity for errors to be introduced. In addition, most claims can be automatically adjudicated by the computer, rather than being processed by a claims analyst.
- Errors can be corrected faster. If errors are found on claims by carriers or the claim is denied, the office is notified immediately and medical assistants can begin work on resolving the issue.
- Payment is faster. Payment can be transferred electronically to the provider's bank, eliminating delays in cash flow. These payments are referred to as electronic remittances. Medicare is required by law to process electronic

claims in 14 days, and is prohibited from processing paper claims for at least 28 days after receipt.

Electronic claims also have disadvantages:

- Claims transmission can be disrupted occasionally due to power failures, or computer hardware or software problems that might require claims to be resubmitted.
- Many patient billing programs cannot create an electronic attachment, so when a claim attachment is required, the electronic claim must be sent separately from mailed attachments, which sometimes causes problems for the payer in matching up the two. In some cases, the claim must instead be submitted on paper when it must be accompanied by a claim attachment.

Electronic claims, which are the leading method of claims submission by providers, are submitted through a clearinghouse, a billing service, or directly to the carrier. A physician who plans to use electronic billing must contact all major insurers and carriers for a list of the vendors approved to handle electronic claims, and must have a signed agreement with each. Each carrier has special electronic billing requirements and is knowledgeable in which systems meet their criteria and which are compatible in format. The field data that is requested by the carriers is almost identical to the information on the CMS-1500 claim form. Insurance carriers also provide information about how to submit an electronic bill for patients who have secondary coverage. Medicare provides the software and training for electronic submissions. Medicare, Medicaid, TRICARE, and many private insurance carriers allow providers to submit insurance claims directly to them with no "middle man." In this type of system, the medical practice must have special software or the physician must lease a terminal from the carrier to key in claims data. The data is transmitted via modem (dedicated telephone line) directly to the carrier's computer for processing.

If the physician is not sending the data directly to the carrier, a clearinghouse may be used. A clearinghouse is a company that receives claims from providers, puts them through a series of audits to check for errors, and then forwards them to the appropriate insurance carrier in the carrier's required data format. Clearinghouses may charge a flat fee per claim or charge a percentage of the claim's dollar value. It is very important for physicians' practices to negotiate the best possible fee for using a clearinghouse's services.

The clearinghouse conducts an audit to determine if any data on the claim is incorrect or missing; such a claim is referred to as a dirty claim. The results of the audit are sent back to the provider from the clearinghouse in the form of an audit/edit report. The medical assistant will need to correct any claims with incorrect data (as indicated on the audit/edit report) and resubmit them to the clearinghouse. Dirty claims, those with errors, will not be transmitted to the carriers. When the claims are corrected and resubmitted to the clearinghouse, they are considered **clean claims**, which are then formatted and forwarded to the carrier. Each time the claim is returned there is an

(1500)

HEALTH INSURANCE CLAIM FORM
APPROVED BY NATIONAL UNIFORM CLAIM COMMITTEE 08/05

BLUE CROSS BLUE SHIELD
379 BLUE PLZ
CAPITAL CITY NY   12345

CARRIER

| | | PICA | | | | | | PICA | | |

1. MEDICARE	MEDICAID	TRICARE CHAMPUS	CHAMPVA	GROUP HEALTH PLAN	FECA BLK LUNG	OTHER	1a. INSURED'S I.D. NUMBER	(For Program in Item 1)
☐ (Medicare #)	☐ (Medicaid #)	☐ (Sponsor's SSN)	☐ (Member ID#)	☐ (SSN or ID)	☐ (SSN)	☒ (ID)	YYJ744258013	

2. PATIENT'S NAME (Last Name, First Name, Middle Initial)	3. PATIENT'S BIRTH DATE MM DD YY	SEX	4. INSURED'S NAME (Last Name, First Name, Middle Initial)
ABNER AARON	01 28 1976	M ☒ F ☐	ABNER MELISSA

5. PATIENT'S ADDRESS (No, Street)	6. PATIENT RELATIONSHIP TO INSURED	7. INSURED'S ADDRESS (No, Street)
98 N ROSEWOOD DR	Self ☐ Spouse ☒ Child ☐ Other ☐	SAME

CITY	STATE	8. PATIENT STATUS	CITY	STATE
TOWNSHIP	NY	Single ☐ Married ☒ Other ☐		

ZIP CODE	TELEPHONE (Include Area Code)		ZIP CODE	TELEPHONE (Include Area Code)
12345	(555) 5558552	Full-Time ☐ Part-Time ☐ Employed ☒ Student ☐ Student ☐		( )

9. OTHER INSURED'S NAME (Last Name, First Name, Middle Initial)	10. IS PATIENT'S CONDITION RELATED TO:	11. INSURED'S POLICY GROUP OR FECA NUMBER 015386
a. OTHER INSURED'S POLICY OR GROUP NUMBER	a. EMPLOYMENT? (Current or Previous) ☐ YES ☒ NO	a. INSURED'S DATE OF BIRTH MM DD YY 08 04 1974 SEX M ☐ F ☒
b. OTHER INSURED'S DATE OF BIRTH MM DD YY SEX M ☐ F ☐	b. AUTO ACCIDENT? PLACE (State) ☐ YES ☒ NO	b. EMPLOYER'S NAME OR SCHOOL NAME PASTA USA
c. EMPLOYER'S NAME OR SCHOOL NAME	c. OTHER ACCIDENT? ☐ YES ☒ NO	c. INSURANCE PLAN NAME OR PROGRAM NAME BLUE CROSS BLUE SHIELD
d. INSURANCE PLAN NAME OR PROGRAM NAME	10d. RESERVED FOR LOCAL USE	d. IS THERE ANOTHER HEALTH BENEFIT PLAN? ☐ YES ☒ NO *If yes,* return to and complete item 9 a-d

READ BACK OF FORM BEFORE COMPLETING & SIGNING THIS FORM.

12. PATIENT'S OR AUTHORIZED PERSON'S SIGNATURE I authorize the release of any medical or other information necessary to process this claim. I also request payment of government benefits either to myself or to the party who accepts assignment below.

SIGNED SOF   DATE

13. INSURED'S OR AUTHORIZED PERSON'S SIGNATURE I authorize payment of medical benefits to the undersigned physician or supplier for services described below.

SIGNED SOF

14. DATE OF CURRENT MM DD YY	◄ ILLNESS (First symptom) OR INJURY (Accident) OR PREGNANCY (LMP)	15. IF PATIENT HAS HAD SAME OR SIMILAR ILLNESS, GIVE FIRST DATE MM DD YY	16. DATES PATIENT UNABLE TO WORK IN CURRENT OCCUPATION MM DD YY MM DD YY FROM TO
17. NAME OF REFERRING PHYSICIAN OR OTHER SOURCE	17a. 17b. NPI		18. HOSPITALIZATION DATES RELATED TO CURRENT SERVICES MM DD YY MM DD YY FROM TO
19. RESERVED FOR LOCAL USE			20. OUTSIDE LAB? $ CHARGES ☐ YES ☒ NO

21. DIAGNOSIS OR NATURE OF ILLNESS OR INJURY (Relate Items 1,2,3 or 4 to Item 24E by Line)

1. 300   01   3. V17   3
2. 305   1   4. V17   5

22. MEDICAID RESUBMISSION CODE   ORIGINAL REF. NO.

23. PRIOR AUTHORIZATION NUMBER

24. A. DATE(S) OF SERVICE From MM DD YY	To MM DD YY	B. PLACE OF SERVICE	C. EMG	D. PROCEDURES, SERVICES, OR SUPPLIES (Explain Unusual Circumstances) CPT/HCPCS	MODIFIER	E. DIAGNOSIS POINTER	F. $ CHARGES	G. DAYS OR UNITS	H. EPSDT Family Plan	I. ID. QUAL.	J. RENDERING PROVIDER ID. #
12 01 XX	12 01 XX	11		99203		1234	85 00	1		NPI	1234567890
12 01 XX	12 01 XX	11		85025		123	95 00	1		NPI	1234567890
12 01 XX	12 01 XX	11		93000		123	75 00	1		NPI	1234567890
12 01 XX	12 01 XX	11		80053		123	75 00	1		NPI	1234567890
12 01 XX	12 01 XX	11		36415		123	15 00	1		NPI	1234567890
										NPI	

25. FEDERAL TAX ID NUMBER SSN EIN	26. PATIENT'S ACCOUNT NO.	27. ACCEPT ASSIGNMENT? (For govt. claims, see back)	28. TOTAL CHARGE	29. AMOUNT PAID	30. BALANCE DUE
750246810 ☐ ☒	B2	☐ YES ☐ NO	345 00	$	$

31. SIGNATURE OF PHYSICIAN OR SUPPLIER INCLUDING DEGREES OR CREDENTIALS (I certify that the statements on the reverse apply to this bill and are made a part thereof)

PHIL WELLS MD 12/01/XX

SIGNED   DATE

32. SERVICE FACILITY LOCATION INFORMATION
CAPITAL CITY MEDICAL
123 UNKNOWN BLVD
CAPITAL CITY NY 12345
a. 1513171216   b.

33. BILLING PROVIDER INFO & PH. # (555) 5551234
CAPITAL CITY MEDICAL
123 UNKNOWN BLVD
CAPITAL CITY NY 12345
a. 1513171216   b.

NUCC Instruction Manual available at: www.nucc.org
WCMS-1500CS

APPROVED OMB 0938-0999 FORM CMS-1500 (08/05)

PATIENT AND INSURED INFORMATION

PHYSICIAN OR SUPPLIER INFORMATION

Figure 16-18 ◆ A completed CMS-1500 claim form.

additional charge, so the medical assistant should ensure that clean claims are transmitted initially.*

Working with Fee Schedules

Providers have different methods in determining their fee structure (the amount charged for each procedure performed). As stated by the American Medical Association (AMA), "Physicians have the right to establish their fees at a level which they believe fairly reflects the costs of providing a service and the value of the professional judgment." Two main methods are used for determining fees: charge-based and resource-based fee structures.

Charge-Based Fee Structures

Charge-based fees are the fees that many providers charge for similar services. To set their fees, providers begin with an analysis of their procedure codes. To determine if their fees are in range with other providers of the same specialty they may research a nationwide fee database. This information can be purchased by the provider to ascertain how fees compare to national averages. The database is divided into categories to indicate fees that are 25%, 50%, 75%, and 90% higher based on fees charged throughout the nation. A provider can decide if his usual fees should be on the high, low, or midpoint range.

Resource-Based Fee Structures

Resource-based fees are based on the following three factors:

1. How difficult it is for the provider to perform the procedure (work).
2. How much office overhead the procedure involves (practice expense).
3. The relative risk that the procedure presents to the patient and the provider (malpractice).

Third-party payers also establish the amount they will reimburse providers. Each payer will determine the usual, customary, and reasonable (UCR) fee they feel should be charged by the provider by determining the percentage of the published fee in the national database that they will pay.[†]

Medicare's Resource-Based Relative Value Scale

Medicare bases its payment system on the **resource-based relative value scale** (**RBRVS**), which assigns a unit of relative value for provider's services based on the amount Medicare believes those services actually cost to provide.

The RBRVS has three parts: (1) national relative value (**RVU**), (2) **geographic adjustment factor** (**GAF**), and (3) na-

tional uniform **conversion factor** (CF). The national relative value is based on the type of work a physician does, the cost of practicing (overhead), and the cost of the provider's medical malpractice insurance. For example, the relative value for a basic office visit is lower than the value of a surgical procedure. The second part of RBRVS, the geographic adjustment factor, considers the area of the country in which a physician practices, adjusting higher or lower based on that area's cost of living. The third and final RBRVS part, the national uniform conversion factor, is a dollar amount used to determine the payment amount for a service. Each year, Medicare adjusts this factor according to the cost-of-living index.

Before agreeing to participate with any plan, health care providers should carefully review the fee schedules the managed care companies provide. Once contracts are in place, physicians have little leverage to adjust fee schedules and may find some, or all, fees are lower than they can afford to accept.

Posting Payments

Once an insurance carrier has processed a claim, a check is sent to the health care provider with an **Explanation of Benefits** (**EOB**) statement (Figure 16-19 ◆). With large insurance carriers, providers may receive one EOB and check as payment for several patients. The EOB lists the name of the patient, the name of the insured, the date of service, the amount billed, the amount allowed (should it be a managed care insurance carrier), the amount paid, and the amount the provider may bill the patient. Medical assistants must check EOBs to ensure all services that were billed are accurately listed and that service payment matches the amount in the insurance company contract.

An explanation will not always be accompanied by payment, but it will state the status of the claim. The claim may be pending waiting for additional information. A pending claim is one that is received but not processed by the carrier because additional information is needed or there is an error. For claims submitted electronically, the EOB is referred to as the Electronic Remittance Advice (ERA). The EOB lists the patient, dates of services, types of service, and the charges filed on the insurance claim form. The EOB also describes how the amount of the benefit payment was determined. If claim forms were filed for more than one patient with the same insurance carrier at the same time, the provider's EOB may include information on more than one patient.

The format and contents of each EOB vary based on the benefit plan and the services provided. No universal form for explaining benefits is available. It has been a point of debate that all providers are required to use the CMS-1500 and the UB-04 standardized forms, yet carriers can customize their EOBs in any way. Terminology is also different on various EOBs. For example, some EOBs show the "Allowed Amount or Charge" and some EOBs read "Deducted Amount." The medical assistant will eventually become accustomed to the carriers with whom the provider contracts, but should always review all EOBs carefully prior to entering data.

However, many terms and categories are common to all carriers. Insurance carriers often use codes on the EOB to refer

---

*Source: Vines, Deborah, Braceland, Ann, Rollins, Elizabeth, and Miller, Susan. *Comprehensive Health Insurance: Billing, Coding, and Reimbursement.* © 2008, pp. 215–216. Reprinted by permission of Pearson Education, Inc. Upper Saddle River, NJ.

[†]Source: Vines, Deborah, Braceland, Ann, Rollins, Elizabeth, and Miller, Susan. *Comprehensive Health Insurance: Billing, Coding, and Reimbursement.* © 2008, p. 419. Reprinted by permission of Pearson Education, Inc. Upper Saddle River, NJ.

Uniform Medical Plan
Your Health, Your Plan Your Choice

Explanation of Benefits
This is not a bill.
06/08/2007

CHRIS R LONEMA
3160 GRAND AVE
EVERETT WA 12345

Your UMP ID Number: W125370058
Subscriber Name: CHRIS R LONEMA
Patient Name CHRIS R LONEMA
Claim Number: K100925-0038

Provider Information
CATHERINE N DORTON ARNP
7620 44TH ST NE
MARYSVILLE WA 12345

If you have questions, contact us:

By Mail:
Uniform Medical Plan
PO Box 84578
Seattle, WA 98124-1578

By Phone/E-mail:
Local: 425-555-3000
Toll Free: 1-800-555-6004
E-mail: www.ump.hca.wa.gov

Provider Name:	Date(s) of Service	Service(s) Provided	Amount Charged	UMP Allowed	PPO Savings	Non-Cov'd Amount	Deductible	Copay	Co-Ins. %	UMP Paid	Patient's Responsibility	See Notes Section
CATHERINE N DORTON ARNP	05/07/07 - 05/07/07	87621 90 PATHOLOGY-PHYS CHGS	125.00	66.94	58.06			6.69	90	60.25	6.69	PPU
CATHERINE N DORTON ARNP	05/07/07 - 05/07/07	88142 90 PATHOLOGY-PHYS CHGS	72.00	28.31	43.69			2.83	90	25.48	2.83	PPU
		TOTALS	197.00	95.25	101.75	0.00	0.00	9.52		85.73	9.52	

Other Insurance Paid Amount 0.00
(*) See Notes Adjustment 0.00
UMP Final Paid Amount/Check 85.73   # 4398431

Total Payment to Provider: ******85.73   **Total Payment to Enrollee:** ********0.00

NOTES:

THANK YOU FOR USING A UNIFORM MEDICAL PLAN PARTICIPATING PROVIDER

PPU   THIS IS YOUR PLANS PARTICIPATING PROVIDERS CONTRACTUAL ALLOWANCE FOR THIS SERVICE. PROVIDER AGREES TO REDUCE THE FEE TO THE AMOUNT ALLOWED.

DEDUCTIBLE
YOU HAVE MET 200.00 OF YOUR 200.00 DEDUCTIBLE FOR 01/01/2007 - 12/31/2007

Figure 16-19 ◆ Explanation of Benefits (EOB).

to these terms or situations. These codes are called reason codes and remark codes. Usually these codes are explained on the face or back of the EOB. If one line is read at a time, the descriptions and calculations for each patient are easily understood. An EOB statement has three sections that explain how a claim was processed:

1. Service Information. Identifies the provider (hospital or other facility, doctor, specialist, or clinic), dates of service, and charges from the provider.
2. Coverage Determination. Summarizes the total deductions, charges not covered by the plan, and the amount the patient may owe the provider.
3. Benefit Payment Information. Indicates who was paid, how much, and when.

Information on an EOB

The following information appears on an EOB:

1. Account name: company name
2. Date the EOB statement was finalized
3. Member's or insured's name and ID number
4. Patient's identification number as it appears on his ID card
5. Number assigned to the claim
6. Name of the person who received the service (the patient)
7. Provider's name
8. Service description column, which indicates:
   - Dates of the services provided (DOS)
   - Procedures performed (CPT codes)
   - Total charge for each procedure
   - The portion of the bill not covered by the plan
   - The contractual allowed amount
   - Patient's copay
   - Patient's deductible or noncovered procedures or amounts
   - Patient's coinsurance
9. Total payment to the provider
10. The total amount that is the patient's responsibility to the provider of services.

After posting the payment to the specific date and procedure, an adjustment may be needed. An adjustment is a positive or negative change to a patient's account balance. Corrections, changes, and write-offs to patients' accounts are made by means of adjustments to the existing transactions. The medical assistant will also adjust a patient's bill as a result of any discounts given. If the provider is a PAR provider, the difference between the billed amount (the provider's UCR fee) and the allowed amount is adjusted from the amount the patient owes. Also note whether a balance is due from the patient, or whether a refund is due the patient or insurance carrier. For example, if a patient paid for a service in advance and was reimbursed by the carrier or if the patient or insurance carrier overpaid on an account, then a refund is due.*

*Source: Adapted from Vines, Deborah, Braceland, Ann, Rollins, Elizabeth, and Miller, Susan. *Comprehensive Health Insurance: Billing, Coding, and Reimbursement.* © 2008. Reprinted by permission of Pearson Education, Inc. Upper Saddle River, NJ.

In addition to sending EOBs to providers, insurance carriers send EOB copies to the insured. When providers contract with insurance carriers, they must accept the allowed amount of the claim as payment in full. Billing the patient for the difference between the billed amount and the allowed amount, a practice called **balance billing,** violates the health care provider's contract with the insurance carrier. Figure 16-20 ◆ shows how this works. If providers are not contracted with the carriers, they should balance bill.

When patients have set copayments, those copays should be collected at the time of service. When patients owe coinsurance or deductible amounts, medical assistants must bill patients once the insurance carriers send notification.

Tracing Claims

Each state has its own guidelines that outline the timeframe within which an insurance carrier must pay or deny a claim. In Washington State, for example, that timeframe is 30 days. Any claims that have not been processed within that timeframe are subject to interest in the amount allowed by state law. As a general rule, any claim that has not been paid or denied within 45 days of submission on paper, or 20 days of submission electronically, may be considered past due and warrants a telephone call to the insurance carrier. Most medical office software can print a list of past due claims, making it easy to identify the claims that require further investigation.

When a claim is past due, the medical assistant should call the insurance carrier to follow up on or trace the claim. During this call, the medical assistant may be told that the insurance carrier does not have the claim on file. If this is the case,

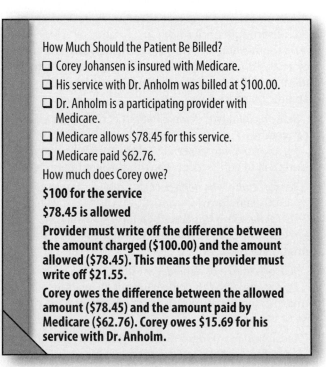

How Much Should the Patient Be Billed?
❑ Corey Johansen is insured with Medicare.
❑ His service with Dr. Anholm was billed at $100.00.
❑ Dr. Anholm is a participating provider with Medicare.
❑ Medicare allows $78.45 for this service.
❑ Medicare paid $62.76.
How much does Corey owe?
$100 for the service
$78.45 is allowed
Provider must write off the difference between the amount charged ($100.00) and the amount allowed ($78.45). This means the provider must write off $21.55.
Corey owes the difference between the allowed amount ($78.45) and the amount paid by Medicare ($62.76). Corey owes $15.69 for his service with Dr. Anholm.

Figure 16-20 ◆ Sample billing when provider is contracted with the insurance carrier.

the medical assistant can request a fax number to send the claim to the customer service representative for processing personally. The medical assistant may also be told that there was an error on the claim. Sometimes, the medical assistant may be able to clarify the error over the phone; other times, the claim will need to be resubmitted. The medical assistant should always document any phone call made to an insurance carrier, noting the date and time of the call, the name of the person spoken to, and the results of the call.

Reconciling Payments and Rejections

Claims are sometimes denied or rejected, many times for errors the medical office made. Incorrect identification numbers, incorrect birthdates, missing diagnosis codes, and missing supporting documentation all delay payment of insurance claims.

Keys to Success
QUICK REFERENCES FOR REASONS FOR DENIED CLAIMS

Reason claim was denied: Need supporting documentation

Tip for avoiding this denial: When calling for preauthorization of any procedure, ask the insurance company customer service representative if supporting documentation will be required. If so, copy the chart notes, operative report, laboratory report, or other documentation and send it in with the CMS-1500 billing form.

Reason claim was denied: Diagnosis code does not match procedure performed

Tip for avoiding this denial: Before sending the claim, look at the diagnosis codes the physician assigns to the patient in the *ICD-9* coding book to verify that the code matches the procedure.

Reason claim was denied: Patient is no longer eligible for coverage

Tip for avoiding this denial: Before scheduling any procedure, call to verify coverage with the insurance carrier.

Reason claim was denied: Missing information on the CMS 1500 claim form

Tip for avoiding this denial: Quickly scan all CMS 1500 claim forms prior to sending to determine any missing information or blank boxes.

Reason claim was denied: Past timely filing limits

Tip for avoiding this denial: Submit all insurance claim forms in a timely manner, usually within 30 days of the date of the procedure.

Reason claim was denied: Preauthorization was not obtained before performing the service

Tip for avoiding this denial: Before scheduling any procedure, call to verify coverage with the insurance carrier.

Attention to detail in the claim submission process saves time and effort in the end.

A **rejected** claim is one that never entered the carrier's system due to an incorrect identification number or similar technical problem. These are often returned to the provider during the EMC process. Rejected claims should be corrected and resubmitted as a new claim. A **denied** claim is one the carrier received and processed but did not pay due to benefits or coverage issues. The reason for denial is usually listed on the EOB. Be careful to differentiate between denials of total charges and disallowances. Disallowances represent partial payment on claims because they are above the maximum allowable fee. If the reason cannot be determined or the medical assistant or patient disagrees with the reason, a telephone call should be placed to the insurance company. Often denials can be handled on the phone. If a corrected claim needs to be resubmitted, the carrier should provide specific directions on how to do this. Denied claims that are resubmitted as new claims, rather than corrected claims, will usually be rejected due to a duplicate date of service.

Submitting a formal **appeal** is very different from submitting a new claim because an appeal involves extra time and paperwork. Additional information and paperwork must be supplied, and detailed clinical information that may involve the physician might also be requested by the carrier. The appeals process involves a lot of administrative work by the medical assistant and other staff members. Because the appeals process is time consuming, it is often not done properly or consistently. Rather than appeal, some facilities take the "easy road" by submitting a statement to the patient and requiring the patient to deal with the carrier, instead of doing so themselves.

If the decision is made to go ahead with an appeal, the first step is to know and follow the appeals policy of the payer. For example, medical assistants must register the appeal in a timely manner because there is often a cutoff date for doing so. Most practices learn about the appeals policies of the major plans they work with by referring to physician administrative manuals, contracts, and newsletters. Plan representatives may also be contacted to learn about specific policies. In general, an appeal includes writing a letter that clearly states why the provider believes the denial was not justified. It is best to be clear and factual rather than emotional, angry, or threatening when writing appeal letters. Attach the EOB and any additional supporting documentation to the letter. Be aware that some plans are instituting paperless review procedures, which will decrease the time spent gathering and documenting detailed information.*

Assistants should also send a copy to the patients. Because health care coverage is an agreement between the patient and the insurance carrier, the patient often gets better results when requesting an appeal. For this reason, the medical assistant should always ask the patient to become involved in any appeal process.

*Source: Adapted from Vines, Deborah, Braceland, Ann, Rollins, Elizabeth, and Miller, Susan. *Comprehensive Health Insurance: Billing, Coding, and Reimbursement.* © 2008, p. 473. Reprinted by permission of Pearson Education, Inc. Upper Saddle River, NJ.

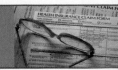

PROCEDURE 16-5 Abstract Data to Complete a Paper CMS-1500 Claim Form

Theory and Rationale

Even though few offices still complete CMS-1500 forms manually and without the aid of a computer, some small offices do. Proper completion of a paper CMS-1500 claim acquaints medical assistants with the form locator fields and data requirements, all of which will be required when using a computer program. This procedure allows medical assistants to focus on how to abstract or locate required information from the source documents without learning a computer software program at the same time.

Materials

- Klaus Davies patient registration form (Figure 16-21 ◆)
- Insurance ID card (Figure 16-22 ◆)
- Encounter form (Figure 16-23 ◆)
- Capital City Medical fee schedule (Figure 16-24 ◆)
- Table 16-2: Instructions on Completing the CMS-1500 Claim Form
- blank CMS-1500 form (photocopy Figure 16-16 or obtain from instructor)
- black ink pen
- calculator

Competency

(**Conditions**) With the necessary materials, you will be able to (**Task**) abstract data from the medical record to complete a CMS-1500 form (**Standards**) correctly within the time limit set by the instructor.

Refer to Table 16-1 to identify how each field is to be completed and where to find the information. Print all information neatly, in capital letters, with a pen. Erasing, crossouts, write-overs and white-out may not be used. You may wish to fill in a draft form in pencil, then recopy it in ink when finished.

1. Enter the insurance company name and mailing address in the carrier area.
2. Check the correct box in FL 1.
3. Enter the insured's ID number in FL 1a.
4. Enter the patient's name in FL 2.
5. Complete FL 3.
6. Complete FL 4.
7. Enter the patient's address and phone in FL 5. Note there are 3 lines of information to complete.
8. Complete FL 6.
9. Leave FL 7 blank.
10. Complete FL 8 for marital status and employment status.
11. Leave FL 9a to 9d blank.
12. Complete FL 10a, 10b, and 10c.
13. Leave FL 10d blank.
14. Enter the group number in FL 11.
15. Leave FL 11a blank.

16. Enter the employer in FL 11b.
17. Enter the insurance plan name in FL 11c.
18. Mark NO in Fl 11d.
19. Enter "SOF" in FL 12.
20. Enter "SOF" in FL 13.
21. Leave FL 14 to FL 19 blank.
22. Mark NO in FL 20.
23. Enter the first diagnosis code in FL 21, line 1.
24. Enter the second diagnosis code in FL 21, line 2.
25. Leave Fl 22 to FL 23 blank.
26. In FL 24A, line on, enter the date of service in both the FROM and TO fields.
27. Enter the code number for place of service in FL 24B.
28. Leave FL 24C blank.
29. Enter the first CPT code in FL 24D.
30. In FL 24E enter "1 2" to designate that both diagnoses 1 and 2 relate to this service.
31. Look on the encounter form to find the description for CPT code 99231. Then look on the fee schedule to find the fee for this service and enter it in FL 24F.
32. Enter 1 for units in FL 24G.
33. Leave blank FL 24H and FL 24I.
34. Enter the physician's NPI number on the unshaded portion of 24J. You will find this on the encounter form.
35. Repeat these steps for lines 2 through 6. In FL 24E be certain you designate the correct diagnoses reference for each service, as some lines will be only "1" or only "2".
36. When all services are completed, enter the EIN in FL 25 and mark X in the appropriate box. You will find this on the patient registration form.
37. Enter the patient's account number in FL 26. You will find this on the patient registration form.
38. Leave FL 27 blank.
39. Add up the total charges in column 24F. Write the total in FL 28.
40. Leave FL 29 and FL 30 blank.
41. Enter the physician's signature, credentials, and the date in FL 31. Be certain to stay within the lines of the box.
42. Enter the name and address of the clinic in FL 32.
43. Enter the clinic's group NPI number in 32a. You will find this on the patient registration form.
44. Leave FL 32b blank.
45. In FL 33, enter the clinic's phone number in the top right corner.
46. Enter the clinic's name and address in FL 33.
47. Enter the clinic's NPI number in FL 33a.
48. Leave FL 33b blank.
49. Proofread your work. Check all spelling and numbers against your source documents.
50. Check your claim against the sample CMS-1500 form in Figure 16-25 ◆.

continued

PROCEDURE 16-5 Abstract Data to Complete a Paper CMS-1500 Claim Form (continued)

Capital City Medical—123 Unknown Boulevard, Capital City, NY 12345-2222 (555)555-1234 Phil Wells, MD, Mannie Mends, MD, Bette R. Soone, MD	Patient Information Form Tax ID: 75-0246810 Group NPI: 1513171216

Patient Information:

Name: (Last, First) <u>Davies, Klaus</u>   ☒ Male ❑ Female   Birth Date: <u>10/24/1965</u>

Address: <u>19 Willow Rd. Capital City, NY 12345</u>   Phone: (555) <u>555-1276</u>

Social Security Number: <u>631-03-4305</u>   Full-Time Student: ❑ Yes   ☒ No

Marital Status: ❑ Single   ☒ Married   ❑ Divorced   ❑ Other

- -

Employment:

Employer: <u>Organic Food Mart</u>   Phone: ( ) <u>(555) 555-5619</u>

Address: <u>13 Mile Blvd, Township, NY 12345</u>

Condition Related to: ❑ Auto Accident   ❑ Employment   ❑ Other Accident

Date of Accident: _____ State _____

Emergency Contact: _____   **Phone: ( )** _____

- -

Primary Insurance: <u>Blue Cross Blue Shield PPO</u>   Phone: ( ) _____

Address: <u>379 Blue Plaza, Capital City, NY 12345</u>

Insurance Policyholder's Name: <u>Same</u>   ❑ M ❑ F DOB: _____

Address: _____

Phone: _____ Relationship to Insured: ☒ Self ❑ Spouse ❑ Child ❑ Other

Employer: _____   Phone: _____

Employer's Address: _____

Policy/ID No: <u>YYZ8436489</u>   Group No: <u>326463</u> Percent Covered: ___%, Copay Amt: $<u>35.00</u>

- -

Secondary Insurance: _____   Phone: ( ) _____

Address: _____

Insurance Policyholder's Name: _____   ❑ M ❑ F DOB: _____

Address: _____

Phone: _____ Relationship to Insured: ❑ Self ❑ Spouse ❑ Child ❑ Other

Employer: _____   Phone: ( ) _____

Employer's Address: _____

Policy/ID No: _____   Group No: _____ Percent Covered: ___%, Copay Amt: $_____

- -

Reason for Visit: <u>Need my blood pressure and cholesterol checked today</u>

Known Allergies: _____

Were you referred here? If so, by whom?: _____

Figure 16-21 ◆ Klaus Davies sample patient registration form.

PROCEDURE 16-5 **Abstract Data to Complete a Paper CMS-1500 Claim Form** *(continued)*

  BlueCross BlueShield | **PPO**

Group Name **ORGANIC FOOD MART**

ID **YY28436489**   Group **32643**   BC Plan **252** BC Plan **353**

Subscriber/Dependents   M RX
01: KLAUS DAVIES   Y Y
02: SARA DAVIES   Y Y

Card Issue Date   10/09/XX

An independent License of the Blue Cross and Blue Shield Association

Provider: Please submit medical and/or vision claims to your local Blue Cross and/or Blue Shield plan in whose Service Area the Member received services. Submit all other claims to 379 BLUE PLZ CAPITAL CITY NY 12345

Member: To locate a preferred or participating Blue Provider outside your service area please call 1 (555) 810-BLUE (2583). For all other questions, please call 1-555-9978 This card is not an authorization for services or a guarantee of payment.

PPP Network   DED $300: COMP CARE $35 COPAY
                           IN-NTWK 20%/OUT-NTWK 40%

REGENCE RX BIN **09870**   PCN **246800**

OV $35   ER $100 $10 GEN
SP $50 $35   FORM
                       $50   NON-FORM

Figure 16-22 ◆ Klaus Davies sample insurance ID card.

continued

Patient Name <u>Klaus Davies</u>

Capital City Medical
123 Unknown Boulevard, Capital City, NY 12345-2222
Physician: Phil Wells, MD NPI 1234567890

Date of Service
10-26-20XX

New Patient					Laboratory		
Problem Focused	99201	Arthrocentesis/Aspiration/Injection			Amylase	82150	
Expanded Problem, Focused	99202	Small Joint		20600	B12	82607	
Detailed	99203	Interm Joint		20605	CBC & Diff	85025	X
Comprehensive	99204	Major Joint		20610	Comp Metabolic Panel	80053	
Comprehensive/High Complex	99205	**Other Invasive/Noninvasive**			Chlamydia Screen	87110	
Well Exam Infant (up to 12 mos.)	99381	Audiometry		92552	Cholesterol	82465	
Well Exam 1–4 yrs.	99382	Cast Application			Digoxin	80162	
Well Exam 5–11 yrs.	99383	Location Long Short			Electrolytes	80051	
Well Exam 12–17 yrs.	99384	Catheterization		51701	Ferritin	82728	
Well Exam 18–39 yrs.	99385	Circumcision		54150	Folate	82746	
Well Exam 40–64 yrs.	99386	Colposcopy		57452	GC Screen	87070	
		Colposcopy w/Biopsy		57454	Glucose	82947	
		Cryosurgery Premalignant Lesion			Glucose 1 HR	82950	
		Location (s):			Glycosylated HGB A1C	83036	
Established Patient		Cryosurgery Warts			HCT	85014	
Post-Op Follow Up Visit	99024	Location (s):			HDL	83718	
Minimum	99211	Curettement Lesion			Hep BSAG	87340	
Problem Focused	99212	Single		11055	Hepatitis panel, acute	80074	
Expanded Problem Focused	99213 X	2–4		11056	HGB	85018	
Detailed	99214	>4		11057	HIV	86703	
Comprehensive/High Complex	99215	Diaphragm Fitting		57170	Iron & TIBC	83550	
Well Exam Infant (up to 12 mos.)	99391	Ear Irrigation		69210	Kidney Profile	80069	
Well exam 1–4 yrs.	99392	ECG		93000	Lead	83655	
Well Exam 5–11 yrs.	99393	Endometrial Biopsy		58100	Liver Profile	80076	X
Well Exam 12–17 yrs.	99394	Exc. Lesion Malignant			Mono Test	86308	
Well Exam 18–39 yrs.	99395	Benign			Pap Smear	88155	
Well Exam 40–64 yrs.	99396	Location			Pregnancy Test	84703	
Obstetrics		Exc. Skin Tags (1–15)		11200	Obstetric Panel	80055	
Total OB Care	59400	Each Additional 10		11201	Pro Time	85610	
Injections		Fracture Treatment			PSA	84153	
Administration Sub. / IM	90772	Loc			RPR	86592	
Drug		w/Reduc		w/o Reduc	Sed. Rate	85651	
Dosage		I & D Abscess Single/Simple		10060	Stool Culture	87045	
Allergy	95115	Multiple or Comp		10061	Stool O & P	87177	
Cocci Skin Test	86490	I & D Pilonidal Cyst Simple		10080	Strep Screen	87880	
DPT	90701	Pilonidal Cyst Complex		10081	Theophylline	80198	
Hemophilus	90646	IV Therapy—To One Hour		90760	Thyroid Uptake	84479	
Influenza	90658	Each Additional Hour		90761	TSH	84443	
MMR	90707	Laceration Repair			Urinalysis	81000	
OPV	90712	Location Size Simp/Comp			Urine Culture	87088	
Pneumovax	90732	Laryngoscopy		31505	Drawing Fee	36415	X
TB Skin Test	86580	Oximetry		94760	Specimen Collection	99000	
TD	90718	Punch Biopsy			**Other:**		
Unlisted Immun	90749	Rhythm Strip		93040			
Tetanus Toxoid	90703	Treadmill		93015			
Vaccine/Toxoid Admin <8 Yr Old w/ Counseling	90465	Trigger Point or Tendon Sheath Inj.		20550			
Vaccine/Toxoid Administration for Adult	90471	Tympanometry		92567			
Diagnosis/ICD-9: **401.9, 272.0**							
					Lipid Panel	80061	X

I acknowledge receipt of medical services and authorize the release of any medical information necessary to process this claim for healthcare payment only. I do authorize payment to the provider.

Patient Signature *Klaus Davies*

Total Estimated Charges: _____

Payment Amount: _____

Next Appointment: _____

Figure 16-23 ◆ Klaus Davies sample encounter form.

continued

Capital City Medical
Fee Schedule

New Patient OV		Laceration Repair various codes	$60
Problem Focused 99201	$45	Punch Biopsy various codes	$80
Expanded Problem Focused 99202	$65	Nebulizer various codes	$45
Detailed 99203	$85	Cast Application various codes	$85
Comprehensive 99204	$105	Laryngoscopy 31505	$255
Comprehensive/High Complex 99205	$115	Audiometry 92552	$85
Well Exam infant (less than 1 year) 99381	$45	Tympanometry 92567	$85
Well Exam 1–4 yrs. 99382	$50	Ear Irrigation 69210	$25
Well Exam 5–11 yrs. 99383	$55	Diaphragm Fitting 57170	$30
Well Exam 12–17 yrs. 99384	$65	IV Therapy (up to one hour) 90760	$65
Well Exam 18–39 yrs. 99385	$85	Each additional hour 90761	$50
Well Exam 40–64 yrs. 99386	$105	Oximetry 94760	$10
Established Patient OV		ECG 93000	$75
Post Op Follow Up Visit 99024	$0	Holter Monitor various codes	$170
Minimum 99211	$35	Rhythm Strip 93040	$60
Problem Focused 99212	$45	Treadmill 93015	$375
Expanded Problem Focused 99213	$55	Cocci Skin Test 86490	$20
Detailed 99214	$65	X-ray, spine, chest, bone—any area various codes	$275
Comprehensive/High Complex 99215	$75	Avulsion Nail 11730	$200
Well exam infant (less than 1 year) 99391	$35	**Laboratory**	
Well Exam 1–4 yrs. 99392	$40	Amylase 82150	$40
Well Exam 5–11 yrs. 99393	$45	B12 82607	$30
Well Exam 12–17 yrs. 99394	$55	CBC & Diff 85025	$95
Well Exam 18–39 yrs. 99395	$65	Comp Metabolic Panel 80053	$75
Well Exam 40–64 yrs. 99396	$75	Chlamydia Screen 87110	$70
Obstetrics		Cholestrerol 82465	$75
Total OB Care 59400	$1700	Digoxin 80162	$40
Injections		Electrolytes 80051	$70
Administration 90772	$10	Estrogen, Total 82672	$50
Allergy 95115	$35	Ferritin 82728	$40
DPT 90701	$50	Folate 82746	$30
Drug various codes	$35	GC Screen 87070	$60
Influenza 90658	$25	Glucose 82947	$35
MMR 90707	$50	Glycosylated HGB A1C 83036	$45
OPV 90712	$40	HCT 85014	$30
Pneumovax 90732	$35	HDL 83718	$35
TB Skin Test 86580	$15	HGB 85018	$30
TD 90718	$40	Hep BSAG 83740	$40
Tetanus Toxoid 90703	$40	Hepatitis panel, acute 80074	$95
Vaccine/Toxoid Administration for Younger		HIV 86703	$100
Than 8 Years Old w/ counseling 90465	$10	Iron & TIBC 83550	$45
Vaccine/Toxoid Administration for Adult 90471	$10	Kidney Profile 80069	$95
Arthrocentesis/Aspiration/Injection		Lead 83665	$55
Small Joint 20600	$50	Lipase 83690	$40
Interm Joint 20605	$60	Lipid Panel 80061	$95
Major Joint 20610	$70	Liver Profile 80076	$95
Trigger Point/Tendon Sheath Inj. 20550	$90	Mono Test 86308	$30
Other Invasive/Noninvasive Procedures		Pap Smear 88155	$90
Catheterization 51701	$55	Pap Collection/Supervision 88142	$95
Circumcision 54150	$150	Pregnancy Test 84703	$90
Colposcopy 57452	$225	Obstetric Panel 80055	$85
Colposcopy w/Biopsy 57454	$250	Pro Time 85610	$50
Cryosurgery Premalignant Lesion various codes	$160	PSA 84153	$50
Endometrial Biopsy 58100	$190	RPR 86592	$55
Excision Lesion Malignant various codes	$145	Sed. Rate 85651	$50
Excision Lesion Benign various codes	$125	Stool Culture 87045	$80
Curettement Lesion		Stool O & P 87177	$105
Single 11055	$70	Strep Screen 87880	$35
2–4 11056	$80	Theophylline 80198	$40
>4 11057	$90	Thyroid Uptake 84479	$75
Excision Skin Tags (1–15) 11200	$55	TSH 84443	$50
Each Additional 10 11201	$30	Urinalysis 81000	$35
I & D Abscess Single/Simple 10060	$75	Urine Culture 87088	$80
Multiple/Complex 10061	$95	Drawing Fee 36415	$15
I & D Pilonidal Cyst Simple 10080	$105	Specimen Collection 99000	$10
I & D Pilonidal Cyst Complex 10081	$130		

Figure 16-24 ◆ Capital City Medical fee schedule.

continued

(1500)

HEALTH INSURANCE CLAIM FORM
APPROVED BY NATIONAL UNIFORM CLAIM COMMITTEE 08/05

BLUE CROSS BLUE SHIELD
379 BLUE PLZ
CAPITAL CITY NY   12345

☐☐ PICA | CARRIER | PICA ☐☐

1. MEDICARE ☐(Medicare #) MEDICAID ☐(Medicaid #) TRICARE CHAMPUS ☐(Sponsor's SSN) CHAMPVA ☐(Member ID#) GROUP HEALTH PLAN ☐(SSN or ID) FECA BLK LUNG ☐(SSN) OTHER ☒(ID)

1a. INSURED'S I.D. NUMBER (For Program in Item 1)
YYZ8436489

2. PATIENT'S NAME (Last Name, First Name, Middle Initial)
DAVIES KLAUS

3. PATIENT'S BIRTH DATE   SEX
MM DD YY
10 24 1965   M☒ F☐

4. INSURED'S NAME (Last Name, First Name, Middle Initial)
SAME

5. PATIENT'S ADDRESS (No, Street)
19 WILLOW RD

6. PATIENT RELATIONSHIP TO INSURED
Self☒ Spouse☐ Child☐ Other☐

7. INSURED'S ADDRESS (No, Street)

CITY
CAPITAL CITY

STATE
NY

8. PATIENT STATUS
Single☐ Married☒ Other☐

CITY

STATE

ZIP CODE
12345

TELEPHONE (Include Area Code)
(555) 5551276

Full-Time Part-Time
Employed☒ Student☐ Student☐

ZIP CODE

TELEPHONE (Include Area Code)
( )

9. OTHER INSURED'S NAME (Last Name, First Name, Middle Initial)

10. IS PATIENT'S CONDITION RELATED TO:

11. INSURED'S POLICY GROUP OR FECA NUMBER
326463

a. OTHER INSURED'S POLICY OR GROUP NUMBER

a. EMPLOYMENT? (Current or Previous)
☐YES ☒NO

a. INSURED'S DATE OF BIRTH   SEX
MM DD YY
04   M☐ F☐

b. OTHER INSURED'S DATE OF BIRTH   SEX
MM DD YY   M☐ F☐

b. AUTO ACCIDENT?   PLACE (State)
☐YES ☒NO

b. EMPLOYER'S NAME OR SCHOOL NAME
ORGANIC FOOD MART

c. EMPLOYER'S NAME OR SCHOOL NAME

c. OTHER ACCIDENT?
☐YES ☒NO

c. INSURANCE PLAN NAME OR PROGRAM NAME
BLUE CROSS BLUE SHIELD PPO

d. INSURANCE PLAN NAME OR PROGRAM NAME

10d. RESERVED FOR LOCAL USE

d. IS THERE ANOTHER HEALTH BENEFIT PLAN?
☐YES ☒NO If yes, return to and complete item 9 a-d

READ BACK OF FORM BEFORE COMPLETING & SIGNING THIS FORM.
12. PATIENT'S OR AUTHORIZED PERSON'S SIGNATURE I authorize the release of any medical or other information necessary to process this claim. I also request payment of government benefits either to myself or to the party who accepts assignment below.

SIGNED SOF   DATE

13. INSURED'S OR AUTHORIZED PERSON'S SIGNATURE I authorize payment of medical benefits to the undersigned physician or supplier for services described below.

SIGNED SOF

14. DATE OF CURRENT ILLNESS (First symptom) OR INJURY (Accident) OR PREGNANCY (LMP)
MM DD YY

15. IF PATIENT HAS HAD SAME OR SIMILAR ILLNESS, GIVE FIRST DATE MM DD YY

16. DATES PATIENT UNABLE TO WORK IN CURRENT OCCUPATION
FROM MM DD YY   TO MM DD YY

17. NAME OF REFERRING PHYSICIAN OR OTHER SOURCE

17a.
17b. NPI

18. HOSPITALIZATION DATES RELATED TO CURRENT SERVICES
FROM MM DD YY   TO MM DD YY

19. RESERVED FOR LOCAL USE

20. OUTSIDE LAB? $ CHARGES
☐YES ☒NO

21. DIAGNOSIS OR NATURE OF ILLNESS OR INJURY (Relate Items 1,2,3 or 4 to Item 24E by Line)
1. 401 9   3.
2. 272 0   4.

22. MEDICAID RESUBMISSION
CODE   ORIGINAL REF. NO.

23. PRIOR AUTHORIZATION NUMBER

24. A. DATE(S) OF SERVICE						B. PLACE OF SERVICE	C. EMG	D. PROCEDURES, SERVICES, OR SUPPLIES (Explain Unusual Circumstances)		E. DIAGNOSIS POINTER	F. $ CHARGES	G. DAYS OR UNITS	H. EPSDT Family Plan	I. ID. QUAL.	J. RENDERING PROVIDER ID. #
From MM	DD	YY	To MM	DD	YY			CPT/HCPCS	MODIFIER						
1 10	26	XX	10	26	XX	11		99213		12	55 00	1		NPI	1234567890
2 10	26	XX	10	26	XX	11		85025		1	95 00	1		NPI	1234567890
3 10	26	XX	10	26	XX	11		80061		2	95 00	1		NPI	1234567890
4 10	26	XX	10	26	XX	11		80076		2	95 00	1		NPI	1234567890
5 10	26	XX	10	26	XX	11		36415		12	15 00	1		NPI	1234567890
6														NPI	

25. FEDERAL TAX ID NUMBER   SSN EIN
750246810   ☐☒

26. PATIENT'S ACCOUNT NO.
A8

27. ACCEPT ASSIGNMENT? (For govt. claims, see back)
☐YES ☐NO

28. TOTAL CHARGE
$ 355 00

29. AMOUNT PAID
$

30. BALANCE DUE
$

31. SIGNATURE OF PHYSICIAN OR SUPPLIER INCLUDING DEGREES OR CREDENTIALS (I certify that the statements on the reverse apply to this bill and are made a part thereof)
Phil Wells MD   10/26/XX
SIGNED   DATE

32. SERVICE FACILITY LOCATION INFORMATION
CAPITAL CITY MEDICAL
123 UNKNOWN BLVD
CAPITAL CITY NY 12345
a. 1513171216   b.

33. BILLING PROVIDER INFO & PH. # (555) 5551234
CAPITAL CITY MEDICAL
123 UNKNOWN BLVD
CAPITAL CITY NY 12345
a. 1513171216   b.

NUCC Instruction Manual available at: www.nucc.org
WCMS-1500CS

APPROVED OMB 0938-0999 FORM CMS-1500 (08/05)

Figure 16-25 ◆ Klaus Davies completed CMS-1500 form.

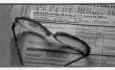

PROCEDURE 16-6 Complete a Computerized Insurance Claim Form

Theory and Rationale

Proper completion of the CMS-1500 insurance claim form is vital to prompt payment of claims in the medical office. So that forms print properly, medical assistants must accurately enter necessary patient data in the computer system.

Materials

- Computer with medical billing software
- Patient medical chart
- Fee slip for patient's visit

Competency

(**Conditions**) With the necessary materials, you will be able to (**Task**) complete an insurance claim form (**Standards**) correctly within the time limit set by the instructor.

1. Choose the patient's account ledger in the computer billing software.
2. Verify that the fee slip is for the patient with the account opened on the computer.
3. Enter the charges and coding as appropriate.
4. Complete the patient insurance information field.
5. Enter the patient's information, including address, telephone number, and birth date.
6. Enter the insured's information, including address, telephone number, and birth date.

7. Enter the patient's relationship to the insured.
8. Enter the insured's identification and group number.
9. Check the appropriate box to indicate the patient has authorized the release of information to the insurance company.
10. Check the appropriate box to indicate the patient has assigned the benefits (payment) to the provider.
11. Check the appropriate boxes to indicate if the visit was related to an accident.
12. If the visit was due to an accident, enter the accident's date.
13. Enter any information regarding a referring physician, if applicable.
14. Enter any information regarding the patient's need for hospitalization for these charges, if applicable.
15. Enter the treating provider's name, address, telephone number, national provider identification (NPI) number, and Internal Revenue Service (**IRS**) tax identification number.
16. Enter information regarding the facility where the services were performed if not performed in the provider's office.
17. Check the appropriate box to indicate the provider accepts assignment.
18. Print the patient's insurance claim form.
19. Review the form for accuracy and completeness.
20. Send the claim to the insurance company.

Sending Supporting Documentation

Many insurance plans require supporting documentation, things like chart notes, surgical/operative reports, laboratory reports, pathology reports, before they will pay for certain, usually high-cost services, like surgeries (Figure 16-26 ◆). When calling insurance carriers to obtain preauthorization for services, medical assistants should ask customer service representatives if they need supporting documentation with the insurance claim forms. Sending proper documentation with the CMS-1500 billing form often avoids claims return and therefore delayed payment.

At other times, the insurance will ask for additional documentation while reviewing the claim. The request usually comes in the form of a letter. When replying to such requests, medical assistants should be certain to identify exactly what information is being requested and respond specifically. It is not necessary to send a voluminous amount of records when only one or two specific items are being requested.

With worker's compensation and TPL claims, carriers may request a progress report. A written progress report clearly describes the extent of the patient's recovery since the injury, what further treatment is needed, and the expected result. Include any test results such as X-rays, lab tests, or physical function tests, such as range of motion or lifting capacity, to document the patient's status. Medical assistants should respond to such requests immediately because no further payment will be made on the claim until the report is received. Medical assistants may have the responsibility of abstracting the pertinent information from the medical record, drafting the report and presenting it to the provider for review and signature.

The Office of the Insurance Commissioner

Each state has an Office of the Insurance Commissioner, a valuable resource for both the medical office and the patient. When medical assistants or patients believe claims were incorrectly processed and appeal attempts have been fruitless, assistants may file formal written complaints with the state's insurance commissioner. It is important to involve patients in this process because they are the consumer the insurance commissioner is charged with protecting. Patients may be reluctant to appeal to the commissioner on their own initiative because they are unfamiliar with the process. One good approach is for medical assistants to write a letter on behalf of the patient and ask the patient to sign it. Sometimes, the threat of complaint alone can inspire insurance carriers to review denied claims.

OPERATION DATE: 10/7/08

SURGEON: GREGORY PROVENCE, MD

PREOPERATIVE DIAGNOSIS:

Right parotid mass.

POSTOPERATIVE DIAGNOSIS:

Same.

PROCEDURE:

Right deep lobe parotid resection, removal of right parotid tumor with facial nerve preservation and with facial nerve monitoring.

DESCRIPTION OF PROCEDURE:

The patient is a 54-year old female who noted a growing mass in the right parotid area. Fine needle biopsy reported benign cells and CT scan confirmed a large bilobed cystic lesion. Risks, expectations, complications, procedure and alternative treatment measures were discussed prior to consent.

FINDINGS:

A bilobed tumor extending medial to the facial nerve branches into the "turquoise" space superior to the thyroid process and most of the deep lobe parotid were absent. Facial nerve was preserved with the facial nerve monitoring.

General endotracheal anesthesia was given. 1% Xylocaine was used for facial skin infiltration. Incision was drawn with an ink pen and incision was carried along the preauricular crease around the "yellow" lobule to the upper neck along the skin crease. Incision carried through the platysmas and the sternomastoid muscle and the external ear canal. The posterior facial vein was identified and dissected laterally, lifting the gland away from the facial vein for the purpose of identifying the lower branch of the facial nerve. Superiorly, the facial branch was identified. It was then carefully preserved and as the parotid gland was lifted, the superficial lobe of the parotid gland was lifted laterally and anteriorly. The lower division of the facial nerve was found and medial to the nerve was the tumor. The tumor was then gently grasped with forceps and the lower division was carefully lifted and shifted superiorly as the tumor was shifted inferiorly for excision. Blunt and sharp dissection was made to free the nerve from surrounding tissue. The deep lobe of the parotid was generally absent because of the size of the mass. The mass was cynlindrical bilobed-shaped, and extending beyond the styloid process, placed superior to the styloid process into the "turquoise" space.

Finally the entire tumor was isolated and removed. Bleeding was controlled with bipolar cautery. An Avitene sheet was used for hemostasis. A 15 Blake drain was inserted, secured with 3-0 nylon. The skin incision was closed with 4-0 chromic and 5-0 nylon. Blood loss was about 25 cc. Dressing applied. Antiobiotic ointment was placed on the incision.

The patient was then extubated and sent to the recovery room in good condition. Postop facial nerve function was intact. She was given Keflex for prophylaxis and Lortab 7.5 mg for pain. She will be seen as needed and drain will be removed in the next 48 hours.

GREGORY PROVENCE, MD

Figure 16-26 ◆ Sample operative report.

Projecting Health Insurance Costs in the Future

With the cost of health care and health insurance coverage rising far beyond the rate of inflation in America, most experts would agree that the U.S. health care system will differ dramatically in the future. In the past, many employees were covered by health insurance plans that covered 100 percent of all health care expenses. These plans are few and far between today; the vast majority of employer-provided health insurance policies require patients to share in the cost of their health care in the form of deductibles, coinsurance, and copays.

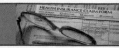

PROCEDURE 16-7 Handle a Denied Insurance Claim

Theory and Rationale

Even after taking care to enter all information into the computer system management software program, insurance claims will occasionally be returned to the medical office. To determine the cause of the denial and the proper action to take, denied claims must be acted on in a timely fashion.

Materials

- Patient insurance information (i.e., ID number, birth date of the insured, name and provider customer service telephone number of insurance company)
- Paper and pen
- Copy of the explanation of benefits (EOB) received
- Description of the procedure the doctor has performed, including CPT code
- Patient's diagnosis pertaining to the procedure performed
- Location where procedure was performed (e.g., office, outpatient surgery, inpatient hospitalization)
- Date the procedure was performed
- Any documentation of the service having been preauthorized by the office

Competency

(**Conditions**) With the necessary materials, you will be able to (**Task**) handle a denied insurance claim (**Standards**) correctly within the time limit set by the instructor.

1. Organize all materials.
2. Call the insurance company's provider customer service phone number as listed on the patient's insurance identification card.
3. Write down the date and time of the telephone call, the number called, and the name of the customer service representative on the phone.
4. Self-identify to the customer service representative, and provide the patient's identification number and date of service.
5. If the service was preauthorized, give that information to the customer service representative.
6. Ask the customer service representative why the procedure was not paid as anticipated.
7. If there was an error in processing the service for payment, ask the customer service representative if any other information is needed to process the claim correctly. Ask the customer service representative when the office can expect payment for the procedure.
8. If the customer service representative says the claim was correctly processed, request the reason for the denial.
9. If the reason for the denial was lack of supporting documentation, ask the customer service representative if faxing the information is a solution. If the answer is yes, get the customer service representative's direct fax line and fax the needed documentation.
10. If the reason for the denial requires an appeal be filed, ask the customer service representative to explain the insurance company's process for appeals.
11. Write down any pertinent information, such as where to mail the appeal and what information the appeal should contain.
12. Call the patient with the findings and get the patient involved as needed.

One possibility for the future is for employers to offer employees vouchers for health insurance coverage. Employees could use these vouchers to purchase plans that suit their needs. In an attempt to find ways to cover the 47 million Americans currently without health insurance coverage, experts studying these types of plans believe all Americans could be offered tax incentives or rebates for purchasing health insurance coverage. Whatever the future may bring, the administrative medical assistant should stay current on the legislation that affects health care and health insurance coverage, both locally and nationally.

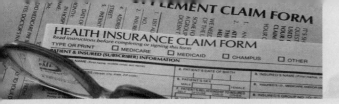

Chapter Summary

- Medical assistants play a central role in insurance claim processing and are responsible for accuracy and responsiveness as well as patient relations.
- Health insurance in the United States began in the mid-1800s. The first group policy giving comprehensive benefits was offered by Massachusetts Health Insurance of Boston in 1847. Insurance companies issued the first individual disability and illness policies around 1890. Hospital insurance coverage began in 1929. During World War II, when wages froze, employers began offering their employees group health insurance as a benefit. Employee benefit plans became popular in the 1940s and 1950s. During the 1950s and 1960s government programs began to cover healthcare costs. Social security coverage included disability benefits for the first time in 1954 and the government created the Medicare and Medicaid programs in 1965. By the end of 1995, individuals and companies paid for about one-half of the health care received in the United States, with the government paying for the other half. The 1980s and 1990s saw a rapid rise in the cost of health care. During this time, the majority of employer-sponsored group insurance plans moved to less expensive managed care plans.
- Americans obtain health insurance from a variety of sources. Medical assistants need to be knowledgeable about the rules and requirements of each. They must understand insurance terminology in order to help patients utilize their health insurance. Patients are often unfamiliar with their insurance benefits and may not understand the terms they hear. MAs who understand insurance terms can advocate for patients and communicate in ways that patients understand.
- A number of national commercial insurance carriers offer health insurance coverage. Examples include Blue Cross/Blue Shield, Aetna, and Cigna. Policies might be purchased by employers for a group of employees or by individuals who lack health insurance through their places of employment. Coverage amounts and premiums vary according to policy type.
- The most common sources of private health insurance are group insurance, self-insured plans, and individual insurance.
- The federal Consolidated Omnibus Reconciliation Act (COBRA) requires employers to extend health insurance coverage at group rates, usually for up to 18 months, to any employee who is laid off, quits, or is fired, except under certain circumstances.
- The HMO Act of 1973 and the Tax Equity and Fiscal Responsibility Act (TEFRA) introduced health insurance plans that allow patients a variety of ways to access providers and share in the cost of care. These various plans differ in how insurance companies pay providers.
- Managed care plans control the costs associated with plan purchase by controlling the amounts they reimburse healthcare providers. MCOs contract with healthcare providers to provide care for a certain group of patients. Managed care plans are divided into the following types: Health Mainte-

- nance Organizations (HMOs), Preferred Provider Organizations (PPOs), Exclusive Provider Organizations (EPOs), and Point of Service Plans (POS). These healthcare plans all support the insurance needs of patient populations, but in varying ways and at varying levels of cost and coverage.
- It is important for the medical assistant to be familiar with all aspects of the Medicare program, divided into Parts A, B, C, and D, as more and more patients will be covered by this type of insurance as the U.S. population ages.
- Medicare and Medicaid both provide vital services such as hospitalization, physician visits, and prescription drug coverage to substantial patient populations.
- Medigap or Medicare supplemental plans are insurance plans offered by private companies to reimburse patients for the out-of-pocket expenses they incur with Medicare.
- In 1997, the State Children's Health Insurance Program (SCHIP) was created to cover children who do not have another form of health insurance coverage. It is similar to Medicaid, in that SCHIP was designed to function as a federal/state joint program.
- The TRICARE and CHAMPVA programs deliver insurance coverage to patients who are in the military or families of military members.
- Worker's compensation is a program designed to provide employees who are injured on the job with an insurance safety net.
- It is important for medical assistants to understand how reimbursement affects the practice. Insurance companies reimburse providers using a variety of methods; however, the most traditional method is a usual, customary, and reasonable (UCR) fee schedule. Other reimbursement methods include a negotiated fee schedule, capitation, per-diem payment method, or per-case payments. When Medicare uses a per case form of reimbursement, it is called Diagnosis Related Groups (DRG).
- Health care claim preparation is an involved process that requires attention to detail, knowledge of health care regulations, and the ability to interface with a broad array of healthcare entities.
- The CMS-1500 claim form is used by all health insurance carriers, including Medicare, Medicaid, and worker's compensation carriers, to complete paper billed claims. The form is divided into two major sections and includes 33 form locators (boxes to be completed on the form).
- Electronic claims are submitted to the insurance carrier via a central processing unit (CPU), tape diskette, direct data entry, direct wire, telephone line via modem, or personal computer. Medicare requires electronic transmission of claims for providers with ten or more employees or facilities with 25 or more employees.
- Providers have different methods for determining their fee structure. Two main methods used for determining fees are charge-based and resource-based fee structures.

Chapter Summary (continued)

- Once an insurance carrier has processed a claim, a check is sent to the healthcare provider with an Explanation of Benefits (EOB) statement. Medical assistants must check EOBs to ensure all services that were billed are accurately listed and that service payment matches the amount in the insurance company contract.
- Medical assistants should call insurance carriers to follow up on or trace claims that are past due. Each state has its own guidelines that outline the timeframe within which an insurance carrier must pay or deny a claim.
- Claims can be rejected or denied for errors made by the medical office. Attention to detail in the claim submission process saves time and effort in the end.

- The Office of the Insurance Commissioner is a valuable resource for both the medical office and the patient. Assistants may file formal written complaints with the state's insurance commissioner.
- Many experts believe that due to the rising costs of health care and health insurance coverage, the U.S. healthcare system will differ dramatically in the future. Today, the vast majority of employer-provided health insurance policies require patients to share in the cost of their health care in the form of deductibles, coinsurance, and copays.

Chapter Review

Multiple Choice

1. Typically, the most expensive health plans to buy are:
   a. Employer provided
   b. Individual
   c. Medicare Part B
   d. Medicare Part A

2. With most insurance carriers, timely filing limits refer to submitting claims within _____ days from the date of service.
   a. 365
   b. 120
   c. 45
   d. 30

3. The best way to trace an overdue insurance claim is to:
   a. Send another copy of the original claim
   b. Send a bill to the patient
   c. Call the insurance company regarding the claim
   d. Call the state's Office of the Insurance Commissioner

4. Which of the following might be eligible for COBRA benefits?
   a. Recently fired employee
   b. Recently laid off employee
   c. Employee who recently quit
   d. All of the above

5. Consumer-directed health care plans:
   a. Offer patients a wide variety of in-network physicians
   b. Cause patients to be more aware of health care costs
   c. Are offered by Medicare
   d. Are called "capitated plans"

6. Balance billing occurs when the physician:
   a. Bills the secondary insurance company after receiving payment from the primary insurance company
   b. Bills the primary insurance company
   c. Bills Medicare
   d. Bills the patient an amount that should be written off under the preferred provider contract

7. Using the birthday rule, the parent who is usually primary when billing for a child's services is the parent who:
   a. Has a birthday earlier in the year
   b. Has birthday later in the year
   c. Is older
   d. Is younger

8. Many insurance plans exclude coverage for:
   a. Routine hearing tests
   b. Elective surgery
   c. Plastic surgery
   d. All of the above

9. HIPAA requires medical offices to give patients:
   a. Copies of the office's privacy practices
   b. Access to their medical records on request
   c. Accounts of any disclosures of their medical records on request
   d. All of the above

True/False

T F   1. Many managed care plans require the medical office to obtain preauthorization before rendering certain services to patients.

T F   2. When insurance companies deny payment for services, the only recourse is to bill the patient for the fee directly.

T F   3. Medicare fee schedules are the same wherever physicians practice.

T F   4. Medicaid is funded entirely by each state.

T F   5. Sending any information to an insurance company without the patient's permission violates HIPAA.

Short Answer

1. Explain the term *pre-existing condition* as it applies to health care.

2. Why is it a good idea to start a new file for an existing patient who has just recently been involved in a worker's compensation claim?

Chapter Review (continued)

3. Which other terms mean the same as "subscriber" with regard to health insurance coverage?

4. What is another term for the Medicare advance beneficiary notice?

5. List two reasons a claim might be denied by an insurance company, and suggest how to avoid those denials.

6. What does CMS stand for, and what is its role?

Research

1. Interview a person who works in a medical office. How does that office handle insurance authorizations for patients with managed care?

2. Look at the Medicare Web site. Where is the office for providers in your state to call for help with claims processing or questions?

3. Look at your state's Medicaid Web site. What telephone number do providers in your state call in order to obtain authorization for procedures on a Medicaid-covered patient?

Externship Application Experience

Phyllis Allen is a patient of Dr. King's. The physician would like to have Phyllis scheduled for a biopsy procedure to be performed in the office. What information should the medical assistant gather before calling the insurance carrier? What information should the assistant write down during the telephone call?

Resource Guide

Centers for Medicare and Medicaid Services
7500 Security Boulevard
Baltimore, MD 21244
Phone: (877) 267-2323
www.cms.hhs.gov/

U.S. Department of Defense Military Health System
Skyline 5, Suite 810
5111 Leesburg Pike
Falls Church, VA 22041-3206
http://www.tricare.org/

U.S. Department of Health and Human Services
200 Independence Avenue, SW
Room 509F, HHH Building
Washington, DC 20201
Phone: (800) 368-1019
http://www.hhs.gov/ocr/hipaa/

U.S. Department of Labor
Frances Perkins Building, 200 Constitution Ave., NW
Washington, DC 20210
Phone: (866) 4-USA-DOL
www.dol.gov

 MedMedia

http://www.MyMAKit.com

More on this chapter, including interactive resources, can be found on the Student CD-ROM accompanying this textbook and on http://www.MyMAKit.com.

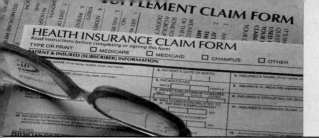

Objectives

After completing this chapter, you should be able to:

- Define and spell the key terminology in this chapter.
- Define the medical assistant's role in diagnostic coding.
- Explain the history of diagnostic coding.
- Describe the function and layout of the ICD-9 coding book.
- List the steps to correctly choose diagnosis codes.
- Explain how to code for various special situations.
- Describe how the medical assistant might purse professional certification.

ICD-9-CM Coding

Case Study

Recently hired in the billing department of Dr. Johnson's medical office, Mary is asked to assign a diagnostic code to a patient's visit and bill for the charges. Unfortunately, Mary has a difficult time deciphering Dr. Johnson's handwriting. After deciding she cannot read the writing in the patient's chart, she says, "Well, it looks like the visit has something to do with the patient's ear, so I'll just code the visit as an earache."

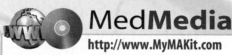

MedMedia
http://www.MyMAKit.com

Additional interactive resources and activities for this chapter can be found on http://www.MyMAKit.com. For a video, tips, audio glossary, legal and ethical scenarios, on-the-job scenarios, quizzes, and games related to the content of this chapter, please access the accompanying CD-ROM in this book.

Video: *Insurance Coding*
Legal and Ethical Scenario: *ICD-9-CM Coding*
On the Job Scenario: *ICD-9-CM Coding*
Tips
Multiple Choice Quiz
Audio Glossary
HIPAA Quiz
Games: Spelling Bee, Crossword, and Strikeout

Key Terminology

adverse reaction—unexpected or dangerous reaction to a drug

and—interpreted as *either/and/or* in a diagnostic code description

category—a three-digit code in ICD-9-CM tabular list

chapter—one of 17 major sections of ICD-9-CM Volume I tabular list, organized by body system and etiology

chief complaint—statement in the patient's own words of the reason for seeking medical care

combination code—a single code that describes two or more conditions that frequently occur together

conventions—ICD-9-CM coding rules, abbreviations, symbols, or formatting intended to ensure consistency in coding

E codes—codes that indicate the external cause of an illness or condition

etiology—cause of a disease or an illness

first listed—the diagnosis that is chiefly responsible for the outpatient services provided; formerly called *primary diagnosis*

late effect—current condition that results from a previous, resolved condition

M codes—identify neoplasm type and tumor behavior; used by tumor registries

main term—words by which conditions and diseases are alphabetized in ICD-9-CM Volume II; may be name of condition, eponym, acronym, or synonym, but not an anatomical site

manifestation—outward or associated condition resulting from an underlying disease

morbidity—cause of illness or injury

mortality—cause of death

multiple coding—a diagnosis that requires more than one ICD-9-CM code to completely describe it; often indicated by a second code in slanted brackets

neoplasm—the medical term for an abnormal growth of new tissue; often referred to as a tumor

---

⊕ MEDICAL ASSISTING STANDARDS

CAAHEP ENTRY-LEVEL STANDARDS	ABHES ENTRY-LEVEL COMPETENCIES
■ Describe how to use the most current diagnostic coding classification system (cognitive) ■ Perform diagnostic coding (psychomotor) ■ Work with physician to achieve the maximum reimbursement (affective)	■ Conduct work within scope of education, training, and ability ■ Monitor legislation related to current health care issues and practices ■ Apply managed care policies and procedures ■ Obtain managed care referrals and precertification ■ Exercise efficient time management ■ Analyze and use current third party guidelines for reimbursement ■ Perform diagnostic coding ■ Implement current procedural terminology and ICD-9 coding

---

✓ COMPETENCY SKILLS PERFORMANCE

1. Perform diagnostic coding.

Introduction

Diagnostic coding is the process of assigning a number to a description of the patient's condition, illness, or disease as it appears in the health care provider's listing in the patient's medical chart. Procedure codes, discussed in ∞ Chapter 18, describe services performed on patients; diagnostic codes outline the reasons services were needed. Diagnostic codes are used to group and identify diseases and illnesses and to track causes of **morbidity** and **mortality.** Diagnostic codes must be accurate, because they inform insurance companies of the severity of patients' conditions and therefore the need for services, procedures, or tests.

The History of Diagnostic Coding

Diagnostic coding has existed for more than a century, beginning in 1893 with French physician Jacques Bertillon. Dr. Bertillon composed the Bertillon Classification of Causes of Death, which the American Public Health Association (**APHA**) adopted in 1898. At the time, the classification contained an alphabetic index and a tabular list, and was quite small compared to coding references used today. The APHA recommended the classification be revised every ten years to ensure it was current.

   In 1901, the APHA published a coding book called the *International Classification of Diseases (ICD), Volume I.* The *ICD-1* was used until 1910, when the second volume, *ICD-2,* was published. Volume updates continued to be published approximately every ten years until the *International Classification of Diseases, Volume 9, Clinical Modification* (ICD-9-CM) was published in 1979.

   ICD-10 was completed in 1999 and has replaced the *ICD-9-CM* in all major countries except the United States. An implementation date for the United States has not been established, but it is expected that there will be a transition period of at least two years. The ICD-10 will

Key Terminology   *(continued)*

nonessential modifiers—words in parentheses after a main term in the ICD-9-CM, clarifying the main term, but need not be present in the medical record

not elsewhere classified (NEC)—code that cannot be found elsewhere in the coding book

not otherwise specified (NOS)—a general code used when details are not available in the medical record

primary diagnosis—patient's chief complaint or reason for visit

principal diagnosis—the reason determined, after study, to be responsible for an inpatient stay

qualified—diagnosis statement accompanied by terms such as possible, probable, suspected, rule out (R/O), or working diag-

nosis, indicating the physician has not determined the root cause

secondary diagnoses—conditions, diseases, or reasons for seeking care in addition to the first-listed diagnosis; they may or may not be related to the first-listed diagnosis

section—an organizational division of a chapter that groups together multiple categories

sequelae—an abnormal condition resulting from a previous injury, condition, or disease

sign—a physical sign of a condition that can observed or measured by a physician

subcategory—a four-digit code in ICD-9-CM tabular list

subclassification—a five-digit code in ICD-9-CM tabular list

subterm—indented two spaces under the boldfaced main term in the ICD-9-CM; further describes the condition, in terms of etiology, co-existing conditions, anatomic site, episode, or similar descriptor

symptom—indication of a condition reported by the patient that the physician cannot observe or measure

synonyms—words of equivalent meaning

tabular list—Volume I of ICD-9-CM which lists all diagnostic codes in numerical order

uncertain—see *qualified*

V codes—codes for visits' reasons, other than disease or illness

with—interpreted as *both, together with* in a diagnostic code description

Abbreviations

AAPC—American Academy of Professional Coders

AHIMA—American Health Information Management Association

APHA—American Public Health Association

CCS-P—Certified Coding Specialist-Physician based

CPC—Certified Professional Coder

DM—diabetes mellitus

ICD-9-CM—*International Classification of Diseases,* 9th Rev., *Clinical Modification*

NEC—not elsewhere classified

NOS—not otherwise specified

TBSA—total body surface area, of burns

provide a revised and expanded code structure that will incorporate updated terminology, make it easier to add codes, such as for new technologies, allow for greater specificity and consistency, and comply with code set standards outlined by HIPAA.

Table 17-1 compares the *ICD-9-CM* and *ICD-10* coding manuals. Once *ICD-10* is incorporated into common use, the *ICD-9-CM* will become obsolete, and physicians, clinics, and hospitals will have to change their electronic and manual coding systems to reflect the new coding structure.

Coding with the *ICD-9-CM* Book

The *ICD-9-CM* book lists the codes to use for any diagnoses physicians give patients. The challenge is to find appropriate codes. Diagnostic codes describe the medical need of visits. If, for example, a patient presents in the office complaining of a headache and sore throat and the physician orders a throat culture, the medical assistant must ensure the claim form carries a diagnostic code that relates to a sore throat. If instead the

TABLE 17-1 COMPARISON OF ICD-9 AND ICD-10

ICD-9-CM	ICD-10
Title: *International Classification of Diseases,* 9th Rev., *Clinical Modifications*	Title: *International Statistical Classification of Diseases and Related Health Problems*
Contains a chapter titled, "Diseases of the Nervous System and Sense Organs"	Divides the chapter into three chapters titled: "Diseases of the Nervous System" "Diseases of the Eye and Adnexa" "Diseases of the Ear and Mastoid Process"
Contains a chapter titled "Mental Disorders"	Renames this chapter "Mental and Behavioral Disorders"
Contains a supplement titled "V Codes"	"V Codes" becomes a chapter rather than a supplement
Contains a supplement titled "E Codes"	"E Codes" becomes a chapter rather than a supplement
Contains numeric codes that require four and five digits	Contains alphanumeric codes that require up to 7 digits and letters
Contains two volumes for diagnosis coding	Contains three volumes for diagnosis coding

medical assistant codes only for a headache, the office will not likely be paid for the throat culture.

Incorrect diagnostic coding may not only impede the office's ability to get paid by the insurance carrier, it may adversely affect the patient's ability to obtain health insurance coverage in the future. Assume the medical assistant incorrectly assigns a patient a diagnostic code for acute myocardial infarction when that patient was treated for chest pain due to heartburn. That patient might be incorrectly perceived as having heart disease and therefore experience insurance coverage issues, such as denial of coverage in the future.

?—Critical Thinking Question 17-1–

Referring to the case study at the beginning of the chapter, what is the potential harm in Mary's guessing at the patient's diagnostic code?

The *ICD-9-CM* lists over 10,000 diagnostic codes in three volumes. ICD-9-CM codes are updated annually and take effect October 1 of each year. Medical assistants should use the edition of the ICD-9-CM that was in effect on the date of service. For example, patients seen on September 30, 2009 would be coded using the 2009 coding manual while those seen on October 1, 2009 would be coded using the 2010 coding manual. The transition date for diagnosis coding differs from the one used for procedural coding, January 1, which will be addressed in Chapter 18. *ICD-9-CM* updates are needed to amend current listings and reflect new diseases or illnesses. The World Health Organization (WHO) has updated ICD codes since 1948. Code changes are published by the National Center for Health Statistics and the Centers for Medicare and Medicaid Services (CMS), in conjunction with the WHO.

The Volumes of ICD-9-CM

Each of the three *ICD-9-CM* volumes has a distinct purpose. Volume I is a tabular list of diseases, Volume II is an alphabetic index of diseases, and Volume III is a tabular list and alphabetic index of hospital procedures. Physicians use Volumes I and II of *ICD-9-CM;* hospitals use all three volumes.

In the physical organization of the manual, Volume II appears first, followed by Volume I, then Volume III. Many publishers print ICD-9-CM manuals for physician offices that contain only Volumes I and II, in order to save on cost. We will first provide an overview of each volume, in the order it appears in the book. Later in the chapter, detailed coding instructions will be presented. Each volume also uses a number of specialized rules, abbreviations, formatting, and symbols called **conventions.** These are described at the beginning of the manual. A key to selected symbols usually appears at the bottom of each page. The conventions and symbols are specific to each volume.

Volume II

Volume II, which appears first in the coding manual, contains two sections.

■ **Section 1: Alphabetic Index to Diseases**—This is the section of the ICD-9-CM that medical assistants need to utilize as the first step in coding. Conditions, diseases, and reasons for seeking medical care are listed alphabetically by **main term** and **subterms** that aid in locating the most appropriate code. After identifying potential codes in the index, they are verified in Volume I, the Tabular List. Final code selection should never be done based only on the index. Section 1 also contains two tables that have cross-tabbed index entries for hypertension and neoplasms. Detailed use of the index and tables will be described later.

■ **Section 2: Alphabetic Index to External Causes of Adverse Effects of Drugs and Other Chemical Substances, Injuries and Poisonings**—When a condition is caused by an accident or poisoning, there are supplemental codes used to describe the circumstances. The first part of this section is the Table of Drugs and Chemicals. This table contains an alphabetical list of drugs and other chemical substances, cross tabbed with a list of causes, to identify poisonings and external causes of drug-related adverse effects, such as drug-induced attempted suicide or an adverse reaction to penicillin. This is followed by an alphabetic index used to locate the external cause of an injury, such as a fall or motor vehicle accident. Detailed use of this will be described later.

Volume I

After locating the diagnosis in the appropriate index in Volume II, it will be verified by referencing the tabular list in Volume I. Volume I is a numerically-sequenced list of all diagnosis codes, divided into 17 chapters based on cause, or **etiology**, of the disease or injury, as well as by location of the disease or injury on or in the body. Every chapter title describes the conditions within, followed by the range of three-digit codes within. Table 17-2 gives an overview of Volume I chapters.

In addition to a title, each Volume I chapter has a subtitle in large print followed by a range of three-digit codes in that category. Each three-digit code combination describes a general disease; subsequent fourth and fifth digits add more specificity. Five-digit codes confer the highest level of definition. Volume I indicates the number of digits needed for coding: three, four, or five. Figure 17-1 ◆ shows sample 3, 4, and 5 digit codes from the ICD-9-CM coding book.

Supplementary Code Listings

Following the 17 chapters listing codes 000-999, there are two sections with supplemental codes. The first of these, Supplementary Classification of Factors Influencing Health Status and Contact with Health Services, are commonly referred to as **V codes,** because these codes begin with the letter "V" and range from V01 to V83 (Figure 17-2 ◆). These codes classify the reason for care, other than an active illness. V codes are located through the alphabetical index in Volume II, Section 1. The second supplementary classification in Volume I is the Supplementary Classification of External Causes of Injury and

TABLE 17-2 CONTENTS OF THE ICD-9-CM VOLUME I

Chapter Number	Chapter Name	Code Numbers Included
1	Infectious and Parasitic Diseases	001–139
2	Neoplasms	140–239
3	Endocrine, Nutritional, and Metabolic Diseases and Immunity Disorders	240–279
4	Diseases of the Blood and Blood-Forming Organs	280–289
5	Mental Disorders	290–319
6	Diseases of the Nervous System and Sense Organs	320–389
7	Diseases of the Circulatory System	390–459
8	Diseases of the Respiratory System	460–519
9	Diseases of the Digestive System	520–579
10	Diseases of the Genitourinary System	580–629
11	Complications of Pregnancy, Childbirth, and the Puerperium	630–677
12	Diseases of the Skin and Subcutaneous Tissue	680–709
13	Diseases of the Musculoskeletal System and Connective Tissue	710–739
14	Congenital Anomalies	740–759
15	Certain Conditions Originating in the Perinatal Period	760–799
16	Symptoms, Signs, and Ill-Defined Conditions	780–799
17	Injury and Poisoning	800–999
	Supplementary	V01–V83
	Classification of Factors Influencing Health Status and Contact with Health Services	
	Supplementary	E800–E999
	Classification of External Causes of Injury and Poisoning	
Appendix A	Morphology of Neoplasms	
Appendix B	Glossary of Mental Disorders	
Appendix C	Classification of Drugs by American Hospital Formulary Service	
Appendix D	Classification of Industrial Accidents	

Poisoning, commonly called **E codes**, because these codes begin with the letter "E" and range from E800-E899 (Figure 17-3 ◆). E codes classify causes of injury and poisoning. E codes are located through the index in Volume I, Section 2.

ICD-9-CM Appendices

Volume I of the ICD-9-CM book has four appendices. These appendices are used as a reference to the user in order to provide a clinical picture or further information about the patient's diagnosis. The appendices are used to further define the diagnosis, to classify new drugs, or to reference the type and cause of on-the-job injury the patient has sustained.

■ **Appendix A: Morphology of Neoplasms**—This appendix provides "M" codes that indicate how neoplasms (tumors)

have morphed to other body areas. **M codes** are not used for billing; they are used only by tumor registries.
■ **Appendix B: Glossary of Mental Disorders**—Appendix B was officially deleted from the ICD-9-CM coding manual on October 1, 2004.
■ **Appendix C: Classification of Drugs by American Hospital Formulary Service**—Each drug currently on the market appears here. This appendix is used to code any adverse effects of drugs on the patient.
■ **Appendix D: Classification of Industrial Accidents**—This appendix describes on-the-job accidents. This list contains codes to describe accidents according to the type or place of accident. The following list shows the categories of on the job accidents and an example of a code found under each list.

3-digit code: 037 Tetanus
4-digit code: 245.0 Acute thyroiditis
5-digit code: 372.05 Acute atopic conjunctivitis

Figure 17-1 ◆ Sample 3-, 4-, and 5-digit codes from the ICD-9-CM coding book.

V61.3 Problems with aged parents or in-laws
V21.0 Period of rapid growth in childhood
V65.44 HIV counseling

Figure 17-2 ◆ Sample V codes.

E836 Machinery accident in water transport

E878.3 Surgical operation with formation of external stoma

E904.0 Abandonment or neglect of infants and helpless persons

Figure 17-3 ◆ Sample E codes.

00.02 Therapeutic ultrasound of the heart

53.61 Incisional hernia repair with prosthesis

87.43 X-ray of ribs, sternum, and clavicle

Figure 17-4 ◆ Sample hospital procedure codes.

■ **Appendix E: List of Three-Digit Categories**—All three-digit categories in the ICD-9-CM book appear here.

Volume III

Because Volume III of *ICD-9-CM* is for inpatient procedure coding, medical assistants will only use it if working in hospital settings. Though medical assistants may be hired by hospital-owned physician practices, the majority of hospitals hire professional certified coders to code inpatient charts.

Volume III contains an Index to Procedures, followed by the Tabular List of Procedures. Hospital procedure codes are three or four digits long and range from 00.01 to 99.99 (Figure 17-4 ◆). Physicians use the CPT manual to code for procedures and services, which will be discussed in Chapter 18.

Determining the Correct Diagnosis Code

Coding begins and ends with the patient's medical record. Medical assistants abstract information from the medical record in order to code for services and the reasons they were provided. Coding is to be done to the highest level of certainty, meaning that all relevant information in the chart should be coded, but missing information should not be assumed or coded. Only

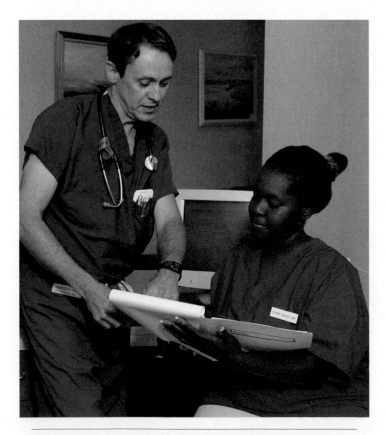

Figure 17-5 ◆ The medical assistant may need to consult the physician in order to obtain the correct code to use.

conditions, diseases, and symptoms documented in the medical record can be coded and billed. If the medical record is incomplete or inaccurate, it should be corrected or amended before attempting to code (Figure 17-5 ◆).

In Practice

Sharon is the administrative medical assistant who completes billing work in the office. One day when she receives a patient file for billing, Sharon notices that the fee slip the physician completed indicates that he drained a cyst on the patient's wrist. When Sharon reviews the chart notes to assign a diagnosis code, she finds that the physician has written nothing in the chart about the cyst or the procedure. In situations like these, Sharon usually just "jots something" in the chart. What might be wrong with this scenario?

—Critical Thinking Question 17-2—
When Mary cannot decipher the physician's handwriting, what should she do?

HIPAA Compliance

Some physicians outsource their billing services. Because the information needed to process insurance claims is confidential, offices using outside billing services must sign a Business Associates Agreement, which verifies that those services are **HIPAA** compliant and will keep patient information confidential.

There are a number of documents within the medical record that may contain needed information. When coding for office-based or other outpatient services, medical assistants will refer to the patient registration form, the encounter form, visit notes, lab and radiology reports, and operative reports for outpatient procedures. When coding for services physicians provide to inpatients, medical assistants will refer to the admitting history and physical (H&P), daily progress notes, operative reports, lab and radiology reports, and the discharge summary.

It is important to keep in mind that when performing diagnosis coding in order to bill for services, the diagnosis must describe the reasons the specific service was provided and related medical conditions that may affect the specific service. Diagnosis codes should not repeat patients' entire problem list, which is a comprehensive list of all active conditions that often appears in the front of the medical record.

For example, assume a patient is seen for a sinus infection, and she also has chronic gastric reflux. An antibiotic is prescribed for the sinus infection and the physician inquires how the gastric reflux is doing, but does not actively treat it. Only the sinus infection would be coded.

In another example, assume a patient is seen for a burn on the hand, and he also has diabetes. The physician indicates that the diabetes may slow the healing process and requires more frequent followup visits due to the diabetes impact. Therefore, both the burn and the diabetes would be coded.

The following coding steps provide the practical details medical assistants need to patiently and accurately execute the process. The majority of this discussion will be oriented toward office-based coding. Inpatient coding guidelines have some variations, and these will be highlighted at the end of the chapter.

1. **Identify the first-listed diagnosis as stated in the medical record.** Often the physician will indicate a diagnosis code on the encounter form, but it is wise to verify it against the medical record. Look for a definitive diagnostic statement by the physician for reason for the visit. The diagnosis may be indicated with the word *impression* or, in SOAP notes, it will be under *A (Assessment)*. This will be the **first-listed** or **primary diagnosis,** the reason chiefly responsible for the services provided.

Uncertain or **qualified** diagnoses are those accompanied by terms such as *possible, probable, suspected, rule out (R/O),* or *working diagnosis,* indicating the physician has not determined the root cause. For outpatient coding, do not use uncertain diagnoses. Instead, look for the patient's **signs** or **symptoms** that are part of the patient's **chief complaint.** The chief complaint is a statement in the patient's own words of the reason for the visit. Signs are indications of a condition that the physician can observe or measure, such as a rash. Symptoms are indications reported by the patient that the physician cannot observe or measure, such as a headache.

Additional conditions or complaints will become **secondary** diagnoses, which will be coded in the same way as the primary, but listed after them on the CMS-1500 billing form. Signs and symptoms that are routinely associated with the first-listed diagnosis are not coded as secondary diagnoses.

The following sample patient scenarios illustrate the difference between a definitive diagnosis and signs and symptoms. These same scenarios will be developed throughout each step in the coding process discussed.

Sample Patient Scenario
Selecting the First-Listed Diagnosis

Scenario 1—A patient presents with difficulty breathing and fever. The physician takes a sputum culture and diagnoses acute pneumonia. The first-listed diagnosis is pneumonia, acute. Difficulty breathing and fever are commonly associated symptoms of pneumonia, so they would not be coded.

Scenario 2—A patient presents with difficulty breathing and fever. The physician orders a chest X-ray for "suspected pneumonia." The first-listed diagnosis would be difficulty breathing and the secondary diagnosis would be fever.

2. **Locate the main term in the alphabetic index, Volume II.** Identify the word(s) from the first-listed diagnosis to be looked up under the main term in the index (Figure 17-6 ◆). It may be the name of a *condition,* such as "Fracture"; a *disease,*

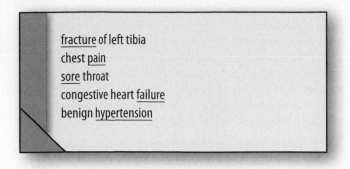

fracture of left tibia

chest pain

sore throat

congestive heart failure

benign hypertension

Figure 17-6 ◆ Examples of diagnostic statements with main term underlined.

such as "Pneumonia"; or *reason* for a visit, such as "Screening." The main term may also be located by *eponym* (a disease or condition named after an individual) such as "Colle's fracture"; an abbreviation or *acronym,* such as "AIDS"; a nontechnical *synonym* (a word similar in meaning) such as "broken" instead of fracture; and, occasionally, an *adjective,* such as "twisted." Some main terms are rather generic with pages of subterms, such as "Disease," while others are quite specific with only a single code, such as "Duroziez's disease." It is helpful to note that diagnoses usually cannot be located by looking up the anatomic site. The main term is always boldfaced with an initial capital letter. After locating the main term, the tentative code(s) will be verified in Volume I. Never code from the index. The steps for verifying codes will be described later.

Exercise
Getting Acquainted with the Alphabetical Index

Look at the first few pages of your ICD-9-CM Volume II index. Find examples of each the following types of main terms:

condition _____

disease _____

reason for visit _____

eponym _____

acronym _____

synonym _____

Sample Patient Scenario
Identifying the Main Term

Scenario 1—*Diagnosis:* Acute pneumonia. *Main term:* Pneumonia.

Scenario 2—*Diagnosis:* Difficulty breathing. Fever. Suspected pneumonia. *Main term:* Breathing, for the first-listed diagnosis. Fever would be the main term for a secondary diagnosis. "Suspected" pneumonia is a qualified or uncertain diagnosis and should not be coded.

3. Review any modifiers, instructional notes or subterms associated with the main term. Subterms are indented two spaces under the boldfaced main term and further describe the condition, in terms of etiology, such as *Pneumonia, allergic;* coexisting conditions, such as *Pneumonia, with influenza;* anatomic site, such as *Pneumonia, interstitial;* episode, such as *Pneumonia, chronic,* or similar descriptors. Subterms often have additional layers of one or more of their own subterms, each of which are indented another two spaces.

Carry over lines are indented more than two spaces from the level of the preceding line. If the main term or subterm is too long to fit on one line, a carry over line is used. It is important to read carefully to distinguish between carry over lines and subterms.

Main terms may also have **nonessential modifiers**, words that appear in parentheses immediately after the main term. These words do not have to be present in the medical record in order to use the code, but if they are present, it confirms the user has located the appropriate code. For example, *Pneumonia* has many nonessential modifiers including *(acute), (Alpenstich), (benign),* and others.

Main terms or subterms may contain instructional notes, such as *see* or *see also,* which direct the user to other entries. For example, *Pneumonia, alveolar—see Pneumonia, other.* This instructs the user where to look for the code needed. Terms may also contain special formatting, such as slanted brackets, indicating that **multiple coding** may be required. For example, *Pneumonia, anthrax* is followed by the codes "022.0 *[484.5]*" The second code in slanted brackets is required in addition to the first code to completely describe the condition.

Exercise
Identifying Conventions in Volume II

Look up the main term *Pneumonia* in the alphabetical index and locate examples of the following:

nonessential modifier _____

subterms _____

subterms of a subterm _____

instructional note _____

multiple coding _____

The acronym NEC (not elsewhere classified) means that a more specific code is not available for a certain variation of a condition.

Sample Patient Scenario
Using Volume II Conventions

Scenario 1—*Main term:* Pneumonia. *Nonessential modifier:* (acute) *Subterm:* No further description is provided, so no subterms are required.

Scenario 2—*Main term:* Breathing. *Nonessential modifier:* None. *Subterm:* The word "difficulty" is not listed as a subterm, but the synonym "labored" appears and would be an appropriate choice.

4. Identify the tentative code(s) associated with the most appropriate subterm(s). When the appropriate subterms are located, the tentative code(s) is printed immediately to the right. It is helpful to jot down the potential appropriate codes before verifying in the tabular list. Never use the index to make the final code selection.

Sample Patient Scenario
Selecting the Tentative Code(s)

Scenario 1—Pnemonia (acute) 486
Scenario 2—Breathing, labored 786.09

5. Locate the tentative code(s) in the tabular list of Volume I. Look for the tentative code number in the tabular list where codes are arranged in numerical order. Volume I is organized into 17 **chapters** based on etiology or the body system. The chapter numbers do not correlate directly with the code numbers. Refer back to Table 17-2. Chapters are divided into **sections** with boldfaced or highlighted headings. Within the sections, the actual code numbers are tabulated in three levels: **category** (three-digit codes), **subcategeory** (four-digit codes), and **subclassification** (five-digit codes) (Figure 17-7 ◆). It is helpful to learn the specific meanings of these designations, because the terms are used frequently in coding instructions.

6. Interpret the Volume I conventions used with the category. Before verifying and finalizing the code, the MA must interpret the conventions presented with the code and its category. Volume I conventions include punctuation, instructional notes and symbols and may appear on the same line with the code, above it, below it, or at the beginning of a subcategory, category, section, or chapter. Look carefully for any information that may be relevant to your tentative code selection, as the additional information may direct you when to use a different code or an additional code, depending on your original diagnostic statement.

In Volume I, the way in which punctuation is used has meaning (Figure 17-8 ◆). Medical assistants should become familiar with these meanings:

:	Colons are used after an incomplete phrase or term that requires one or more of the modifiers indented under it to make it assignable to a given category.
[ ]	Square brackets are used to enclose **synonyms**, alternate wordings, or explanatory phrases
( )	Parentheses are used to enclose optional or supplementary words that may be present or absent in a physician's statement of condition without affecting the code assignment.

Instructional notes are used to define terms, provide coding instructions, and provide fifth-digit information.

Use Additional Code or *Code Also* This instruction is placed in the tabular list in the categories where the coder may wish to add further information, by means of an additional code, to give a more complete picture of the diagnosis or procedure.

Code First Underlying Disease As Used for those codes not intended to be used as the first-listed diagnosis. These codes are for symptoms only (**manifestation**) and never for causes. The codes and their descriptions are in italic type, meaning that the code cannot be listed first, even if the diagnostic statement is written that way.

Includes Indicates separate terms, such as modifying adjectives, sites, conditions entered under a subdivision (such as a category), to further define or give examples of the content of the category.

Excludes Exclusion terms are enclosed in a box and are printed in italics to draw attention to their presence. The importance of this instructional term is its use as a guideline to direct the coder to the proper code assignment. In other words, all terms following the word *Excludes:* are to be coded elsewhere as indicated in each instance.

Level	Code	Description
Chapter	None	3. Endocrine, Nutritional and metabolic diseases, and immunity disorders (240–279)
Section	None	Diseases of other endocrine glands (250–259)
Category	250	Diabetes mellitus
Subcategory	250.0	Diabetes mellitus without mention of complication
Subclassification	250.00	Diabetes mellitus without mention of complication, type II, not stated as uncontrolled

Figure 17-7 ◆ Example of Volume I tabulation levels.

482.82 Escherichia coli [E. coli]
490 Bronchitis, not specific as acute or chronic
Bronchitis NOS:
catarrhal
with tracheitis NOS

Figure 17-8 ◆ Examples of punctuation conventions.

NOS (**not otherwise specified**) means unspecified. This acronym refers to a lack of sufficient detail in the diagnostic statement to be able to assign it to a more specific subdivision within the classification.

NEC (**not elsewhere classified**) is used to alert coders that some forms of the condition may be classified differently, but there is not a more specific code for their condition. In other words, the coder may have more specific information than what the codes provide for. An everyday example would be if a friend were to ask you, "What is your favorite color: red, yellow, blue, or other?" Perhaps your favorite color is purple, so you would respond "Other." You have a more specific response than what your friend provided. In coding, NOS and NEC should be used with caution, only as a last resort if no more appropriate code exists.

Symbols are used to alert the coder that something is different with the code.

▲ ▶ ◀ upright or sideways triangles mean that there is a revision to the description of an existing code number

● a round bullet means that the code number is new to this revision.

⬤ an octagon, or a number within a circle (❹ ❺), depending on the publisher, means that the code must be coded either to the fourth level or the fifth level of specificity.

✖ a "x" or ☐ empty box, depending on the publisher, indicates a nonspecific (NEC or NOS) code. These should be used only when absolutely necessary because doing so may delay payment on the claim.

Certain words also have special meaning in Volume I. For example, *and* is interpreted as *either/and/or* in a diagnostic code description; *with* is interpreted as *both, together with* in a diagnostic code description (Figure 17-9 ◆).

787.0 Nausia **and** vomiting → codes for both
    symptoms are included in this subcategory
  787.01 Nausia **with** vomiting → patient with
      both symptoms
  787.02 Nausea **alone** → patient presents with
      only nausea
  787.03 Vomiting **alone** → patient presents with
      only vomiting

Figure 17-9 ◆ Example of usage of words "and" and "with."

Sample Patient Scenario
Interpreting Volume I Conventions

Scenario 1—Tentative code 486 is designated as an "Unspecified Code." Review the documentation for any additional specific information. None appears. Because the index directed us to this code for acute pneumonia, this choice is acceptable. Also note that the category contains an "excludes" statement that redirects the coder to more specific codes for specific types of pneumonia. None of these apply.

Scenario 2—Tentative code 786.09 is a subclassification. First locate the subcategory (786.0 Dyspnea and respiratory abnormalities) and category (786 Symptoms involving respiratory systems and other chest symptoms) headings for conventions. The only convention is a symbol indicating that five digits must be used. Going back to 786.09 we find some explanatory notes with synonyms and "excludes" notes. Read these. None apply to our patient. We also note that 786.09 is designated as an "Unspecified Code," but since we cannot code any more certainty based on the documentation, use of the code is acceptable.

---

7. **Select the code with the highest level of specificity.** There is no general rule regarding how many digits any given code will have. This is determined only after reading all the instructional notes and conventions available in the category. Assign a three-digit code if there are no four-digit codes in that category. Assign a four-digit code if there are no five-digit codes in the subcategory. Fourth- and fifth-digit codes may be found in one of several possible locations, depending on the number of options available. They may be located sequentially in the **tabular list**, at the beginning of the category, section, or chapter. Fifth digits may be found sequentially in the tabular list, or at the beginning of the subcategory, category, section, or chapter. Be certain to review these areas thoroughly to locate the correct fourth and fifth digits when required. It sometimes requires a little detective work and reviewing several pages of codes to locate the appropriate listing.

Sample Patient Scenario
Selecting the Code with the Highest Level of Specificity

Scenario 1—Pneumonia, organism unspecified, 486. This code matches the physician's diagnostic statement and there are no subcategories or subclassifications available. This is an example of a final code with only three digits.

Scenario 2—Dyspnea and respiratory abnormalities, other, 786.09. This is a five-digit subclassification so no additional digits are required. While there are other subclassifications in this category for more specific variations of the condition, none accurately describe this patient.

8. Review the code for appropriate age, gender, and reimbursement edits. The bottom of the page in the *ICD-9-CM* manual contains additional symbols that indicate codes that should be used only with specific age groups and genders, as well as those that may contain reimbursement alerts. The symbols used vary by publisher and are usually described in a key at the bottom of each page or two-page spread.

Exercise
Identifying Volume I Conventions and Edits

The following is a sample entry from the *ICD-9-CM* manual. How many conventions and edits can you identify? Circle each one and write next to it the meaning of the punctuation, symbol, or instruction.

❹ **600 Hyperplasia of prostate**
      INCLUDES enlarged prostate
❺ **600.0 Hypertrophy (benign) of prostate**
      Benign prostatic hypertrophy
      Enlargement of prostate
      600.00 Hypertrophy (benign) of prostate without urinary obstruction and other lower urinary tract symptoms (LUTS) ♂ 𝔸
          Hypertrophy (benign) of prostate NOS
      600.01 Hypertrophy (benign) of prostate with urinary obstruction and other lower urinary tract symptoms (LUTS) ♂ 𝔸
          Hypertrophy (benign) of prostate with urinary retention
          Use additional code to identify symptoms:
              nocturia (788.43)
              straining on urination (888.65)
              urinary urgency (788.63)

♂ Male   𝔸 Adult (15+) years   𝕄 Maternity (12–55 yr)   ℕ Newborn (0 yr)

Sample Patient Scenario
Reviewing the Code for Age, Gender, or Reimbursement Edits

Scenario 1—486 There are no age, gender, or reimbursement edits for this code.
Scenario 2—786.09 There no age, gender, or reimbursement edits for this code.

9. Verify the final code against the documentation. As a final check, with coding manual instructions fresh in your mind, refer back to the original documentation and verify that all conditions of the code agree with the medical record. If a discrepancy arises, work through the process again from the beginning.

Sample Patient Scenario
Verifying the Final Code Against Documentation

Scenario 1—Pneumonia, organism unspecified, 486. The final code matches the documentation.
Scenario 2—Dyspnea and respiratory abnormalities, other, 786.09
You would repeat this entire process to code for the other symptom, fever.

10. Assign the code. Write down the final code where indicated on your worksheet or documentation. Be certain to proofread the number as you wrote or keyboarded it to avoid transcription errors that are easy to make.

11. Repeat this process for any additional codes required by the medical record. Selecting a diagnosis code may seem like a long and tedious process at first. As medical assistants become familiar with the services and codes used by their medical office, coding becomes faster and easier, but accuracy and attention to detail is always paramount. Taking time and care to learn the fundamentals correctly will help create long-term success in the medical assistant's coding role.

Coding for Special Situations

As with any activity, there are always special situations that require additional information and knowledge. Diagnosis coding is the same. There are a number of conditions and circumstances that have unique tables, codes, and guidelines. An overview of these are provided in the remainder of the chapter.

Secondary Diagnoses

Patients may present with more than one complaint or condition that needs to be treated. Up to four diagnosis codes may be entered on the CMS-1500 form. As discussed earlier, the main reason for the visit is the first-listed diagnosis. Other conditions may be listed as secondary diagnoses, in the priority documented in the medical record. If two complaints are equal in priority, either can be listed first. If signs and symptoms are common to the diagnosed condition, only the condition is coded, not the signs and symptoms.

Keys to Success
MEDICAL BILLING SOFTWARE UPDATES

Medical billing software typically comes programmed with ICD-9-CM codes. To keep current and insert accurate diagnosis code information in insurance claims, it is crucial that such software be updated regularly. Claims with outdated or expired codes will likely experience delays or denials by insurance carriers.

PROCEDURE 17-1 **Perform Diagnostic Coding**

Theory and Rationale

Proper diagnostic coding is key to proper reimbursement from insurance carriers. The medical assistant must know precisely where to look in the ICD-9-CM coding book in order to obtain proper codes, as well as which steps to take when unsure of the proper code.

Materials

- Patient's medical chart
- Current ICD-9-CM coding book
- Superbill with doctor's written diagnosis

Competency

(**Conditions**) With the necessary materials, you will be able to (**Task**) perform diagnostic coding (**Standards**) correctly within the time limit set by the instructor.

1. Locate the patient's diagnostic code(s) or description on the superbill or in the chart notes.
2. Verify that the diagnostic code(s) or description on the superbill also appear in the patient's chart in the form of a patient complaint (subjective finding) or a test finding (objective finding).
3. Using Volume II (the Alphabetic Index) of the ICD-9-CM coding book, find the diagnostic code(s).
4. Using Volume I (the Tabular Index), confirm that the written description matches the chart notes. If in doubt, check with the physician.
5. Read and defer to the conventions in the Tabular List.
6. Assign the code for each diagnosis, beginning with the appropriate first-listed diagnosis.

EXAMPLE: The patient presents to the office with complaints of a sore throat. The physician finds upon examination that the patient has an abscess on his tonsil. In addition, the physician assigns diagnoses for this patient for ringing in the ears and sinus infection. The first-listed diagnosis is 475 peritonsillar abscess, followed by 388.31 subjective tinnitus, followed by 473.1 frontal sinusitis.

Combination Coding

Some conditions that frequently occur together may be described with a **combination code**. Careful reading of subterms in the index and category *includes* and *excludes* notes in the tabular list will guide the medical assistant as to when a combination code is available. Combination code descriptions frequently contain specific words that indicate more than one condition is covered, such as *associated with, due to, secondary to, without, with, complicated by,* and *following.* In Figure 17-9, code *787.1 Nausea with vomiting* is a combination code.

Multiple Coding

Multiple coding is when a condition requires two or more codes to fully describe it. In the index, multiple coding may be indicated by a second code in slanted brackets. In the tabular list, it is indicated by the instructional note *Code also (condition)* or *Code first (condition)* or *Use additional code.* Omission of the additional codes could result in denial or delay of payment.

In the earlier example of *600.01 Hypertrophy (benign) of prostate with urinary obstruction and other lower urinary tract*

symptoms (LUTS), there was an instructional note to *Use additional code to identify symptoms* followed by commonly paired conditions. This is an example of multiple coding.

Multiple codes are also used when an underlying condition (etiology) causes a second condition (manifestation). For example, *Diabetes, type II, with renal manifestations* (250.40) requires a second code for the specific kidney disease, such as *Chronic kidney disease, stage III* (585.3).

Signs and Symptoms Codes

When a definitive diagnosis is not yet available, the medical assistant may assign a sign or symptom diagnosis code. Assume, for example, the physician suspects pneumonia is the patient's diagnosis but will be unsure until an X-ray is taken and read. The medical assistant can assign diagnoses related to the patient's symptoms, such as wheezing, fever, cough, and shortness of breath. Signs, symptoms, and ill-defined conditions are found in the ICD-9-CM code book under codes 780.56 to 781.1.

EXAMPLE: 780.6 fever, 786.07 wheezing, 786.2 cough, 785.05 shortness of breath.

Hypertension

Hypertension in medical terms refers to a condition of elevated blood pressure regardless of the cause. It has been called "the silent killer" because it usually does not cause symptoms for many years—often not until a vital organ has been damaged.

When blood pressure is checked, two values are recorded. The higher one occurs when the heart contracts (systole); the lower occurs when the heart relaxes between beats (diastole). Blood pressure is written as the systolic pressure followed by a slash and the diastolic pressure, for example, 120/80 mm Hg (millimeters of mercury). This reading would be referred to as "one twenty over eighty." Hypertension is defined in adults as 140 mm Hg systolic or 90 mm Hg diastolic on three separate readings recorded several weeks apart.

Figure 17-10 ◆ provides a complete listing of all conditions associated with hypertension. Four columns are shown:

- Condition (not titled as such in the excerpt)
- Malignant
- Benign
- Unspecified.

The first column identifies the hypertensive condition, such as:

Accelerated
Cardiovascular disease
Renal involvement
Heart involvement

The last three columns identify the subcategories of the disease as malignant, benign, or unspecified. Do not select a code from the malignant or benign category unless the documentation indicates the specific type of hypertension. When the documentation does not indicate the type of hypertension, ask the physician to specify the type. If that alternative is not available, select "unspecified."

EXAMPLE

Hypertension (arterial) (essential) (primary) (systemic) NOS to Category 401 with the appropriate fourth digit. Do not use either .0 (malignant) or .1 (benign) unless the medical record documentation supports it. Otherwise assign .9 (unspecified).*

As with any other code, after the tentative code has been identified in the hypertension table, it should be verified in the tabular list.

Neoplasms

Neoplasm is the medical term for an abnormal growth of new tissue, often referred to as a tumor. Neoplasms can occur in any type of tissue anywhere in the body, and they can be either malignant or benign. Tumors that have cellular characteristics that cause them to invade adjacent healthy tissue or spread to distant sites are malignant, or life threatening. The spreading of malignant neoplasm is called metastasis. Tumors that do not have these characteristics are benign. The neoplasm table in Volume II provides the index to the behaviors and anatomic sites of neoplasms (Figure 17-11 ◆).

The neoplasm table lists the anatomical sites alphabetically. For each site, there are six possible codes, depending on the type of neoplasm behavior. Malignant neoplasms will be identified as primary (site of origin), secondary (site of metastasis), or ca in situ (cells that have begun to change but have not yet invaded normal tissue). Malignant neoplasms are coded as primary unless the medical record indicates secondary (metastasis) or ca in situ (preinvasive carcinoma). Benign neoplasms will be stated as such in the medical record. "Uncertain behavior" refers to situations in which the pathologist clearly indicates that further study is needed before determining the benign or malignant behavior. "Unspecified" is used when the medical record does not contain adequate description of the neoplasm,

*Source: Vines, Deborah, Braceland, Ann, Rollins, Elizabeth, and Miller, Susan. *Comprehensive Health Insurance: Billing, Coding, and Reimbursement.* © 2008, p. 92. Reprinted by permission of Pearson Education. Upper Saddle River, NJ.

ICD-9-CM Index to Diseases Addenda (FY08) Effective October 1, 2007

Hypertension Table	Malignant	Benign	Unspecified
Hypertension, hypertensive (arterial) (arteriolar) (crisis) (degeneration) (disease) (essential) (fluctuating) (idiopathic) (intermittent) (labile) (low renin) (orthostatic) (paroxysmal) (primary) (systemic) (uncontrolled) (vascular)	401.0	401.1	401.9
cardiorenal (disease)	404.00	404.10	404.90
with			
heart failure	404.01	404.11	404.91
and chronic kidney disease	404.01	404.11	404.91
stage I through stage IV or unspecified	404.01	404.11	404.91
venous, chronic (asymptomatic) (idiopathic)	—	—	459.30

Figure 17-10 ◆ Conditions due to or associated with hypertension.
Source: International Classification of Diseases, Ninth Revision, Clinical Modification (2008). Reprinted from National Center for Health Statistics, http://www.cdc.gov/nchs/datawh/ftpserv/ftpicd9/ftpicd9.htm guidlines.

	Malignant			Benign	Uncertain Behavior	Unspecified
	Primary	Secondary	Ca In situ			
Neoplasm, neoplastic	199.1	199.1	234.9	229.9	238.9	239.9
abdomen, abdominal	195.2	198.89	234.8	229.8	238.8	239.8
cavity	195.2	198.89	234.8	229.8	238.8	239.8
organ	195.2	198.89	234.8	229.8	238.8	239.8
viscera	195.2	198.89	234.8	229.8	238.8	239.8
acoustic nerve	192.0	198.4	–	225.1	237.9	239.7
acromion (process)	170.4	198.5	–	213.4	238.0	239.2
adenoid (pharynx) (tissue)	147.1	198.89	230.0	210.7	235.1	239.0

Figure 17-11 ◆ Sample entries for neoplasm table.

such as a patient who has relocated and whose previous medical records are not yet available.

After determining the anatomic site and the type of behavior, select the code from the appropriate column, then verify it in the tabular list. For example, primary carcinoma of the anal canal, 154.2.

V Codes

Not all patients who seek healthcare services have a specific disease or condition. They may receive services such as preventive care, therapy, followup, suture removal, or pregnancy supervision. They may have problems that require screening. They may carry certain risk factors or have a certain health status that may affect treatment and require coding. All of these are examples of situations that require V codes.

V codes can be used in many different ways. Depending on the encounter, the V code could be primary or supplemental. Usually, if the V code is primary, the reason for this encounter was not due to an injury or illness. That is, V codes are mainly used for encounters other than disease or injury such as annual checkups, physical exams, and immunizations. The V code would be the primary reason for the encounter since there is no chief complaint at these types of visits. These visits are also referred to as *well check-ups*. There are three exceptions in which the V code is used as the primary code when there is a disease:

1. Chemotherapy
2. Radiation
3. Rehabilitation

EXAMPLE

HIV/AIDS—the code must distinguish between exposure and/or testing positive for the presence of the acquired immunodeficiency syndrome (AIDS) virus.

The question that must be asked is "Why is the patient here today?" Although the patient may have cancer for which he is receiving chemotherapy or radiation, the encounter today is not for the disease but for the treatment. In this case, the V code is primary and the disease is secondary.

V codes fall into one of three categories: problems, services, or factual.

1. **Problems:** V codes identify a problem that could affect a patient's overall health status but is not itself a current illness or injury. The V code in this example is supplemental.

EXAMPLE

Allergy to drug

2. **Services:** As mentioned, a V code can be used to describe circumstances other than an illness or injury that prompted the patient's visit. This is an exception to the rule for coding V codes. Although there is a disease, the V code is coded primary because it is the main reason for the encounter. The disease would be coded supplemental to the V code.

EXAMPLE

Chemotherapy
Radiation
Rehabilitation

3. **Factual:** V codes are used to describe certain facts that do not fall into the "problem" or "service" categories. For example, coding the type of birth, look under "Outcome of Delivery."

EXAMPLE

Single liveborn to indicate birth status.

V codes indicate a reason for an encounter—*they are not diagnosis codes.* A corresponding diagnosis code must accompany a V code to describe the reason the procedure was

Admission for	Dialysis	Maladjustment
Aftercare (of)	Donor	Observation
Attention to	Examination	Problem (with)
Care (of)	Fitting of	Prophylactic
Carrier	Follow-up	Replacement (by) (of)
Checking/checkup	Health or healthy	Screening
Contact	History (of)	Transplant
Contraception	Maintenance	Vaccination
Counseling		

Figure 17-12 ◆ Key words in diagnostic statements that may result in selection of a V code.
Source: Vines, Deborah, Braceland, Ann, Rollins, Elizabeth, and Miller, Susan. Comprehensive Health Insurance: Billing, Coding, and Reimbursement. p. 85.

performed. Key words found in diagnostic statements that may result in selection of a V code are shown in Figure 17-12 ◆.

EXAMPLE

A patient who has a family history of colon cancer presents with rectal bleeding (569.3).
Alphabetic index: History (personal) of Family malignant neoplasm (of) colon
Tabular List: V16.0
Correct code: V16.0
Correct code sequence: 569.3, V16.0

EXAMPLE

A patient presents to a healthcare facility for care after having unprotected sex with a partner who has tested positive for human immunodeficiency virus (HIV).
Alphabetic index: Exposure to HIV
Tabular list: V01.7, contact with or exposure to other viral diseases
Correct code: V01.79*

V codes are indexed in the alphabetical index of Volume II. The V code tabular list appears in Volume I after category 999.

E Codes

E codes are a supplementary classification that describes the external cause of illness or injury. They are never the first-listed diagnosis and are never used alone. They must be preceded by a diagnostic code from 001 to 999. For example, if a patient is being treated for a fractured ulna because he fell off a ladder, a code from category 813 would describe the fracture and E881.0 would describe the cause, fall from ladder.

In the event medical treatment is due to a drug overdose, whether accidental or due to attempted suicide, E codes are mandatory. Figure 17-13 ◆ lists other rules for E code use.

*Source: Vines, Deborah, Braceland, Ann, Rollins, Elizabeth, and Miller, Susan. *Comprehensive Health Insurance: Billing, Coding, and Reimbursement.* © 2008, pp. 83–85.

Some examples of when E codes would be used are as follows:

- A patient was involved in a motor vehicle accident.
- A patient was a pedestrian who was struck by a car while crossing the street.
- A patient fell off a ladder at home.
- A patient has accidentally ingested rat poison.
- A patient was injured as a result of a medical mistake, such as the physician operating on the wrong limb.
- A patient was bitten by a poisonous spider.
- A patient was knocked down at a sporting event.
- A patient was assaulted by another person.

E codes have a separate index in Volume II, which begins after the alphabetic index and after the table of drugs and chemicals. E codes also have a separate tabular list, which appears in Volume I after the V codes.

Poisonings and Adverse Effects

The Table of Drugs and Chemicals is a cross-tabulated index to poisoning and external causes of adverse effects of drugs and other chemical substances.

Never use as primary diagnostic codes.
Use does affect reimbursement from insurance carriers.
Can hasten reimbursement by providing the insurance carrier information.
Child abuse codes have top priority.
After child abuse codes, cataclysmic events take priority.
After cataclysmic events and child abuse codes, transportation codes take priority.

Figure 17-13 ◆ Rules for E code use.

When coding for drugs or chemicals that have caused poisonings or **adverse reactions,** the medical assistant will need to determine the type of drug or chemical involved, if the event was accidental or purposeful, and whether the substance was prescribed by a health care provider. Table 17-3 outlines external causes, event descriptions, and ranges where codes can be found.

If the adverse reaction is due to therapeutic use of a drug, code the adverse reaction first, followed by the appropriate E code from the table. For example, rash due to adverse reaction to initial dose of penicillin, 693.0, E930.0. A poisoning code from column 1 is never used with a therapeutic use code from column 3.

Any situation other than therapeutic use will be coded with first, a poisoning code from column 1; second, a code for the adverse effect from 000 to 999; and third, an E code for the intent, from the columns *accident, suicide attempt, assault,* or *undetermined.* If more than one adverse effect is present, multiple codes may be used.

Coding for Fractures

When coding fractures, the medical assistant will need to know the type of fracture and whether that fracture is open or closed. The ICD-9-CM coding book contains codes to indicate fractures in the following categories:

- **Spiral**—typically occurs due to twisting
- **Fissure or hairline**—usually imposes minimal trauma to the bone and tissues
- **Comminuted**—Has more than two fragments of bone that have been broken off, are unstable, and include tissue damage.
- **Linear**—Runs the length of the bone.
- **Closed**—Keeps the skin intact.
- **Double**—Refers to multiple fractures of the same bone.
- **Simple**—Does not break the skin and has little tissue damage.
- **Greenstick**—Is bend-like fracture in which the bone is not broken through; mostly found in children.
- **Infected**—Is in an infected area.
- **Compound/Open**—Breaks the skin.
- **Depressed**—Is a skull fracture with the bone broken inward.
- **Oblique**—Presents as an oblique break in the bone; very rare.

- **Pathological**—Caused by disease.
- **Impact/Compression**—Refers to a situation in which the vertebral (spinal) column is compressed and then breaks under the pressure.
- **Complex**—severely damages the tissue around the fracture site
- **Stress**—Caused by repeated stress to the bone.
- **Impacted**—Diagnosed when bones are broken and the ends smash together.
- **Fragmented**—Occurs when trauma breaks many bones inside the patient.

Coding for fractures requires specific identification of the exact bone fractured and, often, the location of the fracture on the bone. For example, Closed fracture of the humerus, upper end, surgical neck 812.01. Fifth digits are required on most fracture codes and are often located at the beginning of the category or section rather than in the sequential tabular listing. Fractures of the skull, neck, and trunk include combination codes for associated conditions. For example, Fracture of base of the skull, closed with subarachnoid, subdural, and extradural hemorrhage, with moderate loss of consciousness 801.23. In this code, 801 category describes Fracture of base of skull. The fourth digit .2 describes closed with subarachnoid, subdural, and extradural hemorrhage. The fifth digit subclassfication 3, which appears at the beginning of the section Fracture of the skull (800-804), describes moderate (1–24 hours) loss of consciousness.

Coding Burns

When coding for burns (codes 940-948), the medical assistant must know the depth and extent of the burn, as well as the burn-causing agent. Burns are classified by depth as first degree (redness of the skin), second degree (blistering of the skin), and third degree (full thickness of skin involved). To code burns, first code the site(s) and degree of the burn, with the most severe first; second, code the percentage of total body surface area (TBSA) with third-degree burns, based on the rule of nines; third, if the burn is infected, use code 958.3; finally, use an E code to describe the cause of the burn. With multiple burns, the first code should indicate the highest burn degree. If a patient has a first, second, or third degree burn in the same body area, the highest degree code is given to that burn. In other words, if a patient sees the physician for first and second degree burns of the right hand, the medical assistant will only

TABLE 17-3 DRUG AND CHEMICAL POISONING OR ADVERSE EFFECT CODE

External Cause	Code Description	Code Range
Poisoning	Assigned to a patient according to the classification of the drug or chemical in the poisoning	960–989
Accidental	Used for accidental overdose, wrong substance given or taken, drug taken accidentally, or accidental use of a drug or chemical during a medical procedure	E850–E869
Therapeutic use	Used for the external effect caused by a correct substance properly administered that caused an adverse or allergic reaction	E930–E952
Suicide attempt	Used to report attempted suicide via drugs or chemicals	E950–E952
Assault	Used to report a poisoning that was inflicted on another person with the intent to harm or kill	E961–E962
Unknown	Used when the medical record is unclear whether the poisoning was intentional or accidental	E980–E982

code for the second-degree burn since it is the highest degree of burn. If that same patient also has a first-degree burn on the lower leg, the medical assistant would code for the second-degree burn of the right hand and the first-degree burn of the lower leg.

Using the Rule of Nines in Coding Burns

The medical assistant should assign codes from category 948 when coding burns according to the extent of the total body surface area (**TBSA**) involved, or when the site of the burn is not specified. Category 948 codes are based on the "rule of nines" in estimating the body surfaces involved. The head and neck are assigned 9%, each arm is assigned 9%, each leg is assigned 18%, the anterior and posterior trunk are each assigned 18%, and the genitalia are assigned 1%. Physicians may change these percentages when treating infants or children in order to accurately describe the amount of skin that has been burned, or when treating larger adults who may have more body surface area (Figure 17-14 ◆).

For example, assume a patient suffered third-degree burns to the back and back of the left arm, and second-degree burns to the back of the right arm when she fell into a campfire. The third-degree burn of back is coded as 942, burn of trunk, plus fourth digit .3 for third degree and fifth digit 4 for back, creating the code 942.34; third degree burn of left back upper arm and forearm is 943 upper extremities, fourth digit .3 for third degree, fifth digit 9 for multiple sites (upper arm and forearm), arriving at the code 943.39; the second-degree burn of right back upper arm and forearm is similar, but uses a fourth digit of .2 for second degree burn, for a code of 943.29. To code for TBSA, first add up the percentage of each body area: 18% for the back and 9% for each arm totaling 36%. This gives a

subcategory code of 948.3. The fifth digit describes the TBSA with third-degree burns, which is 27% for the back and back of left arm, for a final code 948.32. To code for the cause of the burn, use E897, accident caused by controlled fire not in building or structure, including bonfire. Total coding for this patient is 942.34, 943.39, 943.29, 948.32, E897.

Late Effects

Late effects are conditions that arise from acute illnesses, old injuries, or previous conditions that have been resolved. There is no specific guideline for how much time must pass between the original event and its manifestation or **sequela** for it to be classified as a late effect. It is largely dependent on the physician's judgment, which should be documented in the medical record.

Key words that indicate a late effect include *due to (an old injury), late, following (previous condition)*. For example, a malunion due to a previous fracture, hemiplegia following a stroke, or scarring due to a burn. First code the current condition or sequelae; second, assign a late effect code from categories 905 through 909; third, assign a late effects E code from category E929 late effects of accidental injury, if applicable. For example, Malunion of fracture of the humerus, 733.11, Late effect of fracture of upper extremities, 905.2.

Obstetrics

Obstetric coding is one of the more complex areas of coding because multiple codes are required for anything other than a normal delivery of a single liveborn infant. All visits for supervision of a pregnancy require a V code from the category V22 for a normal pregnancy or V23 for a high-risk pregnancy. These codes can be located in the index under *Pregnancy, supervision.*

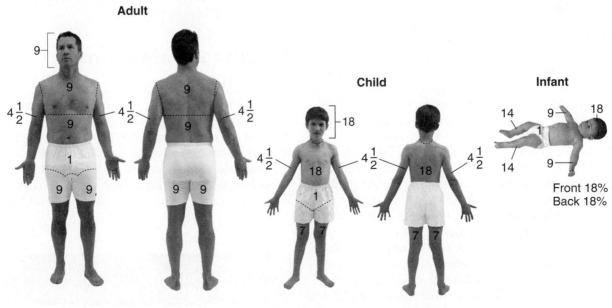

Adult

Child

Infant

Front 18%
Back 18%

Note: Each arm totals 9% (front of arm $4\frac{1}{2}$ %, back of arm $4\frac{1}{2}$ %)

Figure 17-14 ◆ Rule of nines.

Carefully review the subcategories to ensure correct code selection. Complications of pregnancy are located in the index under *Pregnancy, complicated by* or *Pregnancy, management affected by.* Chapter 11 of the tabular list (630-677) contains the codes for complications of pregnancy, childbirth and the puerperium (six weeks after delivery). These codes are used only on the record of the mother. Most complications of pregnancy have a unique code from Chapter 11 that is to be used in place of, or in addition to, a code for the same condition in a non-pregnant person. For example, when pregnancy causes diabetes, called gestational diabetes, a code from the subcategory 648.8 is used, rather than a code from the diabetes category, 250. When a woman with pre-existing type I or type II diabetes becomes pregnant, a code from the subcategory 648.0 is used in addition to a secondary code from the category 250. For example, DM complicating pregnancy, 648.03, 250.00.

The birth itself will include codes for the delivery, any complications, and the outcome of delivery. A normal delivery is defined as a vaginal delivery needing minimal or no assistance, resulting in a single liveborn infant. In addition, the code V27.0 is required to indicate the outcome of delivery.

Multiple births, caesarean sections, and complicated deliveries require multiple codes that describe all the circumstances. In addition, codes from the range V27.1 to V27.9 are used to indicate the number of liveborn infants and stillborn fetuses. For example, delivery of twins by vaginal delivery with no antepartum or postpartum complication, both liveborn, 651.01, V27.2.

A separate medical record is opened for all liveborn infants. The record will have a code from the range V30-V39, which describes the location of birth and the existence of multiple liveborn or stillborn mates. Any other medical conditions of the infant are separately coded. For example, Twin, mate liveborn, V31.

Diabetes

Not only is diabetes mellitus (**DM**) a common condition, it causes and impacts many other conditions, so medical assistants will frequently encounter the need to code for it. Category 250 Diabetes Mellitus is the category used. It excludes gestational diabetes, neonatal DM, nonclinical diabetes, and hyperglycemia that has not been diagnosed as DM.

DM is always coded to the fifth digit and frequently involves combination coding as well as multiple coding. Medical assistants need to thoroughly review the medical record to abstract certain facts about patients' DM: whether it is type I, type II, or unspecified; whether it is stated as being uncontrolled; what complications exist. If no complications exist, subcategory 250.0 is used, and the fifth digit is assigned based on the type of DM and whether it is uncontrolled or not. Acute manifestations or complications are coded with subcategories 250.1 to 250.3, and the fifth digit is assigned based on the type of DM and whether it is uncontrolled or not. Chronic manifestations are coded with subcategories 250.4 through 250.9, based on body system affected. Again, the fifth digit is assigned based on the type of DM and whether it is uncontrolled or not. If more than one body system is affected, use a code from each body system, and be certain the fifth digit is the same for all. For each body system with manifestation(s), an additional code is required to specify the nature of the manifestation. The most common manifestations are listed in the instructional notes within each subcategory. Verify the manifestation code where it originally appears within the tabular list. If a type II diabetic requires long-term insulin use, assign the additional code V58.67 to report this information.

For example, type II DM, with long-term insulin use and associated glaucoma. The first code is 250.50 for DM. The fourth digit ".5" indicates ophthalmic manifestations. The fifth digit "0" indicates type II, not stated as uncontrolled. The second code is 365.44 for Glaucoma associated with systemic disorders. Note that this is a different code in the tabular list category, 365 Glaucoma, than if the glaucoma had developed independent of DM. Finally, assign V58.67 to report long-term insulin use by a type II diabetic. The complete coding would be 250.50, 365.44, V58.67.

Inpatient Services

When coding for services provided by the physician in the inpatient setting, a few guidelines are different. The patient will be assigned an admitting diagnosis code, which describes the reason for the admission. After all tests and studies are completed and results reported, a **principal diagnosis** is assigned based on these results. The principal diagnosis must be assigned prior to final billing. Uncertain conditions, which are not coded in the outpatient setting, are coded "as though they exist" in the inpatient setting. Patients may have multiple diagnoses for co-existing conditions, so physicians should report only the diagnoses that pertain to their services. For example, if a patient has a fractured leg and is also diabetic, the orthopedic surgeon would report the fracture as the diagnosis while the endocrinologist would report the DM.

Pursuing Professional Certification

Medical assistants who enjoy the problem-solving and detective work involved in diagnostic coding often choose to pursue certification as a professional coder. This career path allows them to use their clinical knowledge to enhance their coding skills. While many organizations offer certifications, the most widely recognized are the Certified Professional Coder (**CPC**), offered by the American Academy of Professional Coders (**AAPC**), and

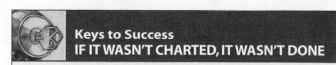

Keys to Success
IF IT WASN'T CHARTED, IT WASN'T DONE

The saying in the medical office, "If it wasn't charted, it wasn't done," holds true for coding. A provider can only charge for items noted in patients' charts.

the Certified Coding Specialist-Physician based (**CCS-P**), offered by the American Health Information Management Association (**AHIMA**). Both certifications require an in-depth knowledge of both diagnostic and procedural coding, as well as reimbursement basics. Certification is obtained by passing a written examination that is several hours long. Both organizations offer entry-level apprentice options for graduating students, as well as certification for hospital-based coders and advanced certification for a variety of physician and administrative specialties. Local chapter meetings provide opportunities for professional networking, education, and employment

searches. Their Web sites, listed at the end of the chapter, provide more detailed information and requirements.

Whether medical assistants decide to become certified professional coders or remain in a largely clinical role, diagnostic coding skills are important to their career. Some medical assistants may perform hands-on coding, while others review encounter forms or serve as an interpreter or communication link for other coders. Understanding how to abstract diagnostic information from the medical record and accurately translate it into codes that justify reimbursement will enable medical assistants to play a vital role in supporting both patients and their medical office.

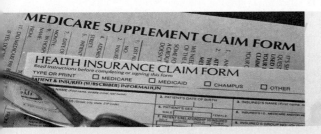

REVIEW

Chapter Summary

- The medical assistant's role in diagnostic coding must be done with the utmost attention to detail. The physician is responsible for assigning diagnoses to patients; however, the MA is responsible for applying the correct code to match the diagnosis the physician provides.
- Proper coding and health insurance reimbursement are tightly linked. If coded incorrectly, procedures may not be reimbursed at the proper level.
- Diagnostic coding has existed for more than a century. French physician Jacques Bertillon composed the Bertillon Classification of Causes of Death in 1893, which the American Public Health Association (APHA) adopted in 1898. In 1901, the APHA published a coding book called the *International Classification of Diseases (ICD), Volume I*, which was used until 1910, when the second volume was published. Volume updates continued to be published every ten years until the ICD-9-CM was published in 1979.

- ICD-10 was complete in 1999 and has replaced ICD-9-CM in all major countries except the United States.
- Proper prioritization of diagnosis codes helps ensure both proper documentation and appropriate insurance reimbursement.
- To choose diagnosis codes correctly, medical assistants must follow a number of predefined steps.
- Coding for various special situations must be done accurately in order to properly describe the patients' condition to the insurance carrier.
- Medical assistants may choose to pursue certification as a professional coder. The most widely recognized certifications are the Certified Professional Coder (CPC), offered by the American Academy of Professional Coders (AAPC), and the Certified Coding Specialist-Physician based (CCS-P), offered by the American Health Information Management Association (AHIMA).

Chapter Review

Multiple Choice

1. To locate the proper diagnosis code, which volume of the *ICD-9-CM* coding book should be consulted first?
   a. I
   b. II
   c. III
   d. None of the above

2. The *ICD-9-CM* coding book has how many volumes?
   a. 1
   b. 2
   c. 3
   d. 4

3. ICD-9-CM codes are how many digits?
   a. 3
   b. 4
   c. 5
   d. All of the above

4. Which of the following volumes is the alphabetic index of the ICD-9-CM coding book?
   a. I
   b. II
   c. III
   d. None of the above

Chapter Review (continued)

True/False

T F 1. Volume I is only used for hospital codes.

T F 2. Volume I indicates the number of digits required for coding.

T F 3. V codes indicate the reason for care, other than present illness.

T F 4. V codes cover HIV testing.

T F 5. E codes greatly affect reimbursement by insurance carriers.

T F 6. Diagnosis codes describe the need for medical care.

T F 7. Each visit a patient has with a health care provider can only have one diagnosis code.

Short Answer

1. How do you determine the first-listed diagnosis given to a patient?

2. What is the main concern with outsourced insurance billing services?

3. Explain what coding conventions are and how they are used in coding.

4. Explain how signs and symptoms are coded.

5. Explain a "late effect" diagnosis, and give an example.

6. Why would a physician code a condition as suspected?

7. What does the saying, "If it wasn't charted, it wasn't done," mean?

8. When is the ICD-10 coding book expected to be used in ambulatory care?

9. What is meant by the etiology of a disease?

Research

1. Interview a person who works in the billing department of a local medical office. How does that office handle the process of coding? Do the physicians assign the codes? What is the role of medical assistants in coding?

2. Look at the Medicare Web site. What are some of the rules Medicare applies regarding the use of diagnostic codes?

3. Look at your state's Medicaid Web site. What are some of the rules Medicaid applies regarding the use of diagnostic codes?

Externship Application Experience

Mabel Donchez, a patient of Dr. Bridges, is being seen today for an accidental overdose of a prescription medication Dr. Bridges prescribed. What part of the *ICD-9-CM* coding book would hold the proper code for this diagnosis?

Resource Guide

American Academy of Professional Coders
2480 South 3850 West
Suite B
Salt Lake City, UT 84120
Toll Free Phone: 800-626-CODE (2633)
Phone: 801-236-2200
Fax: 801-236-2258
Email: info@aapc.com
http://www.aapc.com

American Health Information Management Association
233 N. Michigan Avenue, 21st Floor
Chicago, IL 60601-5800
Toll Free Phone: (800) 335-5535
Phone: (312) 233-1100
Fax: (312) 233-1090
Email: info@ahima.org
http://www.ahima.org

American Medical Association
515 N State Street
Chicago, IL 60610
Phone: (800) 621-8335
http://www.ama-assn.org/

Centers for Disease Control and Prevention
1600 Clifton Road
Atlanta, GA 30333
Phone: (800) 311-3435
http://www.cdc.gov

Flash Code (provides information on proper ICD-9-CM coding)
Phone: (800) 711-7873
http://www.icd9coding1.com

Ingenix
12125 Technology Drive
Eden Prairie, MN 55344
Phone: (888) 445-8745
Fax: (952) 833-7079
http://www.ingenix.com/

 MedMedia

http://www.MyMAKit.com

More on this chapter, including interactive resources, can be found on the Student CD-ROM accompanying this textbook and on http://www.MyMAKit.com.

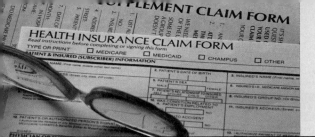

Objectives

After completing this chapter you should be able to:

- Define and spell the key terminology in this chapter.
- Understand the history of procedural coding.
- Describe the layout of the CPT® coding book.
- List the steps to accurate CPT coding, including determining correct codes via chart notes.
- Discuss how modifiers are used in procedural coding.
- Explain the use of the Health Care Common Procedure Coding System (HCPCS) and coding guides for specialized medical practices.
- Explain the relationship between accurate documentation and reimbursement.
- Identify fraudulent practices in coding and billing.
- Describe how bundled codes are used and what it means to unbundle a code.

Procedural Coding

Case Study

At Monday morning's staff meeting, Dr. Anderson mentions she is unhappy with the amount she is being reimbursed for her Medicare patients' office visits. To boost reimbursement, Dr. Anderson asks her medical assistant, Lydia, to use higher codes for those patients.

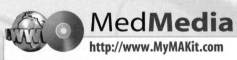

MedMedia

http://www.MyMAKit.com

Additional interactive resources and activities for this chapter can be found on http://www.MyMAKit.com. For a video, tips, audio glossary, legal and ethical scenarios, on-the-job scenarios, quizzes, and games related to the content of this chapter, please access the accompanying CD-ROM in this book.

Video: *Insurance Coding*
Legal and Ethical Scenario: *Procedural Coding*
On the Job Scenario: *Procedural Coding*
Tips
Multiple Choice Quiz
Audio Glossary
HIPAA Quiz
Games: Spelling Bee, Crossword, and Strikeout

Key Terminology

abuse—improper behavior and billing practices that result in financial gain but are not fraudulent

add-on code—a CPT code designated by the plus sign (+) that cannot be used alone; must be used with another CPT code

alphabetical index—alphabetical listing of CPT codes by procedure name, condition, eponym, and acronym

audit—a review process that verifies that every detail of a CPT code is clearly documented in the medical record

bilateral—on both sides of the body

bundling—combining multiple services under a single, all-inclusive CPT code and one charge

category—a division of a subheading within the tabular index

Category I codes—CPT codes numbered 00100 to 99999 representing widely used services and procedures approved by the FDA

Category II codes—supplemental tracking codes that can be used for performance measurement; four numbers followed by the letter F, such as 1002F

Category III codes—temporary codes for data collection and tracking the use of emerging technology, services, and procedures; four numbers followed by the letter T, such as 0162T

common descriptor—the portion of a standalone code before the semicolon that is shared with the indented codes that follow

contributing factors—three secondary criteria, in addition to the key components, that may influence the selection of an E&M code; include presenting problem, counseling/coordination of care, and physicians' face-to-face time with patients and families

coordination of care—a contributory factor in E&M coding that describes physicians' work in arranging care with other providers

counseling—a contributory factor in E&M coding that describes physicians' discussion with patients and family members regarding diagnosis, treatment options, instructions, and followup

CPT-4 manual—procedural coding book used in all U.S. health care settings

 MEDICAL ASSISTING STANDARDS

CAAHEP ENTRY-LEVEL STANDARDS	ABHES ENTRY-LEVEL COMPETENCIES
■ Describe how to use the most current procedural coding system (cognitive) ■ Define upcoding and why it should be avoided (cognitive) ■ Describe how to use the most current HCPCS coding (cognitive) ■ Perform diagnostic coding (psychomotor) ■ Work with physician to achieve the maximum reimbursement (affective)	■ Conduct work within scope of education, training, and ability ■ Monitor legislation related to current healthcare issues and practices ■ Apply managed care policies and procedures ■ Obtain managed care referrals and precertification ■ Receive, organize, prioritize, and transmit information expediently ■ Analyze and use current third-party guidelines for reimbursement ■ Use physician fee schedule ■ Implement current procedural terminology and ICD-9 coding

✓ **COMPETENCY SKILLS PERFORMANCE**

1. Code for a procedure.

Introduction

Procedural coding is the act of assigning a code to a patient's procedure or service. Since 1966, procedure codes have been **standardized,** which has rendered coding both more efficient and more accurate. Accuracy in procedural coding is essential, because incorrect or inadequate coding may lead to denial or delay of insurance claims.

The History of Procedural Coding

Before the mid-1960s, health care providers used the **usual, customary, and reasonable (UCR)** system to determine fair charges for their services. The UCR system was designed by insurance carriers to determine what the usual, customary and reasonable fee was for providers of health care services. In other words, insurance companies would look at billing records to see what providers in a certain geographic area charged for any given procedure code. The average of those charges was taken and then called the usual, customary, and reasonable charge for that service in that geographic area by that type of provider. Insurance companies would reimburse charges based on what they believed to be usual, customary, and reasonable. Most patients paid for their services, and when they had health insurance, they submitted their own reimbursement claims. There were no standard medical billing forms or procedure codes.

To standardize medical fees and increase the accuracy of the coding process, in 1992 the U.S. Congress developed a system that assigned a **relative value unit (RVU)** to every health care procedure or treatment. ∞ Chapter 16 details how RVUs are used to determine fee schedules.

Key Terminology *(continued)*

downcode—to assign a code for a lower level of service than was actually performed; done by some insurance companies to save money; done by some physicians to avoid fraud or abuse charges

established patient—patients who have seen the same provider, or another provider of the same specialty in the same practice within the past three years

Evaluation and Management (E&M)—CPT codes used for billing physician services to evaluate and manage patient care, such as office visits

examination—a key component of E&M coding that describes the complexity of the physical assessment of the patient

face-to-face time—a contributory factor in E&M coding that measures the amount of time the provider spent in the presence of the patient and/or family, as opposed to time spent documenting the visit or arranging referrals

fraud—to intentionally bill for services that were never given, including billing for a service that has a higher reimbursement than the service provided

global period—refers to the number of days surrounding a surgical procedure during which all services relating to that procedure—preoperative, during the surgery, and postoperative—are considered part of the surgical package

global surgical concept—see *global period*

guidelines—specific instructions at the beginning of each section of the CPT manual that define terms and describe specific information about how to use codes in that section

Health Care Common Procedure Coding System (HCPCS)—process for coding procedures and services

history—a key component of E&M coding that describes the background, onset, and progression of the patient's current condition

indented code—a CPT code whose description is indented 3 spaces under another (standalone) code and whose definition includes the portion before the semicolon (;) in the standalone code; done to save space in the CPT manual

inpatient—patient who has been formally admitted to a facility with written admission orders from a physician

instructional notes—directions in the tabular index, which appear in parentheses before or after a code entry, to point the user to alternative codes for closely-related procedures or to codes that must or must not be used together

key component—three primary determining criteria in selecting an E&M code; include history, examination, and medical decision making

Level I codes—same as CPT

Level II codes—HCPCS alphanumeric codes created by CMS to bill supplies, drugs, and certain services

Level III codes—HCPCS alphanumeric codes created by regional Medicare carriers; being phased out under HIPAA

main term—words by which procedures and services are alphabetized in the CPT index; may be a procedure, service, anatomic site, condition, synonym, eponym, or abbreviation

medical decision making (MDM)—a key component of E&M coding that describes the complexity of establishing a diagnosis and/or selecting a management option

modifier—two-digit alphanumeric codes appended to CPT or Level II codes to further describe circumstances

modifying term—descriptive words in the alphabetic index that appear indented under the main term to further describe the service or procedure

new patient—patients who have not seen the same provider, or another provider of the same specialty in the same practice, for more than three years

observation status—a designated type of care in which a patient is hospitalized for monitoring, but not formally admitted

outpatient—patient who has not been formally admitted to a facility, such as office visits, emergency department, and observation status

parent code—see *standalone code*

patient status—classification of patients as new or established

physical status modifier—2-digit alphanumeric codes (P1 to P6) appended to anesthesia codes, which indicate the health status of the patient at the beginning of the procedure

postoperative period—the number of days following a procedure during which

followup visits are bundled with the primary procedure and are not billed separately

presenting problem—a contributory factor in E&M coding that consists of a disease, condition, illness, injury, symptom, sign, finding complaint, or other reason for the encounter, as stated by the patient

procedural coding—process of assigning codes to health care services and procedures

procedures—services health care providers perform on patients

relative value unit (RVU)—unit of measure assigned to medical services based on the resources required to provide it; includes work, practice expense, and liability insurance

section—one of six major divisions of the CPT manual: evaluation and management; anesthesia; surgery; radiology; pathology and laboratory; medicine

semicolon (;)—a punctuation mark in a standalone code; the part of the definition before the semicolon is used by the indented codes that follow

special instructions—directions within each section describing specific rules and definitions for use of codes within a particular category or subcategory

standalone code—a CPT code that contains a full description and is not dependent on another code for complete meaning

standardized—uniform practice

subcategory—a division of a category within the tabular index

subheading—a division of a subsection within the tabular index

subsection—subdivisions within a CPT section of the tabular index

tabular index—the numerical listing of all CPT codes, accompanied by guidelines and notes

unbundling—billing multiple services with separate CPT codes and separate charges that should be combined under a single CPT code and one charge

upcode—to code and bill for a higher level of service than was actually provided

usual, customary, and reasonable (UCR)—reimbursement method in which insurance companies compare provider's charges against their normal charge, other providers' charges, and unusual circumstances

Abbreviations

AMA—American Medical Association

ASA—American Society of Anesthesiologists

B*T*M—Basic unit, Time, Modifying circumstances; formula for anesthesia reimbursement

CMS—Centers for Medicare and Medicaid Services

cm—centimeters

CPT—Current Procedural Terminology

DME—durable medical equipment

E/EX—examination (component of E&M codes)

E&M—evaluation and management

FDA—Food and Drug Administration

H—history (component of E&M codes)

HCPCS—Health Care Common Procedure Coding System

MDM—medical decision making (component of E&M codes)

POS—place of service

RVU—relative value unit

UCR—usual, customary, and reasonable

Coding with the CPT-4 Manual

Today, the **CPT-4 manual** covers all procedures approved by the Federal Drug Administration (**FDA**). When it was first published in 1966, however, the book focused mainly on surgical procedures. Some codes covered radiology, laboratory, and pathology services. Although the book is updated annually, the last major revision, the fourth, occurred in 1977.

In an effort to establish industry standards, in the 1980s the U.S. Congress began requiring providers to use CPT codes for all services Medicare patients receive. The codes, which are five digits long, must now appear on the CMS-1500 insurance claim form. ∞ Chapter 16 explains how to complete the CMS-1500 insurance claim form.

Procedures and services performed by physicians are reported using codes from the *Current Procedural Terminology, Fourth Edition*, which is published by the American Medical Association (AMA). The purpose of CPT® is to provide uniform language that will accurately describe medical, surgical, and diagnostic services so that those involved with health management and reimbursement will have an effective means of communication.

As with diagnostic coding, the challenge is to find the most appropriate and accurate code. Patient encounters for what is commonly referred to as an "office visit," for example, may be reported with any of 30-plus codes, depending on a number of circumstances surrounding the visit, but only one of these code choices is correct in any given situation. Likewise, more than 50 codes exist for a patient who receives sutures for a wound, depending on location, length and depth of the wound. Medical assistants need to be familiar with all the criteria for coding services offered by their office to be certain they select the most accurate code. When uncertain of the best code, it may be tempting to **upcode**, that is, to code for a higher level of service than what was actually provided in order to gain higher reimbursement, or **downcode**, to code for a lower level of service than what was actually provided in order to avoid potential **fraud** or **abuse**. *Fraud* is to intentionally bill for services that were never given, which includes upcoding. *Abuse* is improper behavior and billing practices that result in financial gain but are not fraudulent. As in all areas of health care, "ignorance is no excuse." When medical assistants are unsure regarding a coding issue, they may consult with the physician, a colleague, or a professional organization.

The CPT lists over 8,800 procedural codes. They are updated every year and take effect January 1. Medical assistants should use the edition of the CPT that was in effect on the date of service. For example, patients seen on December 31, 2009, would be coded using the 2009 coding manual while those seen on January 1, 2010, would be coded using the 2010 coding manual. The transition date for diagnosis coding differs from the one used for procedural coding, which is October 1. This is addressed in ∞ Chapter 17. CPT updates are needed to amend current listing and reflect new technologies and equipment. Code changes are published by the AMA in conjunction with CMS.

CPT is a registered trademark of the American Medical Association.

Organization of the CPT Manual

The organization of the 2008 CPT manual appears in Figure 18-1 ◆. The content and labeling of the many appendices sometimes changes when the manual is updated.

While it may seem unusual to discuss the covers of a manual, the inside front and back covers contain helpful information for medical assistants. Inside the front cover is a list of commonly used symbols, **modifiers**, and place-of-service codes. These will be discussed in detail later. Inside the back cover are commonly used medical abbreviations. Following the covers is a section of introductory matter that presents the table of contents by page number, instructions for use of the codebook, and other valuable information, depending on the publisher. Possible inclusions are a review of medical terminology and anatomical plates.

Tabular Index

The **tabular index** is a numerical listing of all CPT codes, divided into **Category I**, **Category II** and **Category III**. Category I codes, which comprise the bulk of the CPT, are numbered 00100 to 99999. They describe widely-used services and procedures approved by the FDA and are organized into six **sections** (see Table 18-1). While most of the codes are in numeric order, the codes 99201 through 99499 appear in the first section: Evaluation and Management. This is done for ease of use because these codes

Inside covers
Introductory matter
Tabular index
    Category I
    Category II
    Category III
Appendices
    A — Modifiers
    B — Summary of Additions, Deletions and Revisions
    C — Clinical Examples
    D — Summary of CPT Add-on Codes
    E — Summary of CPT Codes Exempt from Modifier 51
    F — Summary of CPT Codes Exempt from Modifier 63
    G — Summary of CPT Copes That Include Moderate (Conscious) Sedation
    H — Alphabetic Index of Performance Measures by Clinical Conditions or Topic
    I — Genetic Testing Code Modifiers
    J — Electrodiagnostic Medicine Listing of Sensory, Motor, and Mixed Nerves
    K — Product Pending FDA Approval
    L — Vascular Families
    M — Crosswalk to Deleted CPT Codes
Alphabetical index

Figure 18-1 ◆ Organization of the CPT manual.
CPT only copyright 2008 American Medical Association. All rights reserved.

TABLE 18-1 SECTIONS OF THE CPT-4 CATEGORY I CODES

Section	Code Range(s)
Evaluation and Management (E&M)	99201–99499
Anesthesiology	00100–01999
	99100–99140
Surgery	10021–69990
Radiology	70010–79999
Laboratory/Pathology	80048–89356
Medicine	90281–99199
	99500–99602

are the most frequently used and are used by all medical specialties. Other codes are used more selectively, based on the specific services provided by each office. The majority of this chapter will discuss category I codes in detail.

Category II codes are supplemental tracking codes and can be used for performance measurement. The use of these codes is optional and should not be used to replace category I codes. They are four numbers followed by the letter F, such as 1002F. Most medical assistants will likely not use these codes often.

Category III codes are temporary codes for data collection and tracking the use of emerging technology, services, and procedures. The codes are four numbers followed by the letter T, such as 0162T. If a category III code is available, medical assistants should use it in place of a category I code. Category III technology and procedures may be in the FDA approval process. Services may be items that the AMA is considering adding to category I. For example, online medical evaluation was a temporary code, 0074T, from 2005 to 2007; in 2008, it was assigned to category I as 99444.

Appendices

The CPT manual has several appendices, which provide additional reference information.

> Appendix A—Modifiers presents a complete description of all modifiers applicable to the current year codes. Modifiers are two-digit alphanumeric codes appended to CPT or Level II codes to further describe circumstances. An abbreviated list of commonly used modifiers appears inside the front cover, but medical assistants should develop the habit of referring to Appendix A until they are familiar with the details of how a specific modifier is to be used. Use of modifiers will be introduced later in the chapter.
>
> Appendix B—Summary of Additions, Deletions and Revisions is a valuable reference at the beginning of the year when the new CPT codes are released. Medical assistants can quickly cross reference the CPT codes on encounter forms to Appendix B in order to determine what commonly used codes in their office might be affected by the annual revision.
>
> Appendix C—Clinical Examples provides examples of E&M code scenarios for many medical specialties.

CPT is a registered trademark of the American Medical Association.

These should not be used for coding, but for learning and understanding how various patient encounters might be coded. Every E&M code has at least one example.

> Appendix D—Summary of CPT **Add-on Codes** lists the code numbers for those codes than cannot be used alone. Add-on codes are also designated with a + sign in the tabular index. Use of add-on codes will be described later.
>
> Appendix E—Summary of CPT Codes Exempt from Modifier 51 is a summary, not exhaustive, list of code numbers that do not require modifier 51, multiple procedures. These are codes that are typically performed with another procedure but are not subject to reimbursement reductions that typically accompany multiple procedures performed at the same time. Since multiple procedures usually are billed with modifier 51, these codes do not require modifier 51. Modifier 51 exempt codes are also designated with a ⊘ sign in the tabular index. Use of modifier 51 will be described later.
>
> Appendix F—Summary of CPT Codes Exempt from Modifier 63 lists code numbers that do not require modifier 63 procedure performed on infants less than 4 kg. Modifier 63 exempt codes are also designated with a parenthetical instruction in the tabular index.
>
> Appendix G—Summary of CPT Codes That Include Moderate (Conscious) Sedation is a list of codes in which moderate sedation by the surgeon is an inherent part of the procedure. For these codes, sedation should not be billed separately. Moderate sedation codes are also designated with a ⊙ symbol in the tabular index.
>
> Appendix H—Alphabetic Index of Performance Measures by Clinical Condition or Topic is a cross reference between Category II codes and situations in which they might be used. Most medical assistants will likely not use this appendix often.
>
> Appendix I—Genetic Testing Code Modifiers lists modifiers for reporting molecular laboratory procedures related to genetic testing. This enables providers to be more precise in coding without altering the test description. Only medical assistants working in the area of genetic testing will use these modifiers.
>
> Appendix J—Electrodiagnostic Medicine Listing of Sensory, Motor, and Mixed Nerves is used in accurately coding nerve conduction studies with CPT codes 95900, 95903, and 95904. Only medical assistants who work in an office performing nerve conduction studies will use this appendix.
>
> Appendix K—Product Pending FDA Approval lists CPT Category I codes for vaccines expected to be approved by the FDA at some point after the CPT manual is published, often in July. This enables a code to be immediately available once approval is granted. These codes are also designated with a dagger symbol ⫫ in the tabular index.

Appendix L—Vascular Families depicts the structure of first, second, and third order vascular branches. It aids medical assistants in coding for catheterization of the aorta.

Appendix M—Crosswalk to Deleted CPT Codes cross references codes from the previous year that have been deleted with suggested replacement codes in the current year's manual. Medical assistants can quickly cross reference the CPT codes on encounter forms that were deleted in the annual revision to Appendix M in order to determine what codes they can consider using instead.

Alphabetical Index

As in the ICD-9-CM manual, CPT coding begins with the **alphabetical index**. All procedures and services in the CPT manual are listed alphabetically by **main term** and **modifying terms** that aid in locating the most appropriate code or range of codes. After identifying potential codes in the index, they are verified in the tabular index. Final code selection should never be done based only on the alphabetical index. Detailed use of the index will be described later.

Conventions and Symbols

The CPT manual uses a number of formatting conventions and special symbols to provide information and to use space efficiently. Many of these are printed inside the front cover of the manual. They will be discussed in detail in the next section.

Determining the Correct Procedure Code

As with diagnostic coding, procedure coding also begins and ends with the patient's medical record. Medical assistants abstract information from the medical record in order to code for services and the reasons they were provided. Coding is to be done to the highest level of certainty, meaning that all relevant information in the chart should be coded, but missing information should not be assumed or coded. Only procedures and services documented in the medical record can be coded and billed. If the medical record is incomplete or inaccurate, it should be corrected or amended before attempting to code.

There are a number of documents within the medical record that may contain needed information. When coding for office-based or other outpatient services, medical assistants will refer to the encounter form, visit notes, in-house lab and radiology reports, and operative reports for outpatient procedures. When coding for services physicians provide to inpatients, medical assistants will refer to the daily rounds sheet, which lists the patients seen in the hospital; daily progress notes; and operative reports.

It is important to keep in mind that when performing procedure coding, the MA must code and bill only for the services actually delivered on a specific date by a specific provider. Do not bill for services previously completed, performed by a different provider, or ordered to be completed in the future.

CPT is a registered trademark of the American Medical Association.

A patient, Henry, makes a followup visit to Dr. Jessop related to back pain. Dr Jessop discusses Henry's progress and current condition, performs a physical examination, reviews X-rays taken by the hospital outpatient department, adjusts Henry's medication, provides therapeutic ultrasound, and orders a magnetic resonance imaging (MRI) study. The medical assistant, Heather, codes for the E&M visit and the therapeutic ultrasound, both of which Dr. Jessop performed today. The X-ray was not performed by Dr. Jessop; it was done previously at another location, so Heather doesn't code for the X-ray. Reviewing the X-ray and adjusting the medication are part of the medical decision making in the E&M visit, so there are not separate codes for these activities. The prescription itself is filled by the pharmacy, so she does not code for it. Heather also does not code for the MRI, which will be performed in the future at another location. If Dr. Jessop had a physical therapist on staff who provided the therapeutic ultrasound treatment, Heather would have still coded for it, but when she billed it, she would indicate on the CMS-1500 form (FL 24J) who actually performed that service.

The eleven coding steps described below provide the practical details medical assistants need to patiently and accurately execute the process of procedural coding.

1. Identify the primary and secondary services or procedures performed, as stated in the medical record. Often the physician will indicate procedure codes on the encounter form, but it is wise to verify them against the medical record. When abstracting from the medical record, be certain to not write in the record. Make a photocopy of the pertinent pages that can be annotated and highlighted or keep a separate paper for notes.

Look first for the chief complaint or reason for the visit. Services or procedures may be indicated in SOAP notes, under *O (Observation)*. Identify the primary procedure, or the main service provided during the encounter. Often, this may simply be the E&M encounter, the history, examination, and recommendations. It is common for the E&M to be the only service provided. E&M coding will be discussed in detail later. It may be a treatment, such as an injection, or a minor surgical procedure, such as removal of a lesion or repair of a laceration.

Additional services documented in the medical record should be identified by the medical assistant as secondary procedures. Secondary procedures are coded in the same way as primary procedures and prioritized from highest cost to lowest cost on the CMS-1500 form. This is because many insurance companies pay the first procedure in full, but discount additional procedures performed at the same time. Generally, the E&M is identified first, with additional procedures to follow, but some insurers may request that all services be listed in descending cost order.

Finally, note the quantity of each procedure. For many procedures, such as E&M, the quantity will be one. For services such as removal of lesions, it is important to identify the type and number of lesions removed. For services based on time, such as therapeutic ultrasound, identify the number of minutes spent providing the service.

The following sample patient scenario illustrates how to identify procedures. The same scenario will be developed throughout each step in the coding process discussed. An example of coding for E&M services will be presented later.

Sample Patient Scenario
Selecting the Primary and Secondary Procedures

Patient presents with a lesion on the back. The physician prepares the area, administers local anesthetic, and removes a 0.7 cm benign lesion from the back. The site is closed with simple sutures.

The primary procedure is removal of a lesion on the back.

2. **Locate the main term in the alphabetic index.** The index of the CPT manual lists main terms used to locate procedure codes. The main term may be located in one of four ways. (1) It may be the name of the *procedure* or *service*, such as "Endoscopy" or "Splint"; (2) it may the name of the *organ* or *anatomic* site, such as "Colon" or "Tibia"; (3) it may be the name of a *condition*, such as "Fracture"; a *disease*, such as "Polyp" or "Fracture"; (4) it may also be located by *eponym* (a disease or condition named after an individual) such as "Colle's fracture"; an abbreviation or *acronym*, such as "AIDS"; a nontechnical *synonym* (a word similar in meaning) such as "Removal" instead of "excision." While in many ways these options are similar to those used in the *ICD-9-CM* index, the biggest difference is that in the CPT index, main terms include organs and anatomic sites, whereas in the *ICD-9-CM* anatomical site was not an option (Figure 18-2 ♦). Because there are so many choices of how to locate a main term, a good guideline is to search in this order: eponym or abbreviation; procedure or service; organ or anatomical site; disease or condition; synonym.

Some main terms are rather generic with pages of modifying terms, such as "Excision," while others are quite specific with only a single code, such as "Color Vision Examination." The main term is always boldfaced with each word beginning with a capital letter. After locating the main term, the tentative

code(s) will be verified in Volume I. Never code from the index. The steps for verifying codes will be described later.

Exercise
Getting Acquainted with the Alphabetical Index

Look at the first few pages of your CPT alphabetical index. Find examples of each the following types of main terms:

eponym _____

acronym _____

procedure _____

organ _____

anatomic site _____

condition _____

Sample Patient Scenario
Identifying the Main Term

There is no acronym or eponym for removal of lesions. The first choice is to look under the procedure, Excision. When looking by organ system or anatomic site, the medical assistant remembers that lesions are located on the "skin," not on the back or other body area. In the CPT manual, entries for back procedures reference the internal musculoskeletal structure, not the skin itself. To locate by condition, the medical assistant would look under "Lesion."

3. **Review any modifying terms or instructional notes associated with the main term.** Main terms rarely provide the exact code needed. Frequently main terms function as major headings that have up to three series of modifying terms. Modifying terms are descriptive words in the alphabetic index that appear indented under the main term to further describe the service or procedure (modifying terms different than two-digit modifiers that are appended to Category I codes). When modifying terms appear, it is important to review the entire list, as they do affect the appropriate code selection.

Eponym/ Acronym	Procedure	Anatomic Site	Condition	Synonym
(Eponym) Colles fracture	Repair	Wrist	Fracture	
(Acronym) EKG	Electrocardiogram	Heart		Monitoring
	Excision	Eye	Cataract	Removal

Figure 18-2 ♦ Alternative methods for locating the CPT main term.

CPT is a registered trademark of the American Medical Association.

The first series of modifying terms is aligned on the same margin as the main term, but in smaller, non-boldfaced type. The second and third levels of modifying terms are each indented several spaces beyond the previous level. They further describe the main term, in reference to anatomical site such as *Excision, kidney;* extent, such as *Excision, Clavicle, Partial;* procedure, such as *Electrocardiography, 24-Hour Monitoring;* or similar descriptors.

If the main term or modifying term is too long to fit on one line, a carry over line is used. Carry over lines are indented the same number of spaces as the beginning of the line. It is important to read carefully to distinguish between carry over lines and modifying terms.

Main terms and modifying terms contain instructional notes, such as *see* or *see also,* which direct the user to synonyms. For example, *Pneumonotomy—see Excision, Lung.* This instructs the user where to look for the code needed.

Codes may be listed singly, as a range, or as a nonsequential list. A range of codes is presented with a hyphen "-", such as *Bone Graft, Harvesting 20900-20902.* This indicates that all codes beginning with 20900 and ending with and including 20902 should be reviewed. Nonsequential codes are presented with a comma "," such as *Biopsy, Urethra 52204, 52354, 53200.* This indicates that three codes should be reviewed, but the intervening code numbers are probably not applicable.

Exercise
Identifying Conventions in the CPT Index

Look up the main term Blood in the alphabetical index and locate examples of the following:

Main term _____

Instructional note _____

First-level modifying term _____

Second-level modifying term _____

Third-level modifying term _____

Carry over line _____

Sample Patient Scenario
Using CPT Alphabetical Index Conventions

Main term: Excision
Instructional note: See Debridement; Destruction
First modifying term: Lesion
Second modifying term: Skin
Third modifying term: Benign.

There is not a modifying term for the location of the lesion. This will be identified once the tabular index is consulted.

4. Identify the tentative code(s) associated with the most appropriate modifying term(s). When the appropriate modifying terms are located, the tentative code(s) is printed immediately to the right. It is helpful to jot down the potential appropriate codes before verifying in the tabular list. Never use the index to make the final code selection. Even if only one code appears, it must be verified in the tabular index to be certain the code selection is accurate.

Sample Patient Scenario
Selecting the Tentative Code(s)

Excision
  Lesion
    Benign   *Code range:* 11400-11471

5. Locate the tentative code(s) in the tabular index. Look for the tentative code number in the tabular index where codes are arranged in numerical order. The tabular index contains six sections based on medical specialty. Chapters are divided into **subsections**, **subheadings**, **categories**, and **subcategories** based on anatomy, procedure, condition, or descriptor. The name of each of these divisions is printed with a specific typeface and text formatting, depending on the publisher. Not all of the divisions appear under every subsection; it depends on the amount of information in each specific subsection. All codes appear under the lowest division. It is helpful to learn the specific meanings of these designations, because the terms are used frequently in coding instructions (Figure 18-3 ◆).

6. Interpret the conventions used in the tabular index.[*] Even though you are now eager to verify and finalize your code, you first need to interpret the conventions presented with the code. The codes are presented as a five-digit number with no decimal point, and a description to the right. Tabular index conventions include formatting, punctuation, instructional notes, and symbols and may appear on the same line with the code, above it, below it, or at the beginning of a subcategory, category, subheading, subsection, or section. Look carefully for any information that may be relevant to your tentative code selection, as the additional information may direct you when to use a different code or an additional code, depending on the specific procedure performed.

In the tabular index, the most critical convention is the paired use of the **semicolon** (;) and indents. To conserve space and avoid having to repeat common terminology, some of the procedure descriptors in the tabular index are not printed in their entirety, but rather refer back to a common portion of the procedure descriptor listed in a preceding entry. The **standalone** or **parent code** is the one whose description is left-justified and

---

[*]Adapted from Vines, Deborah, Braceland, Ann, Rollins, Elizabeth, and Miller, Susan. *Comprehensive Health Insurance: Billing, Coding, and Reimbursement,* pp. 133–135.

Level	Description				
Section	**Anesthesia**		**Surgery**		
Subsection	**HEAD**	**NECK**	**CARDIOVASCULAR SYSTEM**		
Subheading	*none*	*none*	**Heart and Pericardium**		**Arteries & Vessels**
Category	*none*	*none*	***Pericardium***	***Cardiac Valves***	***Arterial Grafting***	*multiple*
Subcategory	*none*	*none*	*none*	**Aortic** **Mitral** **Tricuspid** **Pulmonary**	*none*	*multiple*

Figure 18-3 ◆ Example of tabular index organization levels and formatting.

begins with a capital letter. The shared portion of the code before the semicolon is the common descriptor, which is shared with indented codes. The portion after the semicolon is the unique descriptor that applies to only one code number. The **indented code** description is indented three spaces and begins with a small letter. It is only the unique descriptor for that code number. This unique descriptor must be combined with the unique descriptor from the standalone code in order to obtain a full description of the code. Within any series of indented codes, you *must* refer back to the standalone code within that series to determine the common descriptor of the indented code(s). Indented codes describe variations on the standalone code, such as alternative anatomic site, alternative procedure, or extent of services.

Figure 18-4 ◆ illustrates this formatting convention. The standalone code is 27134. The common part of its description is the words before the semicolon ("Revision of total hip arthroplasty"). This **common descriptor** should be considered part of each of the following indented codes in that series. For example, the full procedure descriptor represented by code 27137 is as follows:

27137 Revision of total hip arthroplasty, acetabular component only, with or without autograft or allograft

An indented code does not have to be billed together with the standalone code. They are considered two distinct procedures or services. The common descriptor is simply a space-saving convention in the printed book.

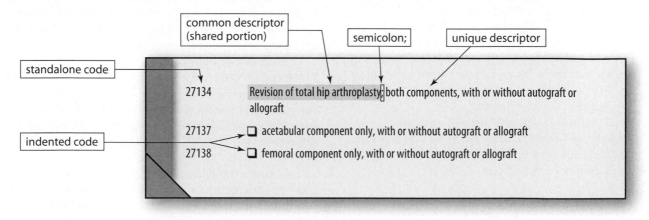

Figure 18-4 ◆ Example of standalone and indented codes.
CPT only copyright 2008 American Medical Association. All rights reserved.

CPT is a registered trademark of the American Medical Association.

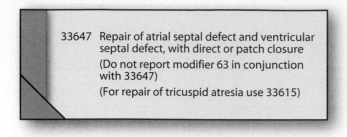

33647	Repair of atrial septal defect and ventricular septal defect, with direct or patch closure
	(Do not report modifier 63 in conjunction with 33647)
	(For repair of tricuspid atresia use 33615)

Figure 18-5 ◆ Example of instructional notes.
CPT only copyright 2008 American Medical Association. All rights reserved.

Instructional notes, which appear in parentheses, are used in the tabular index to point the user to alternative codes for closely-related procedures or to codes that must or must not be used together (Figure 18-5 ◆).

Special instructions are directions within each section describing specific rules and definitions for use of codes within a particular category or subcategory. These also should be read and interpreted before assigning a code, even if it means going back to the top of the page or a previous page to find them. **Guidelines** are instructions that appear at the beginning of each of the six sections and apply to all codes in that section. Guidelines also list commonly used modifiers and provide subsection information.

Symbols are used in the tabular index to alert the user to certain circumstances that may affect use or interpretation of codes. There is a key at the bottom of each page. Medical assistants should become familiar with these meanings:

⊙   Moderate sedation is automatically included in the code description

⊘   Modifier 51 exempt. When billing multiple procedures, a code with this symbol does not require using modifier 51.

\+   Add-on code must be used in conjunction with another CPT code. Frequently, the accepted companion codes are provided in an instructional note.

✗   FDA approval pending. FDA approval of the vaccine described is expected to come during the current year.

( )   Parentheses are used to enclose synonyms, eponyms, or supplementary descriptors that may be present or absent in a physician's statement of condition without affecting the code assignment.

●   New code in this edition of the CPT manual

▲   Revised code—the code number is the same, but the descriptor has been updated

▶◀   Contains new or revised text

New and revised code symbols are an important aid to medical assistants experienced in coding. They alert the user to the fact that a code they may be accustomed to using in a certain manner has been updated and may no longer be appropriate.

CPT is a registered trademark of the American Medical Association.

Exercise
Interpreting Special Instructions

Look up CPT code 11400 in the tabular index. Locate the special instructions under the subheading *Excision—Benign Lesions*. Read the instructions, then write down answers to the questions below:

1. Is anesthesia included? _____
2. Where should one look for codes for shave removal? _____
3. Where should one look for codes for electrosurgical and other methods of removal? _____
4. What is the definition of *excision*? _____
5. What is the margin? _____
6. What is included in the size of the excised lesion? _____
7. What type of closure is included? _____
8. Where should one look for codes for intermediate closures? _____
9. Where should one look for codes for complex closures? _____
10. Where should one look for codes for adjacent tissue transfer? _____
11. What part of the instructions contains new or revised information? _____

Sample Patient Scenario
Interpreting Tabular Index Conventions

The index directed us to Excision, Lesion, Benign 11400-11471. The task now is to look up this range of codes in the tabular index to select the one that best describes the procedure (0.7 cm lesion from the back, closed with simple sutures, benign). First, read the special instructions at the beginning of the subheading *Excision—Benign Lesions* and complete the exercise on interpreting special instructions to help understand what is being said.

Scan all the codes in this range. The last six codes, 11450 to 11471, describe E*xcision of skin and subcutaneous tissue for hidradenetis,* which is not appropriate for this case. You quickly see among codes 11400 to 11446 that there are many indented codes that appear to be the same. For example, 11401, 11421, 11441 all state *excised diameter 0.6 to 1.0 cm.*

To understand the differences between these codes, it is necessary to compare the common portion of the accompanying standalone codes, 11400, 11420, 11440. The first part of the common portion of the standalone codes is also the same *Excision, benign lesion including margins, except skin tag (unless listed elsewhere).* The last half line of the common portion that describes the body area is what varies among the standalone codes.

7. Select the code with the highest level of specificity. There is no universal rule that describes how many codes need to be reviewed before identifying the one with the highest specificity. Sometimes, the best code is the first one listed; other times, there may be a dozen or more codes to review and additional ones to cross-reference. There also is no universal rule that describes how precise the correct code will be in its description. For example, many codes on the integumentary system include the size of the area treated, but the size is usually a range, such as 1.1 cm to 2.0 cm. If a treatment covers 1.5 cm exactly, there is not a more specific code or modifier to describe the exact size. The medical record often contains more detail than what is coded. Only by carefully interpreting the conventions associated with each code, category, and section can one be certain. As medical assistants become experienced in a particular office, they become very familiar with the most frequently used codes.

Sample Patient Scenario
Selecting the Code with the Highest Level of Specificity

First, select the standalone code that contains the description for this patient. The term *back* does not appear, but using knowledge of anatomy, you know that *trunk* includes the back. 11400, *trunk, arms, or legs* is the appropriate standalone code.

Now select the indented code that describes the diameter of 0.7 cm. Code 11401 is *excised diameter 0.6 to 1.0 cm,* so this is the best code.

8. Review the code for appropriate bundling, add on codes and quantity. Carefully review code descriptions, instructional notes, and special instructions one more time to be certain that the code selected is accurate. Pay special attention to **bundling** edits, frequently triggered by the words *includes* and *not separately reportable.* This indicates that multiple services are included in a single code. The words *report separately* or *use in conjunction with* indicate that additional codes should be used. For example, the special instructions for *33510 to 33516 Coronary artery bypass, vein only* include both bundling and multiple coding situations. For bundling, the instructions state *Procurement of the saphenous vein graft is included in the description of the work for 33510-33516 and should not be reported as a separate service or co-surgery.* However, an additional code is needed in other situations: *to report harvesting of an upper extremity vein, use 35500 in addition to the bypass procedure.*

CPT codes also differ regarding how the quantity of procedures is to be reported. This information is provided in the code description or special instructions. For example, to report removal of skin tags, a single code, 11200, describes *up to and including 15 lesions.* While the code is reported with a quantity of *1* on the CMS-1500 form, block 24G, it describes as many as 15 lesions. For shaving of epidermal or dermal lesions (11300-11313), each code describes a single lesion; multiple

CPT is a registered trademark of the American Medical Association.

lesions of the same size and body area are reported by designating the number of lesions in block 24G on the CMS-1500 form. End-stage renal disease services are reported with a single code for the entire month (90918-90921); the special instructions describe the scope of services included. Codes that include a time-based element also vary in how quantity is reported. For example, codes for certain physical therapy treatments (97032-97039) describe 15 minutes of treatment with a quantity of *1* on the CMS-1500 form, block 24G. Thirty minutes of treatment is reported with a quantity of *2* on the CMS-1500 form, block 24G.

Add-on codes should also be verified. Use of add-on codes may be limited to only a few codes that are listed in instructional notes. For example, when coding for discectomy of multiple disks, the code for each additional interspace is reported in addition to a specific primary procedure code. CPT add-on code 63078 should be used in conjunction with 60377.

Sample Patient Scenario
Reviewing the Bundling, Add-on Code and Quantity Edits

The special instructions describe that local anesthesia and simple closure are included (bundled) with the codes in this subheading. No add-on codes apply. No additional coding is required for these services. Only a single lesion was excised, so there are no quantity edits.

Note: If a second lesion in the same location and same size range is performed, the code is reported with a quantity of *2* on the CMS-1500 form, block 24G.

9. Determine if modifiers are required. Modifiers affect the complete description of a service and frequently have a significant impact on reimbursement and coding compliance. Use of modifiers may be described in the instructional notes, special instructions, or guidelines. It is usually dependent on the experience of the coder to determine if the situation calls for any modifiers. Detailed use of modifiers is discussed later in the chapter.

Sample Patient Scenario
Determining if Modifiers Are Required

No modifiers are required for this case. If more than one lesion had been excised, of a different size range or body area, modifier 51, multiple procedures, would be used on the subsequent procedures.

10. Verify the final code against the documentation. As a final check, with coding manual instructions fresh in your mind, refer back to the original documentation and verify that all conditions of the code agree with the medical record. If a discrepancy arises, work through the process again from the beginning.

Sample Patient Scenario
Verifying the Final Code Against Documentation

11401 Excision, benign lesion including margins, except skin tag, trunk arms or legs, excised diameter 0.6 cm to 1.0 cm accurately matches our description of excision of 0.7 cm lesion from the back, closed with simple sutures, benign.

11. Assign the code. Write down the final code where indicated on your worksheet or documentation. Be certain to proofread the number as you wrote or keyboarded it to avoid transcription errors that are easy to make.

Repeat this process for any additional codes required by the medical record.

Selecting a procedure code may seem like a long and tedious process at first. As medical assistants become familiar with the services and codes used by their medical office, coding becomes faster and easier, but accuracy and attention to detail is always paramount. Taking time and care to learn the fundamentals correctly will help create long-term success in your coding role.

Using CPT Modifiers*

Modifiers are two-digit suffixes used with CPT codes to report a service or procedure that has been modified by some specific circumstance without altering or modifying the basic definition or CPT code (Table 18-2). The proper use of modifiers can speed up claims processing and increase reimbursement, whereas the improper use of CPT modifiers may result in claim delays or denials. A complete list of modifiers can be found in the CPT book in Appendix A with their full definitions. Modifiers may be used for these reasons:

- To report only the professional component of a procedure or service
- To report a service mandated by a third-party payer

*Source: Adapted from Vines, Deborah, Braceland, Ann, Rollins, Elizabeth, and Miller, Susan. *Comprehensive Health Insurance: Billing, Coding, and Reimbursement,* pp. 135–140.

TABLE 18-2 CPT MODIFIERS

Modifier	Use
21	Prolonged Evaluation and Management Services
22	Unusual Procedural Services
23	Unusual Anesthesia
24	Unrelated Evaluation and Management Service by the Same Physician during a **Postoperative** Period
25	Significant, Separately Identifiable Evaluation and Management Service by the Same Physician on the Same Day of the Procedure or Other Service
26	Professional Component
32	Mandated Services
47	Anesthesia by Surgeon
50	Bilateral Procedure
51	Multiple Procedures
52	Reduced Services
53	Discontinued Procedure
54	Surgical Care Only
55	Postoperative Management Only
56	Preoperative Management Only
57	Decision for Surgery
58	Staged or Related Procedure or Service by the Same Physician during the Postoperative Period
59	Distinct Procedural Service
62	Two Surgeons
63	Procedure Performed on Infants
66	Surgical Team
76	Repeat Procedure by Same Physicians
77	Repeat Procedure by Another Physician
78	Return to the Operating Room for a Related Procedure during the Postoperative Period
79	Unrelated Procedure or Service by the Same Physician during the Postoperative Period
80	Assistant Surgeon
81	Minimum Assistant Surgeon
82	Assistant Surgeon (when qualified resident surgeon is unavailable)
90	Reference (Outside) Laboratory
91	Repeat Clinical Diagnostic Laboratory Test
99	Multiple Modifiers

Source: CPT 2008. Copyright 2008 American Medical Association. All rights reserved.

CPT is a registered trademark of the American Medical Association.

- To indicate that a procedure was performed **bilaterally**
- To report multiple procedures performed at the same session by the same provider
- To report a portion of a service or procedure that was reduced or eliminated at the physician's discretion
- To report assistant surgeon services.

The most commonly used modifiers are discussed next.

22 Unusual Procedural Service—This modifier is used when the service provided is higher than that usually required for the listed procedure. A special report should be submitted with the claim. A special report is a report that details the reasons for a new, variable, or unlisted procedure or service; it explains the patient's condition and justifies the procedure's medical necessity. An unlisted procedure is a service or procedure that is not listed in the CPT codebook. Each section's guidelines have codes for unlisted procedures.

47 Anesthesia by Surgeon—Regional or general anesthesia provided by the surgeon may be reported by adding modifier 47 to the basic service. This does not include local anesthesia.

50 Bilateral Procedure—Bilateral means pertaining to two sides. Unless otherwise identified in the descriptor, bilateral procedures that are performed at the same operative session should be identified by appending modifier 50 to the procedure.

51 Multiple Procedures—When multiple procedures are performed, other than evaluation and management (E&M) services, at the same session by the same provider, the primary procedure may be listed first. The additional procedures may be identified by appending modifier 51 to the additional procedure. Modifier 51 has four applications, namely, to identify:
- multiple medical procedures performed at the same session by the same provider.
- multiple, related operative procedures performed at the same session by the same provider.
- operative procedures performed in combination, at the same operative session, by the same provider, whether through the same or another incision or involving the same or different anatomy.
- a combination of medical and operative procedures performed at the same session by the same provider.

Many insurers reimburse a lesser amount for procedures using modifier 51, because there is a potential cost savings for the surgeon performing multiple procedures at one session, compared to performing only a single procedure. Modifier 51 should not be appended to designated add-on codes or those with the symbol ⊘, which means "exempt from modifier 51."

53 Discontinued Procedure—Under certain circumstances, the physician may elect to terminate a surgical or diagnostic procedure. Due to extenuating circumstances or those that threaten the well-being of the patient, it may be necessary to indicate that a surgical or diagnostic procedure was started but discontinued. This circumstance may be reported by adding the modifier 53 to the code reported by the physician for the discontinued procedure.

54 Surgical Care Only—When one physician performs a surgical procedure and another provides preoperative and/or postoperative management, surgical services may be identified by adding modifier 54 to the usual procedure number.

55 Postoperative Management Only—When one physician performed the postoperative management and another performed the surgical procedure, modifier 55 is appended to the usual procedure number.

56 Preoperative Management Only—When one physician performed the preoperative care and evaluation and another physician performed the surgical procedure, the preoperative component may be identified by adding modifier 56 to the usual procedure number. Modifier 53 is not used to report the elective cancellation of a procedure prior to the patient's anesthesia induction or surgical preparation in the operating suite. This modifier is not used to report the treatment of a problem that requires a return to the operating room; see modifier 78 instead.

EXAMPLE FOR MODIFIERS 54, 55, AND 56:

A physician may intend to perform all three components of a global service (preoperative management, surgical care, and postoperative management); however, after providing the preoperative management and performing the surgical procedure, he is unexpectedly called out of town. The surgeon in this case reports the surgical procedure with the modifiers 54 and 56 appended. The physician who performed the postoperative management reports the operative procedure code with modifier 55 appended. Reporting the postoperative management indicates that the physician performed all of the postoperative care.

58 Staged or Related Procedure by the Same Physician During the Postoperative Period—The physician may need to indicate that the performance of a procedure or service during the postoperative period was
1. planned prospectively at the time of the original procedure (staged).
2. more extensive than the original procedure.
3. for therapy following a diagnostic surgical procedure. This circumstance may be reported by appending modifier 58 to the staged or related procedure.

59 Distinct Procedural Service—Under certain circumstances, the physician may need to indicate that a procedure or service was distinct or independent from other services performed on the same day. Modifier 59 is used to identify procedures that are not normally reported together, but are appropriate under the circumstances.

CPT is a registered trademark of the American Medical Association.

62 Two Surgeons—When two surgeons work together as primary surgeons performing a distinct part of a procedure, each surgeon should report his or her distinct operative work by adding modifier 62 to the procedure and any associated add-on codes for that procedure as long as both surgeons continue to work together as primary surgeons.

78 Return to the Operating Room for a Related Procedure During the Postoperative Period—The physician may need to indicate that another procedure was performed during the postoperative period of the initial procedure. When this subsequent procedure is related to the first and requires the use of the operating room, it may be reported by adding modifier 78 to the related procedure. If the return is due to a complication, it is eligible for reimbursement, even though it occurs during the postoperative period.

79 Unrelated Procedure or Service by the Same Physician During the Postoperative Period—The physician may need to indicate that the performance of a procedure during the postoperative period was unrelated to the original procedure.

80 Assistant Surgeon—Surgical assistant services may be identified by adding modifier 80 to the usual procedure number.

Coding for Evaluation and Management Services

Evaluation and Management (E&M) codes describe patient encounters with a physician for the evaluation and management of a health problem. Although these codes begin with 99, they are located out of numerical sequence in the CPT manual, at the front of the manual, as the first section. E&M codes are selected based on the category of service, which may be the location or the type of service provided, depending on the category.

Normally, the physician marks the E&M code on the encounter form. Medical assistants need to ensure that documentation in the medical record is consistent with the codes checked off. It is also a good idea to **audit** bills on a regular basis. Auditing is a detailed process that verifies that every detail of the E&M code is clearly documented. E&M coding possesses some differences from the rest of CPT coding. The key steps for E&M coding are described next. Do not be tempted to rush through E&M coding by skipping or abbreviating any of these steps because this could result in inaccurate coding and payment.

1. **Identify the category of service.** When coding for E&M services, it is important to select the category of service first, before trying to determine the specific code. Categories may describe the location of service, such as office visit or hospital inpatient visit, or the type of service, such as consultation, critical care, or preventive care. This can be confusing because not all services provided in the medical office, for example, are coded from the *Office Visit* category. They may be coded from

Consultation, Preventive Care, or several other categories as well. It is important to be familiar with CPT definitions of these services, which are described in special instructions at the beginning of each subsection. Table 18-3 lists the most commonly used categories of E&M service with a brief description of each. To locate codes, look first in the alphabetical index, under the main term *Evaluation and Management,* then select the appropriate category.

2. **Identify the subcategory of service.** Most of the E&M categories are further subdivided based on patient status (new vs. established), location (office vs. inpatient), frequency (initial vs. subsequent), or other relevant characteristic. These criteria are defined in the section guidelines or subsection special instructions. Some of the commonly used terms are discussed in the section that follows.

Medical assistants will frequently need to determine **patient status**; that is, to distinguish between **new patients** and **established patients**, as this criterion is used for office visits and preventive care. A new patient is one who has not received any professional services from the physician, or another physician of the same specialty who belongs to the same group practice, within the past three years. An established patient is one who has received professional services from the physician, or another physician of the same specialty who belongs to the same group practice, within the past three years (Figure 18-6 ◆).

Some codes are determined based on whether the patient is an **outpatient** or an **inpatient**. An inpatient is someone who has been formally admitted to a facility with written admission orders from a physician. All others are considered outpatients, even though they may occupy a hospital bed, for example, on **observation status** and emergency department patients. Observation status is a designated type of care in which a patient is hospitalized for monitoring, but not formally admitted.

3. **Review the reporting instructions for the selected category or subcategory.** Each category and subcategory within the E&M section contains definitions and instructions

TABLE 18-3 COMMONLY USED CATEGORIES OF E&M CODES	
Office (and Other Outpatient) Services	99201–99215
Hospital Observation Services	99217–99220
Hospital (Inpatient) Services	99221–99239
Consultations (Office)	99241–99245
Consultations (Inpatient)	99251–99255
Emergency Department Services	99281–99288
Pediatric Critical Care Patient Transport	99289, +99290
Critical Care Services	99291, +99292
Inpatient Pediatric and Neonatal Critical Care	99293–99300
Nursing Facility Services	99304–99318
Rest Home, Custodial Care, Domiciliary	99324–99337
Oversight Services for Domiciliary, Rest Home or Home	99339–99340
Home Services	99341–99350

Source: CPT 2008. Copyright 2008 American Medical Association. All rights reserved.

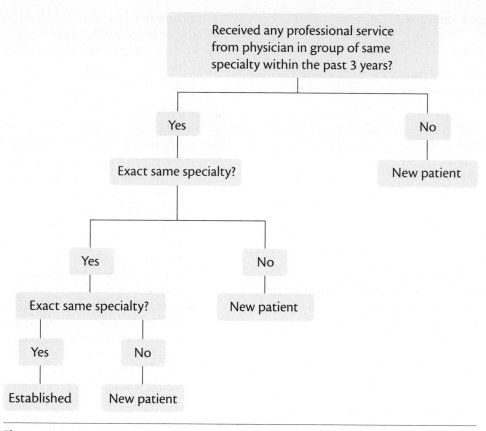

Figure 18-6 ◆ Decision tree for new versus established patients.
Source: CPT 2008, Professional Edition, p. 2. American Medical Association. Reprinted with permission.

that describe key terms, how the codes are to be reported, and what may be bundled into the code description. Even though this can sometimes be lengthy, take time to read and understand what is being said. For example, when reporting critical care services, lengthy examples are provided of what comprises critical care, where it can be provided, and the age of the patient appropriate for the codes. In addition, a list of bundled CPT codes is provided, which cannot be reported separately.

4. **Determine the key components.** Within each subcategory, there are three to five levels of codes, in increasing order of complexity. It is necessary to determine the **key components** or other criteria used for code selection within each subcategory of E&M codes. Many codes are based on the extent of the history (H), the examination (E), and the medical decision making (MDM). Other codes are based on time or age. A summary of the three key components (H, E, MDM) follows. More detailed guidelines can be found in the CPT guidelines and reference texts.

a. **History (H)** To determine the proper level of history for the E&M code, the following descriptions are used:

Problem focused—patient's problem is small; he has only one chief complaint and gives a brief history of his present illness or problem

Expanded problem focused—patient's problem is mild to moderate; he has more than one chief com-

plaint and/or a more extensive history of his present illness or problem.

Detailed—patient's problem is moderate to severe and he has pertinent past, family and/or social history that is directly related to his current problem.

Comprehensive—patient's problem is moderate to severe; he has a more extensive history and needs a complete review of all additional body systems.

b. **Examination (E/Ex)** To determine the proper level of examination for the E&M code, the following descriptions are used:

Problem focused— A limited examination of the affected body area is done.

Expanded problem focused— A limited examination of the affected body area is done along with other related organ systems.

Detailed— An extended examination of the affected body area and other related organ systems is performed.

Comprehensive— A general multisystem examination is performed.

For the purposes of determining a body area, the CPT-4 code book lists the following body areas to be recognized:

• Head, including the face
• Neck
• Chest, including breasts and axilla
• Abdomen

CPT is a registered trademark of the American Medical Association.

- Genitalia, groin, buttocks
- Back
- Each extremity

For the purpose of definition of organ systems, the CPT-4 code book lists the following organ systems:

- Eyes
- Ears, nose, mouth and throat
- Cardiovascular
- Respiratory
- Gastrointestinal
- Genitourinary
- Musculoskeletal
- Skin
- Neurologic
- Psychiatric
- Hematologic/Lymphatic/Immunologic

c. **Medical Decision Making (MDM)** In order to determine the proper level of **medical decision making (MDM)** for the E&M codes, the medical assistant should consider the following:

- The number of possible diagnoses the patient has
- The amount or complexity of the medical records the provider must go through to treat the patient
- The risk of significant complications as a result of this treatment.

There are four types of medical decision making recognized by the CPT-4. These are listed as: straightforward; low complexity; moderate complexity; and high complexity. Straightforward is listed as minimal diagnoses, minimal complexity, and minimal risk of complications. Low complexity is listed as limited diagnoses, limited complexity, and low risk of complications. Moderate complexity is listed as multiple diagnoses, moderate complexity, and moderate risk of complications. High complexity is listed as extensive diagnoses, extensive complexity, and high risk of complications.

The specific E&M code is selected based on how it meets the criteria of the key components. The criteria for each component are described in the code definition in the CPT manual. Some categories of E&M codes require that all three key components be at the level specified in the code description or a higher level in order to assign the code. Other categories require that only two of the key components be at the level specified in the code description or a higher level in order to assign the code. The number of components required is stated in the code description.

5. **Identify the contributing factors.** E&M codes that contain the three key components H, E, and MDM also have three **contributing factors**: counseling, coordination of care, and nature of the **presenting problem**. These factors rarely determine the code, but should be consistent with the code selected.

Counseling is defined as a discussion with the patient and/or a family concerning the patient's diagnosis, test results, impressions, prognosis, risks and benefits of treatment options, and instructions for management of the condition.

Coordination of care is the task of working with other providers or agencies to provide the patient with needed care, such as referral to home healthcare.

E&M codes take the following into consideration in determining the nature of the presenting problem:

- **Minimal**—The problem may not require the presence of the physician, but service is provided under the physician's supervision.
- **Self-limited or minor**—The problem runs a definite and prescribed course, is temporary, and is not likely to permanently alter the patient's health status.
- **Low severity**—The problem has a low risk of causing the patient's death without treatment and full recovery is expected.
- **Moderate severity**—The problem has a risk of death without treatment, there is an uncertain prognosis, or an increased likelihood the problem will cause permanent health problems for the patient.
- **High severity**—The problem has a high risk of causing the patient's death without treatment, or there may be a high probability of prolonged functional impairment to the patient as a result of this condition.

Finally, time is a consideration in E&M coding. Codes with the three key components also include an indication of the amount of time the physician typically spends **face-to-face** with the patient and/or family. While these E&M codes should never be selected based on time, there are unusual situations in which a code level can be increased. If the time spent in counseling and coordination of care is more than 50 percent of total visit time, time may be considered a controlling factor to qualify for a higher level E&M code. In order to do this, documentation needs to indicate the total amount of time spent with the patient and/or family, the amount of time spent in counseling and coordination of care, and a description of why the additional time was required.

6. **Verify and assign the code.** After verifying documentation against CPT guidelines, special instructions, and code descriptions, determine the appropriate code and write it on your coding worksheet or enter it into the computer system. Be certain to verify the accuracy of the code number, as transpositions easily occur.

7. **Identify bundled and separately billable services.** Certain services are included in the E&M code: discussions with patients and their families about the current problem; physical examination; reviewing test results, reports from other providers, and records of outside services; ordering tests and services; writing prescriptions; scheduling procedures; providing instructions and education to patients and their families. Certain codes, such as critical care, include a more specific list of bundled services. If a visit is related to postoperative followup, it should not be billed separately. If an office or emergency department encounter develops into another E&M service on the same date, such as inpatient admission, the first E&M is bundled into the hospital admission.

CPT is a registered trademark of the American Medical Association.

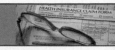

PROCEDURE 18-1   Code for a Procedure

Theory and Rationale

Proper procedure coding in the medical office facilitates timely payment of providers' claims. Therefore, medical assistants must be familiar with the steps involved in locating and assigning proper procedure codes.

Materials

- CPT-4 coding book
- Superbill/encounter form
- Patient's chart

Competency

(**Conditions**) With the necessary materials, you will be able to (**Task**) assign a procedure code (**Standards**) correctly within the time limit set by the instructor.

1. On the superbill, locate the procedure code the physician has circled.

2. Identify the primary and secondary services or procedures performed, as stated in the medical record.
3. Locate the main term in the alphabetic index.
4. Review any modifying terms or instructional notes associated with the main term.
5. Identify the tentative code(s) associated with the most appropriate modifying term(s).
6. Locate the tentative code(s) in the tabular index.
7. Interpret the conventions used in the tabular index.
8. Select the code with the highest level of specificity.
9. Review the code for appropriate bundling, add-on codes, and quantity.
10. Determine if modifiers are required.
11. Verify the final code against the documentation.
12. Assign the code.

Identify as separately billable any other services provided in the office such as venipuncture, immunizations, EKGs, X-rays, and lab tests performed in the office and proceed with the coding of these services.

8. Identify modifiers. * Certain modifiers are used specifically for E&M coding. It is important to assign modifiers correctly to ensure appropriate reimbursement. Commonly used modifiers for E&M codes include the following:

21 Prolonged Evaluation and Management Service. Used when the service provided is greater than the highest level described for the code range.

24 Unrelated Evaluation and Management Service by the Same Physician During a Postoperative Period. Used when the E/M service is not related to the reason for surgery and is provided within the postoperative time period (global period) in the payer's reimbursement; for example, during a postoperative period for an appendectomy, patient sprains an ankle.

25 Significant, Separately Identifiable Evaluation and Management Service by the Same Physician on the Same Day of the Procedure or Other Service. Used when the physician provides an E&M service in addition to another E&M service or procedure on the same day; for example, during a preventive care visit, a heart problem is identified and the physician does a cardiac work up

in addition to the preventive care visit. The cardiac workup is billed with an office visit E&M (99212-99215) with modifier 25 in addition to the code for preventive care.

32 Mandated Services. Used when the encounter is requested by the payer; for example, a second opinion required or independent medical examination in a liability case.

52 Reduced Service. Used when an E&M service is less extensive than the descriptor indicates.

57 Decision for Surgery. Used to indicate a decision for major surgery within 24 hours was made during the visit. The modifier indicates that this visit was more than the preoperative assessment that is included in the surgical code.

9. Identify place of service code for the CMS-1500. While not a direct component of CPT coding, medical assistants who are responsible for completing the CMS-1500 billing form need to assign a place of service (POS) code in block 24B that is consistent with the place of service defined in the CPT code (Table 18-4). These codes can also be found inside the front cover of many CPT manuals. For example, if using CPT code 99213 for a new patient office visit, the POS code on the CMS-1500 cannot be 21 inpatient hospital.

—Critical Thinking Question 18-1—

What should Lydia tell Dr. Anderson about the relationship between appropriate codes and medical chart documentation?

---

*Adapted from Vines, Deborah, Braceland, Ann, Rollins, Elizabeth, and Miller, Susan. *Comprehensive Health Insurance: Billing, Coding, and Reimbursement,* pp. 112–113.

CPT is a registered trademark of the American Medical Association.

TABLE 18-4 CURRENT PLACE OF SERVICE CODES TO BE USED IN BILLING FOR HEALTH CARE SERVICES

Place of Service Code	Place of Service Name	Place of Service Description
01	Pharmacy	A facility where drugs are sold, dispensed, or provided directly to patients
02	Unassigned	Not currently used
03	School	An educational facility
04	Homeless Shelter	A temporary housing facility
05	Indian Health Service Free-Standing Facility	A facility owned and operated by the Indian Health Service to provide services to American Indians and Alaskan Natives who do not require hospitalization
06	Indian Health Service Provider-Based Facility	A facility owned and operated by the Indian Health Service to provide services to American Indians and Alaskan Natives who are admitted as inpatients or outpatients
07	Tribal 638 Free-Standing Facility	A facility owned and operated by a federally recognized American Indian or Alaskan Native tribe to provide services to tribal members who do not require hospitalization
08	Tribal 638 Provider-Based Facility	A facility owned and operated by a federally recognized American Indian or Alaskan Native tribe to provide services to tribal members who are admitted as inpatients or outpatients
09	Prison-Correctional Facility	A prison or jail maintained by federal, state, or local authorities
10	Unassigned	Not currently used
11	Office	An ambulatory care clinic where the physician sees the patient
12	Home	The patient's private residence
13	Assisted Living Facility	A residential facility that provides on-site support 24 hours every day
14	Group Home	A residence with shared living areas where the patient receives supervision
15	Mobile Unit	A facility that moves from place to place to provide preventive, treatment or screening services
16–19	Unassigned	Not currently used
20	Urgent Care Facility	A location other than the hospital emergency room where patients are seen for unscheduled emergency care
21	Inpatient Hospital	A hospital facility where the patient is admitted for 24 hours or more
22	Outpatient Hospital	A portion of a hospital facility where the patient is seen for care as an outpatient
23	Emergency Room—Hospital	The Emergency Room of a Hospital
24	Ambulatory Surgical Center	A free-standing facility, other than the physician's office, where the patient is seen for surgical and diagnostic services on an ambulatory basis
25	Birthing Center	A facility, other than a hospital's maternity facility, which provides a setting for labor and delivery
26	Military Treatment Facility	A medical facility operated by a branch of the United States military
27–30	Unassigned	Not currently used
31	Skilled Nursing Facility	A facility that provides inpatient skilled nursing care but does not provide the level of care available in the hospital
32	Nursing Facility	A facility that provides care to patients who require care above the level of custodial care
33	Custodial Care Facility	A facility that provides supervision of patients who requires assistance that is not medically related
34	Hospice	A facility other than the patient's home where palliative care is given to terminally ill patients
35–40	Unassigned	Not currently used
41	Ambulance—Land	A land vehicle used for transporting the sick or injured
42	Ambulance—Air or Water	An air or water vehicle used for transporting the sick or injured
43–48	Unassigned	Not currently used
49	Independent Clinic	A location, other than a hospital, that is operated to provide medical services to outpatients only
50	Federally Qualified Health Center	A facility located in a medically underserved area that provides Medicare patients preventive medical care under the direction of a physician
51	Inpatient Psychiatric Facility	A facility that provides inpatient psychiatric services supervised by a physician
52	Psychiatric-Facility Partial Hospitalization	A facility that provides treatment for mental illnesses for patients who do not require full-time hospitalization
53	Community Mental Health Center	A facility that provides mental health benefits on an outpatient basis
54	Intermediate Care Facility/Mentally Retarded	A facility that provides custodial care to mentally retarded individuals

TABLE 18-4 CURRENT PLACE OF SERVICE CODES TO BE USED IN BILLING FOR HEALTH CARE SERVICES

Place of Service Code	Place of Service Name	Place of Service Description
55	Residential Substance Abuse Treatment Facility	A facility that provides treatment for substance abuse
56	Psychiatric Residential Treatment Center	A facility that provides 24-hour psychiatric care
57	Nonresidential Substance Abuse Treatment Facility	A facility that provides treatment for substance abuse on an ambulatory basis
58–59	Unassigned	Not currently used
60	Mass Immunization Center	*A facility where providers administer vaccines*

Source: http://www.cms.gov/placeofservicecodes

In addition to leveraging documentation to code properly, medical assistants must remember that codes and the physician's time are sometimes indirectly related. Some patients simply take more of the physician's time. When, however, patients require longer visits because they need translators or are severely disabled, codes that reflect extended visits are appropriate.

Coding for Special Situations*

Coding for Anesthesia

Anesthesia codes have their own section, which is located before the Surgery section. Basic anesthesia administration services are those services provided by or under the responsible supervision of a physician. These services include general and regional anesthesia, as well as supplementation of local anesthesia. Anesthesia is coded and reimbursed according to the formula B*T*M. B is basic unit, the relative value assigned by the American Society of Anesthesiologists (**ASA**). The relative value is a number that reflects how complicated a particular procedure is compared to others. T stands for time, reported as the minutes from when the anesthesiologist begins

*Adapted from Vines, Deborah, Braceland, Ann, Rollins, Elizabeth, and Miller, Susan. *Comprehensive Health Insurance: Billing, Coding, and Reimbursement,* pp. 141–153.

preparing the patient until the patient is no longer under the care of the anesthesiologist. Depending on the insurer, the minutes may be reported on the CMS-1500 form as total minutes, 15-minute units, or 30-minute units. M is the modifying unit, for the **physical status modifier**, which indicates the condition of the patient at the time anesthesia is administered (Table 18-5).

In the case of difficult and/or extraordinary circumstances such as extreme youth or age (under 1 year of age or over 70 years) or other unusual risk factors, it may be appropriate to report one or more of the qualifying circumstances by using an add-on code listed in Figure 18-7 ◆ addition to the anesthesia services.

The index is researched for the procedure under the main term Anesthesia. The section's subsections are organized by body site. Under each subsection the codes are arranged by procedures. For example, under the heading "Neck," codes for procedures performed on various parts of the neck, the esophagus, thyroid, larynx, trachea; lymphatic system; and the major vessels are listed.

Coding for Surgery

The Surgery section is the largest section in CPT. The subsections found in the Surgery section and how they are broken down into the body systems is shown in Figure 18-8 ◆.

TABLE 18-5 P CODE MODIFIERS FOR ANESTHESIA BILLING

P Code	Patient Condition	Description
P1	Normal and healthy	Modifier indicates the patient is normal and healthy
P2	Mild systemic disease	Modifier indicates the patient has some form of mild systemic disease, such as hypertension
P3	Severe systemic disease	Modifier indicates the patient has a severe systemic disease that could affect the care of the patient. May be used for a patient who has congestive heart failure or uncontrolled diabetes.
P4	Severe systemic disease that threatens life	Modifier indicates the patient has a severe systemic disease that is a threat to life, such as a patient with a life-threatening blood clot
P5	Expected to die without the procedure	Modifier used for patients who are critically injured and require emergency surgery
P6	Brain-dead and being prepped to remove organs for transplant	Modifier used for a patient who is brain dead and being maintained on life support for organ removal

Source: CPT 2008. Copyright 2008 American Medical Association. All rights reserved.

CPT is a registered trademark of the American Medical Association.

+99100	Anesthesia for patient of extreme age; younger than 1 one year and older than 70
+99116	Anesthesia complicated by utilization of total body hypothermia
+99135	Anesthesia complicated by utilization of controlled hypotension
+99140	Anesthesia complicated by emergency conditions (specify) (list separately in addition to code for primary anesthesia procedure)

Figure 18-7 ◆ Qualifying circumstances for anesthesia.
CPT only copyright 2008 American Medical Association. All rights reserved.

The anatomic arrangement of each subsection is as follows:

- Head
- Neck (Soft Tissue) and Thorax
- Back and Flank
- Spine (Vertebral Column)
- Abdomen
- Shoulder
- Humerus (Upper Arm) and Elbow
- Forearm and Wrist
- Hand and Fingers
- Pelvis and Hip Joint
- Femur (Thigh Region) and Knee Joint
- Leg (Tibia and Fibula) and Ankle Joint
- Foot and Toes
- Application of Casts and Strapping
- Endoscopy/Arthroscopy.

Within each heading there is also a consistent theme of procedures described such as:

- Incision
- Excision

Integumentary System	10021–19499
Musculoskeletal System	20000–29999
Respiratory System	30000–32999
Cardiovascular System	33010–39599
Digestive System	40490–49999
Urinary System	50010–53899
Male Genital System	54000–55980
Female Genital System	56405–58999
Maternity Care and Delivery	59000–59899
Endocrine System	60000–60699
Nervous System	61000–64999
Eye and Ocular Adnexa	65091–68899
Auditory System	69000–69979
Operating Microscope	69990

Figure 18-8 ◆ The subsections found in the Surgery section.
CPT only copyright 2008 American Medical Association. All rights reserved.

CPT is a registered trademark of the American Medical Association.

- Introduction or Removal
- Repair, Revision, and/or Reconstruction
- Fracture and/or Dislocation
- Arthrodesis/Amputation.

A surgical CPT code is a bundled code. As mentioned earlier, a *bundled code* is a single CPT code used to report a group of related procedures as in the surgical package. **Unbundling** occurs when separate procedures are reported that should have been included under a bundled code. This practice will result in denial of a claim.

A surgical package includes specific services in addition to the operation, including these:

- One related E/M encounter on the date immediately prior to or on the date of procedure, subsequent to the decision for surgery
- Preparing the patient for surgery including local infiltration, topical anesthesia
- Performing the operation, including normal additional procedures, such as debridement
- Immediate postoperative care, including dictating operative notes, talking with the family and other physicians
- Writing orders
- Evaluating the patient in the postanesthesia recovery area
- Typical postoperative followup.

The typical postoperative care includes follow up visits for normal uncomplicated care. Each third-party payer determines the number of days in which this followup care may take place. Therefore, it is important when certifying for surgery to ask the global period of the third-party payer. The **global period** refers to the number of days surrounding a surgical procedure during which all services relating to that procedure—preoperative, during the surgery, and postoperative—are considered part of the surgical package. This is also referred to as the **global surgical concept**. To determine global days, information from the insurance carrier or other payers may need to be obtained. Many publications and software packages on the market address global days for most carriers and unbundling.

Third-party payers have varying definitions of what constitutes a surgical package and varying policies about what is to be included in the surgical package. Because surgical package rules define what is or is not included in addition to the surgical procedure, the surgery also defines the services for which additional charges can or cannot be submitted.

Two types of services are not included in surgical package codes. These services are reported separately and reimbursed in addition to the surgical package fee:

- Complications, exacerbations, recurrence, or the presence of other diseases or injuries requiring additional services should be reported separately.
- Care for the condition for which a diagnostic surgical procedure was performed or of other coexisting conditions is not included and may be reported separately.

An area of great concern in medical billing is inaccurately billing separately for procedures considered incidental to the major procedure. Many CPT surgical narratives in the CPT book include "with or without" or other language to include or exclude incidental services. Numerous procedures are done in conjunction with other procedures, and often the CPT code subsection notes and guidelines will indicate that a particular code includes a variety of the supporting procedures.

The CPT book further states that followup care for complications, exacerbations, recurrence, and the presence of other diseases that require additional services is not included in the surgery package. General anesthesia for surgical procedures is not part of the surgical package, and the anesthesiologist bills general anesthesia services separately.

Supplies and materials provided by the physician (e.g., sterile trays/drugs) over and above those usually included with procedures rendered are listed separately.*

Wound repair is coded according to wound size and location. The *CPT-4* describes three types of wound repair: (1) simple, (2) intermediate, and (3) complex. Simple wound repairs involve closing partial or full-thickness wounds to the skin and subcutaneous tissues with no deep structure involvement. Intermediate repairs impact one or more deep layers of subcutaneous tissue and nonmuscle fascia, as well as the skin. Complex repairs are closures of layered wounds that require such added work as scar revision, debridement, or retention sutures.

To bill for wounds appropriately, health care providers must measure and record all repairs in centimeters. When more than one wound classification is repaired, the most complicated should be listed as the primary procedure and the less complicated should appear as secondary. When wound repair involves nerves, blood vessels, and/or tendons, medical assistants should locate codes from the proper surgery sections of the CPT-4 code book.

EXAMPLE
A patient presents to the medical office with a laceration on his scalp. The laceration measures 2 cm and is therefore coded with CPT code 13120—Repair, complex, scalp, arms and/or legs; 1.1 cm to 2.5 cm.

When providers complete multiple procedures on the same day, they must code those procedures separately and order them on the CMS-1500 claim form from major to minor. Major

*Vines, Deborah, Braceland, Ann, Rollins, Elizabeth, and Miller, Susan. *Comprehensive Health Insurance: Billing, Coding, and Reimbursement,* pp. 143–149.

CPT is a registered trademark of the American Medical Association.

Keys to Success
BILLING FOR MEDICARE PATIENTS

For Medicare patients, avoid billing for injections on the same day as exams. Medicare will not pay visit codes and injections on the same visits. When offices accidentally bill for both, Medicare throws out the visit code and funds the injection only. As a result, the office receive the lesser of two fees.

procedures are complex, "serious" surgeries, while minor procedures are simpler ones. Assume, for example, a patient has a tonsillectomy, a chin wound repair, and a small mole removed from the nose all on the same day. For this patient, the medical assistant would place the most important surgery, the tonsillectomy, at the top of the claim form, and the least serious one, the small mole removal, at the bottom.

EXAMPLE
Coding for the above patient would be listed as follows: 42826—Tonsillectomy, primary or secondary; age 12 or over, followed by code 12011—Simple repair of superficial wound of face, ears, eyelids, lips and/or mucous membranes; 2.5 cm or less, followed by code 11400–Excision, benign lesion including margins, trunk, arms, or legs; excised diameter 0.5 cm or less.

Coding for Radiology
The codes in the Radiology section are used to report radiological services performed by or supervised by a physician. Radiology codes may have two parts:

1. Results are the technical component of a service. Testing leads to results. The technical component is the part of the relative value associated with the procedure that reflects the test, technologist, the equipment, and processing including preinjection and postinjection services such as local anesthesia, placement of a needle or catheter, and injection of contrast material. The technical component of taking the X-ray would be reported with the procedure code and the modifier "-TC" attached to the procedure.
2. Results lead to interpretation. Reports are the work product of the interpretation of numerous test results. The professional component is the part of the relative value associated with a procedure that represents a physician's skill, time, and expertise used in performing it, as opposed to the technical component. The reading, interpretation, and the written report of the radiological examination by the physician would be the professional component and the modifier "-26" would be attached to the procedure.

These modifiers are to be used only when the physician's office states that only part of the radiological procedure was done; otherwise, the descriptor remains as stated with no modifier.†

†Vines, Deborah, Braceland, Ann, Rollins, Elizabeth, and Miller, Susan. *Comprehensive Health Insurance: Billing, Coding, and Reimbursement,* pp. 149–150.

Contrast material is commonly used for imaging enhancement. Contrast material improves visualization and evaluation of the body structure or organ studied. Some of the procedures listed in the Radiology section of the CPT book may be performed with or without the use of contrast material for imaging enhancement. The phrase "with contrast" used in the codes for procedures using contrast for imaging enhancement represents contrast material administered intravascularly, intra-articularly, or intrathecally. When contrast materials are only administered orally and/or rectally, the study does not qualify as "with contrast" and should be coded "without contrast."

Coding for Pathology and Laboratory

The codes in the Pathology/Laboratory section cover services provided by physicians or by technicians under the supervision of a physician. A complete procedure includes:

- Ordering the test
- Taking and handling the sample
- Performing the actual test
- Analyzing and reporting on the test results.

The 8000 series codes are used to report the performance of specific laboratory tests only and do not include the collection of the specimen via venipuncture (or finger/heel/ear stick), arterial puncture, or other collection methodology (e.g., lumbar puncture). The collection of the specimen by venipuncture or by arterial puncture is not considered an integral part of the laboratory procedure(s) performed. Codes in the 36400-36425 series are used to report venipuncture for obtaining blood samples.

Organ or disease-oriented panels are reported with the codes from the 80048-80076 series. These panels were developed for coding purposes and should not be interpreted as clinical standards for testing. A *panel* is a group of tests ordered together to detect particular diseases or malfunctioning organs. When a panel is reported, all of the listed tests must have been performed with no substitution. If fewer tests are performed than those listed in the panel code (unbundling), then the individual code number(s) for each test should be listed rather than the panel code.

EXAMPLE

80051 Electrolyte Panel
  This panel must include the following:

Carbon dioxide	(82374)
Chloride	(82435)
Potassium	(84132)
Sodium	(84295)

Procedures and services are listed in the index under the following types of main terms:

- Name of the test, such as urinalysis, drug test
- Procedure such as hormone assay
- Abbreviations such as CBC, RBS, TLC
- Panel of tests, under Blood Tests.

CPT is a registered trademark of the American Medical Association.

Some medical practices have laboratory equipment and perform their own testing. In-office labs must be certified by the Clinical Laboratory Improvement Amendment (CLIA) of 1988, which awards three levels of certification. The lowest level for an in-office certified lab can perform dipstick urinalysis and urine pregnancy. If the medical practice does not have a lab but obtains the specimen for the lab, the venipuncture code 36415 may be billed for obtaining the blood sample. As in every medical setting, the Occupational and Safety and Health Administration (OSHA) regulates safety.

Although Medicare does not allow physicians to bill for lab work they did not perform, other third-party payers do. When a medical practice has a contract with a lab (pays the lab for the work), it may bill for the tests reported. The modifier 90 is attached to the code for the lab test. On the CMS-1500, form locator 20 must say "yes" and the fee the medical practice pays the lab must be entered under "Charges." Also, form locator 32 must report the name and address of the lab.

Coding for Medicine

The Medicine section of the CPT book contains a variety of listings for reporting procedures and services provided by many different types of healthcare providers. In addition, many services and procedures provided by nonphysician practitioners can be found in the Medicine section. For example, codes in the physical medicine and rehabilitation subsection are often used to report the services and procedures provided by physical and occupational therapists. Audiologists and speech therapists find listings in the special otorhinolaryngologic services subsection that describes some of the technical procedures and services they provide.

Codes from the Medicine section may be used with codes from any other section. Add-on codes and separate procedure codes are included in the Medicine section.

Immunizations require two codes, one for administering the immunization and the other for the particular vaccine or toxoid that is given (Figure 18-9 ◆).

The descriptors for injections require two codes, one for administering the immunization and the other for the particular vaccine or toxoid that is given.

Cardiac catheterizations are the most commonly performed surgical procedure, with more than 1 million performed each year. Complete coding of cardiac catheterization requires at least three codes: a code for the catheterization procedure itself, a code for the injection procedure, and a code for the imaging supervision and interpretation. Each of these has a professional and a technical component. Unless the physician owns the laboratory, those codes are billed using modifier 26.*

Unlisted Procedure Codes

When physicians perform procedures not in the coding book, medical assistants must use "unlisted procedure codes" and submit copies of procedure reports with claims. When procedure reports are not submitted, claims may be denied or delayed. To

*Source: Vines, Deborah, Braceland, Ann, Rollins, Elizabeth, and Miller, Susan. *Comprehensive Health Insurance: Billing, Coding, and Reimbursement*, pp. 151–153.

| 90471 | Immunization administration |
| 90710 | Measles, mumps, rubella, and varicella vaccine (MMRV), live, for subcutaneous use |

Figure 18-9 ◆ Coding for immunizations.

ensure timely, accurate processing, procedure reports should contain the following:

■ Reason the procedure was needed
■ Time the procedure took
■ Complexity of patient's symptoms
■ Patient's final diagnosis
■ Examination findings pertinent to the procedure
■ Diagnostic or therapeutic procedures that led to the procedure
■ Any concurrent patient problems
■ Any needed followup care

The Health Care Common Procedure Coding System (HCPCS)

The **Health Care Common Procedure Coding System (HCPCS)**, called "Hick Picks" in the industry, is a set of codes developed and maintained by CMS for the reporting of professional services, nonphysician services, supplies, durable medical equipment (**DME**), and injectable drugs. Historically, HCPCS has had three levels.

CPT codes are **Level I** HCPCS **codes** for professional services.

Level II codes are alphanumeric codes that begin with a letter, followed by four numbers, for example, A4356. Typically, when professionals refer to "HCPCS codes," they are referring to Level II codes. Level II codes cover supplies, DME, drugs, nonphysician providers, and certain physician services for Medicare and Medicaid. When CPT and HCPCS codes exist for the same service, use the CPT code. When procedure descriptions differ, HCPCS Level II codes have priority. They are required by Medicare and Medicaid. They have been mandated as a HIPAA uniform code set for all insurance carriers, but implementation is in progress. Be sure to check with private carriers to verify if they accept HCPCS Level II codes. Reimbursement for supplies and equipment is usually faster when HCPCS codes are used, because they are more specific than using the generic CPT code for supplies, 99070. A list of the categories in Level II appears in Table 18-6. Level II codes are updated on a quarterly basis; the manual is published annually in October. Quarterly updates are available on the CMS Web site at www.cms.gov.

Level III HCPCS **codes** were developed by regional Medicare carriers, but are being phased out under HIPAA's administrative simplification provision, which requires uniform code sets.

CPT is a registered trademark of the American Medical Association.

The HCPCS Level II coding manual contains an alphabetical index and a tabular listing. As with the other coding manuals, use the alphabetical index first to locate the item or service, then refer to the tabular list to verify. Many DME manufacturers print a suggested HCPCS code on the item packaging. This is a useful aid, but the code should always be verified in the manual. Many entries in the manual also contain cross-reference information to Medicare reimbursement rules for the specific item or service.

HCPCS Level II also contains alphanumeric modifiers that can be used with either Level I CPT codes or Level II codes. The most commonly used modifiers are those that designate specific anatomical sites of procedures and nonphysician provider types (Table 18-7). Many additional modifiers exist for specific Medicare and Medicaid reimbursement situations. One of the most important of these is the modifier GA that indicates a Medicare Advanced Beneficiary Notice (ABN) form was signed by the patient when a covered service is expected to be denied (see ∞ Chapter 16). Through experience, medical assistants become familiar with the specific requirements for their medical office.

TABLE 18-6 LEVEL II HCPCS CODES

Transportation services	A0000–A0999
Medical and surgical supplies	A4000–A7509
Miscellaneous and experimental	A9000–A9999
Enteral and parenteral therapy	B0000–B9999
Temporary hospital outpatient PPS	C0000–C9999
Dental procedures	D0000–D9999
Durable medical equipment (DME)	E0000–E9000
Procedures and services, temporary	G0000–G9999
Rehabilitative services	H0000–H9999
Drugs administered other than oral method	J0000–J8999
Chemotherapy drugs	J9000–J9999
Temporary codes for DMERCS	K0000–K9999
Orthotic procedures	L0000–L4999
Prosthetic procedures	L5000–L9999
Medical services	M0000–M9999
Pathology and laboratory	P0000–P9999
Temporary codes	Q0000–Q9999
Diagnostic radiology services	R0000–R9999
Private payer codes	S0000–S9999
State Medicaid agency codes	T0000–T9999
Vision	V0000–V2999
Hearing services	V5000–V5999

TABLE 18-7 COMMON HCPCS MODIFIERS

Modifier	Description
AH	Clinical psychologist
AJ	Clinical social worker
AS	Assistant at surgery service
CC	Procedure code change
E1	Upper left eyelid
E2	Lower left eyelid
E3	Upper right eyelid
E4	Lower right eyelid
F1	Left hand, second digit
F2	Left hand, third digit
F3	Left hand, fourth digit
F4	Left hand, fifth digit
F5	Right hand, thumb
F6	Right hand, second digit
F7	Right hand, third digit
F8	Right hand, fourth digit
F9	Right hand, fifth digit
FA	Left hand, thumb
GA	Signed advance beneficiary notice (ABN) form on file (for Medicare patients)
LT	Left side
PC	Professional courtesy
Q6	Locum tenens medical doctor (MD) service
QW	Clinical Laboratory Improvement Amendments Act (CLIA) waived test
RT	Right side
SA	Nurse practitioner with physician
SB	Nurse midwife service
TC	Technical component

Source: www.cms.gov

Ensuring Proper Reimbursement

To receive proper payment for medical services, health care teams must keep adequate, accurate, and complete patient medical and billing records. The adage, "If it isn't charted, it wasn't done," applies.

CPT is a registered trademark of the American Medical Association.

To keep proper medical records, medical offices must undertake accurate and comprehensive procedure coding. Proper coding begins with the right tools: an up-to-date *CPT-4* coding book, a HCPCS book, and a medical dictionary. Outdated coding tools can provide outdated codes, and outdated codes risk claim delay or denial. Once the right tools are on hand, every service or procedure must be documented in electronic or paper form, and before any claims are sent to insurance companies.

When medical assistants are asked to code charts with incomplete service or procedure documentation, those assistants must route the charts back to the health care providers who performed the services. While rerouting may delay insurance claim submission, in the long run it proves faster, and more effective than inaccurate or incomplete claims.

?—Critical Thinking Question 18-2—
Assuming Lydia complied with Dr. Anderson's request to bill Medicare for higher codes, what might Medicare do, and why?

?—Critical Thinking Question 18-3—
How would Lydia describe upcoding to Dr. Anderson?

In Practice

During the 5 years Audrey has worked for Dr. Suarez, the physician has often asked her to bill for services he did not perform. Audrey has never objected, in part because she feels patients are unharmed by the practice. She also believes she is blameless, because she receives no additional money from the process.

One day Audrey arrives at work to find that Dr. Suarez has been arrested. Later, the physician is convicted and sentenced to 2 years in jail. The office closes, and Audrey loses her job. Audrey begins a job search but finds that her association with Dr. Suarez is affecting her negatively. In fact, several potential employers have turned her away as a result. One of those employers said, "I'm sorry, but we just can't trust someone who worked for a doctor involved in insurance fraud." How could Audrey have avoided this situation?

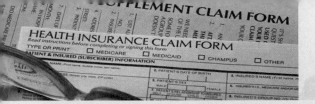
Chapter Summary

- The CPT coding book is designed to standardize the coding process by requiring healthcare providers to choose a procedure code based on the explicit description.
- Accurate CPT coding involves a number of steps, including determining correct codes via chart notes.
- Modifiers are an integral part of procedural coding, serving to add detail to procedure codes. By using modifiers, the coder is able to further identify any special circumstances that surround that particular service for that patient.
- The Health Care Common Procedure Coding System (HCPCS) provides codes for reporting nonphysician services, supplies, or durable medical equipment (DME), and certain physician services for Medicare and Medicaid.
- In all forms of coding, accurate documentation and reimbursement are tightly linked. Insurers will often request copies of patient health care records in order to determine the necessity of care rendered. Having accurate records of the services provided is helpful in timely and accurate payment of claims.
- Coding and billing fraud impose severe penalties. It includes falsifying medical records, billing for services not performed, and intentionally charging incorrect patients. Providers who are caught intentionally submitting fraudulent claims may be arrested and charged with crimes. In addition, they risk the loss of their licenses, practices and preferred provider status.
- Bundling of services is the process of charging one procedure code for a group of charges that typically are performed at the same time. For bundled procedures, coders may not unbundle the charges, or charge for each procedure individually. This would be unbundling and insurance carriers consider this practice to be fraudulent.

Chapter Review

Multiple Choice

1. Procedure codes are always _____ digits long.
   a. three
   b. four
   c. five
   d. six

2. Anesthesia codes begin with:
   a. 0
   b. 1
   c. 2
   d. 3

3. "Standardized" procedural coding means that every health care provider:
   a. uses the same code to describe the same service
   b. references the same book to look up codes
   c. employs only registered or certified medical assistants as coders
   d. all of the above

4. The "CPT" acronym in the *CPT-4* code book stands for:
   a. Correct Procedural Terminology
   b. Current Procedural Terminology
   c. Causal Procedural Terminology
   d. none of the above

True/False

T F 1. E&M codes are rarely used in health care.

T F 2. All insurance carriers today reimburse health care providers based on UCR charges.

T F 3. The time a physician spends with a patient is the most important factor in code selection.

T F 4. All insurance companies have the same number of followup days in their fee schedules.

T F 5. Wound repair is coded depending on the wound's location and size.

Short Answer

1. When a physician performs a procedure not found in the *CPT-4* coding book, how is that procedure billed?

2. What are the four classifications of history and physical examinations for E&M codes?

3. What are the four classifications of decision making for E&M codes?

4. Define a physical status modifier and how it is used for coding.

5. What does it mean to "unbundle" codes?

6. What are the three types of wound repairs in the CPT-4 coding book?

7. When multiple procedures are performed on the same day, how should they appear on the CMS-1500 billing form?

8. What are the four classifications of radiology codes?

9. Explain what is meant by "upcoding."

10. Describe three patient-billing situations that require modifiers.

11. Describe the relationship between accurate documentation and proper reimbursement.

Research

1. Interview a person who works in the billing office of a local medical office. How does that office handle the process of procedural coding? Do the physicians assign the codes? Do the medical assistants assign the codes?

Chapter Review (continued)

2. Go to your state's Department of Health Web site. What resources are available for providers who have questions about proper coding?

3. Look at your state's Medicaid Web site. What are some of the rules Medicaid applies regarding the use of procedure codes?

Externship Application Experience

Willie Harrison, a Medicare-covered patient, arrives at Dr. Annissette's office, and the physician removes two skin flaps from Willie's neck. After the procedure, the physician circles one procedure code on the superbill and writes "× 2" next to it to indicate the medical assistant should charge for two procedures. What is the proper way for the medical assistant to indicate to Medicare that the patient had two skin flaps removed?

Resource Guide

American Medical Association
515 N. State Street
Chicago, IL 60610
Phone: (800) 621-8335
http://www.ama-assn.org

Center for Medicare and Medicaid Services
7500 Security Boulevard
Baltimore, MD 21244
Phone: (877) 267-2323
http://www.cms.hhs.gov

MedMedia

http://www.MyMAKit.com

More on this chapter, including interactive resources, can be found on the Student CD-ROM accompanying this textbook and on http://www.MyMAKit.com.

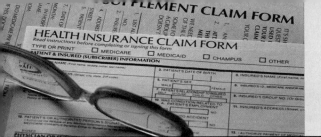

Objectives

After completing this chapter, you should be able to:

- Define and spell the key terminology in this chapter.
- Describe the functions of a manual billing system, including the use of day sheets and charge slips.
- Identify the three types of payment typically made in the medical office.
- Discuss how computers are used for billing in the medical office.
- List desired features in a computerized medical billing system.
- Post payments to manual and computerized billing systems.
- Prepare an accounts receivable trial balance.
- Outline how professional fees are determined, and create a fee schedule.
- Review a managed care contract, and determine if participating would benefit the practice.
- Review the medical office's accounts receivables, and manage those accounts effectively.
- Verify patient identification.
- Create coherent collection policies in the medical office, and explain them to patients.
- Describe the various types of collection issues in managed care.
- Research collection agencies, and describe their pros and cons.
- Describe the medical assistant's role when account overpayments are made.
- Describe how small claims court works for the medical office, and discuss the pros and cons of using this method to collect past-due accounts.

Billing, Collections, and Credit

Case Study

Millie Alonso owes $550 for services her young son received, but she has made no payments for 2 months. As a result, her account now appears as past due. The medical assistant must call Millie to determine when she will send payment, either in full or by installment.

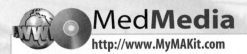

MedMedia
http://www.MyMAKit.com

Additional interactive resources and activities for this chapter can be found on http://www.MyMAKit.com. For a video on collecting money, tips, audio glossary, legal and ethical scenarios, on-the-job scenarios, quizzes, and games related to the content of this chapter, please access the accompanying CD-ROM in this book.

Video: *Collecting Money*
Legal and Ethical Scenario: *Billing, Collections, and Credit*
On the Job Scenario: *Billing, Collections, and Credit*
Tips
Multiple Choice Quiz
Audio Glossary
HIPAA Quiz
Games: Spelling Bee, Crossword, and Strikeout

Key Terminology

accounts receivables (AR)—money owed the medical practice

aging report—documentation of the money owed the medical office and how long accounts have been outstanding

certified letter—postal service letter that the recipient must sign for upon receipt

collection agency—company that pursues overdue accounts for a fee

community property laws—legislation that deems one spouse financially responsible for the other spouse's debts

day sheet—used with a manual pegboard system to document and track the charges and payments within the medical office

dual fee schedule—facility or health care provider with two fees for the same service

Fair Debt Collection Act—law that dictates how debts may be collected

fee schedule—list of services and their fees

geographical practice cost index (GPCI)—Medicare system of adjusting fees based on the area in which the health care provider practices

hardship agreement—agreement a patient signs to indicate an inability to pay full health care costs due to financial hardship

insurance fraud—illegal act by a healthcare provider involving an insurance company

ledger card—document used to track services rendered and payments made; used with manual pegboard systems

national conversion factor—number released by Medicare each year that determines fee schedules for all health care services

national standard—point of reference for developing charges for healthcare services used throughout the United States

Omnibus Budget Reconciliation Act (OBRA)—legislation passed by Congress in 1989 to calculate health care service fees by formula

patient billing statements—monthly statements sent to patients who have an outstanding balance

pegboard accounting system—manual bookkeeping system

✚ MEDICAL ASSISTING STANDARDS

CAAHEP ENTRY-LEVEL STANDARDS	ABHES ENTRY-LEVEL COMPETENCIES
■ Compare manual and computerized bookkeeping systems used in ambulatory healthcare (cognitive) ■ Explain both billing and payment options (cognitive) ■ Identify procedure for preparing patient accounts (cognitive) ■ Discuss procedures for collecting outstanding accounts (cognitive) ■ Discuss precautions for accepting checks (cognitive) ■ Compare types of endorsements (cognitive) ■ Differentiate between accounts payable and accounts receivable (cognitive) ■ Describe the impact of both the Fair Debt Collection Act and the Federal Truth in Lending Act of 1968 as they apply to collections (cognitive) ■ Discuss types of adjustments that may be made to a patient's account (cognitive) ■ Perform accounts receivable procedures, including: a. Post entries on a daysheet; b. Perform billing procedures; c. Perform collection procedures; d. Post adjustments; e. Process a credit balance; f. Process refunds; g. Post non-sufficient fund (NSF) checks; h. Post collection agency payments (cognitive) ■ Utilize computerized office billing systems (cognitive) ■ Demonstrate sensitivity and professionalism in handling accounts receivable activities with clients (affective)	■ Adapt to change ■ Maintain confidentiality at all times ■ Use appropriate guidelines when releasing records or information ■ Project a positive attitude ■ Be cognizant of ethical boundaries ■ Evidence a responsible attitude ■ Conduct work within scope of education, training, and ability ■ Professional components ■ Monitor legislation related to current healthcare issues and practices ■ Orient patients to office policies and procedures ■ Adapt what is said to the recipient's level of comprehension ■ Adaptation for individualized needs ■ Locate resources and information for patients and employers ■ Use proper telephone techniques ■ Application of electronic technology ■ Apply computer concepts for office procedures ■ Apply managed care policies and procedures ■ Obtain managed care referrals and precertification ■ Follow established policy in initiating or terminating medical treatment ■ Establish and maintain a petty cash fund ■ Perform basic secretarial skills ■ Prepare a bank statement ■ Reconcile a bank statement ■ Maintain records for accounting and banking purposes ■ Post entries on a day sheet ■ Prepare a check ■ Post collection agency payments ■ Use manual and computerized bookkeeping systems ■ Manage accounts payable and receivable ■ Be courteous and diplomatic

Key Terminology *(continued)*

posting—process of adding charges or payments to a patient's account

professional courtesy—to give a patient a discount, or free service, due to the fact that the patient is a healthcare professional

relative value unit (RVU)—numeric value assigned by Medicare to formulate fee schedules for health care providers

superbill—document that indicates the services performed with a patient on a given visit; also called an encounter form

tickler file—tool for tracking future events, such as patient appointments

uncollectible—account believed never to be paid

write off—to remove a balance from a patient account

Abbreviations

AR—accounts receivable

CMS—Center for Medicare and Medicaid Services

CPT—Current Procedural Terminology

GPCI—geographic price cost index

HIPAA—Health Insurance Portability and Accountability Act

NCR—no carbon required

NSF—nonsufficient funds

OBRA—Omnibus Budget Reconciliation Act

RBRVS—resource-based relative value scale

RVU—relative value unit

✓ COMPETENCY SKILLS PERFORMANCE

1. Post an entry on a day sheet.
2. Prepare an accounts receivable trial balance.
3. Explain professional fees to a patient.
4. Call a patient regarding an overdue account.
5. Send a patient a billing statement.
6. Post a nonsufficient funds check.
7. Post an adjustment to a patient account.
8. Post a collection agency payment.
9. Process a patient refund.
10. Process an insurance company overpayment.

Introduction

To stay in business, the medical office must be financially sound. Service fees, a vital facet of an office's success, must be in line with federal and local laws, as well as consistent from patient to patient. **Dual fee schedules**, which impose different fees on different patients, are fraudulent. In health care, billing, collections, and credit are best undertaken equitably and communicated about openly.

Identifying Payment Basics

Patients typically make three types of payment in the medical office: (1) cash, (2) check, and (3) debit or credit card. With cash payments, medical assistants should write receipts as documents both for patients and the office. Keeping a copy of the receipt in the medical office helps discourage stealing by the office staff. With a paper trail, medical assistants or office managers can easily track all office cash.

When patients offer personal checks as payment, medical assistants must verify that the check's written amount matches the check's number amounts. Assistants must also ensure that checks are dated and signed. When assistants take checks from parties other than patients, those assistants should request the check writers' photo identification to verify the writers' identities. Many medical offices do not accept third party checks. When checks are suspicious or for large amounts, assistants should call the issuing banks to ensure funds are available. When checks are marked "Payment in Full," assistants must verify that the checks are for the full amount owed by the patient. When they are not, patients may later argue that no additional payment is required.

For the third and final payment type, debit or credit cards, providers pay bank fees in the amount of 1 to 3 percent of charges, depending on providers' credit card use when they accept credit card payments from patients. Some offices use check-verification systems that, while costly, guarantee checks. Some of these systems simply check to see if patients have written bad checks. Others are more sophisticated, holding the patient's bank funds until the check clears. As such systems become more sophisticated, however, their costs increase.

Manual Billing Systems

As most medical offices adopt computerized accounting systems, manual billing systems, also called **pegboard accounting systems**, have been losing popularity in health care. With pegboard systems, staff responsible for **posting** charges place **day sheets** on pegboards at the start of each business day (Figure 19-1 ◆). The day sheet is a document where the administrative medical assistant records the charges for services and payments received throughout the day. Patients' **ledger cards**, which carry information including patients' current and previous balances, are placed on the day sheets under **superbills**. Staff write patients' charges and payment information on the ledger card, being sure to press hard enough on the no carbon required (**NCR**) paper to impact all copies. At the end of the day, or the end of the sheet if more than one sheet is used in a day, staff must total all columns to calculate the day's charges and collections. The collection total must match the bank deposit amount.

Computerized Billing Systems

With the decline of manual billing systems in the medical office, computerized systems have become the norm. While computerized systems vary, most allow staff to:

- Post charges and payments to patient accounts
- Print insurance billing forms and patient billing forms
- Create **aging reports** (documentation of the money owed the medical office and how long the account has been outstanding) that detail patients' owed amounts

Most medical billing programs offer a wide variety of reports. Such reports can list information like all patients with birthdays in any given month or all female patients over age 40 who have not had a mammogram in the past year.

Billing systems with basic features like reports are affordable for most medical offices. Higher level features increase systems' prices. Some systems, for example, offer integrated electronic appointment books. Others send insurance claims electronically and receive insurance payments electronically. Some systems even allow remote access, which means health care teams can access their billing systems when out of their offices. To ensure that the office receives the software package it needs, the medical assistant or office manager should research a number of options. Online, the Web site www.2020software.com lists the most popular medical billing programs on the market and allows users to order demo CDs of programs at no charge.

Fee Schedules

In 1989, the U.S. Congress passed the **Omnibus Budget Reconciliation Act (OBRA)**, in part to require that physician reimbursement for Medicare services be based on a **fee schedule** (Figure 19-2 ◆). Fee schedules set maximum amounts for services using the resource-based relative value scale (**RBRVS**), which is designed to reduce Medicare costs and establish a **national standard** for physician payment. This national standard is itself based on the Current Procedural Coding (**CPT**) codes used for patient visits.

Medicare service fees are calculated based on the five following factors:

- Service intensity
- Time needed for the service
- Skills needed to perform the service
- Practice's overhead
- Practice's malpractice premiums

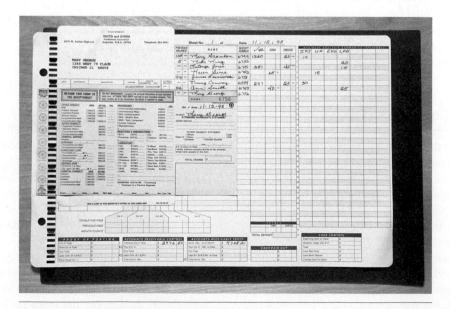

Figure 19-1 ◆ Pegboard accounting system.

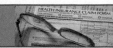

PROCEDURE 19-1 Post an Entry on a Day Sheet

Theory and Rationale

Proper use of the pegboard accounting system includes strict attention to details, such as numbers and letters. Medical assistants using the pegboard system must be able to write legibly and use a ten-key calculator skillfully.

Materials

- Pegboard
- Day sheet
- Patient ledger card
- Superbill
- Blue or black ink pen
- Calculator

Competency

(**Conditions**) With the necessary materials, you will be able to (**Task**) post an entry on a day sheet (**Standards**) correctly within the time allowed by the instructor.

1. Place the patient's ledger card on the day sheet.
2. Place the patient's superbill on top of the ledger card.
3. Pressing hard enough to impact all copies, enter the date, procedures, charges, and any payment in the appropriate boxes.
4. In the appropriate box, enter the new balance.
5. Verify that the entry appears on all copies.
6. File the patient's ledger card.

Physicians' fees are adjusted according to a **geographical practice cost index (GPCI)**, which factors in the differing health care costs across the United States. Together, these factors determine a health care provider's **relative value unit (RVU)**. The RVU was devised by the Centers for Medicare and Medicaid Services (**CMS**) as a way for physicians to create a fee schedule for the services they render. RVUs take into account three factors: how much work by the physician is involved in performing the service, what sort of expertise the physician needs to have in order to perform the service, and the cost of the physician's malpractice insurance policy.

Each year, Medicare assigns a **national conversion factor** that is added to the RVU. The national conversion factor is a number released by Medicare each year that determines fee schedules for all health care services. The national conversion factor is multiplied by the physician's RVU for any given service or procedure to determine the allowed fee for that service.

For example, imagine CPT code 99205 has an RVU of 4.78 for a health care provider practicing in the Los Angeles area, and the national conversion factor is 37.5623. This would make the Medicare allowed charge for this service $179.55 (4.78 × 37.5623 = $179.55). Because most health insurance plans base their fee schedules on the Medicare fee schedule, the Medicare allowed charge is typically considered the maximum charge any insurance plan will allow for any given service or procedure.

In Practice

Dr. Bowman wants to raise his prices for certain services. He tells his medical assistant he fails to understand why insurance companies do not pay him more simply because he has begun charging more. What can the medical assistant say about fee schedule determination?

Participating Provider Agreements

Most patients with private health insurance are covered by managed care plans, which are detailed in ∞ Chapter 16. As a condition of participation, managed care plans credential health care providers and require those providers to apply. When providers agree to participate in managed care plans, they agree to accept predetermined fee schedules. Some managed care plans also dictate the type of medications providers can prescribe and the types of specialist referrals those providers are allowed to make.

Participating provider agreements range from several pages long to small-book size. Though it may be time consuming, physicians should read their agreements in full. Once providers have signed with plans, they are obligated to see patients with that coverage for the agreed-upon fees, which may be lower than providers are willing to accept.

AUDIOLOGY SERVICES		
Screening audio air only	92551	$38.00
Pure tone air	92552	$37.00
Pure tone air and bone	92553	$50.00
Comprehensive audio	92557	$101.00
Loudness balance test	92562	$38.00
Tone decay	92563	$41.00
Tympanography	92567	$40.00
Acoustic reflex	92568	$42.00
Reflex decay	92569	$43.00
Visual reinforced audio	92579	$78.00
Brain stem audiogram	92585	$327.00

Figure 19-2 ◆ Sample fee schedule.

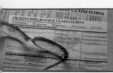

PROCEDURE 19-2 Prepare an Accounts Receivable Trial Balance

Theory and Rationale

By preparing an accounts receivable trial balance, the medical assistant is able to determine if there is any discrepancy between the daily journal and the ledger or the patient accounts.

Materials

- Patient accounts in computerized or paper ledger format
- Computer, if using a computerized billing system
- Fee slips for services rendered to the patients for the day
- Calculator
- Pegboard system, if using a manual billing system
- Pen

Competency

(**Conditions**) With the necessary materials, you will be able to (**Task**) prepare an accounts receivable trial balance (**Standards**) correctly within the time limit set by the instructor.

1. Calculate the total of the charges on the fee slips for the day.
2. Using the computer or the manual ledger card system, calculate the total of the charges posted to patient accounts for the day.
3. Compare the total of the charges from the fee slips to the total of the charges in the computer or on the manual ledger card system.
4. If the balances do not match, calculate the totals a second time to verify you added them correctly.
5. If the balances continue to differ, go through the fee slips to see where the error in entry has occurred.
6. Correct the entry error and calculate the totals again.
6. If the balances continue to differ, go through the above steps until they match.

The best way to review participating provider agreements is with a highlighter. Medical assistants should highlight all areas of interest or concern, especially any details about fee schedules or provider care restrictions, and then review the highlighted areas with the physicians. Objections to any item may be grounds for declining plan participation.

Credit and Collections

The best way to ensure that patients pay their bills properly is to discuss the medical office's credit and collection policies before services are rendered. Medical assistants should discuss all fees and outline all payment policies. When patients will make regular payments on their balances, for example, medical assistants should provide written contracts that stipulate the payment amounts and due dates (Figure 19-3 ◆). Such contracts avoid confusion and reduce or eliminate patient questions.

To further help ensure payment terms are clear, many medical offices include important financial information in their office brochures and send these brochures, along with registration paperwork and fee and credit policies, before patients arrive for their first visits. Figure 19-4 ◆ identifies some items that should be included in introductory brochures. Well informed patients help avoid collection problems. Copayments, for example, should be paid at visit check-in.

Each state has a statute of limitations that sets the maximum time in which health care providers can collect patient debts. Because Medicare and many managed care insurance companies prohibit providers from billing patients until insurance companies have issued explanations of benefits outlining

---

May 21, 2009

I, [patient's name], agree to pay Monroe Family Practice $100 every 2 weeks until my $800 balance is paid in full. I understand that finance charges will not accrue while I am making these payments and that if I stop making payments before my balance is paid in full finance charges will begin to accrue on the remaining balance.

Patient Signature   Date

_____

Witness Signature   Date

_____

Figure 19-3 ◆ Sample payment contract.

- ❏ Requirement for payment at the time of service, if any
- ❏ Allowable time frame for payment (e.g., "within 30 days")
- ❏ Guidelines for insurance claim submission on patients' behalf
- ❏ Time the medical office will carry an outstanding balance
- ❏ Credit limit extended to patients
- ❏ Percentage of finance charges that will accrue on a balance and when starting (e.g., after 30 days, after 60 days)
- ❏ Point at which accounts are turned over to collection agencies
- ❏ Process for assigning benefits to the provider

Figure 19-4 ◆ Payment policies in an office brochure.

the amounts patients owe, it is crucial to bill insurance providers soon after the service is provided so that the patient portion can be billed in a timely manner. Table 19-1 outlines the number of years from the patient's last date of service or last billing statement that a health care provider may send a bill to a patient.

? —Critical Thinking Question 19-1—
Would Millie be more or less likely to have a balance due if someone in the medical office had discussed a payment plan when services were rendered? Why?

TABLE 19-1 STATUTES OF LIMITATIONS ON HEALTH CARE DEBTS

State	Number of Years	State	Number of Years
AL	6	MT	8
AK	6	NE	5
AZ	6	NV	6
AR	5	NH	3
CA	4	NJ	6
CO	6	NM	6
CT	6	NY	6
DE	3	NC	3
D.C.	3	ND	6
FL	5	OH	15
GA	6	OK	5
HI	6	OR	6
ID	5	PA	6
IL	10	RI	15
IN	10	SC	10
IA	10	SD	6
KS	5	TN	6
KY	15	TX	4
LA	10	UT	6
ME	6	VA	5
MD	3	VT	6
MA	6	WA	6
MI	6	WI	6
MN	6	WV	10
MS	3	WY	10
MO	10		

In terms of credit, medical offices should predetermine the amounts they are willing to extend to patients, document those amounts in policies, and apply the policies equitably. The health care provider may not pick and choose the patients who

PROCEDURE 19-3 Explain Professional Fees to a Patient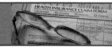

Theory and Rationale

Patients who clearly understand fees for physician services are better equipped to make health care choices, as well as understand their bills. When a patient does not understand the fees they incur in the medical facility, this confusion can lead to nonpayment of the bill.

Materials

- Patient medical record
- Copy of office fee schedule
- Blue or black pen
- Payment contract

Competency

(**Conditions**) With the necessary materials, you will be able to (**Task**) explain the physician's professional fees to a patient

(**Standards**) correctly within the time limit set by the instructor.

1. Find a private location to sit with the patient.
2. Explain to the patient the procedure the physician has prescribed.
3. Explain to the patient the fee for the procedure.
4. Explain to the patient any insurance coverage for the fee.
5. Explain to the patient the payment amount and deadline.
6. Secure an agreement from the patient about the payment date.
7. Enter the payment agreement and arrangements on the payment contract.
8. On the payment contract, obtain the patient's signature and sign as the witness.
9. Answer any questions the patient may have about the fee or the procedure.
10. Place the payment agreement in the patient's financial record.

Keys to Success
INFORMATION REQUIRED ON PATIENT REGISTRATION FORMS

Medical offices should request certain pieces of information on their patient registration forms to make tracking patients, and therefore debt collection, easier. For example, offices should request patients' employers' names and telephone numbers, as well as the names and numbers of emergency contacts who do not live with the patients. Emergency contact information helps provide options for contacting the patient when patients' accounts become past due and medical assistants cannot reach patients at home.

will receive an extension of credit. The credit extension policy must apply to every patient in the facility.

Verifying Patient Identification

When new patients visit the medical office, medical assistants must copy those patients' driver's licenses and insurance cards, front and back (Figure 19-5 ◆). Such documentation confirms the patient's identity and can help the assistant track the patient for collection purposes.

Managing Accounts Receivables

Any successful medical office must manage its **accounts receivables (AR)**, which is the money owed the office from all sources, including patients, insurance companies, worker's compensation, Medicare, and Medicaid. AR management, which entails documenting how much money is owed the office, by whom, and for how long, is a weighty task and so must be done regularly and thoroughly.

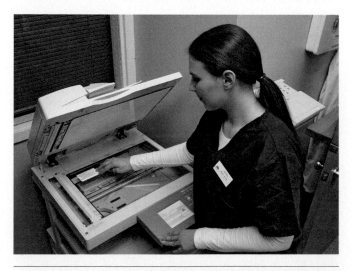

Figure 19-5 ◆ The medical assistant should make a copy of both sides of the patient's insurance card.

As mentioned earlier, medical billing programs can run reports, some on AR accounts. Aging reports are important to AR management for a number of reasons. When physicians wish to take business loans, for example, banks will request documentation on AR accounts. Some malpractice insurance companies are beginning to examine physicians' AR before extending policies. Physicians with high or old AR are considered greater risks to insure.

The most effective way to collect money on past due accounts is to speak with patients while they are in the office. When face-to-face communication is not possible, the next most effective method is calling patients, but from private office locations to safeguard patient confidentiality. Medical assistants making such calls must pay strict attention to the law regarding collections and document all calls and conversations, as well as any patient messages, in patients' financial records. Table 19-2 outlines procedures for telephone collection calls.

Collection in Managed Care

Some medical offices collect entire first-day visit fees from patients, but the practice is not recommended if the patient is covered by managed care. Some managed care plans strictly govern how much money, if any, providers may collect from patients. When offices participate with Medicare, for example, providers are disallowed from charging patients for covered services at the time of service. Instead, those providers must bill Medicare and then bill the patients for the portions Medicare states those patients owe.

When speaking with patients about fees or payments, it is important to remember that people tend to associate payment with value. When medical assistants act embarrassed about fees, or fail to ask for payment, they give the impression that the physician's services lack value.

Forgiving Deductibles or Copayments

It is illegal, and in fact considered **insurance fraud**, for health care providers to forgive patients' deductibles or copayments. When patients cannot pay their bills and physicians agree to treat them for lesser or no fees, those patients must sign and date **hardship agreement** letters for their file (Figure 19-6 ◆). Hardship letters become part of patients' permanent medical records.

Patients Who File for Bankruptcy

Patients who are unable to pay their medical bill may file for bankruptcy. A Harvard study performed in 2005 found that inability to pay medical bills is the leading cause of bankruptcy filings, affecting nearly 2 million Americans each year. Depending upon the type of bankruptcy the patient files, the medical office may or may not be repaid any of the amount outstanding on the patient's account. Since bankruptcy is designed to protect debtors from further collection activity, the medical office

TABLE 19-2 DOs AND DON'Ts FOR COLLECTION TELEPHONE CALLS

Do	Don't
Call the patient from a private location in the medical office.	Call the patient from a location where other patients can over hear.
Call the patient between 8 A.M. and 9 P.M.	Call the patient despite the patient's wishes.
Verify the patient's identity.	Speak with anyone except the patient or the patient's parent or guardian about the patient's bill.
Be respectful, polite, and professional.	
Tell the patient the reason for the call.	Call repeatedly if the patient fails to answer or return messages.
Keep the conversation short and to the point.	Become angry if the emotion arises.
Document any promises the patient makes.	Make promises that cannot be kept, such as reducing the bill.
Follow up on any of the patient's promises.	Converse about topics other than the subject of the call.
	Neglect to document all parts of the conversation with the patient.

may no longer contact the patient for payment of their account once the patient has filed a bankruptcy claim.

Patients may file bankruptcy in one of the following chapters:

1. **Chapter 7**—All nonexempt patient assets are sold and the proceeds distributed to creditors. Secured creditors, like mortgage or car loans, are paid first; unsecured creditors, like medical providers, are paid last. This type of bankruptcy is considered complete in that most or all patient debt dissolves. If the patient's assets are less than their debts, the medical office may not receive any of the amount outstanding and may have to write off the patient's balance.

2. **Chapter 13**—Protects debtors from creditors while the debtors arrange to repay all or some of their debts over 3- to 5-year periods. When those periods end, the balances on most debts dissolve.

Professional Courtesy

Physicians who treat other physicians for free or at greatly reduced fees extend what is called **professional courtesy**. Such courtesy is often extended to family or friends of the physician, to the family of other physicians, or even to such professional associates as the physician's attorney or accountant.

In cases of professional courtesy, accurate patient charts are vital to avoid the appearance of fraud or impropriety. Medical assistants should have any patients in these situations sign professional courtesy agreements, such as, "I understand Dr. Jones is giving me a professional courtesy discount for services rendered."

Patient Billing Statements

Medical offices should set aside a day each month to send **patient billing statements** to patients with balances due (Figure 19-7 ◆), preferably after the first of the month when rent and mortgages are typically due. Patient billing statements that arrive mid- to late month are more likely to be paid in a timely fashion.

While patient billing statements are one means of securing patients' payment, collecting patient copays at the time of office visit is far more cost effective. Monthly billing statements have been shown to cost about $8 per month per bill. To provide incentive, health care providers can offer discounts, called "cash discounts," to patients who pay their bills in full. However, such discounts should not exceed 5 percent of total fees or the provider may be accused of having a dual fee schedule, which is considered insurance fraud.

> "I am receiving treatment with Dr. Josephine Smith. Due to my financial hardship, Dr. Smith is giving me a discount for her services. I understand that the fee I am receiving is not Dr. Smith's conventional charges for these services."
>
> Patient Signature   Date
>
> _____   _____

Figure 19-6 ◆ Sample hardship agreement.

?—Critical Thinking Question 19-2—
Should medical offices have policies to offer discounts to patients like Millie when those patients agree to pay their full bills via credit card during collection calls? Why?

Heritage Park Women's Clinic
14 Heritage Way
Heritage Park, IN 12345

STATEMENT

CLOSING DATE	PREVIOUS BALANCE	BALANCE DUE
10/2/09	0	20.00

NOTE: ALL PAYMENTS AND CHARGES POSTED AFTER THE ABOVE CLOSING DATE WILL APPEAR ON THE NEXT STATEMENT.

AMOUNT PAID $ _____

BANKCARD PAYMENT AUTHORIZATION	☐ VISA	☐ M/C
VISA M/C ACCOUNT NUMBER		
CARDHOLDER SIGNATURE		EXP. DATE

Lillian Vidali
2715-16th Drive SW
Heritage Park, IN 12345

PLEASE DETACH AND **RETURN** THIS STUB WITH YOUR PAYMENT TO INSURE PROPER CREDIT

RETAIN THIS PORTION FOR YOUR RECORDS.

DATE OF SERVICE	DOCTOR / CPT CODE	DESCRIPTION	CHARGES	CREDITS
9/7/09	Wilson/99211	Office Visit	62.00	
9/20/09	Wilson	Insurance payment 9/7/09		42.00

PAST DUE				CURRENT		BALANCE DUE
0	0	0	0	20.00	▶	20.00
OVER 120 DAYS	OVER 90 DAYS	OVER 60 DAYS	OVER 30 DAYS	0 - 30 DAYS		

COMMENTS: Payment due by 11/10/09

Figure 19-7 ◆ Sample patient billing statement.

Collecting from patients while those patients are in the office is the most effective way to collect payment. When patients with past due accounts are due in for appointments, medical assistants should ask the receptionist to route those patients to the billing department before those patients receive treatment. In private areas out of other patients' hearing range, the assistants can then remind the patients of their balances. When patients cannot provide payment in full, the assistants should make payment arrangements with the patient.

Dismissing Patients Due to Nonpayment

When patients are chronically late with payments or refuse to pay at all, providers can dismiss those patients from care via **certified letter**. Figure 19-8 ◆ provides an example of a dismissal letter to a patient. Providers must give patients at least 30 days to receive care, but after that period providers are no longer bound to provide treatment. Physicians who do not honor this commitment

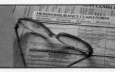

PROCEDURE 19-4 Call a Patient Regarding an Overdue Account

Theory and Rationale

Even with the most efficient administrative staff, every medical office has patients who are slow to pay and long overdue accounts. These accounts require medical assistants to act, such as call the patients. These telephone calls must be made professionally and documented appropriately.

Materials

- Telephone
- Patient's ledger information
- Blue or black pen

Competency

(Conditions) With the necessary materials, you will be able to **(Task)** call a patient regarding an overdue account **(Standards)** correctly within the time limit set by the instructor.

1. Dial the patient's home telephone number.

2. If you reach the patient:
   a. Identify yourself and the name of your clinic and state the reason for the call.
   b. Ask the patient when payment on the outstanding bill will be made.
   c. If the patient agrees to pay via credit card, take the credit card information over the telephone, verify the amount to be charged, charge the credit card, and mail the patient a receipt.
   d. If the patient agrees to mail payment to the office, secure a date by which the payment is to be received and note the date in the patient's billing ledger.
   e. If the patient expresses an inability to make a payment at this time, secure a date by which the patient expects to be able to make a payment and note the date in the patient's billing ledger.
3. If unable to reach the patient, leave a message that discloses no personal information about the patient's care in the office.
4. Note the message in the patient's billing ledger.

---

may be sued for patient abandonment. Patients should be dismissed only after physicians have given their consent, and a signed receipt verifying that the patient received the certified letter has been filed in the patient's permanent medical records.

Charging Interest on Medical Accounts

Medical providers who wish to charge interest on past due balances must be sure to check the laws in their states. Any changes in financial policy, including the decision to charge interest on accounts, requires providers to post written notices in prominent office locations at least 30 days before the financial changes occur.

Addressing Checks That Fail to Clear

When patients provide "bounced" or nonsufficient funds (**NSF**) checks, which are checks drawn on insufficient funds, most banks charge the medical office a fee. As a result, offices can legally charge patients a fee in return. Most banks redeposit NSF checks only once, so when checks cannot be redeposited, medical assistants must contact the patients to inform them of their checks' return and communicate the fee charged by the office. In such conversations, assistants should determine the date by which the patient will send a replacement payment. At the end of the interaction, assistants should make any relevant notations in the patient's billing ledger.

Contacting Nonpaying Patients

When patients fail to pay their monthly billing statements by the date due, medical assistants should try to contact the patients regarding payment. Unless patients have instructed otherwise, it is legal to contact patients at their places of employment. Once assistants reach patients, they should communicate the outstanding balance and ask when payment may be expected. When patients agree to dates and amounts, assistants should make notations in a **tickler file**. Serving as a reminder, a tickler file facilitates followup should payment fail to arrive when expected. Tickler files can be manual, as in index cards in a small box, or electronic. Many medical software programs have such reminder mechanisms.

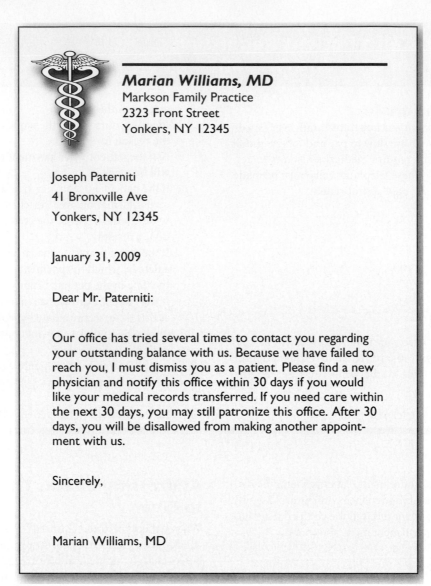

Marian Williams, MD
Markson Family Practice
2323 Front Street
Yonkers, NY 12345

Joseph Paterniti
41 Bronxville Ave
Yonkers, NY 12345

January 31, 2009

Dear Mr. Paterniti:

Our office has tried several times to contact you regarding your outstanding balance with us. Because we have failed to reach you, I must dismiss you as a patient. Please find a new physician and notify this office within 30 days if you would like your medical records transferred. If you need care within the next 30 days, you may still patronize this office. After 30 days, you will be disallowed from making another appointment with us.

Sincerely,

Marian Williams, MD

Figure 19-8 ◆ Sample dismissal letter.

In addition to making notes in tickler files, assistants should follow up with patients in writing. Letters should outline conversation details, including the amount owed on the account, the agreed-upon payment amount and due date, and any followup actions in the event of nonpayment. Many medical offices send a return envelope with these letters to give the patient an easy way to mail the payment to the office.

HIPAA Compliance

HIPAA regulations prevent members of the health care team from leaving messages with live parties or on voice mail when those messages may violate patient confidentiality. It is inappropriate, for example, to mention that a message is about a past due balance. An appropriate message is, "This is Ceila from Dr. Stewart's office. I need to leave a message for John Cooper to call me at (425) 555-9899." Document all phone calls in the patient's financial ledger.

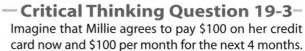
?─Critical Thinking Question 19-3─
Imagine that Millie agrees to pay $100 on her credit card now and $100 per month for the next 4 months. What is the best means the medical assistant has for tracking this agreement?

Sending Patients Collection Letters

When patients continue to be delinquent in their accounts, medical assistants can send those patients letters stating the amounts owed and any requested payment terms. Figure 19-9 ◆ gives an example. Some offices have their office managers, clinic directors, or health care providers try to contact the patients. Whatever procedure an office follows, the medical assistant must be sure to consistently and carefully apply the same guidelines to all patients.

When patients ignore medical offices' efforts to collect their accounts, offices may send those patients' accounts to

PROCEDURE 19-5   Send a Patient Billing Statement

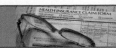

Theory and Rationale

Nearly every medical office sends monthly billing statements to patients with outstanding balances. These billing statements must be Health Insurance Portability and Accountability Act (**HIPAA**)–compliant and sent on or near the same day each month. In order to be HIPAA compliant, the statement must be sent in a security envelope (one that does not allow for the contents to be viewed without opening the envelope).

Materials

- Computer with medical billing software
- Printer (computerized billing)
- Patient ledger card (manual billing)
- Copy machine (manual billing)

Competency

(**Conditions**) With the necessary materials, you will be able to (**Task**) send a patient billing statement (**Standards**) correctly within the time limit set by the instructor.

1. Manual billing: Make a photocopy of the patient's ledger card.
   - Make a notation on the ledger card of the date and write "Bill to Patient" on the ledger.
   - Verify that the information on the ledger is correct, including that the balance has been correctly totaled.
   - Photocopy the ledger.
   - Place the copy of the ledger card in an envelope.
   - Stamp the envelope, and place it in the mail.
2. Computerized billing: Within the billing software, follow the appropriate steps to print a patient billing statement.
   - Once printed, verify the information on the bill is correct.
   - Place the copy of the ledger card into an envelope.
   - Stamp the envelope and place it in the mail.

PROCEDURE 19-6   Post a Nonsufficient Funds Check

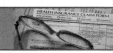

Theory and Rationale

When medical offices receive nonsufficient (NSF) checks from patients, those checks must be handled according to office policy and with respect for the patients. As with any patient conversations about finances, NSF check discussions must be clearly noted in patients' financial records.

Materials

- Check returned due to NSF
- For manual billing:
  - Patient billing ledger
  - Day sheet
  - Blue or black pen
- For computerized billing:
  - Computer with medical billing software

Competency

(**Conditions**) With the necessary materials, you will be able to (**Task**) post an NSF check (**Standards**) correctly within the time limit set by the instructor.

1. Verify that you have the correct patient ledger.
2. When billing manually:
   - Place the patient's ledger on the day sheet.
   - On the ledger card, record the NSF check and any applicable fees.
   - Calculate the new total on the account.

   When using computer billing software:
   - Enter the NSF check and any fees into the patient's ledger.
3. Notify the patient via phone that the check was returned. Indicate any corresponding fees.
4. Secure a date by which a replacement payment will be received.
5. In the patient's financial record or ledger, note the outcome of the conversation.

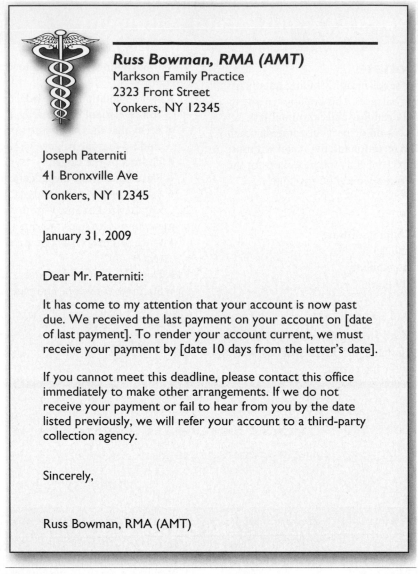

Russ Bowman, RMA (AMT)
Markson Family Practice
2323 Front Street
Yonkers, NY 12345

Joseph Paterniti
41 Bronxville Ave
Yonkers, NY 12345

January 31, 2009

Dear Mr. Paterniti:

It has come to my attention that your account is now past due. We received the last payment on your account on [date of last payment]. To render your account current, we must receive your payment by [date 10 days from the letter's date].

If you cannot meet this deadline, please contact this office immediately to make other arrangements. If we do not receive your payment or fail to hear from you by the date listed previously, we will refer your account to a third-party collection agency.

Sincerely,

Russ Bowman, RMA (AMT)

Figure 19-9 ◆ Sample collection letter to a patient.

collection agencies, write off the balances, or take the patients to small claims court. All these options require the physicians' consent, however.

When offices choose **collection agencies** to collect past due accounts, those collection agencies must be reputable. Other medical offices are good sources for agency references. Collection companies should actively pursue accounts, not harass or offend patients. Such agencies must also abide by federal guidelines for debt collection (Figure 19-10 ◆). The **Fair Debt Collection Act** was enacted to eliminate abusive, deceptive, and unfair collection practices. This law applies to all consumer debt for personal, family, or household purposes.

Once accounts go to collections, offices typically write off the balances owed. Collection agencies typically charge percentage fees for their services. The standard rate is 33 percent of the amount owing. Therefore, if a patient owes $99 when the office sends the account to collections, the provider is paid $66.00 when the collection agency collects the account in full ($99.00 − $33.00). Some collection agencies charge flat dollar

Medical offices must:

❏ Threaten to take only action that is legal or intended to come to fruition. For example, offices that threaten to sue patients for nonpayment must file lawsuits or face harassment accusations.

❏ Accurately represent themselves and the amounts patients owe.

❏ Make collection phone calls before 9 p.m. or after 8 a.m. unless directed by patients.

❏ Stop calling about accounts upon patients' requests. Continued calling would be considered harassment.

Figure 19-10 ◆ Highlights of the federal Fair Debt Collection guidelines.

PROCEDURE 19-7 Post an Adjustment to a Patient Account

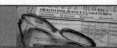

Theory and Rationale

Once medical offices have sent accounts to collection agencies, the balances of those accounts are typically written off. To effect this change, medical assistants must post adjustments to those accounts.

Materials

■ For manual billing:
  • Patient's ledger
  • Day sheet
  • Blue or black pen
  • Calculator
■ For computerized billing:
  • Medical billing software

Competency

(**Conditions**) With the necessary materials, you will be able to (**Task**) post an adjustment to a patient account (**Standards**) correctly within the time limit set by the instructor.

1. When billing manually:
   • Place the patient's billing ledger on the day sheet.
   • Pressing hard enough to impact all layers of paper, enter the type of adjustment on the ledger card.
   • Add or subtract adjustments as appropriate.
   • Calculate the new balance.
   • Enter the new balance on the ledger card.

   When billing via computer:
   • Locate the correct patient ledger in the computer.
   • Enter the adjustment as a debit or a credit.
2. In the patient's financial record, note the reason for the adjustment.

PROCEDURE 19-8 Post a Collection Agency Payment

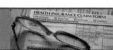

Theory and Rationale

When collection agencies send medical offices payments on accounts, medical assistants must properly post the payments and make appropriate debit adjustments.

Materials

■ For a manual posting system:
  • Day sheet
  • Ledger card
  • Pegboard
  • Calculator
  • Blue or black pen
  • Collection agency payment
■ For a computerized posting system:
  • Calculator
  • Computer
  • Collection agency payment

Competency

(**Conditions**) With the necessary materials, you will be able to (**Task**) post a collection agency payment (**Standards**) correctly within the time limit set by the instructor.

When using a manual system:

1. Verify which patient account will receive the payment.

2. Align the patient's ledger card with the next line on the day sheet.
3. In the appropriate columns, enter the patient's name, previous balance, payment date, payment amount, and name of the collection agency.
4. In the checks column of the day sheet's deposit section, enter the payment amount.
5. Subtract the payment from the previous patient balance.
6. Record the new balance on the patient's ledger card.
7. When an adjustment is to be made to the account due to collection agency fee, record the amount in brackets [ ] in the adjustment column of the ledger card and enter as the description "collection agency fee."
8. Subtract the amount of the adjustment from the previous patient balance, and record the new balance on the patient's ledger card.

   When using a computerized system:

1. Find the patient's account in the computer.
2. Verify the patient account is correct.
3. Post the payment, choosing "collection payment" as the payment source.
4. If applicable, enter any adjustment due to collection agency fee.
5. Verify the payment amount and adjustment.
6. Save all changes.

amounts to collect accounts, which is most cost effective for large accounts. To maximize their collections efforts, medical offices can use multiple collection agencies.

Uncollectible Accounts

Some offices choose to **write off** accounts deemed **uncollectible** to maintain patient relations. Patients may have legitimate reasons for nonpayment, such as the death of a spouse or the loss of a job. Writing off the account balance is legal and should only be done with the physician's approval. When medical offices choose to write off patients' owed balances, medical assistants must send the patients letters to that effect (Figure 19-11 ◆). Copies of the letters should reside in the patients' files.

Collecting from Estates

Patients sometimes die with balances owed the medical office. Providers may choose to forgive the balances when the deceased were unmarried, for example, or lacked assets. When providers choose to pursue the amounts, however, medical assistants should send statements to the deceased's estates in the following format:

> Estate of [patient's name]
> c/o [name of patient's spouse or next of kin]
> Patient's last known address

In return, the person handling the deceased's estate should contact the medical office to arrange for payment. If the office receives no response, the medical assistant can contact the County Recorder's Office in the Probate Department of the Superior Court in the county where the deceased resided. This office should provide the name of the estate's executor. If the office receives no response from the estate's executor, the assistant should gather the proper forms from the County Clerk's office to file a claim against the estate for the amount owing. In general, medical offices have from 2 to 36 months to act depending upon state law. While a claim remains

---

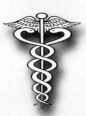

Adam Nichols, CMA (AAMA)
Markson Family Practice
2323 Front Street
Yonkers, NY 12345

Joseph Paterniti
41 Bronxville Ave
Yonkers, NY 12345

January 31, 2009

Dear Mr. Paterniti:

Our medical office has been unable to collect the $55 outstanding on your account. At this time, we are forgiving that balance and bringing your account balance to zero.

If you should again seek care in this office, you will be required to pay any patient portion of your bill at the time of service.

Sincerely,

Adam Nichols, CMA (AAMA)

Figure 19-11 ◆ Sample letter forgiving a patient balance.

PROCEDURE 19-9 Process a Patient Refund

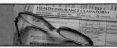

Theory and Rationale

When patient balances are overpaid, credit balances result. Research is needed to return credit balances to the appropriate parties. When patients are owed refunds, medical assistants must know how to post those refunds.

Materials

■ For manual billing:
  • Patient ledger card
  • Day sheet
  • Blue or black pen
  • Calculator
■ For computerized billing:
  • Computer with medical billing software

Competency

(**Conditions**) With the necessary materials, you will be able to (**Task**) process a refund to a patient (**Standards**) correctly within the time limit set by the instructor.

1. When billing manually:
   • Place the patient's ledger card on the day sheet.
   • Pressing hard enough to impact all copies, enter "Patient Refund" on the line.
   • Enter the dollar amount of the refund being sent to the patient.
   • Add the refund amount to the patient's balance.
   • Enter the new balance in the proper box.

   When billing via computer:
   • Locate the proper patient ledger in the billing software.
   • Enter the refund amount.
   • Choose the adjustment code for "Refund to Patient."
2. Obtain a refund check from the physician or office manager.
3. Send the refund check to the patient.
4. In the patient ledger, note the party receiving the refund and the number of the refund check.

PROCEDURE 19-10 Process an Insurance Company Overpayment

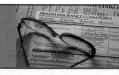

Theory and Rationale

When credits appear on patient accounts due to insurance company overpayment, medical assistants must process refunds to those companies. The medical assistant must carefully review the file to determine the appropriate insurance company to receive the refund.

Materials

■ For manual billing:
  • Patient ledger card
  • Day sheet
  • Blue or black pen
  • Copies of insurance companies' explanations of benefits
■ For computerized billing:
  • Computer with medical billing software
  • Copies of insurance companies' explanations of benefits

Competency

(**Conditions**) With the necessary materials, you will be able to (**Task**) process a refund to an insurance company (**Standards**) correctly within the time limit set by the instructor.

1. Using the insurance companies' explanations of benefits, determine which company is the patient's primary insurance carrier and which is secondary.
2. When billing manually:
   • Place the patient's ledger card on the day sheet.
   • Pressing hard enough to impact all copies, enter the refund amount and write "refund to insurance company." The refund amount is written in the adjustment column on the patient ledger.
   • Enter the new balance.

   When billing via computer:
   • Find the appropriate patient ledger in the computer.
   • Using the appropriate code, enter the refund to the insurance company.
3. Obtain a refund check from the physician or office manager.
4. Send a note to the insurance company explaining the reason for the refund, as well as copies of the primary and secondary insurance companies' explanations of benefits.

outstanding, the assistant should continue sending the estate's executor monthly billing statements.

Overpaying on Accounts

Account overpayments can occur for a number of reasons, including when patients overpay on their accounts or when insurance policies pay unexpectedly high amounts or when patients have multiple policies that together pay more than owed. When overpayments occur, careful review is needed to identify the party to receive the refund.

Collections Through Small Claims Court

Small claims court is yet another option for collecting on past due accounts. To pursue a small claims suit, the patient's balance owing must fit the "small claim" criteria in the state where the provider's office is located.

Depending on the laws in the states where medical assistants work, those assistants may be able to file claims online or through the mail. Some states require claims to be filed in person at the local county courthouse. All methods incur a cost at the time of filing. Notice of the suit must be served on the patient by someone who does not work in the medical office. Often, offices hire companies specializing in this task.

When small-claims cases enter court, staff from the medical office must appear to testify. The office representative will need a copy of the patient's account ledger and any documentation proving the health care provider treated the patient. Any signed documentation indicating the patient agreed to pay any outstanding bill is also important to bring. Typically, in small claims court, the health care provider's office need only prove that the patient was treated and that the patient knew of the charges for the service. Providers often win judgment in these cases, and patients are ordered to pay their bills.

When patients fail to pay their ordered amounts, physicians may opt to garnish those patients' wages. In states with **community property laws**, patients' spouses are also responsible for the bills. As a result, spouses' wages can also be garnished. To act appropriately, medical assistants must check the laws in their states.

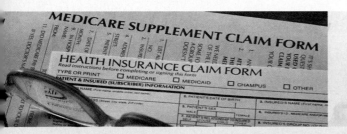

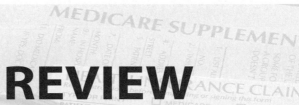

REVIEW

Chapter Summary

- A manual billing system, though used less often in the medical office, employs day sheets and charge slips to secure patient payment.
- Given their ease, accuracy, and cost effectiveness, computers are now predominantly used for medical office billing.
- The best computerized medical billing systems provide basic functionality, like payment posting and reporting, as well as any advanced features that support the office's business objectives.
- Professional fees are determined by a set of defined criteria so medical offices can operate within a fair and consistent fee schedule.
- A medical office's accounts receivables department is vital to securing payment for services rendered.

- Because fees are a crucial facet of an office's business success, collection policies are important.
- Collection agencies should be fair and equitable while being effective.
- Out of professional courtesy, physicians may sometimes treat patients they know personally without charging the patient for the service, or for a reduced fee.
- Hardship discounts are reserved for those who most need them. They are typically given to those patients who need the care but are unable to afford the cost. These cases are typically granted on a case-by-case basis.
- When otherwise able patients fail to honor their financial obligations, small claims courts can help medical offices collect their past-due accounts.

Chapter Review

Multiple Choice

1. A physician might decide to give a professional-courtesy discount to:
   a. another physician
   b. an employee of the physician
   c. the physician's mother
   d. all of the above

2. Each month, each patient statement costs about $_____ to send.
   a. 5
   b. 6
   c. 7
   d. 8

3. Health care providers can discount their services _____ percent for patients who pay in full at the time of service.
   a. 5
   b. 10
   c. 15
   d. 20

4. The most effective way to collect money from patients who owe is:
   a. over the telephone
   b. in person in the office
   c. through the mail
   d. none of the above

5. Which of the following is illegal under the Fair Debt Collection Act?
   a. Refusing to self-identify to patients
   b. Calling patients who have requested no further contact
   c. Threatening to send patients to collections with no intentions of followthrough
   d. All of the above

True/False

T F   1. Pegboard accounting systems are common in health care today.

T F   2. Most health insurance plans base their fee schedules on the Medicare fee schedule.

T F   3. A medical office can choose which patients will receive credit.

T F   4. Legally, health care providers can forgive patients' co-pays or deductibles.

T F   5. Dismissing patients from care due to nonpayment is legal.

T F   6. The interest rate on medical accounts is the same in all states.

T F   7. All collection agencies charge a 33 percent fee to collect accounts.

T F   8. Small claims court cases handle amounts of less than $500.

Short Answer

1. What is an accounts aging report?

2. Why is it important to analyze participating provider agreements before deciding to become a participating provider?

3. What are "accounts receivables" in the medical office?

4. What is a hardship agreement, and how is it used in the medical office?

5. What is a professional courtesy?

6. What is a tickler file, and why would it be useful in a medical office?

7. What is the purpose of sending an office brochure to new patients before those patients first visit the office?

8. How should a medical office handle a situation in which a patient dies while owing an outstanding balance to the office?

Research

1. Interview a person who works in the billing department of a local medical office. What kind of training has the person had before taking the job?

2. Research the various collection agencies in your area that handle medical accounts. How do they compare to one another?

3. Research the laws in your state regarding collecting medical debts.

Externship Application Experience

Martina Sylvan, a patient in Dr. DaSilva's office, owes $652 on her account. The medical assistant must contact Martina regarding her outstanding balance and set up a payment plan.

When the assistant reaches Martina via telephone, she says she has no extra money to pay her bill at this time. How should the medical assistant handle this situation?

Resource Guide

Federal Trade Commission
600 Pennsylvania Avenue, N.W.
Washington, D.C. 20580
Phone: (202) 326-2222
www.ftc.gov

Managed Outsource Solutions (provides both domestic and offshore outsourcing services)
Phone: (918) 451-8175
http://www.managedoutsource.com

Med**Media**

http://www.MyMAKit.com

More on this chapter, including interactive resources, can be found on the Student CD-ROM accompanying this textbook and on http://www.MyMAKit.com.

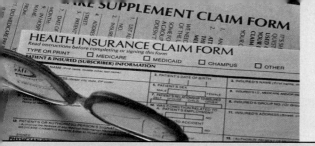

Objectives

After completing this chapter, you should be able to:

- Define and spell the key terminology in this chapter.
- Discuss the payroll function in the medical office.
- List the pros and cons of manual and computerized payroll systems.
- Describe the function of accounts payable in the medical office.
- List the correct procedure for writing a payroll check.
- Differentiate between monthly expenses and one-time expenses.
- Name the steps to creating a deposit of payments collected in the medical office.
- List the steps to endorsing a check for deposit.
- Describe how to access bank accounts via the Internet.
- Give several uses of petty cash in the medical office.
- Describe how to reconcile a monthly bank statement.

Payroll, Accounts Payable, and Banking Procedures

Case Study

Francie, who works as the medical office's receptionist, recently married a man with three children. Francie asks the medical assistant, who is in charge of payroll, to help her change her tax deductions so that fewer taxes are taken from her paycheck.

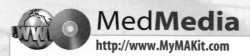

http://www.MyMAKit.com

Additional interactive resources and activities for this chapter can be found on http://www.MyMAKit.com. For a video on the petty cash fund, tips, audio glossary, legal and ethical scenarios, on-the-job scenarios, quizzes, and games related to the content of this chapter, please access the accompanying CD-ROM in this book.

Video: *The Petty Cash Fund*
Legal and Ethical Scenario: *Payroll, Accounts Payable, and Banking* Procedures
On the Job Scenario: *Payroll, Accounts Payable, and Banking Procedures*
Tips
Multiple Choice Quiz
Audio Glossary
HIPAA Quiz
Games: Spelling Bee, Crossword, and Strikeout

Key Terminology

auditors—those who review personal or corporate bank or tax records on behalf of an agency such as the Internal Revenue Service (IRS)

charitable contributions—cash or other donations given to charitable organizations

Circular E—yearly booklet published by the IRS that outlines the federal tax deductions to be taken from individuals' wages depending on marital status and number of exemptions

deductions—number of allowances to be withheld from wages

endorsement stamp—rubber tool that imprints a receiving agency's banking information

Fair Labor Standards Act (FLSA)—law passed by U.S. Congress in 1938 to address employment issues like federal minimum wage

Federal Insurance Contributions Act (FICA)—law that addresses Social Security withholding taxes

Federal Unemployment Tax Act (FUTA)—law that addresses federal unemployment tax withholdings

garnish—to withhold wages from an employee's paycheck due to a court order

gross pay—amount earned before taxes or deductions are subtracted

net pay—amount remaining after deductions and taxes are subtracted

outsource—to send to another business for completion

overtime—wages paid beyond 40 hours in a work week, at a rate 1½ times the normal rate for that employee

payroll—process of calculating the amounts employees receive for their work

payroll taxes—monies withheld from wages for federal income, Social Security, and Medicare obligations

personnel file—set of employment-related documents for an employee, to include an original application, federal withholding requests, and dates and copies of evaluations

quarterly payroll reports—documents that specify the taxes withheld from wages quarterly

security envelope—nontransparent envelope

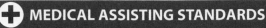

✚ MEDICAL ASSISTING STANDARDS

CAAHEP ENTRY-LEVEL STANDARDS	ABHES ENTRY-LEVEL COMPETENCIES
■ Explain basic bookkeeping computations (cognitive) ■ Differentiate between bookkeeping and accounting (cognitive) ■ Describe banking procedures (cognitive) ■ Differentiate between accounts payable and accounts receivable (cognitive) ■ Compare manual and computerized bookkeeping systems used in ambulatory healthcare (cognitive) ■ Describe common periodic financial reports (cognitive) ■ Prepare a bank deposit (psychomotor)	■ Adapt to change ■ Maintain confidentiality at all times ■ Use appropriate guidelines when releasing records or information ■ Project a positive attitude ■ Be cognizant of ethical boundaries ■ Evidence a responsible attitude ■ Conduct work within scope of education, training, and ability ■ Monitor legislation related to current healthcare issues and practices ■ Application of electronic technology ■ Establish a petty cash fund ■ Perform basic secretarial skills ■ Prepare a bank statement ■ Reconcile a bank statement ■ Maintain records for accounting and banking procedures ■ Prepare a check ■ Use manual and computerized bookkeeping systems ■ Manage accounts payable and receivable ■ Exercise efficient time management ■ Process employee payroll

✓ COMPETENCY SKILLS PERFORMANCE

1. Create a new employee record.
2. Calculate an employee's payroll.
3. Write checks to pay bills.
4. Pay an office supply invoice.
5. Complete a deposit slip.
6. Account for petty cash.
7. Reconcile a bank statement.

Introduction

In health care, payroll, accounts payable, and banking procedures are vital to office functioning. The payroll function involves keeping accurate records on employees. Accounts payable involves paying the office bills for rent, utilities, and supplies. Banking procedures involve balancing the office checking account and filing the appropriate quarterly and yearly statements with state and federal agencies.

Many large medical offices hire outside firms to help them complete their financial procedures; smaller offices tend to rely on their physicians or office managers for these tasks. Whether accounting, banking, and payroll procedures are outsourced or completed in house, medical assistants should understand how those procedures work.

Key Terminology *(continued)*

Social Security Act—law passed by the U.S. Congress in 1935 to provide workers and their families financial security post-retirement

time clock—piece of equipment that records employees' arrival and departure times for payroll purposes

unemployment insurance—program that pays employees who have lost their jobs

W-2 form—U.S. federal form that annually documents the wages employees drew the previous year

W-4 form—U.S. federal form that indicates employees' marital status and federal tax exemptions

wages—monies paid for work performed

withholding allowances—number of exemptions on federal tax forms

Abbreviations

CPR—cardiopulmonary resuscitation

FICA—Federal Insurance Contributions Act

FLSA—Fair Labor Standards Act

FUTA—Federal Unemployment Tax

HIPAA—Health Insurance Portability and Accountability Act

IRS—Internal Revenue Service

Processing Payroll

Given its role in employees' financial stability, payroll in the medical office is vital. As computer technology has advanced, payroll's function has been transformed.

The History of Payroll

When the 16th Constitutional Amendment passed in 1913, the Congress gained the ability to impose a federal income tax on individuals and corporations. Each year when they filed their returns, employees paid the federal government directly. By 1918, the government was collecting just over $1 billion each year as a result. By 1920, that figure had risen to $5.4 billion. When World War II launched and employment increased, taxes climbed to $7.3 billion annually.

In 1935, Congress passed the **Social Security Act** to provide workers and their families financial security. Congress followed that legislation with the **Fair Labor Standards Act (FLSA)** in 1938. This act addressed several worker-related issues, including a federal minimum wage that rises with the inflation rate. As of 2007, the federal minimum wage was $5.15. Many states choose to enforce a minimum wage that is higher than the federal minimum wage. In addition to things like minimum wage, the FLSA requires employers to pay employees **overtime** earnings of 1.5 times normal hourly wages for any work completed beyond 40 hours in 1 week.

As the years passed, the government tried to remain vigilant to workers' needs, but many employees were finding it difficult to keep up with increasing taxes. Many individual taxpayers found it tough to pay their full tax bills at the end of each year. In 1943 withholding taxes on wages was introduced. Under this law, businesses were responsible for collecting employees' income taxes and sending those taxes to the government. Employers had to keep written records of all the taxes they withheld from employee pay, as well as records of those employees' addresses, employment dates, and wages. This legislation boosted the number of taxpayers yet further. By 1945, taxes collected had jumped to $43 billion.

Present-Day Employment Issues

Throughout the decades, the U.S. government has continued to use legislation to address employment issues. For example, the Social Security Act enacted in the mid-1930s has evolved over the years to a system that today has two main parts: (1) elderly, survivors, and disability insurance and (2) hospital insurance, known as Medicare. Two other laws address the payment of Social Security and Medicare taxes: (1) the **Federal Insurance Contributions Act (FICA)** and (2) the **Federal Unemployment Tax Act (FUTA).** Still other laws require **unemployment insurance,** a program for which employers make quarterly payments to their state and federal governments. Employees who lose their jobs may be eligible to collect from the unemployment insurance fund while they seek new employment.

When the FICA tax started, it was set at 1 percent. In 2007, given rising inflation, it rests at 7.65 percent. Of that 7.65 percent FICA tax, employees pay 6.2 percent of their gross income for Social Security and 1.45 percent for Medicare. All employers must match the 7.65 percent amount, creating a deposit for each employee of 15.3 percent of their gross payrolls. Not all income is subject to FICA tax, however. As of 2007, only the first $90,000 of an individual's wages is subject to FICA tax. The Medicare tax has no wage limit.

The federal agency responsible for enforcing income tax laws is the Internal Revenue Service (IRS). This agency has offices in every major city and employs over 15,000 **auditors.** Auditors are responsible not only for conducting tax audits but also for giving taxpayers federal tax advice. The federal income taxes an employer withholds from employees' pay must be paid to the IRS each month. FICA taxes, like IRS taxes, must be deposited monthly. Every business must file quarterly payroll reports to the IRS in which they account for all monies withheld as taxes and deposits made to the IRS of those taxes (Figure 20-1 ◆).

Many states have income taxes that are separate from the federal income tax. States laws are similar to federal ones with regard to tax deductions and deposits. To comply with state tax laws, employers must withhold specified amounts and file reports quarterly.

Form **941** for **2008**: Employer's QUARTERLY Federal Tax Return
(Rev. October 2008)   Department of the Treasury — Internal Revenue Service

950108

OMB No. 1545-0029

(EIN)
Employer identification number

Name *(not your trade name)*

Trade name *(if any)*

Address
Number   Street   Suite or room number
City   State   ZIP code

Report for this Quarter of 2008
(Check one.)

☐ **1:** January, February, March
☐ **2:** April, May, June
☐ **3:** July, August, September
☐ **4:** October, November, December

Read the separate instructions before you complete Form 941. Type or print within the boxes.

Part 1: Answer these questions for this quarter.

1 Number of employees who received wages, tips, or other compensation for the pay period
   including: *Mar. 12* (Quarter 1), *June 12* (Quarter 2), *Sept. 12* (Quarter 3), *Dec. 12* (Quarter 4) **1**

2 Wages, tips, and other compensation **2**

3 Income tax withheld from wages, tips, and other compensation **3**

4 If no wages, tips, and other compensation are subject to social security or Medicare tax . . ☐ Check and go to line 6.

5 Taxable social security and Medicare wages and tips:

	Column 1		Column 2
5a Taxable social security wages		× .124 =	
5b Taxable social security tips		× .124 =	
5c Taxable Medicare wages & tips		× .029 =	

5d Total social security and Medicare taxes (*Column 2*, lines 5a + 5b + 5c = line 5d) . **5d**

6 Total taxes before adjustments (lines 3 + 5d = line 6) **6**

7 **TAX ADJUSTMENTS.** Read the instructions for line 7 before completing lines 7a through 7g.

7a Current quarter's fractions of cents . . . .

7b Current quarter's sick pay . . . .

7c Current quarter's adjustments for tips and group-term life insurance

7d Current year's income tax withholding. Attach Form 941c . .

7e Prior quarters' social security and Medicare taxes. Attach Form 941c

7f Special additions to federal income tax. Attach Form 941c . . .

7g Special additions to social security and Medicare. Attach Form 941c

7h **TOTAL ADJUSTMENTS.** Combine all amounts on lines 7a through 7g **7h**

8 Total taxes after adjustments. Combine lines 6 and 7h **8**

9 Advance earned income credit (EIC) payments made to employees **9**

10 Total taxes after adjustment for advance EIC (line 8 – line 9 = line 10) **10**

11 Total deposits for this quarter, including overpayment applied from a prior quarter . . . **11**

12 **Balance due.** If line 10 is more than line 11, write the difference here. **12**
    For information on how to pay, see the instructions.

13 **Overpayment.** If line 11 is more than line 10, write the difference here   Check one ☐ Apply to next return. ☐ Send a refund.

▶ You **MUST** complete both pages of Form 941 and **SIGN** it.   Next ➡

For Privacy Act and Paperwork Reduction Act Notice, see the back of the Payment Voucher.   Cat. No. 17001Z   Form **941** (Rev. 10-2008)

Figure 20-1 ◆ A 941 payroll tax reporting statement.

In addition to income taxes, most states have laws that require employers to provide employees with coverage should those employees become injured on the job. This coverage, known as workers' compensation, is used for medical care, lost wages, or death benefits. In many states, the employee pays a portion of the workers' compensation premium, but the employer generally funds the larger share. Employers in high-injury-risk industries like construction or mining pay higher premiums than those in low-risk businesses like insurance processing or data entry. However, even employers in low-risk industries will pay higher premiums if many of their employees are injured on the job.

Payroll Processing

Today, **payroll** processing involves far more than paycheck issuance. Various laws and regulations govern just about every phase of payroll, from calculating employees' deductions and the

Name *(not your trade name)*	Employer identification number (EIN)

Part 2: Tell us about your deposit schedule and tax liability for this quarter.

If you are unsure about whether you are a monthly schedule depositor or a semiweekly schedule depositor, see *Pub. 15 (Circular E)*, section 11.

14 ☐☐ Write the state abbreviation for the state where you made your deposits OR write "MU" if you made your deposits in *multiple* states.

15 Check one: ☐ Line 10 is less than $2,500. Go to Part 3.

☐ You were a monthly schedule depositor for the entire quarter. Enter your tax liability for each month. Then go to Part 3.

Tax liability: Month 1 ☐ .

Month 2 ☐ .

Month 3 ☐ .

Total liability for quarter ☐ . Total must equal line 10.

☐ You were a semiweekly schedule depositor for any part of this quarter. Complete *Schedule B (Form 941): Report of Tax Liability for Semiweekly Schedule Depositors,* and attach it to Form 941.

Part 3: Tell us about your business. If a question does NOT apply to your business, leave it blank.

16 If your business has closed or you stopped paying wages . . . . ☐ Check here, and

enter the final date you paid wages ☐ / / .

17 If you are a seasonal employer and you do not have to file a return for every quarter of the year . . ☐ Check here.

Part 4: May we speak with your third-party designee?

Do you want to allow an employee, a paid tax preparer, or another person to discuss this return with the IRS? See the instructions for details.

☐ Yes. Designee's name and phone number ☐ ( ) –

Select a 5-digit Personal Identification Number (PIN) to use when talking to the IRS. ☐☐☐☐☐

☐ No.

Part 5: Sign here. You MUST complete both pages of Form 941 and SIGN it.

Under penalties of perjury, I declare that I have examined this return, including accompanying schedules and statements, and to the best of my knowledge and belief, it is true, correct, and complete. Declaration of preparer (other than taxpayer) is based on all information of which preparer has any knowledge.

X **Sign your name here** ☐ Print your name here ☐

Print your title here ☐

Date / / Best daytime phone ( ) –

Paid preparer's use only Check if you are self-employed . . . . ☐

Preparer's name		Preparer's SSN/PTIN	
Preparer's signature		Date	/ /
Firm's name (or yours if self-employed)		EIN	
Address		Phone	( ) –
City	State	ZIP code	

Page **2** Form **941** (Rev. 10-2008)

Figure 20-1 ◆ (Continued)

taxes to be withheld from employees' **gross pay** to maintaining and reporting payroll records. The local and national laws impacting payroll practices can continue to change, so it is crucial for the staff member responsible for the medical office's payroll function to track those changes.

Many large offices now use computer software for their payroll functions, but some still calculate payroll manually. Still other offices **outsource** their payroll function to parties like accountants. In large and small medical offices alike, the member of the health care team who processes payroll is assigned a wide range of duties, including:

- Staying current with state and federal laws for **payroll taxes**
- Keeping written records of employees' hours and wages
- Computing the taxes and other **deductions** to be taken from employees' paychecks

PROCEDURE 20-1 Create a New Employee Record

Theory and Rationale

As each new staff member is added to the medical facility, a new employee record must be created. Much of what is contained in the record is mandated by local and federal law. The medical assistant must be aware of the paperwork needed and must comply with all laws regarding the maintenance of these records.

Materials

- Pen
- Paper
- Employee file
- Copy machine

Competency

(**Conditions**) With the necessary materials, you will be able to (**Task**) create a new employee record (**Standards**) correctly within the time limit set by the instructor.

1. Ask the new employee to bring the following items with them on their first day of employment:
   a. Picture identification or other proof of ability to work in the United States.
   b. Social security card.
   c. Copies of any certifications or professional licenses.
2. Photocopy any documents the employee has brought for the employee record.
3. Give the employee a W-4 IRS form to complete to indicate the number of exemptions to be claimed.
4. Place the employee's resume and application into the employee record.
5. Give the employee an I-9 form to complete to verify citizenship.

- Documenting the **wages**, deductions, and **net pay** for each employee
- Preparing and distributing paychecks to employees
- Calculating payroll taxes and depositing the funds
- Preparing **quarterly payroll reports**

Creating New Employee Records

For each new employee, the medical office should create a **personnel file** with all of the employee's employment-related documentation, such as the job application, resume, credentials, licensing and insurance information, I-9, and references. To prove their identities at hire, all new employees must provide copies of their drivers' licenses or other photo identification, as well as copies of their Social Security cards.

Updating Employee Records

Personnel records should reflect all changes to employee employment status, such as pay raises, evaluations, disciplinary actions, marital status changes, tax exemptions, and continuing education credits, as those changes occur. Employee records should also include copies of such items as employees' cardiopulmonary resuscitation (**CPR**) certifications and malpractice insurance documents. In short, personnel records should be accurate, up-to-date pictures of employees.

According to the Health Insurance Portability and Accountability Act (**HIPAA**), all personal employee information in the medical office, including payroll information, must be kept confidential and in places where only health care staff can access it. Under no circumstances should unauthorized parties be allowed access to personal employee information. Employ-

ees, however, must be allowed to view their personnel files and to request corrections as needed.

─Critical Thinking Question 20-1─

What should the medical assistant do with Francie's employee file now that she has provided new information?

The W-4 Form

Every new employee must complete an **IRS W-4 form,** or Employee's Withholding Allowance Certificate, which shows the employer the number of **withholding allowances** the employee is claiming (Figure 20-2 ◆). This number determines the amount, if any, to be withheld from the employee's earnings each payroll period.

─Critical Thinking Question 20-2─

What does the office manager need to do to help Francie ensure that withholding allowances are processed properly?

To ensure timely payroll processing, employees must complete and sign their W-4 forms before their first payroll period. As employees experience life changes, such as marriage or children, those employees' withholding allowances will change. To keep their payrolls up to date, medical offices should require employees to notify their personnel departments or payroll staff of any such changes.

Form W-4 (2008)

Purpose. Complete Form W-4 so that your employer can withhold the correct federal income tax from your pay. Consider completing a new Form W-4 each year and when your personal or financial situation changes.

Exemption from withholding. If you are exempt, complete **only** lines 1, 2, 3, 4, and 7 and sign the form to validate it. Your exemption for 2008 expires February 16, 2009. See Pub. 505, Tax Withholding and Estimated Tax.

Note. You cannot claim exemption from withholding if (a) your income exceeds $900 and includes more than $300 of unearned income (for example, interest and dividends) and (b) another person can claim you as a dependent on their tax return.

Basic instructions. If you are not exempt, complete the **Personal Allowances Worksheet** below. The worksheets on page 2 adjust your withholding allowances based on itemized deductions, certain credits,

adjustments to income, or two-earner/multiple job situations. Complete all worksheets that apply. However, you may claim fewer (or zero) allowances.

Head of household. Generally, you may claim head of household filing status on your tax return only if you are unmarried and pay more than 50% of the costs of keeping up a home for yourself and your dependent(s) or other qualifying individuals. See Pub. 501, Exemptions, Standard Deduction, and Filing Information, for information.

Tax credits. You can take projected tax credits into account in figuring your allowable number of withholding allowances. Credits for child or dependent care expenses and the child tax credit may be claimed using the **Personal Allowances Worksheet** below. See Pub. 919, How Do I Adjust My Tax Withholding, for information on converting your other credits into withholding allowances.

Nonwage income. If you have a large amount of nonwage income, such as interest or dividends, consider making estimated tax

payments using Form 1040-ES, Estimated Tax for Individuals. Otherwise, you may owe additional tax. If you have pension or annuity income, see Pub. 919 to find out if you should adjust your withholding on Form W-4 or W-4P.

Two earners or multiple jobs. If you have a working spouse or more than one job, figure the total number of allowances you are entitled to claim on all jobs using worksheets from only one Form W-4. Your withholding usually will be most accurate when all allowances are claimed on the Form W-4 for the highest paying job and zero allowances are claimed on the others. See Pub. 919 for details.

Nonresident alien. If you are a nonresident alien, see the Instructions for Form 8233 before completing this Form W-4.

Check your withholding. After your Form W-4 takes effect, use Pub. 919 to see how the dollar amount you are having withheld compares to your projected total tax for 2008. See Pub. 919, especially if your earnings exceed $130,000 (Single) or $180,000 (Married).

Personal Allowances Worksheet (Keep for your records.)

A Enter "1" for **yourself** if no one else can claim you as a dependent . . . . A _____

B Enter "1" if:
  - You are single and have only one job; or
  - You are married, have only one job, and your spouse does not work; or
  - Your wages from a second job or your spouse's wages (or the total of both) are $1,500 or less. B _____

C Enter "1" for your **spouse**. But, you may choose to enter "-0-" if you are married and have either a working spouse or more than one job. (Entering "-0-" may help you avoid having too little tax withheld.) . . . . C _____

D Enter number of **dependents** (other than your spouse or yourself) you will claim on your tax return . . . . . . D _____

E Enter "1" if you will file as **head of household** on your tax return (see conditions under **Head of household** above) . E _____

F Enter "1" if you have at least $1,500 of **child or dependent care expenses** for which you plan to claim a credit . . F _____
  (**Note.** Do **not** include child support payments. See Pub. 503, Child and Dependent Care Expenses, for details.)

G **Child Tax Credit** (including additional child tax credit). See Pub. 972, Child Tax Credit, for more information.
  - If your total income will be less than $58,000 ($86,000 if married), enter "2" for each eligible child.
  - If your total income will be between $58,000 and $84,000 ($86,000 and $119,000 if married), enter "1" for each eligible child plus "1" **additional** if you have 4 or more eligible children. G _____

H Add lines A through G and enter total here. (**Note.** This may be different from the number of exemptions you claim on your tax return.) ▶ H _____

For accuracy, complete all worksheets that apply.	• If you plan to **itemize or claim adjustments to income** and want to reduce your withholding, see the **Deductions and Adjustments Worksheet** on page 2.
	• If you have **more than one job** or are **married and you and your spouse both work** and the combined earnings from all jobs exceed $40,000 ($25,000 if married), see the **Two-Earners/Multiple Jobs Worksheet** on page 2 to avoid having too little tax withheld.
	• If **neither** of the above situations applies, **stop here** and enter the number from line H on line 5 of Form W-4 below.

-------------------- Cut here and give Form W-4 to your employer. Keep the top part for your records. --------------------

Form **W-4**
Department of the Treasury
Internal Revenue Service

Employee's Withholding Allowance Certificate
▶ Whether you are entitled to claim a certain number of allowances or exemption from withholding is subject to review by the IRS. Your employer may be required to send a copy of this form to the IRS.

OMB No. 1545-0074
20 08

1 Type or print your first name and middle initial.	Last name	2 Your social security number

Home address (number and street or rural route)	3 ☐ Single ☐ Married ☐ Married, but withhold at higher Single rate. **Note.** If married, but legally separated, or spouse is a nonresident alien, check the "Single" box.
City or town, state, and ZIP code	4 If your last name differs from that shown on your social security card, check here. You must call 1-800-772-1213 for a replacement card. ▶ ☐

5 Total number of allowances you are claiming (from line **H** above **or** from the applicable worksheet on page 2) **5** _____

6 Additional amount, if any, you want withheld from each paycheck . . . . **6** $ _____

7 I claim exemption from withholding for 2008, and I certify that I meet **both** of the following conditions for exemption.
  - Last year I had a right to a refund of **all** federal income tax withheld because I had **no** tax liability **and**
  - This year I expect a refund of **all** federal income tax withheld because I expect to have **no** tax liability.
  If you meet both conditions, write "Exempt" here . . . . ▶ **7**

Under penalties of perjury, I declare that I have examined this certificate and to the best of my knowledge and belief, it is true, correct, and complete.
Employee's signature
(Form is not valid unless you sign it.) ▶   Date ▶

8 Employer's name and address (Employer: Complete lines 8 and 10 only if sending to the IRS.)	9 Office code (optional)	10 Employer identification number (EIN)

For Privacy Act and Paperwork Reduction Act Notice, see page 2.   Cat. No. 10220Q   Form **W-4** (2008)

Figure 20-2 ◆ W-4 form.

When employees wish to change their withholding allowance, they must complete and sign new W-4 forms. W-4 changes should take effect in the next payroll period. When medical offices outsource their payroll functions, W-4 changes may be delayed. When this is the case, offices should notify the affected employees.

?—Critical Thinking Question 20-3—

Because the medical assistant, and not an outside agency, handles the medical office's payroll, what can the assistant tell Francie about the time it will take to change her payroll deductions?

Recording Employees' Work Hours

To meet FLSA requirements for overtime pay, employers must accurately record the hours their employees work. For all employees, salaried and hourly, employers must also send their states premiums to cover workers' compensation insurance. Such premiums are based on the number of hours all covered employees worked in each quarter.

Calculating Payroll

Employers have varied ways to track employees' work hours. Some employers use **time clocks** that stamp employees' cards at the beginning and end of shifts (Figure 20-3 ◆). Other

Form W-4 (2008)   Page **2**

Deductions and Adjustments Worksheet

Note. Use this worksheet *only* if you plan to itemize deductions, claim certain credits, or claim adjustments to income on your 2008 tax return.

1   Enter an estimate of your 2008 itemized deductions. These include qualifying home mortgage interest, charitable contributions, state and local taxes, medical expenses in excess of 7.5% of your income, and miscellaneous deductions. (For 2008, you may have to reduce your itemized deductions if your income is over $159,950 ($79,975 if married filing separately). See *Worksheet 2* in Pub. 919 for details.) . .   **1** $ _____

2   Enter:
- $10,900 if married filing jointly or qualifying widow(er)
- $ 8,000 if head of household
- $ 5,450 if single or married filing separately   . . . .   **2** $ _____

3   **Subtract** line 2 from line 1. If zero or less, enter "-0-" . . . .   **3** $ _____

4   Enter an estimate of your 2008 adjustments to income, including alimony, deductible IRA contributions, and student loan interest   **4** $ _____

5   **Add** lines 3 and 4 and enter the total. (Include any amount for credits from *Worksheet 8* in Pub. 919)   **5** $ _____

6   Enter an estimate of your 2008 nonwage income (such as dividends or interest) . . . .   **6** $ _____

7   **Subtract** line 6 from line 5. If zero or less, enter "-0-" . . . .   **7** $ _____

8   **Divide** the amount on line 7 by $3,500 and enter the result here. Drop any fraction . . . . . .   **8** _____

9   Enter the number from the **Personal Allowances Worksheet,** line H, page 1 . . . .   **9** _____

10 **Add** lines 8 and 9 and enter the total here. If you plan to use the **Two-Earners/Multiple Jobs Worksheet,** also enter this total on line 1 below. Otherwise, **stop here** and enter this total on Form W-4, line 5, page 1   **10** _____

Two-Earners/Multiple Jobs Worksheet (See *Two earners or multiple jobs* on page 1.)

Note. Use this worksheet *only* if the instructions under line H on page 1 direct you here.

1   Enter the number from line H, page 1 (or from line 10 above if you used the **Deductions and Adjustments Worksheet**)   **1** _____

2   Find the number in **Table 1** below that applies to the **LOWEST** paying job and enter it here. **However,** if you are married filing jointly and wages from the highest paying job are $50,000 or less, do not enter more than "3." . . . .   **2** _____

3   If line 1 is **more than or equal to** line 2, subtract line 2 from line 1. Enter the result here (if zero, enter "-0-") and on Form W-4, line 5, page 1. **Do not** use the rest of this worksheet   **3** _____

Note. If line 1 is *less than* line 2, enter "-0-" on Form W-4, line 5, page 1. Complete lines 4–9 below to calculate the additional withholding amount necessary to avoid a year-end tax bill.

4   Enter the number from line 2 of this worksheet . . . .   **4** _____

5   Enter the number from line 1 of this worksheet . . . .   **5** _____

6   **Subtract** line 5 from line 4 . . . .   **6** _____

7   Find the amount in **Table 2** below that applies to the **HIGHEST** paying job and enter it here . . . .   **7** $ _____

8   **Multiply** line 7 by line 6 and enter the result here. This is the additional annual withholding needed . .   **8** $ _____

9   Divide line 8 by the number of pay periods remaining in 2008. For example, divide by 26 if you are paid every two weeks and you complete this form in December 2007. Enter the result here and on Form W-4, line 6, page 1. This is the additional amount to be withheld from each paycheck . . . .   **9** $ _____

Table 1					Table 2			
Married Filing Jointly		**All Others**			**Married Filing Jointly**		**All Others**	
If wages from **LOWEST** paying job are—	Enter on line 2 above	If wages from **LOWEST** paying job are—	Enter on line 2 above		If wages from **HIGHEST** paying job are—	Enter on line 7 above	If wages from **HIGHEST** paying job are—	Enter on line 7 above
$0 - $4,500	0	$0 - $6,500	0		$0 - $65,000	$530	$0 - $35,000	$530
4,501 - 10,000	1	6,501 - 12,000	1		65,001 - 120,000	880	35,001 - 80,000	880
10,001 - 18,000	2	12,001 - 20,000	2		120,001 - 180,000	980	80,001 - 150,000	980
18,001 - 22,000	3	20,001 - 27,000	3		180,001 - 310,000	1,160	150,001 - 340,000	1,160
22,001 - 27,000	4	27,001 - 35,000	4		310,001 and over	1,230	340,001 and over	1,230
27,001 - 33,000	5	35,001 - 50,000	5					
33,001 - 40,000	6	50,001 - 65,000	6					
40,001 - 50,000	7	65,001 - 80,000	7					
50,001 - 55,000	8	80,001 - 95,000	8					
55,001 - 60,000	9	95,001 - 120,000	9					
60,001 - 65,000	10	120,001 and over	10					
65,001 - 75,000	11							
75,001 - 100,000	12							
100,001 - 110,000	13							
110,001 - 120,000	14							
120,001 and over	15							

Figure 20-2 ◆ (Continued)

employers direct employees to track their hours on timesheets they submit when each pay period ends.

Employees Paid on an Hourly Basis

The gross earnings of an employee paid hourly are calculated by multiplying the number of regular hours worked by the employee's hourly rate. Any overtime hours are calculated by multiplying the overtime hours worked by 1.5 times the employee's hourly rate. When employees work partial hours, some employers round those hours to the nearest half hour; others round to the nearest quarter hour. Figure 20-4 ◆ shows how hourly payroll is calculated.

Salaried Employees

The gross earnings of a salaried employee remain the same each pay period, no matter how many hours are worked, up to 40 hours in 1 week. In general, when salaried employees work more than 40 hours in a week, they must be paid overtime for each hour over 40. Overtime pay is calculated based on an hourly rate, which is calculated by dividing the employee's

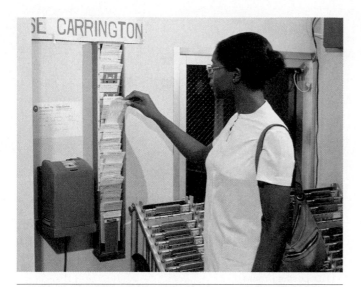

Figure 20-3 ◆ An employee uses a time clock to document the time she arrives at work.

Molly is a salaried employee paid $1,000.00 for each 2-week payroll period. In this pay period, Molly worked 85 hours. Calculating Molly's overtime pay entails first determining her normal hourly wage by dividing her $1,000.00 salary by the 80 hours in the 2-week pay period ($1,000.00/80 hours = $12.50 per hour). Next, determine Molly's overtime rate by multiplying 1.5 by her normal hourly rate (1.5 × $12.50 = $18.75) and then multiplying that figure by the 5 extra hours she worked during the pay period ($18.75 × 5 hours = $93.75). Finally, add Molly's base salary to her overtime hours to determine her gross earnings total for the pay period ($1,000.00 + $93.75 = $1093.75).

Figure 20-5 ◆ Salaried payroll calculation.

salaried amount by the number of hours in the pay period. Figure 20-5 ◆ provides an example of how salaried payroll is calculated.

Computing Payroll Deductions

Some payroll deductions, like the federal withholding and FICA taxes discussed earlier, are mandated by law. Other deductions, like those for health and life insurance or disability policies, are voluntary. Medical offices should give new employees lists of voluntary deductions so those employees can choose to participate if desired.

The Circular E

When employers calculate payroll manually, medical assistants need an IRS publication called the **Circular E** (Figure 20-6 ◆). This publication, revised annually, tells employers how much federal tax to withhold for each employee. Married and single

Ortiz's regular hourly rate is $15.00, and his regular hours per week are 40. In the past 2-week payroll period, Ortiz worked 84 hours. To calculate Ortiz's gross earnings, multiply his regular hours by his hourly wage (80 × $15.00 = $1,200.00). Next, calculate his overtime earnings by calculating his overtime hourly rate (1.5 × $15.00 = $22.50) and then multiply his overtime rate by his overtime hours ($22.50 × 4 = $90.00). Finally, add the amount Ortiz earned in regular hours with the amount he earned in overtime hours to determine his gross earnings for the payroll period ($1,200.00 + $90.00 = $1,290.00).

Figure 20-4 ◆ Hourly payroll calculation.

employees appear in separate tables, as do weekly, biweekly, semi-monthly, and monthly pay periods. To use the Circular E form properly, medical assistants need employees' completed W-4 forms. Table 20-1 describes how to use the Circular E tables.

To determine employees' FICA withholding amounts, medical assistants must first multiply the employees' gross earnings from regular and overtime pay by 6.2 percent for Social Security. Next, the assistants must multiply the employees' gross earnings by 1.45 percent for Medicare withholding. When assistants work in states with state and local income taxes, they will consult state and local reference tables to determine state and local taxes.

Other Deductions

To determine total deductions from employees' payrolls, amounts for items like worker's compensation insurance, health insurance, retirement plans, and **charitable contributions** must be calculated and added to federal and state or local taxes. Once all deductions are subtracted, the balance, called the net payroll or "take-home pay," is the amount the employee will receive in a check.

Using Software to Calculate Payroll

For employers who calculate payroll using computer software, payroll is far simpler than for those who choose the manual option. Although payroll software requires employers to set up

TABLE 20-1 CIRCULAR E USE

Danesha is married and claims four withholding allowances from her payroll. Her gross earnings this biweekly payroll period are $855.00. To determine the federal tax to withhold from Danesha's earnings, consult the married persons, biweekly payroll period chart (Figure 20-7 ◆). Move down the left column to Danesha's wages, and then move across the row to the number for people claiming four exemptions. This amount is the federal tax to withhold from Danesha's earnings.

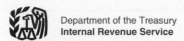

Department of the Treasury
Internal Revenue Service

Publication 15
Cat. No. 10000W

(Circular E), Employer's Tax Guide

(Including 2008 Wage Withholding and Advance Earned Income Credit Payment Tables)

For use in **2008**

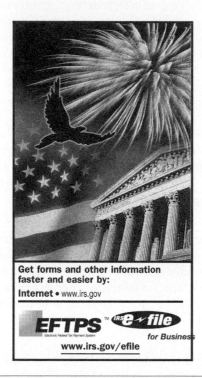

Get forms and other information faster and easier by:

Internet • www.irs.gov

EFTPS ™ IRS *e-file*
Electronic Federal Tax Payment System
for Business
www.irs.gov/efile

Contents

What's New

Social security and Medicare tax for 2008. Do not withhold social security tax after an employee reaches $102,000 in social security wages. There is no limit on the amount of wages subject to Medicare tax. Social security and Medicare taxes apply to the wages of household workers you pay $1,600 or more in cash. Social security and Medicare taxes apply to election workers who are paid $1,400 or more.

Disregarded entities and qualified subchapter S subsidiaries (QSubs). The IRS has published final regulations (T.D. 9356) under which QSubs and eligible single-owner disregarded entities are treated as separate entities for employment tax purposes. For more information, see *Disregarded entities and qualified subchapter S subsidiaries* in the Introduction.

Figure 20-6 ◆ The Circular E IRS table is used to find the correct amount of federal withholding tax for an employee.

each new employee, it streamlines the process of entering employees' hours and calculating employees' withholdings. Many such software packages also print payroll checks, quarterly payroll tax reports, and **W-2 forms.**

W-2 forms (Figure 20-8 ◆) outline employees' payroll information for the previous year. Because employees need these forms to file their personal taxes, federal law requires employers to send these forms to employees with no later than a January 31 postmark.

Garnishing Wages

Employees' wages may be **garnished,** or taken, for many reasons. Wages may be garnished to repay loans, honor child or spousal support, or pay monetary judgments against employees. Medical assistants who handle payroll must keep accurate records of all garnishment requests, which arise from court orders. These court orders specify the amounts to be taken from employees' gross wages, as well as the parties who are to receive those

MARRIED Persons—**BIWEEKLY** Payroll Period
(For Wages Paid in 2008)

If the wages are—		And the number of withholding allowances claimed is—										
At least	But less than	0	1	2	3	4	5	6	7	8	9	10
		The amount of income tax to be withheld is—										
$1,380	$1,400	$132	$112	$92	$72	$54	$41	$27	$14	$1	$0	$0
1,400	1,420	135	115	95	75	56	43	29	16	3	0	0
1,420	1,440	138	118	98	78	58	45	31	18	5	0	0
1,440	1,460	141	121	101	81	61	47	33	20	7	0	0
1,460	1,480	144	124	104	84	64	49	35	22	9	0	0
1,480	1,500	147	127	107	87	67	51	37	24	11	0	0
1,500	1,520	150	130	110	90	70	53	39	26	13	0	0
1,520	1,540	153	133	113	93	73	55	41	28	15	1	0
1,540	1,560	156	136	116	96	76	57	43	30	17	3	0
1,560	1,580	159	139	119	99	79	59	45	32	19	5	0
1,580	1,600	162	142	122	102	82	61	47	34	21	7	0
1,600	1,620	165	145	125	105	85	64	49	36	23	9	0
1,620	1,640	168	148	128	108	88	67	51	38	25	11	0
1,640	1,660	171	151	131	111	91	70	53	40	27	13	0
1,660	1,680	174	154	134	114	94	73	55	42	29	15	2
1,680	1,700	177	157	137	117	97	76	57	44	31	17	4
1,700	1,720	180	160	140	120	100	79	59	46	33	19	6
1,720	1,740	183	163	143	123	103	82	62	48	35	21	8
1,740	1,760	186	166	146	126	106	85	65	50	37	23	10
1,760	1,780	189	169	149	129	109	88	68	52	39	25	12
1,780	1,800	192	172	152	132	112	91	71	54	41	27	14
1,800	1,820	195	175	155	135	115	94	74	56	43	29	16
1,820	1,840	198	178	158	138	118	97	77	58	45	31	18
1,840	1,860	201	181	161	141	121	100	80	60	47	33	20
1,860	1,880	204	184	164	144	124	103	83	63	49	35	22
1,880	1,900	207	187	167	147	127	106	86	66	51	37	24
1,900	1,920	210	190	170	150	130	109	89	69	53	39	26
1,920	1,940	213	193	173	153	133	112	92	72	55	41	28
1,940	1,960	216	196	176	156	136	115	95	75	57	43	30
1,960	1,980	219	199	179	159	139	118	98	78	59	45	32
1,980	2,000	222	202	182	162	142	121	101	81	61	47	34
2,000	2,020	225	205	185	165	145	124	104	84	64	49	36
2,020	2,040	228	208	188	168	148	127	107	87	67	51	38
2,040	2,060	231	211	191	171	151	130	110	90	70	53	40
2,060	2,080	234	214	194	174	154	133	113	93	73	55	42
2,080	2,100	237	217	197	177	157	136	116	96	76	57	44
2,100	2,120	240	220	200	180	160	139	119	99	79	59	46
2,120	2,140	243	223	203	183	163	142	122	102	82	62	48
2,140	2,160	246	226	206	186	166	145	125	105	85	65	50
2,160	2,180	249	229	209	189	169	148	128	108	88	68	52
2,180	2,200	252	232	212	192	172	151	131	111	91	71	54
2,200	2,220	255	235	215	195	175	154	134	114	94	74	56
2,220	2,240	258	238	218	198	178	157	137	117	97	77	58
2,240	2,260	261	241	221	201	181	160	140	120	100	80	60
2,260	2,280	264	244	224	204	184	163	143	123	103	83	63
2,280	2,300	267	247	227	207	187	166	146	126	106	86	66
2,300	2,320	270	250	230	210	190	169	149	129	109	89	69
2,320	2,340	273	253	233	213	193	172	152	132	112	92	72
2,340	2,360	276	256	236	216	196	175	155	135	115	95	75
2,360	2,380	279	259	239	219	199	178	158	138	118	98	78
2,380	2,400	282	262	242	222	202	181	161	141	121	101	81
2,400	2,420	285	265	245	225	205	184	164	144	124	104	84
2,420	2,440	288	268	248	228	208	187	167	147	127	107	87
2,440	2,460	291	271	251	231	211	190	170	150	130	110	90
2,460	2,480	294	274	254	234	214	193	173	153	133	113	93
2,480	2,500	297	277	257	237	217	196	176	156	136	116	96
2,500	2,520	300	280	260	240	220	199	179	159	139	119	99
2,520	2,540	303	283	263	243	223	202	182	162	142	122	102
2,540	2,560	306	286	266	246	226	205	185	165	145	125	105
2,560	2,580	309	289	269	249	229	208	188	168	148	128	108
2,580	2,600	312	292	272	252	232	211	191	171	151	131	111
2,600	2,620	315	295	275	255	235	214	194	174	154	134	114
2,620	2,640	318	298	278	258	238	217	197	177	157	137	117
2,640	2,660	321	301	281	261	241	220	200	180	160	140	120
2,660	2,680	324	304	284	264	244	223	203	183	163	143	123
2,680	2,700	327	307	287	267	247	226	206	186	166	146	126

$2,700 and over		Use Table 2(b) for a **MARRIED person** on page 38. Also see the instructions on page 36.

Publication 15 (2008)   Page 47

Figure 20-7 ◆ This chart from the Circular E shows the correct amount of withholding tax for this employee.

amounts. Occasionally, percentages of employees' gross wages, rather than set dollar amounts, are garnished. Separate checks for garnished amounts must be sent to the agencies on the court orders. Whenever medical assistants mail checks to agencies, insurance carriers, or patients, they should use **security envelopes** to mask the contents. When wages are garnished, corresponding deductions appear on employees' payroll sheets. The employees receive the balances of their wages, which are less other deductions and taxes.

Accounts Payable

The accounts payable function in the medical office is like the financial function most people have in their homes: Bills come in and must be paid. In the medical office, bills may include those for office rent, utilities, insurance, and supplies. Some accounts are paid in single installments, whereas others are paid monthly or on other, similarly regular schedules. The medical assistant in charge of the accounts payable function must

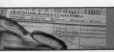

PROCEDURE 20-2 Calculate an Employee's Payroll

Theory and Rationale

Depending on the size of the medical office, the medical assistant may perform the employee payroll function. This function must be performed while paying strict attention to the state and national laws governing payroll.

Materials

■ Calculator
■ Employee's W-4 form
■ IRS Circular E list of federal tax deduction amounts
■ Record of number of hours the employee worked
■ Employee's payroll record

Competency

(**Conditions**) With the necessary materials, you will be able to (**Task**) calculate the amount of an employee's payroll (**Standards**) correctly within the time limit set by the instructor.

1. Calculate the number of hours the employee worked during the payroll period.

2. For an hourly employee, calculate the employee's gross wage by multiplying the number of hours worked in the payroll period by the employee's hourly wage.

3. If the employee worked any overtime hours, first multiply the employee's hourly wage by 1.5 and then multiply that amount by the employee's overtime hours.

4. Consult the employee's W-4 form to determine filing status (i.e., married or single) and the number of deductions.

5. Consult the IRS Circular E form to determine the amount to be withheld from the employee's gross wages.

6. Deduct the federal withholding tax from the Circular E form from the employee's gross payroll.

7. Multiply the employee's gross payroll amount by 6.2 percent to determine the FICA (Social Security) to withhold from the employee's payroll.

8. Multiply the employee's gross payroll amount by 1.45 percent to determine the Medicare tax to withhold from the employee's payroll.

9. Consult the employee's file to determine any other deductions (e.g., health insurance or retirement contributions) to withhold from the employee's payroll.

10. Determine the net payroll by subtracting all deductions from the gross payroll.

Figure 20-8 ◆ W-2 form.

determine the accuracy of bills before making payment and keep accurate records of all checks going out.

Several suppliers offer discounts for bills paid by set dates, which are typically 10, 15, or 30 days after supplies ship. Other suppliers offer discounts when supplies are paid by credit card rather than invoice. To take advantage of such discounts, medical assistants should research suppliers' and vendors' policies.

The Checkbook Register

Whether medical offices keep their checkbook registers electronically or in handwritten form, those registers must be accurate and clear as to payment purpose and receiver. Clarity, like the availability of the information, is especially important when the IRS conducts audits. To ensure clarity, checkbook registers should have columns with labels such as "Utilities," "Payroll," and "Clinical Supplies." Categorized expenditures help offices track their payments. Figure 20-9 ◆ lists some common expenditure categories.

Ordering and Receiving Supplies

Before ordering medical office supplies, the health care team should thoroughly investigate the suppliers and their policies. For example, staff should try to uncover any hidden costs, determine shipping costs, explore the possibility of bulk-rate discounts, and examine companies' return policies. For large purchases, offices may want to ask suppliers for referrals as an added investigative step.

When supplies arrive in the office, staff should check packing slips to verify the orders. Any invoices should be routed

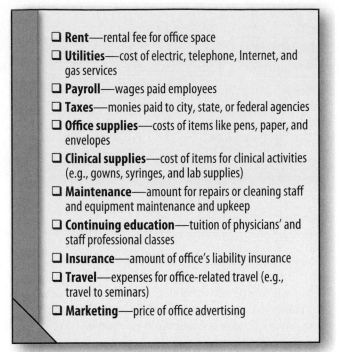

- ❏ **Rent**—rental fee for office space
- ❏ **Utilities**—cost of electric, telephone, Internet, and gas services
- ❏ **Payroll**—wages paid employees
- ❏ **Taxes**—monies paid to city, state, or federal agencies
- ❏ **Office supplies**—costs of items like pens, paper, and envelopes
- ❏ **Clinical supplies**—cost of items for clinical activities (e.g., gowns, syringes, and lab supplies)
- ❏ **Maintenance**—amount for repairs or cleaning staff and equipment maintenance and upkeep
- ❏ **Continuing education**—tuition of physicians' and staff professional classes
- ❏ **Insurance**—amount of office's liability insurance
- ❏ **Travel**—expenses for office-related travel (e.g., travel to seminars)
- ❏ **Marketing**—price of office advertising

Figure 20-9 ◆ Expenditure categories.

to the accounts payable office. ∞ Chapter 13 details the supply inventorying and ordering processes.

Preparing a Deposit Slip

At the end of each business day, medical offices should make deposits of their daily receipts (Figure 20-10 ◆). Such deposits include cash and personal checks collected from patients, usually

---

PROCEDURE 20-3 **Write Checks to Pay Bills**

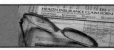

Theory and Rationale
In the medical office, varied bills (accounts payable) must be paid in a timely manner. The medical assistant who performs this function must understand how to use the checkbook register to pay the bills, as well as the importance of accuracy in this function.

Materials
- Office checkbook register
- Bills to be paid
- Blue or black pen
- Calculator

Competency
(**Conditions**) With the necessary materials, you will be able to (**Task**) write checks in payment of office bills (**Standards**) correctly within the time limit set by the instructor.

1. Verify the bill is accurate and that the supplies or services were received.
2. Determine if the company offers a discount if the bill is paid by a certain date. If so, pay the bill by the discount due date to obtain the discount.
3. Complete the check, providing the date, name of the vendor or supplier, and check amount.
4. On the invoice, write the date, check number, and payment amount.
5. File the invoice.
6. Give the check to the physician or office manager for signature.
7. In the checkbook register, note the payment category, date, and amount of the check.

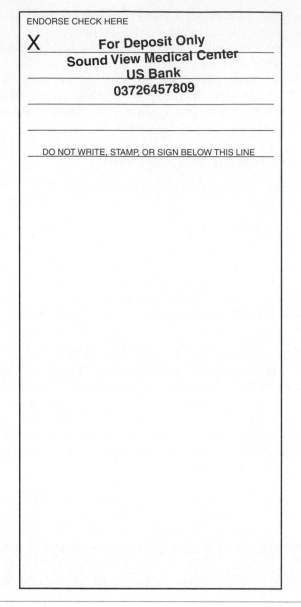

Figure 20-10 ◆ Sample deposit slip.

for copays, and insurance and patient payments received in the mail. Patients may sometimes fund their services through traveler's checks, which are purchased while traveling as a safe alternative to cash. These are deposited with the daily receipts. Computerized offices can print their days' collections via the medical office software. Such reports, which detail the day's receipts, should cross-check against the money to be deposited. In offices using manual bookkeeping systems, like the pegboard, staff must total payment columns and match the amount to be deposited.

The medical assistants who are responsible for preparing deposits must ensure that the amounts the computers or pegboards indicate as the daily collections match the deposit amounts. When these figures fail to match, assistants must search for and rectify the errors. Only when figures match may deposit slips be prepared.

Endorsement Stamps

Medical offices use **endorsement stamps** to endorse the backs of all checks they receive (Figure 20-11 ◆). These stamps list the offices' names, the banks' names, and the banks' account numbers. The phrase "For Deposit Only" should also appear on these stamps. Checks stamped in this manner are difficult to cash by unauthorized parties. The "deposit only" stamp is known as restrictive endorsement.

HIPAA Compliance

Any documents with patient information, including personal checks, are considered confidential. As a result, documents like these must be kept out of the view of other patients or staff who lack the authority to access confidential patient information.

Accessing Bank Accounts via the Internet

Most banks now allow users to access their bank accounts and complete banking functions, like bill paying, via the Internet. These services are convenient, because they are available 24 hours a day, 7 days a week, and medical offices may receive such

Figure 20-11 ◆ Sample endorsed check.

payments from patients via the mail. Medical assistants should post these payments, identified with patient account or identification numbers, as they would post conventional hard-copy checks.

Petty Cash

Most medical offices keep petty cash funds, small amounts of money to fund spur-of-the-moment costs like out-of-stock office supplies or postage. Whenever monies are taken from petty cash, receipts or vouchers in the amounts paid, as well as statements of payments' reasons, should replace the monies in the funds. Each month, petty cash funds should be balanced, which entails ensuring that the total of the receipts for expenditures and the money remaining in the fund equal the petty cash fund's assumed total.

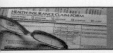

PROCEDURE 20-6 Account for Petty Cash

Theory and Rationale

Most medical offices have petty cash funds for small, unplanned purchases. Medical assistants must know how to balance these funds and should do so regularly. Petty cash funds should be balanced each month. The MA must ensure that the total of the receipts for expenditures and the money remaining in the fund equal the petty cash fund total.

Materials

- Petty cash record
- Receipts for petty cash purchases
- Blue or black pen
- Calculator

Competency

(**Conditions**) With the necessary materials, you will be able to (**Task**) balance the petty cash fund (**Standards**) correctly within the time limit set by the instructor.

1. Verify that all petty cash expenditures have been listed on the petty cash record and that each has a receipt.
2. Subtract all expenditures from the petty cash balance.
3. Enter the new balance on the petty cash record.
4. Count the money in petty cash.
5. Verify that the petty cash amount matches the resulting amount in step 2.
6. If the amounts do not match, verify that all subtraction was done accurately and that all receipts were entered in the petty cash record.
7. Once the account balances, obtain a check for the total expenditures from the physician or office manager.
8. Cash the check at the bank.
9. Enter the money in the petty cash record.

---

in real time. Offices need not wait for statements to arrive or call banks with payment or deposit questions when using online banking.

The reconciliation of medical office bank statements resembles the reconciliation of personal bank statements. Once the office's bank statement arrives from the bank, the staff member in charge of reconciliation must check off on the office's

book register the checks and deposits listed as processed on the statement. Next, staff should add the end-of-month balance on the statement to any outstanding deposits in the office's checkbook register. From that number, any outstanding checks must be deducted. The resulting number should match the amount in the office's checkbook register.

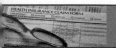

PROCEDURE 20-7 Reconcile a Bank Statement

Theory and Rationale

The medical office's bank statement must be balanced monthly to ensure the account balance is accurate and error free.

Materials

- Bank statement
- Checkbook register
- Calculator
- Blue or black pen

Competency

(**Conditions**) With the necessary materials, you will be able to (**Task**) balance the clinic bank statement (**Standards**) correctly within the time limit set by the instructor.

1. Comparing the bank statement to the checkbook register, make a check mark next to each check processed by the bank.
2. Write the ending balance on the bank statement.
3. Add any deposits made since the bank statement was printed.
4. Subtract any checks not yet processed when the bank statement was printed.
5. Add any interest awarded by the bank.
6. Subtract any bank service fees taken by the bank.
7. If the resulting balance fails to match that in the checkbook register balance, verify that steps 1 through 6 were performed correctly.
8. If the balances still do not match, check for addition or subtraction errors in the checkbook register.

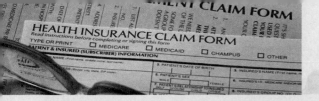

Chapter Summary

- Payroll is a critical function in the medical office. The payroll function involves keeping accurate records on all employees.
- Manual and computerized payroll systems are both employed in health care, though the latter tend to offer greater ease and convenience.
- In the medical office, accounts payable serves to secure the monies that keep the business functioning.
- When it comes time to deposit any payments received, checks must be endorsed properly following a documented procedure.

- Medical office payments are deposited according to a set procedure.
- Petty cash is a valuable tool the medical office can use for unexpected, though minor, purposes.
- The individual charged with reconciling the office's monthly bank statement should do so in a way that ensures an accurate result. The medical office's bank statement should be balanced monthly to ensure that the account balance is accurate and free of errors.

Chapter Review

Multiple Choice

1. In what year did Congress pass legislation requiring that federal income taxes be paid?
   a. 1893
   b. 1903
   c. 1913
   d. 1923

2. As of 2007, the federal minimum wage was:
   a. $3.15
   b. $4.15
   c. $5.15
   d. $6.15

3. Worker's compensation covers:
   a. work time lost due to injury
   b. medical expenses incurred due to injury
   c. a and b
   d. neither a nor b

4. Overtime is to be paid at _____ times the hourly rate.
   a. 1.25
   b. 1.5
   c. 1.75
   d. 2

True/False

T F 1. Employers use the IRS Circular E form to determine the federal withholding taxes to be withheld from employees' wages.

T F 2. Employers must track the hours their employees work, whether those employees are salaried or hourly.

T F 3. Another term for "gross pay" is "net pay."

T F 4. All employers must match the Social Security and Medicare taxes withheld from employees' payrolls.

T F 5. Medical office collections should be deposited daily.

T F 6. All states in America have state income taxes.

Short Answer

1. Name three items that should be in every employee's personnel file.

2. When choosing new suppliers for the medical office, what kinds of questions should be asked?

3. What does it mean to endorse a check?

4. Why is it important to endorse checks soon after they arrive in the medical office?

5. Name a common purchase made with petty cash.

6. Describe some characteristics desired in medical assistants who handle office payroll or accounts payable functions.

7. Why would patients pay for their physician's visits with traveler's checks?

8. Define the term "accounts payable."

9. Explain what it means to garnish an employee's wages.

10. Explain how a time clock is used.

Research

1. Interview the office manager of a local medical office. Ask the manager if the function of payroll is handled within the medical office or if it is handled by an outside firm.

2. Look at the IRS Web site. What information is contained there that might be helpful to the medical office with regard to processing payroll?

3. Research the laws regarding the garnishment of wages in your state.

Externship Application Experience

A recently hired medical assistant has been asked to visit the manager's office on his first day so that the manager can set up an employee file. What type of information should the assistant bring to expedite this task?

Resource Guide

Payroll-Taxes.com
14350 North 87th Street, Suite 170
Scottsdale, AZ 85260
Phone: (480) 596-1500
Fax: (480) 991-0572
http://www.payroll-taxes.com

Quickbooks Payroll
Phone: (888) 729-1996
http://www.quickbooks.com

Med**Media**

http://www.MyMAKit.com

More on this chapter, including interactive resources, can be found on the Student CD-ROM accompanying this textbook and on http://www.MyMAKit.com.

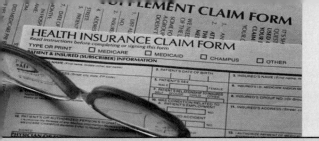

Objectives

After completing this chapter, you should be able to:

- Define and spell the key terminology in this chapter.
- Describe the characteristics and responsibilities of an effective office manager.
- Describe different management leadership styles.
- Explain how to conduct an effective staff meeting, how to write a staff meeting agenda, and discuss items that should be included.
- Explain the importance of a job description.
- Write effective job placement ads.
- List places where a medical office can advertise for staff.
- Describe how to lead an effective interview.
- List appropriate questions for potential employees.
- Name the steps involved in calling for employee references.
- Describe the MA's responsibility in hiring, training, and supervising staff.
- Discuss how to overcome scheduling issues.
- Explain the importance of employee evaluations.
- Discuss the steps to effectively manage medical office staff, including disciplining and terminating staff.
- Discuss the importance of sexual harassment policy in the medical office.
- Describe employment resources available to employees.
- List the steps involved in providing employee references.
- Describe the team effort involved in improving quality and managing risk in the medical office.
- Describe incident reporting in the medical office, including staff training on these procedures.
- Discuss various pieces of personal protective equipment in the medical office.
- Describe the appropriate disposal of hazardous waste.
- Develop employee safety protocol for the medical office.

Managing the Medical Office

Case Study

Juanita Ryan is the office manager at Valley View Medical Clinic, which has three physicians, one of whom arrives late every morning and returns late after lunch. Juanita has spoken with the physician, Dr. Whittier, several times. Patients are angry and frustrated by their long waits.

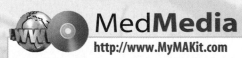

Med**Media**

http://www.MyMAKit.com

Additional interactive resources and activities for this chapter can be found on http://MyMAKit.com. For a video, tips, audio glossary, legal and ethical scenarios, on-the-job scenarios, quizzes, and games related to the content of this chapter, please access the accompanying CD-ROM in this book.

Video
Legal and Ethical Scenario: *Managing the Medical Office*
On the Job Scenario: *Managing the Medical Office*
Tips
Multiple Choice Quiz
Audio Glossary
HIPAA Quiz
Games: Spelling Bee, Crossword, and Strikeout

Key Terminology

adverse outcome—unfavorable treatment result

agenda—list of items to be addressed during a meeting

body language—set of nonverbal actions that communicate what a person is thinking or feeling

chemical waste—wasted drugs, cleaning solutions, germicides

delegate—to assign a task to another individual

Employment Assistance Programs (EAPs)—resources for those in personal crises, such as counseling and drug or alcohol rehabilitation

infectious waste—any garbage exposed to bodily fluids or any laboratory cultures or blood products

radioactive waste—any waste contaminated with radioactive material

sentinel event—in health care, injurious or possibly injurious act

sexual harassment—unwanted sexual attention or comments in the workplace

solid waste—paper, cans, cups and other garbage from nonclinical areas

Abbreviations

ADA—Americans with Disabilities Act

ADEA—Age Discrimination in Employment Act

EAP—Employee Assistant Program

EEOC—Equal Employment Opportunity Commission

✚ MEDICAL ASSISTING STANDARDS

CAAHEP ENTRY-LEVEL STANDARDS	ABHES ENTRY-LEVEL COMPETENCIES
■ Identify nonverbal communication (cognitive) ■ Recognize communication barriers (cognitive) ■ Identify techniques for overcoming communication barriers (cognitive) ■ Discuss the role of assertiveness in effective professional communication (cognitive) ■ Identify time management principles (cognitive) ■ List and discuss legal and illegal interview questions (cognitive) ■ Identify how the Americans with Disabilities Act (ADA) applies to the medical assisting profession (cognitive) ■ Discuss all levels of governmental legislation and regulation as they apply to medical assisting practice, including FDA and DEA regulations (cognitive) ■ Describe the process to follow if an error is made in patient care (cognitive) ■ Respond to issues of confidentiality (psychomotor) ■ Complete an incident report (psychomotor) ■ Demonstrate sensitivity to patient rights (affective) ■ Recognize the importance of local, state, and federal legislation and regulations in the practice setting (affective)	■ Adapt to change ■ Maintain confidentiality at all times ■ Use appropriate guidelines when releasing records or information ■ Project a positive attitude ■ Be cognizant of ethical boundaries ■ Evidence a responsible attitude ■ Conduct work within scope of education, training, and ability ■ Professional components ■ Maintain licenses and accreditation ■ Maintain liability coverage ■ Monitor legislation related to current health care issues and practices ■ Locate resources and information for patients and employers ■ Manage physician's professional schedule and travel ■ Use proper telephone techniques ■ Application of electronic technology ■ Apply computer concepts for office procedures ■ Follow established policy in initiating or terminating medical treatment ■ Exercise efficient time management ■ Receive, organize, prioritize, and transmit information efficiently ■ Fundamental writing skills ■ Orient and train personnel

✓ COMPETENCY SKILLS PERFORMANCE

1. Direct a staff meeting.
2. Write a job description.
3. Conduct an interview.
4. Call employee references.
5. Perform an employee evaluation.
6. Discipline an employee.
7. Terminate an employee.
8. File a medical incident report.
9. Use personal protective equipment.
10. Develop an exposure control plan.
11. Use proper lifting techniques.

Introduction

A skilled office manager is vital to the success of the ambulatory health care office. Often, office managers are medical assistants who prefer to complete administrative tasks, but it is also common to find office managers who lack clinical training. Sometimes, physicians act as their own office managers, but such arrangements fail to use physicians' time most efficiently. In some offices, clinical office managers direct the clinical portions while administrative office managers oversee administrative duties. Whatever the arrangement, as office leader, the office manager oversees and facilitates all office activities.

Characteristics of the Medical Office Manager

Successful office managers know that being a leader involves more than simply telling others what to do. Good leaders lead by example and encourage those they manage to do the best jobs they can do.

As office lead, the medical office manager must be able to multitask, which means being able to manage several people as well as several projects at the same time. Office managers must have excellent communication skills and the ability to project confidence. Figure 21-1 ◆ lists the traits office managers must possess.

Responsibilities of the Office Manager

The office manager may be called on to handle any number of situations in the medical office. Unresolvable disputes between staff are just one example. When such disputes arise, the office manager must remain objective and fair and listen to both parties in an attempt to reach a mutual and fair solution. Office managers may also be called upon to address patient complaints. To address complaints in a fair and timely fashion, the office manager needs top-notch communication skills.

In general, the medical office manager must be able to **delegate** as well as oversee tasks. One person alone cannot complete all tasks in a busy medical practice, so knowing how, and to whom, to hand off tasks is a sign of true efficiency. Figure 21-2 ◆ lists many of the responsibilities that are typically given to the medical office manager. These duties will vary depending upon the type and size of practice.

In Practice

Carrie is an administrative medical assistant working the medical office's reception desk. Mrs. Carnes enters the office and begins to loudly complain about a bill she has received. She demands that Carrie explain why the bill is so high. During the exchange, several other patients in the reception room watch Carrie for her reaction. What should Carrie do to defuse this scene?

❑ Extremely well organized
❑ Flexible
❑ Patient
❑ Honest
❑ Excellent communicator
❑ Good listener
❑ Able to resolve conflict
❑ Supportive of all office personnel

Figure 21-1 ◆ Medical office manager traits.

❑ Supervision of employees
❑ Interviewing and hiring employees
❑ Scheduling staff
❑ Employee evaluations
❑ Disciplining and terminating employees
❑ Tracking the financial flow within the medical office
❑ Handling disputes between staff members
❑ Organizing and leading staff meetings
❑ Handling difficulties with patients
❑ Oversight of the inventory and equipment maintenance within the office
❑ Function as a buffer between the physicians and the staff
❑ Prepare quarterly financial reports
❑ Payroll

Figure 21-2 ◆ Responsibilities of the office manager.

?—Critical Thinking Question 21-1—

As the office manager, how should Juanita address Dr. Whittier's tardiness?

Leadership Styles

Leadership takes one of three basic styles (Figure 21-3 ◆). Managers generally tailor their leadership style to the situation at hand.

It is important for medical office managers to adopt different leadership styles in response to varying situations. Constant use of the autocratic leading style, for example, may inspire staff to resign or resist making decisions on their own. The laissez-faire style, in contrast, may disorganize the office when

Autocratic
The leader makes all decisions without seeking input. This style works best in emergencies, when orders must be given quickly and followed exactly.
Democratic
The leader who tends to ask for opinions and/or advice before making decisions and may seek consensus or retain sole decision-making authority.
Laissez-Faire
The leader tends to allow others to make their own decisions, becoming involved only when absolutely needed.

Figure 21-3 ◆ Leadership styles.

used all the time. The ability to balance all these styles is critical to addressing issues on a case-by-case basis.

Conducting Effective Staff Meetings

Staff meetings should be scheduled regularly in the medical office (Figure 21-4 ◆). During the business day, staff are often too busy to communicate with each other effectively, and miscommunication and errors can result. Regular staff meetings with all staff present can help keep the lines of communication open between coworkers. When staff meetings are scheduled outside normal office hours or during lunch times, all in attendance should be compensated. Such a gesture communicates to staff that the meetings, and their time, are both valuable to the office.

Typically, office managers or physicians lead staff meetings. Some offices find that alternating the staff meeting leader encourages full staff participation, confirms that all staff are members of the health care team, and underscores that each staff member's participation is valuable.

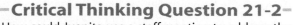

?—Critical Thinking Question 21-2—
How could Juanita use a staff meeting to address the issue of Dr. Whittier's tardiness?

Creating Staff Meeting Agendas

To be maximally effective, staff meetings should have clear start and end times and follow well organized **agendas** that staff receive before the meetings commence (Figure 21-5 ◆). Staff-meeting agendas are designed to notify attendees of discussion topics so those attendees can come prepared to participate. Generally, meeting leaders prepare agendas, which should be followed as strictly as possible to honor time and other commitments.

Occasionally, attendees raise topics not on the agenda. When this occurs, the staff-meeting leader should determine whether there is time to discuss the topic. If not, the topic

> ❑ Report on activities or projects since the last staff meeting
> ❑ Report on upcoming activities or projects
> ❑ Review schedules for the upcoming week/month
> ❑ Review any concerns from staff

Figure 21-5 ◆ Sample staff meeting agenda.

should be deferred to the next staff meeting and listed on the next agenda.

Staff Meeting Minutes

Staff-meeting minutes serve as written accounts of meeting discussions. Such accounts are important for several reasons. First, staff members who cannot attend can review them and catch up on missed material. Second, minutes are written accounts that cannot easily be misinterpreted or forgotten. Finally, staff can use meeting minutes as references when composing the agendas of subsequent meetings. Figure 21-6 ◆ outlines the items that should appear in staff-meeting minutes.

?—Critical Thinking Question 21-3—
Imagine that the chronically late physician, Dr. Whittier, fails to attend the staff meeting at which the issue is addressed. How should Juanita inform him of the staff meeting's discussion?

A person other than the staff-meeting leader should record the meeting's minutes. Like they do with leading the staff meeting, staff should take turns assuming recording duties to encourage full team participation. Whomever records a meeting's minutes should type and distribute those minutes to all staff, including those not in attendance. A copy should also appear in the office notebook as documentation of the meeting's events.

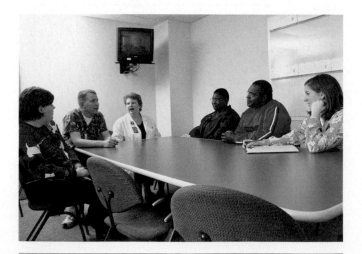

Figure 21-4 ◆ Staff meeting in the medical office.

> ❑ List of all staff members at the meeting
> ❑ List of all staff members absent from the meeting
> ❑ Date and times the meeting began and ended
> ❑ Brief description of each discussed item
> ❑ Brief description of any action taken at the meeting, including any staff member assignments
> ❑ List of any items to be deferred to the next staff meeting
> ❑ Signature of the person taking the minutes

Figure 21-6 ◆ Items to include in staff meeting minutes.

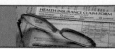

PROCEDURE 21-1 Direct a Staff Meeting

Theory and Rationale

The office manager is often responsible for directing the medical office staff meeting. The office manager should project authority while including all staff.

Materials

- Blue or black pen
- Paper
- Clock or watch to keep time
- Staff meeting agenda

Competency

(**Conditions**) With the necessary materials, you will be able to (**Task**) direct a staff meeting (**Standards**) correctly within the time limit set by the instructor.

1. Before the staff meeting, create an agenda of the meeting's discussion topics.
2. Start the meeting on time.
3. Note staff in attendance and staff who are absent.
4. Discuss the agenda items one at a time, being mindful of the time.
5. When nonagenda items arise, determine if they should be included in this meeting or moved to the next.
6. Address any issues or concerns that arise.
7. End the meeting at the prearranged time.

Staffing the Medical Office

One of the most important parts of the office manager's job is staffing the medical office. Staffing involves discussing staffing needs with physicians, writing job descriptions, recruiting and interviewing candidates, evaluating employees' performances, scheduling staff shifts, and handling any disciplinary or termination actions.

Writing Job Descriptions

Every position in the medical office must have a clear and concise description. A job description outlines the duties and expectations of a position and helps the office manager both interview potential employees and evaluate existing ones. Figure 21-7 ◆ identifies the items every job description should include.

❑ Title of the job
❑ Name of the supervisor for this position
❑ Summary of the position's duties
❑ Required hours for the position
❑ Position's location, when the business has multiple locations
❑ Any employment requirements (e.g., cardiopulmonary [CPR] certification or malpractice insurance)
❑ Any physical requirements (e.g., lifting, standing, sitting, or walking)
❑ Summary of the office's evaluation process

Figure 21-7 ◆ Job description items.

The job-description format may vary from office to office, but within an office that format should be consistent. Figure 21-8 ◆ shows a sample job description.

Creating Job Advertisements

Attracting and hiring the best employees starts with effective job advertisement placement. To be effective, job ads need not include in-depth information about positions. Instead, they should list a handful of the duties required, as well as any certification or experience stipulations. While many employers add terms like "friendly," "team player," and "professional" to their ads, these are characteristics to be uncovered in interviews, not necessarily items that should appear in job ads. Figure 21-9 ◆ is an effective job placement ad.

Recruiting and Interviewing Candidates

Medical offices can recruit new employees in varied ways, but the most common are local employment offices, private job-listing agencies, and local newspapers. Many medical offices post openings with local colleges, especially those with accredited medical assisting programs.

To collect applications from candidates, offices might ask applicants to mail or fax their resumes or submit applications online. Once offices receive applications and resumes, office managers can review them for suitability. Typically, managers will discard any applicants who fail to meet the qualifications. Because resumes and applications reflect the candidates who submit them, office managers also often discard any applications with poor grammar or typographical errors.

Once office managers have identified a pool of potential candidates, they will schedule those applicants for in-person

Administrative Medical Assistant Job Description

Administrative Duties

❑ Answers telephone calls and assesses urgency of call.

- Provides assistance or directs caller to appropriate person, contacting physician/nurse directly for urgent needs.
- Provides assistance to other receptionists in screening patient calls.

❑ Provides specialized information related to section, policies, procedures, insurance and services.

- Assists patients with the completion of forms.
- Builds monthly provider master schedules and clinic calendars from established sources and verifies provider sessions worked. Modifies master schedules to accommodate time off, extra patients, hospital emergencies, etc.
- Creates patient bump lists as necessary due to last-minute provider callouts.
- Schedules patient appointments and resolves scheduling conflicts.
- Notifies patients of changes/cancellations and prioritizes urgency of appointments for rescheduling.
- Receives patients and visitors. Secures names and needs and directs accordingly.
- Updates patient information and verifies insurance information, level of services, and tracks referrals when necessary.
- Initiates billing process by completing patient encounter forms and accepts and processes fee-for-service payments.
- Books diagnostic tests and specialized appointments for patients at hospitals and other medical facilities and ensures that patients are provided with necessary paperwork and specialized instructions for procedures.
- Schedules surgical procedures for patients. Coordinates available dates for surgery and scheduling of pre- and post-operative exams and lab work.
- Obtains and distributes necessary paperwork and maintains system to track completion.
- Coordinates surgery schedule changes as necessary.
- Schedules and coordinates departmental meetings, classes, clinics, conferences, etc.
- Utilizes computer input and retrieves data. Merges and manipulates data to generate complex reports. Compiles and maintains clinical and patient statistical data and produces summaries and reports.
- Keyboards correspondence, clinical information, reports, publicity material, educational handouts, etc. Composes general written material.
- Obtains patient charts, medical records, and lab reports, and verifies for completeness.
- Sorts, screens, and distributes incoming mail. Prioritizes and ensures completion of medical forms by clinical staff.
- Establishes and maintains filing systems.
- Maintains inventory of administrative office supplies and educational material
- Ensures adequate coverage of reception desk.

Figure 21-8 ◆ Sample job description.

Certified or registered medical assistant wanted full time in busy pediatrics office. Two-plus years experience working with children and current CMA (AAMA) or RMA (AMT) certification required. Position includes clinical and administrative duties, as well as laboratory skills. Please e-mail resume to srangel@monroefp.com.

Figure 21-9 ◆ Sample job placement ad.

interviews. Because first impressions are important, office managers use interviews to assess things like applicants' appearance and confidence as well as their professional qualifications. To remain consistent from candidate to candidate, managers should use preprinted lists of questions and tailor any other questions as needed. Figure 21-10 ◆ lists some common questions to ask job candidates.

Because office managers often interview multiple applicants for positions, they should take notes during interviews. In addition to observations about applicants' clothing and appearances, managers should capture applicants' responses and their positive or negative behaviors.

Avoiding Illegal Interview Questions

As the parties in charge of employment practices, office managers must know state and federal laws regulating employees,

PROCEDURE 21-2   Write a Job Description

Theory and Rationale

The medical office manager must compose a job description for every position in the medical office. To avoid confusion between employer and employee, these descriptions must be accurate and thorough.

Materials

- Computer with word-processing software
- List of skills needed for the position
- List of duties required for the position

Competency

(**Conditions**) With the necessary materials, you will be able to (**Task**) write a job description (**Standards**) correctly within the time limit set by the instructor.

1. Create a title for the job position.
2. List the name of the supervisor for the position.
3. Create a summary description of the position's duties.
4. List the hours required of the position.
5. List the location of the position, when it varies.
6. List any employment requirements (e.g., certification, malpractice insurance).
7. List any physical requirements for the position (e.g., lifting, excessive sitting or standing).
8. Describe the evaluation process for the position.
9. Review the job description for accuracy, as well as with the physician if needed.

---

among them Title VII of the Civil Rights Act, the Americans with Disabilities Act (**ADA**), and the Age Discrimination in Employment Act (**ADEA**). According to agencies like the U.S. Equal Employment Opportunity Commission (**EEOC**), which enforces many, similar laws, employers may not discriminate in their hiring, promotion, pay, benefits, retirement plan, discipline, or firing practices. When questions address employee safety or suitability, however, they are appropriate in interviews. For example, when positions will expose medical assistants to medications hazardous to unborn fetuses, employers may ask female candidates about pregnancy. Figure 21-11 ◆ provides questions to avoid in interviews.

Calling for Employment References

Employment references, like employee credentials, are critical tools in the staffing process. During interviews, office managers should ask applicants if they may call previous employers for references. Reference information usually appears on applicants' resumes or applications, but when it does not, managers should ask applicants to supply the information. Applicants who resist such requests may be hiding negative information about previous employment.

> **Keys to Success**
> **CHECKING CREDENTIALS**
>
> Before applicants are offered positions in the medical office, office managers must check their credentials by calling state licensing agencies or certification registries. For example, certified medical assistant (CMA) (AAMA) certification status can be verified by calling (800) ACT-AAMA. Simply asking prospective employees to provide certification information fails to suffice, because some applicants may be dishonest.

- ❑ Why do you want to work in this office?
- ❑ Do you have the skills needed to perform the job?
- ❑ Why did you leave your last position?
- ❑ How do you respond to pressure?
- ❑ What is your desired salary?

Figure 21-10 ◆ Interview questions for job candidates.

- ❑ What is your race or ethnic background?
- ❑ What country are you from?
- ❑ What is/are your religion/religious beliefs?
- ❑ What is your gender?
- ❑ How old are you?
- ❑ Do you have any disabilities? (Note: Disabilities prohibiting job performance are legally addressed.)
- ❑ What is your marital status?
- ❑ What political party do you belong to, or what are your political beliefs?
- ❑ What is your sexual orientation?
- ❑ Are you pregnant or thinking of becoming pregnant? (*Note:* This question may be asked if the employee will be exposed to chemicals hazardous to an unborn child.)

Figure 21-11 ◆ Illegal interview questions.

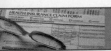

PROCEDURE 21-3 Conduct an Interview

Theory and Rationale

Medical office managers are typically responsible for interviewing prospective employees. Those managers must do so legally and with the aim of finding the best candidates.

Materials

- Pen
- Applicant's resume

Competency

(**Conditions**) With the necessary materials, you will be able to (**Task**) perform an interview (**Standards**) correctly within the time limit set by the instructor.

1. Before meeting the applicant, read the resume.
2. Highlight any areas of concern or interest on the resume.

3. Highlight resume items such as experience that apply to the position being filled.
4. Greet the applicant while making direct eye contact.
5. Use a firm handshake to shake hands with the applicant.
6. Lead the applicant to a private room.
7. Show the applicant where to sit for the interview.
8. Ask the applicant about the potential to perform the job.
9. Review any areas of concern highlighted on the resume.
10. Review the job description
11. Verify the applicant's ability to perform the required tasks.
12. Ask the applicant if he or she has any questions about the office or physicians.
13. Take note of any pertinent information.
14. Provide a decision date for the position.
15. Thank the applicant, and escort the applicant out of the office.

Open-ended questions, not those answered with just "yes" or "no," are appropriate when calling for employment references, because they tend to provide more useful information. For example, office managers might ask former employers to describe employees' work habits rather than simply ask if those employees worked for the organizations.

Hiring New Staff

Once they hire new staff, office managers should create employee files for the new hires. These files, which must be kept

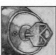

Keys to Success
CALLING THE EMPLOYEE'S CURRENT EMPLOYER

Some applicants are employed when they interview for new positions and do not notify their current employers of their plans to work elsewhere. As a result, office managers should not call applicants' current employers unless those applicants state that doing so is acceptable.

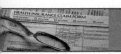

PROCEDURE 21-4 Call Employee References

Theory and Rationale

The medical office manager may uncover useful information from an employee's former employer. The key is to ask the correct questions about the employee's history with his or her previous employer.

Materials

- Telephone
- Employee resume
- Pen

Competency

(**Conditions**) With the necessary materials, you will be able to (**Task**) call for an employee reference (**Standards**) correctly within the time limit set by the instructor.

1. Call the applicant's previous employer.
2. Ask to speak with the office manager or supervisor.
3. Self-identify, and give the reason for the call.
4. Ask the previous employer open-ended questions about the employee.
5. Ask the previous employer if the employee would be eligible for rehire.
6. Ask specifics as to the employee's job duties and job performance.
7. Ask the previous employer for any other, relevant information.
8. Note all of the previous employer's statements.
9. Thank the previous employer.

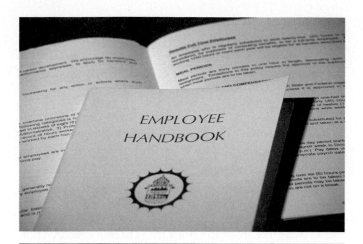

Figure 21-12 ◆ Sample employee handbook.

strictly confidential, will house employees' evaluations and other, work-related documentation. When new staff arrive for work, they should be given copies of their offices' employee handbooks or policy manuals (Figure 21-12 ◆). Such books should outline all office policies, including those for benefits, dress code, and disciplinary action.

Many offices require new employees to sign forms stating they have received copies of their offices' policies and that they agree to abide by those policies. Medical offices also often run criminal background checks on new staff and require those staff to undergo drug testing. For drug testing to occur, applicants must sign consent forms (Figure 21-13 ◆).

Training New Staff

As a lead employee in the medical office, the office manager may be charged with overseeing new staff training. While another staff member typically completes the training, the office manager must ensure that the training has been completed and that the new staff member is clear about employment expectations. A detailed, up-to-date office policy manual facilitates such training (Figure 21-14 ◆). ∞ Chapter 14 details the process behind creating a policy and procedure manual.

Supervising Staff

Well trained employees who clearly understand expectations ease the office manager's task of office supervision. Depending on their work styles and personalities, staff require varying amounts of the manager's time in this arena. Some employees work well with little supervision; others require more oversight. The office manager must determine the best supervision method for each office employee.

Overcoming Scheduling Issues

To ensure staff are scheduled properly, and therefore patient and physician needs are met, the office manager must create and adhere to a fair policy. When employees approach office managers with schedule change requests, those managers must balance the needs of all employees when honoring such requests. To avoid miscommunication, employees should submit their time-off requests in writing within a certain time frame,

I, a current employee of The Marysville Clinic ("the Company"), understand that the use of drugs, alcohol, and other controlled substances by employees creates a dangerous work environment. In consideration for my desire for a safe work environment, I give my consent for the Company to conduct the drug tests it considers necessary as outlined in its Drug Test policy. I hereby allow the Company to take the necessary specimens from me to test for any controlled substance, and I authorize the laboratory or medical personnel retained by the Company for these tests to release the results to the Company for whatever use the Company deems appropriate. Further, I release the laboratory or medical personnel conducting the drug test, the Company, and the Company's employees, directors, officers, and successors from any liabilities, claims, and causes of action, known or unknown, contingent or fixed, that may result from this drug test. I agree not to file any lawsuit or other action to assert a claim.

I have read and understood this agreement, and I sign this without any coercion or duress by any individual or institution.

Print Name   Signature   Date

Figure 21-13 ◆ Sample consent form for drug testing.

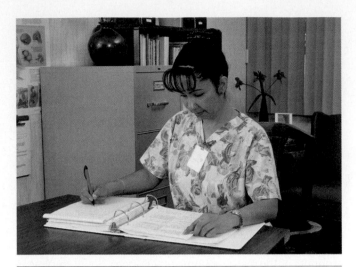

Figure 21-14 ◆ The policy and procedure manual is a valuable resource in the medical office.

such as at least 2 weeks prior to the time requested off. Figure 21-15 ◆ is a sample form for this task.

Performance Evaluations

To monitor employees' job performances and help employees improve as needed, the office manager should evaluate employees yearly. Yearly evaluations help keep employees apprised of job expectations and help to build and maintain confidence and morale.

New employees should be evaluated frequently in their first year, perhaps at 30, 60, and 90 days, and then again on their 1-year anniversaries. Evaluations should be positive experiences for employees, not simply forums for raising new problems or

---

REQUEST FOR TIME OFF

Date: _____

Employee: _____

Request: _____

_____

Figure 21-15 ◆ Time off request.

issues. Well managed offices bring issues to employee attention as soon after those issues arise as is possible.

To lay the groundwork for evaluations, offices should give employees self-evaluation forms to complete before the evaluations occur. Correspondingly, office managers should prepare written evaluations and distribute copies to employees. Originals should reside in employees' files. Once evaluation meetings take place, office managers and employees should review the evaluations and discuss any areas of concern.

Typically, employee evaluations include an assessment of the employee's performance within their position in the office. This will include any attendance or tardiness issues the employee may have had since the last evaluation. The evaluation should include going over the employee's job description and an analysis of how the employee is meeting the expectations outlined within. Any items the employee needs to work on should be noted in writing and the office manager and employee should come up with an agreed-upon time frame for those issues to be resolved. The evaluation should be signed by both the office manager and the employee; a copy is given to the employee and

---

PROCEDURE 21-5 **Perform an Employee Evaluation**

Theory and Rationale
The medical office manager must evaluate all office employees at least once per year. Typically, evaluations fall on or near employees' anniversary dates of hire.

Materials
■ Employee evaluation form
■ Pen

Competency
(**Conditions**) With the necessary materials, you will be able to (**Task**) perform an employee evaluation (**Standards**) correctly within the time allowed by the instructor.

1. Before the evaluation meeting, ask the employee to complete a self-evaluation form on job performance. Be sure to include job performance goals for the next year.

2. Meet with the employee at a prearranged time and in a private room.
3. Compare the employee's self-evaluation form with your evaluation.
4. Address any discrepancies between the two evaluations.
5. Address any areas of concern in performance or behavior.
6. Review the last evaluation's goals, and discuss progress toward those goals.
7. Review the goals set for the next evaluation, and set timelines as needed.
8. Discuss any pay raise associated with employee's performance.
9. Have the employee sign the employee evaluation.
10. Place the evaluation in the employee's personnel file.
11. Raise any concerns about the performance evaluation with the physician.

the original goes into the employee's file. If any issues were brought up in the evaluation, the office manager and employee should meet again after the target date for improvement has passed in order to review the progress that has been made.

Disciplining and Terminating Staff

Employee handbooks should clearly identify situations mandating employee discipline. For example, patient or coworker abuse or use of an illegal substance may be causes for immediate termination. Excessive tardiness or poor job performance, in contrast, may be cause for discipline.

When staff must be disciplined, the office manager should act as soon as possible. Delays may be viewed as endorsements of unacceptable behavior, not only by the employees committing the infractions but by the rest of the staff. Employee morale could plummet as a result. Before disciplining an employee, the office manager should gather all facts relevant to the case. When an employee has been excessively tardy, for example, the office manager should list all the dates the employee has been late.

Meetings on disciplinary issues should occur in private locations, and the office manager should remain professional and calm. First offenses may impose verbal warnings that should be noted in employee files. Serious infractions, like breaching patient confidentiality, require a written warning that outlines the offense and the action the offending employee must take (Figure 21-16 ◆). Employees should sign any written warning and receive a copy. Originals should reside in employee files.

To prepare for the often difficult task of employee termination, office managers should keep clear timelines of warnings and disciplinary actions in employees' files. These types of documents, like clear office policies, both ease the difficult event and help safeguard offices from wrongful termination lawsuits.

When employees are terminated, they should be taken to a private location and advised of the reasons. Managers should regain all keys and other office-owned items and escort employees while they obtain any personal items in the office. When all property has been properly returned, managers should escort the employees from the buildings.

Sexual Harrassment in the Medical Office

Title VII of the Civil Rights Act protects employees against sexual harassment. **Sexual harassment** is legally defined as unwanted sexual advances, requests for sexual favors, and other verbal or physical conduct of a sexual nature, whether intentional or unintentional where:

- An individual's employment hinges upon participating in the sexual activity
- The conduct of an individual causes a hostile, humiliating, or offensive work environment for another individual

Sexual harassment is illegal in all workplaces and the medical office is no exception. In order for the conduct to be considered sexual harassment, it must be unwelcome. While

---

PROCEDURE 21-6 **Discipline an Employee**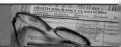

Theory and Rationale
The medical office manager must adhere to office policies for staff discipline. Staff discipline must be done in a private location, and copies of all documents must be signed by the employee and the office manager and placed in the employee's permanent file.

Materials
- Pen
- Paper

Competency
(**Conditions**) With the necessary materials, you will be able to (**Task**) discipline an employee (**Standards**) correctly within the time allowed by the instructor.

1. Verify all facts before meeting with the employee.
2. Write a disciplinary notice that contains the reason for the discipline and the action to be taken by the office and/or by the employee as a result.

3. Request a meeting with the employee.
4. Hold the meeting in a private room.
5. Let the employee know the reason for the meeting.
6. Discuss the disciplinary action being levied on the employee.
7. Discuss your expectations of the employee.
8. Discuss the outcome if the employee's behavior does not change.
9. Ask the employee to sign the disciplinary statement.
10. If the employee refuses to sign the statement, make a note on the statement of "Contents reviewed with employee. Employee refused to sign." Sign your signature and date the document.
11. Place the statement in the employee's personnel record.
12. Agree to a future date on which you will meet with the employee to discuss progress.
13. Inform the physician of the meeting's outcome.

Date: June 21, 2009

Employee: Sara Brown

Infraction: On the following dates, the employee was more than 10 minutes late for her shift:

5/21/09
5/25/09
6/10/09
6/19/09

According to office policy regarding tardiness, any employee who is late four or more times in a month will incur disciplinary action in the form of a written warning. If, after this initial warning, the employee is more than 10 minutes late for a shift in the next 2 weeks, the employee will experience a second disciplinary action of a 1-week, nonpaid employment suspension.

Signature of Employee _____ Date_____

Signature of Office Manager_____ Date_____

Figure 21-16 ◆ Sample warning of disciplinary action.

there are many examples of conduct that could be construed as sexual harassment, examples include:

- Unwelcome sexual advances, including gestures, whistling, or comments
- Sexual jokes, either written or spoken
- Gossip regarding an individual's sex life
- Comments about an individual's body
- Displaying sexually explicit photographs, objects, or cartoons

- Questions about an individual's sexual experiences or activities

If an employee feels he or she has been sexually harassed, he or she must bring the problem to the attention of the office manager or supervisor. The office manager or supervisor must then take immediate action to investigate the claim and take proper action by educating, disciplining, or even terminating the offender. If, after receiving a complaint and verifying the validity of the complaint, the office manager or supervisor does not take action,

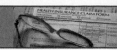

PROCEDURE 21-7 Terminate an Employee

Theory and Rationale
While employee termination is generally difficult, the office manager is obligated to undertake the task professionally, respectfully, and legally.

Materials
- Pen
- Paper

Competency
(**Conditions**) With the necessary materials, you will be able to (**Task**) terminate an employee (**Standards**) correctly within the time allowed by the instructor.

1. Take the employee to a private room.
2. Discuss the reason for termination.
3. Ask the employee to return any office items, such as keys or identification badges.
4. Escort the employee to the workstation to collect personal belongings.
5. Escort the employee from the building.
6. If the employee is loud or abusive, ask the employee to leave immediately and inform the employee that personal belongings will be sent.
7. Note the meeting's outcome in the employee's personnel file.
8. Notify the physician of the meeting's outcome.

---

the complaining employee may then file a lawsuit against the employer for allowing a hostile work environment to continue.

Employment Resources

Employment Assistance Programs (EAPs), resources for those in personal crises, such as counseling and drug or alcohol rehabilitation, are common in large medical offices and hospitals. Any resources should be outlined in office policies. Office managers should keep lists of resources as added reference. While any referrals should appear in employees' personnel files, all such information must be kept confidential.

Providing Employee References

Once staff leave offices' employment, office managers may receive requests from potential employers for those former employees' references. For legal reasons, offices must follow strict, consistent policies in this arena. For example, office managers must give references for all employees, not just a select few, and they must share facts only, not speculations or opinions. Office policy should dictate what information is to be given to potential employers.

References might include only the dates employees worked in the office, the employee's job title, and any proven information in the employee's file. Managers can share when former employees have stolen, for example, but only when such events have been proven. Inaccurate information can damage former employees and subject offices to lawsuits. Similarly, positive references for undeserving employees are grounds for legal action if a potential employer hires an employee with a proven track record for stealing from the office and the office manager did not disclose that information when called for a reference.

Improving Quality and Managing Risk in the Medical Office

As health care consumers, patients face a wide array of choices. As in all other businesses, quality customer service is crucial to medical office success. Patients who are treated respectfully and equitably communicate positive information about the office and will likely stay with those offices long term. Research has shown that patients rate their health care higher simply because they felt staff cared about them and took the time to listen to their concerns. Improving quality in the medical office includes looking for ways to improve the patient's experience in the medical office. This includes making sure patients do not wait for long periods for their appointment, explaining charges to patients prior to services being performed, and maintaining patient confidentiality in all aspects of patient care.

—Critical Thinking Question 21-4—
How could Juanita communicate to the chronically tardy physician the potential impact of his actions on patient care?

Creating a Quality Improvement Program

Quality improvement programs that focus on patients' emotional and physical health are vital to the success of any health care practice. Such programs should be implemented whenever health care employees notice areas or situations that when improved would raise patient satisfaction or safety. When staff members notice broken chairs or hallway carpet that has begun to unravel, they should raise the possible safety hazard with the appropriate parties. Figure 21-17 ◆ identifies other issues that could benefit from quality improvement.

Health care staff should work as a team to solve problems immediately through quality improvement programs, which can be very simple. One common office problem is patient wait time. When offices receive complaints about patient wait times, those offices should mobilize teams quickly to solve the problem by studying appointment times or discussing outcomes with physicians. When patient wait times are allowed to remain long, patients may seek care elsewhere.

Working to Ensure Patient Safety

Every member of the health care team is responsible for patient safety, which means medical assistants should speak up when they see potential risk factors. For example, when physicians order medications that medical assistants believe to be incorrect, those assistants are responsible for clarifying the medication orders before administration. This should only be done outside of the patient's hearing range.

Patient trust is a vital stepping stone to patient safety. Patients who trust their health care providers become partners in their own safety. To participate in the patient partnership, medical assistants should listen to patients' questions and learn to recognize the **body language** that alerts them to patients' unspoken messages. To make these tasks easier, assistants should sit next to patients or their families whenever appropriate (Figure 21-18 ◆) and try to anticipate patient questions. As much as possible, assistants should provide the answers to commonly asked questions. It is also helpful for assistants to use touch appropriately to show concern and to speak in patients' native languages when possible or to arrange for interpreters if needed. To ensure communication is understood, medical assistants should ask patients and their families to repeat discussions in their own words. Respecting patients' decisions and maintaining patients' confidence are parts of advocating for patients in health care.

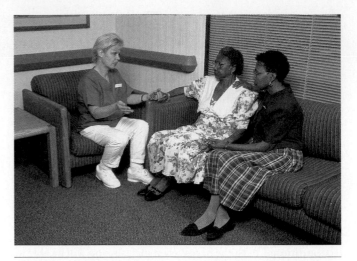

Figure 21-18 ◆ The medical assistant should be ready to speak to the patient's family if necessary.

Reporting Office Incidents

Occasionally, **adverse outcomes,** which are events that were unexpected or that are the result of an error on the part of one or more persons on the healthcare team, occur in the medical office. Adverse outcomes that cause patient injury or could cause patient injury are called **sentinel events.** The Joint Commission on the Accreditation of Healthcare Organizations (JCAHO) describes sentinel events as ones in which injuries occurred, or could have occurred, in a medical setting. Figure 21-19 ◆ lists possible sentinel events in ambulatory care.

When sentinel events occur, the medical office must document and report those events properly, not to blame or punish employees but to aid in prevention. Offices that strive to use errors as learning experiences rather than punishment tools promote a culture in which employees feel safe enough to self-report errors.

To report sentinel events, every office should fully complete sentinel reporting forms or incident report forms, using typed font or blue or black ink (Figure 21-20 ◆). No areas should remain blank. When areas do not apply, medical assistants should write "Not Applicable" or "NA" in them. While sentinel reports should reside in a master incident report file, copies should not appear in employees' files or patients' medical records and copies should not leave the medical office.

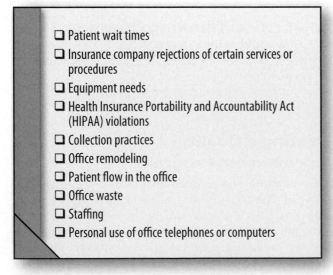

- ❑ Patient wait times
- ❑ Insurance company rejections of certain services or procedures
- ❑ Equipment needs
- ❑ Health Insurance Portability and Accountability Act (HIPAA) violations
- ❑ Collection practices
- ❑ Office remodeling
- ❑ Patient flow in the office
- ❑ Office waste
- ❑ Staffing
- ❑ Personal use of office telephones or computers

Figure 21-17 ◆ Possible issues for quality improvement review.

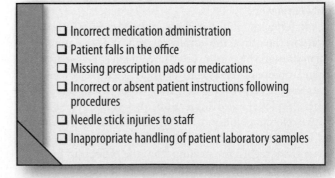

- ❑ Incorrect medication administration
- ❑ Patient falls in the office
- ❑ Missing prescription pads or medications
- ❑ Incorrect or absent patient instructions following procedures
- ❑ Needle stick injuries to staff
- ❑ Inappropriate handling of patient laboratory samples

Figure 21-19 ◆ Possible sentinel events in ambulatory care.

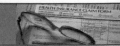

PROCEDURE 21-8   File a Medical Incident Report

Theory and Rationale

In the medical office, staff members must file reports for incidents in which patients or employees are injured or could have been injured. Medical facilities that are JCAHO-certified are required to file incident reports. Medical clinics that are not JCAHO-certified may be required to do so by the Department of Health within the state where the practice is located.

Materials

■ Incident report form
■ Black or blue ink pen
■ Patient's chart

Competency

(**Conditions**) With the necessary materials, you will be able to (**Task**) fill out an incident report (**Standards**) correctly within the time allowed by the instructor.

1. Complete all areas of the incident report form using only facts, not opinions or judgments. For inapplicable areas, enter "NA" or "Not applicable."
2. Sign and date the form.
3. Give the form to the office manager or office director.
4. Participate in any educational meetings to determine how similar events could be avoided.

INCIDENT REPORT

Name of injured party _____ Date _____

Address _____ Telephone _____

_____

The injured party was: ☐ Employee   ☐ Patient   ☐ Other _____

Date of accident/incident _____   Time of incident _____

Where did incident occur? _____

Names of witnesses (include titles):

_____   _____

_____   _____

What first aid/treatment was given at the time of the incident?

_____

_____

Who administered first aid? _____

Briefly describe the incident. _____

_____

_____

_____

Names of employees present at time of incident/injury:

_____

_____

Follow-up: What steps have been taken to prevent a similar accident? _____

_____

_____

Date _____   Employee's signature _____

Date _____   Supervisor's signature _____

Figure 21-20 ◆ Sample incident report.

Martika is a medical assistant in a busy office. On her second day on the job, she slips on her way to the lab on some liquid spilled on the floor. She lands on her back and needs a few moments to catch her breath before rising. Another medical assistant enters the lab just as Martika is getting to her feet. After Martika recounts the events, the medical assistant tells her she must complete an incident report. Martika responds that she believes doing so will jeopardize her new job. What should the second medical assistant do?

Using Protective Equipment

Most medical offices have equipment, or perform procedures, that require staff to use or wear personal protective equipment (Figure 21-21 ◆). For example, whenever health care employees are exposed to patients' bodily fluids those employees must don gloves and possibly eye shields. Employees who X-ray patients must wear radiation badges to assess their possible X-ray exposure (Figure 21-22 ◆). Employers must supply any needed protective equipment, as well as clean and dispose of it per OSHA regulations.

Disposing of Hazardous Waste

Each year, health care facilities create 3.2 million tons of hazardous waste in the four following categories:

- **Solid**—paper, cans, cups, and other garbage from nonclinical office areas.
- **Chemical**—wasted drugs, cleaning solutions, and germicides. These items must be disposed of according to Occupational Safety and Health Association (OSHA) guidelines.
- **Radioactive**—any waste contaminated with radioactive material. Most common in oncology practices, this waste must be disposed of in containers clearly marked "radioactive" and removed only by licensed facilities.

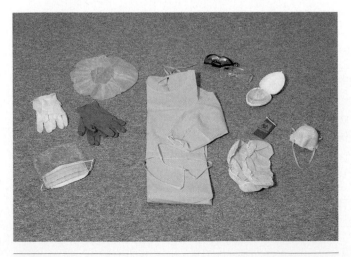

Figure 21-21 ◆ Sample protective equipment found in the medical clinic.

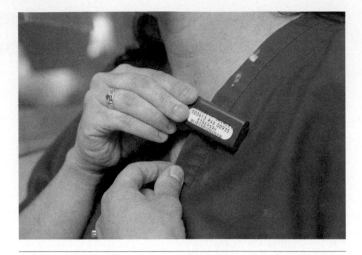

Figure 21-22 ◆ Radiation exposure badge.

- **Infectious**—any garbage exposed to bodily fluids or any laboratory cultures or blood products. These items must be separated from other waste items, placed in bags clearly labeled as "biohazardous waste," and removed by a licensed medical waste removal company.

Though some hazardous waste may be disposed of through local garbage services, all must be disposed of according to federal and local law. On a federal level, medical offices must abide by OSHA guidelines in disposing of hazardous medical waste. These rules are in addition to any state or local laws the medical office must follow. OSHA requires medical offices to dispose of hazardous medical waste in the following manner:

- The waste must be placed into a container that is closable.
- The container must be designed to contain all of the contents and prevent leakage of fluids during handling, storage, transport or shipping.
- The container must be labeled or color-coded noting the contents are hazardous.
- The container must be closed prior to removal to prevent spillage of contents during handling, storage, transport, or shipping.
- If outside contamination occurs, the first container must be placed within a second container that meets all of the listed standards.

Ensuring Employee Safety

Just as patient safety demands constant attention in the medical office, so does employee safety. As a preventive step, all staff must remain vigilant to situations that may lead to employee injury. For example, staff should keep current on the maintenance and repair of office equipment and ensure that all employees are properly trained in the equipment's use. Attention to proper lifting techniques and office ergonomics also helps avoid injuries and lost time in the workplace.

PROCEDURE 21-9   Use Personal Protective Equipment

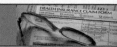

Theory and Rationale

Any employee asked to perform a task that may involve contact with a dangerous material must be given the proper personal protective equipment, as well as instructions on the equipment's proper use.

Materials

■ Latex or nonlatex gloves

Competency

(**Conditions**) With the necessary materials, you will be able to (**Task**) properly don and remove latex or non-latex examination gloves (**Standards**) correctly within the time allowed by the instructor.

1. Wash hands.
2. Holding the rim of the left glove with the right hand, pull on the left glove.
3. Holding the rim of the right glove with the left hand, pull on the right glove.
4. Smooth both gloves onto the hands.
5. If after application the glove rips or is defective, discard the glove and don a new pair. Gloves begin to deteriorate after 15 minutes.
6. To remove the gloves, with the right hand pinch the center of the left glove and pull off the left glove.
7. Hold the left glove in the right hand.
8. With the exposed left hand, cautiously place the first two fingers of the left hand under the rim of the right glove.
9. Push off the right glove and over the left glove, rendering the right glove inside out.
10. Place the removed gloves in the proper disposal container.
11. Wash hands.

PROCEDURE 21-10   Develop an Exposure Control Plan

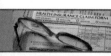

Theory and Rationale

OSHA requires all medical offices to have exposure control plans that list all personal protective equipment in the office and information regarding its use, as well as information on what the employee is to do in the event of an exposure.

Materials

■ List of personal protective equipment within the office
■ Training manual

Competency

(**Conditions**) With the necessary materials, you will be able to (**Task**) develop an exposure control plan (**Standards**) correctly within the time allowed by the instructor.

1. List each piece of personal protective equipment in the office.
2. List the situations when each piece of equipment should/must be used.
3. Hold an in-office training session to review each item and to discuss its use.
4. Demonstrate each item's use.
5. Discuss how the office can reduce or eliminate exposures in the office.
6. Discuss the steps the employees should take in the event of exposure.
7. Document everything discussed at the meeting, and distribute copies to all staff.

PROCEDURE 21-11 **Use Proper Lifting Techniques**

Theory and Rationale

Proper lifting techniques help prevent injuries in the medical office. Any employee who must lift supplies or patients must be properly trained to avoid injury.

Materials

■ Item to lift

Competency

(**Conditions**) With the necessary materials, you will be able to (**Task**) use proper lifting technique (**Standards**) correctly within the time allowed by the instructor.

1. Examine the item to be lifted.
2. While bending at the knees, not the waist, and feet shoulder width apart, grasp the item with both hands (Figure 21-23a ◆).
3. Stand with the item held close to the body (Figure 21-23b).
4. Place the item down, bending at the knees, not at the waist, and keeping the back straight.

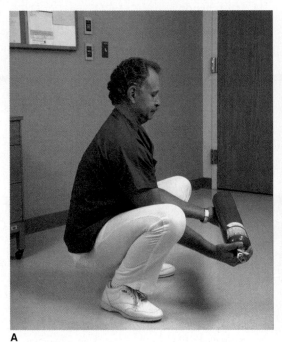
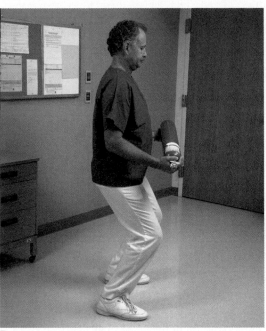

A   B

Figure 21-23 ◆ (a) When picking up a heavy item, the back should remain straight while the knees are bent; (b) keeping the back straight, use the leg muscles to return to a standing position.

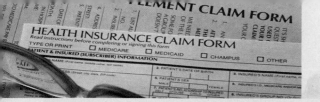

REVIEW

Chapter Summary

- An effective medical office manager demonstrates a range of high-level skills, from communication and organization and possibly clinical aptitude.
- Because health care situations dictate the appropriate management style, office managers must be able to assess situations and adapt accordingly.
- Effective staff meetings, often led by office managers, usually result from planning that includes detailed, accurate agendas.
- Job descriptions are important when medical offices are recruiting staff. Job descriptions include a list of the required duties the employee is expected to perform in addition to the hours and days the employee is expected to work.
- Offices can advertise for staff in a number of places, from conventional newspapers and Web sites to agencies and colleges.
- Effective job placement ads give an overview of job responsibilities.
- Effective interviews uncover the issues and characteristics untouched by resumes. These characteristics might include noticing that an employee is nervous or overly talkative or perhaps an employee who wears unprofessional attire to the interview.
- When interviewing job candidates, employers must be careful to remain within ethical and legal boundaries.

- It is wise for hiring offices to check employees' professional credentials, as well as references.
- Once they are hired, medical office staff are effectively managed with organization, equity, and open communication.
- Employment policies that outline issues such as the terms for employee discipline or termination are valuable tools for offices.
- Employee evaluations are critical ways to ensure employees remain fulfilled and productive as they progress.
- When medical offices must provide employee references, those offices should again defer to legal boundaries to remain professional and appropriate.
- Quality improvement programs are designed to keep the medical office a high-functioning, safe entity. Quality improvement programs include looking for ways to improve patient satisfaction in the medical office.
- All members of the health care team are accountable for quality improvement and patient safety outcomes.
- To help keep patients and health care staff alike safe, offices should report injury incidents properly.
- Medical office protective equipment is designed to safeguard those providing patient care.
- The proper disposal of hazardous waste is just one way to help ensure medical employee safety. This disposal is regulated by OSHA on the federal level and by state and local law.

Chapter Review

Multiple Choice

1. Each year, the United States creates _____ tons of hazardous waste.
   - a. 3,200
   - b. 3.2
   - c. 3.2 million
   - d. 3.2 billion

2. The _____ leader is laid back and becomes involved only when needed.
   - a. Autocratic
   - b. Democratic
   - c. Laissez-faire
   - d. None of the above

3. What is the main purpose of reporting sentinel events in the medical office?
   - a. To fire employees who were involved in the event
   - b. To provide an experience for the office to learn how to prevent a similar event in the future
   - c. To protect the office in the event a patient files a lawsuit
   - d. All of the above

4. Why are employee evaluations necessary?
   - a. To communicate with the employee any areas needing addressed
   - b. To document any agreements made with the employee regarding job performance
   - c. To give the employee a written document outlining their perceived performance within the medical office
   - d. All of the above

5. Before conducting drug testing on employees, employers must do which one of the following?
   - a. Get the employee's written permission
   - b. Not charge the employee for the testing
   - c. Give the employee the result of the testing
   - d. All of the above

True/False

T F 1. Quality improvement programs are used to improve an office's targeted areas.

T F 2. The medical assistant is not responsible for alerting the office to a piece of broken equipment.

Chapter Review (continued)

T F 3. When giving references for former fired employees, the office manager should tell the potential employers why the employees were fired even when lacking proof.

T F 4. To be the most effective, office managers should learn to tailor their leadership styles to situations.

T F 5. Only top-level management should attend staff meetings.

T F 6. In small medical offices, it is appropriate for the physician-employer to require employees to supply their own protective equipment, such as examination gloves.

T F 7. Each job description should outline the duties and physical requirements of the position.

T F 8. Because resumes and applications reflect employees, office managers often discard applications with poor grammar or typographical errors.

T F 9. When giving references for former employees, it is important to have a set policy and to follow it closely.

Short Answer

1. Explain why a medical office manager must have outstanding communication skills.

2. What does it mean to delegate tasks?

3. What is the purpose of a staff meeting agenda?

4. What method might an office manager use to fill a vacant position in the medical office?

5. How can an office check a medical assistant's credentials?

6. Define the term "adverse outcome."

Research

1. What classes might you take at your local community college in order to obtain the skills needed to seek employment as a medical office manager?

2. Looking at Figure 21-10, answer each of those questions as if you were interviewing for a position. How might you improve your answers?

3. Research online for information on how employees in the healthcare setting might work to ensure patient safety.

Externship Application Experience

While patient Monica Schneider is in Dr. Garcia's examination room, she trips over an exposed carpet seam and falls. Afterward, she complains that her knee hurts where it hit the floor.

What should the medical assistant do? What suggestions could the assistant make to prevent similar occurrences?

Resource Guide

Americans with Disabilities Act
Phone: (800) 514-0301
www.ada.gov

Centers for Medicare and Medicaid Services
7500 Security Boulevard
Baltimore, MD 21244
http://www.cms.hhs.gov/HIPAAGenInfo/

Employee Assistance Programs Online (an agency that provides links to employee assistance programs online)
http://www.eap-sap.com/

Joint Commission
One Renaissance Blvd.
Oakbrook Terrace, IL 60181
Phone: (630) 792-5000
http://www.jointcommission.org/SentinelEvents/

U.S. Department of Justice
950 Pennsylvania Avenue, NW
Washington, DC 20530-0001
Phone: (202) 514-2000
http://www.usdoj.gov/

U.S. Department of Labor
Frances Perkins Building,
200 Constitution Avenue, NW
Washington, DC 20210
Phone: (866) 4-USA-DOL
www.dol.gov
http://www.osha.gov/SLTC/healthcarefacilities/index.html

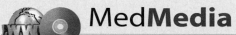

Med**Media**

http://www.MyMAKit.com

More on this chapter, including interactive resources, can be found on the Student CD-ROM accompanying this textbook and on http://www.MyMAKit.com.

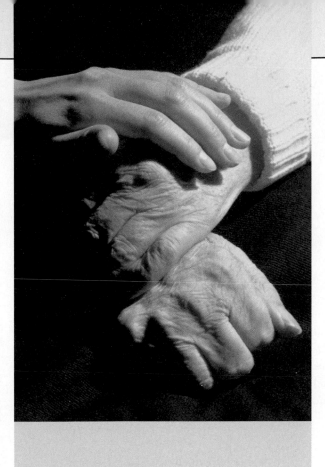

SECTION V

Career Strategies

Chapter 22   Competing in the Job Market

My name is David Jensen. When I decided to become a medical assistant many years ago, I thought that it would be easy to find a job. After I got into the medical assisting program, I found out differently. Being a male, I found it was very difficult to break into the medical assisting field. I talked to many people and ultimately volunteered in a clinic working as an MA. It was a great experience for me, working with patients and doctors who showed me that I was indeed in the field that was right for me.

When I finished the medical assisting program and had volunteered for about 6 months, I started looking for employment in the area clinics. After applying for several positions through the hospital clinics where I had done my volunteer work, I had an interview. I was called back for a second interview and was hired for an on-call position. I was very happy that I was hired, since that was my goal when doing the volunteer work. It is not always easy to land a job right out of school, but hard work does pay off.

Working as a medical assistant is a very rewarding job. I look forward to going to work each day and planning out how I am going to run the doctors' schedules. I get enjoyment out of talking and listening to my patients and relaying that information to the doctors so they may better assess the plan of treatment. The computer is of great importance in the practice of the clinic and doctors; the MA must have a great knowledge of terminology and computer applications to make the day go smoothly.

The best thing about working as a medical assistant is the respect and the trust that comes with the job. The doctors, managers, and rest of the staff depend on the MA to keep the day flowing smoothly. Oftentimes, these team members come to the MA for answers or solutions to problems in the office. Medical assisting is a fast-paced and rewarding field.

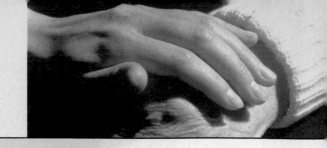

CHAPTER 22

Competing in the Job Market

Case Study

Karim Yousef, a medical assisting graduate seeking employment in health care, lacks personal transportation. Because Karim must rely on public transportation, he has arrived late to a few interviews. As he prepares his cover letter and resume in response to administrative medical assisting job postings, he is trying to determine the most pertinent information to include in these important documents.

Objectives

After completing this chapter, you should be able to:

- Define and spell the key terminology in this chapter.
- Discuss the externship experience, including its benefits for the medical assistant, extern site, and medical assisting program.
- Prepare an attractive and effective resume.
- List several action words that can be used on resumes.
- Write an effective cover letter, and discuss the importance of using cover letters.
- Discuss varied places to look for employment as a medical assistant.
- List the dos and don'ts of an effective interview.
- Discuss the importance of body language and proper dress while interviewing.
- Discuss the importance of following up with a medical office after an interview.
- Develop a plan of action for changing jobs.

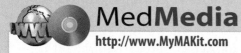

MedMedia

http://www.MyMAKit.com

Additional interactive resources and activities for this chapter can be found on http://www.MyMAKit.com. For a video, tips, audio glossary, legal and ethical scenarios, on-the-job scenarios, quizzes, and games related to the content of this chapter, please access the accompanying CD-ROM in this book.

Video
Legal and Ethical Scenario: *Competing in the Job Market*
On the Job Scenario: *Competing in the Job Market*
Tips
Multiple Choice Quiz
Audio Glossary
HIPAA Quiz
Games: Spelling Bee, Crossword, and Strikeout

MEDICAL ASSISTING STANDARDS

CAAHEP ENTRY-LEVEL STANDARDS	ABHES ENTRY-LEVEL COMPETENCIES
■ Recognize elements of fundamental writing skills (cognitive) ■ List and discuss legal and illegal interview questions (cognitive) ■ Compose professional/business letters (psychomotor) ■ Apply active listening skills (affective) ■ Demonstrate awareness of how an individual's personal appearance affects anticipated responses (affective) ■ Analyze communications in providing appropriate responses/feedback (affective)	■ Adapt to change ■ Project a positive attitude ■ Use proper telephone technique ■ Application of electronic technology ■ Be courteous and diplomatic ■ Fundamental writing skills

COMPETENCY SKILLS PERFORMANCE

1. Write a resume.
2. Compose a cover letter.
3. Follow up with an employer after an interview.

Introduction

The U.S. Department of Labor predicts that medical assisting will be one of the fastest-growing professions between 2004 and 2014, driven largely by the aging "baby boom" generation. Because older patients tend to seek medical care more often than younger patients, medical offices will be expanding. Medical assisting positions, as a result, will be more and more plentiful and the scope of the position will expand. The scope of practice for any health care profession, including medical assisting, consists of the skills and competencies that the professional is licensed, certified, or trained to do. Typically, the scope of practice is defined by the Department of Health within each state. Already, medical assistants are employed in nontraditional organizations, such as insurance companies and inpatient care facilities. The key to finding employment is to make a good impression on potential employers and write cover letters and resumes that stand out.

The Externship Experience

Every accredited medical assisting program ends with a 60- to 240-hour **externship program** that allows students to develop hands-on skills in medical offices. Externship students are guests of the sponsoring medical offices. As such, students should behave as they would when hired: as professionals. In successful externships, extern sites, students, and medical assisting programs work together. Some medical assisting students find they are offered employment at their extern site at the end of the externship. The medical assisting student is not paid for the extern work, but earns credit toward graduation from the medical assisting program.

Understanding the Externship Site's Responsibilities

Extern sites are responsible for giving medical assisting students forums in which to exercise their clinical and administrative skills. During externships, medical assistants who work for the extern sites, called **preceptors** or **mentors**, direct externship students and serve as resources when questions or issues arise. Most extern sites are well versed in the responsibilities of externships and take those responsibilities seriously.

HIPAA Compliance

Before launching externships, medical offices should require students to sign a Health Insurance Portability and Accountability Act (HIPAA) agreement that states the students will share no personal patient information with anyone outside the offices.

Outlining the Student's Responsibilities

Externship programs are excellent places for students to showcase their skills to potential employers. To make their externship experiences as robust as possible, students should actively seek involvement in all their sites' clinical and administrative procedures. While most offices allow externship students to participate in all areas of patient care, patients must give their permission (Figure 22-1 ◆).

Whatever duties they undertake, externship students should remain professional, which means arriving on time, being prepared, and dressing in attire that meets extern sites' requirements. Makeup and jewelry should be minimal, hair should be neat and away from the face, and clothing and shoes should be clean and in good repair.

Sometimes, when externships are particularly successful, extern sites offer students permanent positions upon program completion. When employment is not offered but students are interested in working for their extern sites, those students should advise their preceptors of their desire and leave a copy of their resume.

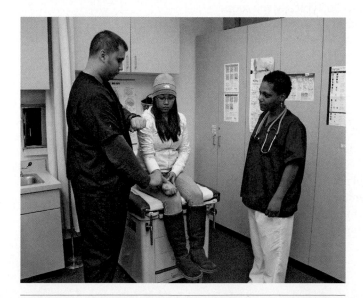

Figure 22-1 ◆ During the externship, the student medical assistant will both observe and participate in caring for patients.

Keys to Success
ASKING QUESTIONS OF THE PHYSICIAN IN FRONT OF THE PATIENT

Medical assisting students should never question the decisions of physicians or other medical assistants in front of patients in the office. Instead, students should pose questions outside patients' hearing range to retain the respect health care professionals command.

The Responsibilities of the Medical Assisting Program

As externship students' **advocates,** medical assisting program directors are primarily responsible for choosing appropriate extern sites for students. With the help of the mentor, program directors should monitor the extern process closely, making sure students succeed in this important last step in their education. To facilitate the monitoring process and observe students in the clinical environment, many program directors visit students on site. Many programs ask externs to log their learning processes in weekly summaries or to meet periodically with the other externs to share their experiences. Students should bring any concerns to the program director's attention. In turn, directors should address student issues as soon as possible.

Writing an Effective Resume

As a first impression of a job applicant, the **resume** is a critical tool in the job market (Figure 22-2 ◆). Poorly written and prepared resumes suggest that their authors will similarly produce poor quality work in the medical office. As a result, many employers discard resumes with poor grammar, typographical errors, or handwritten corrections. When medical assistants change phone numbers, for example, they should revise and reprint their resumes, not hand-mark changes. An applicant may be perfect for the job; however, a sub-par resume will sacrifice employment opportunities.

Ideally, resumes are short, preferably one to two pages, as well as impeccably written and presented. Instead of detailing all duties ever performed, resumes should summarize applicants' qualifications and experience and highlight experience most relevant to the open position. Figure 22-3 ◆ provides a

Keys to Success
ASKING QUESTIONS OR RAISING CONCERNS DURING THE EXTERNSHIP EXPERIENCE

When medical assisting students have questions or concerns during the externship and the mentor cannot address them, those students should raise their issues with the medical assisting program director.

RICHARD CORNELIUS, RMA (AMT)
1234, West Nile Street
Worcester, MA 12345
(808) 555-7890

OBJECTIVE:
To obtain a challenging position in a medical setting that will allow me
to gain experience working with a diverse and challenging population
of patients.

EDUCATION:
**Northridge Community College Medical Assisting Program,
Northridge KY** (September 1999–June 2001)

EXPERIENCE:
Williamsburg Women's Clinic, Northridge, KY (July 2001-
January 2005): Clinical medical assistant

Martinville Pediatrics, Worcester, MA (March 2005–Present):
Clinical medical assistant

ACTIVITIES:
Member of the PTA since 1997
Member of the AAMA

REFERENCES:
Excellent references are available upon request

Figure 22-2 ◆ Sample resume from a medical assistant.

framework of some required resume items. In addition to reviewing work history, the resume should stress an applicant's
skills and accomplishments. Any perceived shortcomings, such
as disabilities or missing skills, should only be raised in the interview. That way, the applicant can point out positive ways in
which to address those issues.

? **─Critical Thinking Question 22-1─**
Should Karim note his lack of personal transportation
on his resume? Why or why not?

Accuracy is also crucial in resume presentation. Applicants should never embellish resume information. Falsifying
applications or resumes is grounds for termination in most organizations. Instead of trying to capture employers' attention
with erroneous information, applicants should focus on top-
notch physical presentation to help get their resumes noticed.
In general, however, applicants should defer to good taste and
judgment. Resumes printed on lime-green paper may get noticed, but they may also give readers the wrong impression. Action words, in contrast, tend to give the right impression and
capture readers' attention in desired ways. Figure 22-4 ◆ lists

❑ Name, address, and telephone number
❑ Educational background
❑ Licensures or certifications
❑ Work experience, including dates of employment and
  brief summaries of duties
❑ Reference information

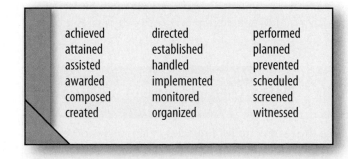

achieved	directed	performed
attained	established	planned
assisted	handled	prevented
awarded	implemented	scheduled
composed	monitored	screened
created	organized	witnessed

Figure 22-3 ◆ Items to include on a resume.

Figure 22-4 ◆ Action words.

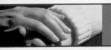

PROCEDURE 22-1 Write an Effective Resume

Theory and Rationale

Every job search starts with a good resume. Many employers see dozens of resumes for one open position in their organizations. To secure interviews, medical assistants need a professional resume with the right information.

Materials

■ Computer with word processing software

Competency

(**Conditions**) With the necessary materials, you will be able to (**Task**) compose your resume (**Standards**) correctly within the time allowed by the instructor.

1. Choose a resume template in the word processing program.
2. Enter your name, address, telephone number, and e-mail address.
3. Enter an objective (e.g., "To obtain a position as a certified medical assistant in a medical practice where my skills can be used to their full potential").
4. Enter your educational background, including degrees.
5. Enter your employment history, including dates.
6. List references or a phrase like, "References available upon request."
7. Review the document for typographical errors.
8. Print the resume on quality paper.
9. Review the resume again for typographical errors.

---

some action words applicants can use to reflect their skills and experiences properly on resumes.

—Critical Thinking Question 22-2—

Karim was fired from his last two jobs due to chronic tardiness. Should he mention those terminations in his cover letter? Why or why not?

Preparing a Cover Letter

Often, **cover letters** help job applicants secure opportunities to **interview.** They are, much like resumes, critical job-searching tools. Because cover letters can be critical to job searches, they should accompany all resumes, even those transmitted via e-mail. In addition, like resumes, they should be error-free and professionally presented.

Cover letters are the links between resumes and open jobs. As such, they should address open positions and explain why applicants are the best candidates for those positions. Figure 22-5 ◆ provides an example of a cover letter. Effective cover letters have headings with applicants' full names, addresses, telephone numbers, fax numbers when appropriate, and e-mail addresses. As much as possible, personal e-mail addresses should be professional. Potential employers are more likely to favor patricialocke12@sample.com over crazypatty@sample.com

Keys to Success
FLUENCIES IN LANGUAGES OTHER THAN ENGLISH

Use the resume to list fluencies in languages other than English. Many medical offices, especially those in diverse neighborhoods, seek employees who are fluent in languages other than English.

Identifying Places to Look for Employment

Employment advertisements may appear in a number of venues, including newspapers and employment agencies. Medical assisting programs may also list job postings, and medical offices often advertise open positions on their Web sites. To cover all bases, medical assistants should send resumes and cover letters to offices that are not currently hiring. Those resumes may arrive just as open positions become available.

—Critical Thinking Question 22-3—

If Karim lacks personal transportation, how should he seek employment?

Completing Employment Applications

Employment applications are an effective way for employers to capture consistent information from all job applicants (Figure 22-6 ◆). As a result, many employers ask applicants to complete employment applications, even when those applicants have submitted resumes.

Before providing any information on job applications, candidates should carefully read all parts of the documents, particularly the instructions. When it comes to entering information, all answers should be well thought out, as well as organized and neatly written in black or blue ink. Every space should contain some type of information. When a section does not apply, applicants should enter "Not applicable" or "N/A." Errors should be neatly crossed through, not scribbled out. Even when applicants have already submitted resumes, they should attach an additional copy to the application they turn in.

Joan Monson, CMA (AAMA)
2121 1st Avenue South
Seattle, WA 12345
Home Phone: (206) 555-9084
Mobile Phone: (206) 555-2434
e-Mail: joanmonson@direct.com

Dear Ms. Nielsen:

I enclose my resume in response to your ad for an administrative medical assistant skilled in pediatric medicine.

After working with children extensively for several years, I recently completed my associate degree and obtained a Certificate in Medical Assisting (CMA) distinction. I completed my externship in a pediatric office, because I wish to continue applying my skills with children in the administrative environment.

As followup to this letter, I will call your office next week to determine if my qualifications meet your needs at this time, and to schedule an interview with you. Thank you for your time and consideration. I look forward to meeting you.

Sincerely,

Joan Monson, CMA (AAMA)

Figure 22-5 ◆ Sample cover letter.

PROCEDURE 22-2 Compose a Cover Letter

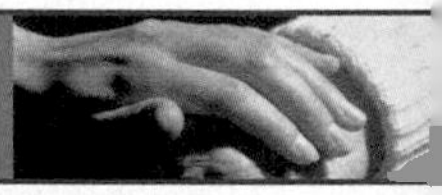

Theory and Rationale
Every resume should include a cover letter. As personalized links between resumes and desired jobs, cover letters allow the medical assistant to tell potential employers why he or she should be chosen for an interview.

Materials
■ Computer with word processing software

Competency
(**Conditions**) With the necessary materials, you will be able to (**Task**) compose a cover letter (**Standards**) correctly within the time allowed by the instructor.

1. Using the word processing software, enter the date and name, company, and address of the letter recipient.
2. Compose a letter that addresses the desired job and the reasons the employer should consider you for the position.
3. List any information that directly relates to your ability to perform the desired job.
4. Request an interview.
5. State that you will call the employer to follow up in a few days.

APPLICATION FOR EMPLOYMENT

Mountain View Health Care Center is an equal opportunity employer and upholds the principles of equal opportunity employment. It is the policy of Mountain View Health Care Center to provide employment, compensation and other benefits related to employment based on qualifications and performance, without regard to race, color, religion, national origin, age, sex, veteran status or disability, or any other basis prohibited by federal or state law. As an equal opportunity employer, Mountain View Health Care Center intends to comply fully with all federal and state laws and the information requested on this application will not be used for any purpose prohibited by law. Disabled applicants may request any needed accommodation. This application is intended to allow you, the applicant, to provide Mountain View Health Care Center with the information and data so that your suitability and qualifications can be fairly determined for the position(s) for which you are applying. Please complete this application and answer all questions completely. Please print clearly in ink.

PLEASE PRINT CLEARLY—BE SURE TO SIGN THIS APPLICATION

Date

Name: Last   First   Middle

Social Security No.:   Home Phone:

Address:

     No.   -   Street

City   State   Zip

Have you been previously employed by Mountain View Health Care Center? ☐ Yes ☐ No
If "Yes", when?   In what capacity?

How did you learn of the position for which you are applying:
☐ Newspaper/Print Advertisement   ☐ Friend/Relative   ☐ Employment Agency   ☐ Job Service   ☐ Radio/TV Advertisement

EMPLOYMENT DESIRED
Position(s) applied for
Shift Preferences: ☐ First Shift – Days   ☐ Second Shift – Evenings   ☐ Third Shift – Nights
☐ Full-time   ☐ Part-time If "Part time", number of shifts/hours desired:
Date available to start   Salary requested

PERSONAL HISTORY
Are you a United States citizen or do you have an entry permit which allows you to lawfully work in the U.S.? ☐ Yes ☐ No
     If applicable, Visa Type: Immigration No.:
Are you at least 18 years old?   ☐ Yes   ☐ No

Are you able to perform all of the duties required by the position for which you are applying, without endangering yourself or compromising the safety, health, or welfare of the Patients or other Staff Persons?   ☐ Yes   ☐ No
     If "No," please explain:

EDUCATION

Name and Location Of School	Graduation Date	Course of Study/ Degree Issued
High School		
College		
Other		

LICENSURE/CERTIFICATION/REGISTRATION

Type of License/Certification	Registration Number

List any special skills or qualifications which you posses and feel are relevant to health care and the position for which you are applying.

Figure 22-6 ◆ Sample employment application.

EMPLOYMENT HISTORY
Please give accurate and complete information. Start with present or most recent employer.

May we contact and communicate with your present employer? ☐ Yes ☐ No

Employer	Telephone No.
Address	Employed from / to /
Name of Supervisor	Hourly Pay: Start Last
Position and Responsibilities	
Reason for Leaving	

- -

Employer	Telephone No.
Address	Employed from / to /
Name of Supervisor	Hourly Pay: Start Last
Position and Responsibilities	
Reason for Leaving	

- -

Employer	Telephone No.
Address	Employed from / to /
Name of Supervisor	Hourly Pay: Start Last
Position and Responsibilities	
Reason for Leaving	

- -

MILITARY SERVICE

Branch   From   To

What were your duties?

Did you receive any specialized training? ☐ Yes ☐ No
If "Yes", describe:

REFERENCES
Names of friends or relatives, if any, currently employed by Mountain View Health Care Center.

Name	Address	Phone
Name	Address	Phone

Names of co-workers (no relatives) you have worked with and whom we may contact for a reference.

Name	Address	Phone
Name	Address	Phone

Please read the following statements completely and carefully before you initial and sign your name.

The Applicant HEREBY CERTIFIES that the answers given on this Application For Employment, including any statements or answers provided by the Applicant during interview, are true and correct. The Applicant fully authorizes Mountain View Health Care Center to contact any references, past and present employers, persons, schools, law enforcement agencies and any other sources of information which may be relevant to the Applicant and this Application For Employment. It is understood and agreed that any misrepresentation, false statement, or omission by the Applicant will be sufficient reason for rejection of the Application For Employment or for dismissal from employment at any time, without recourse or liability to Mountain View Health Care Center.

I have read, understand and agree to the above statement. (Please initial here). _____

SIGN HERE _____ DATE _____

Figure 22-6 ◆ (Continued)

The Successful Interview

When resumes succeed in capturing employers' attention, their applicants are generally called for interviews and asked for references. To facilitate the interview process and prepare their references properly, applicants should get their references' permission before using them for job-search purposes. Applicants can use the cover letter to ask prospective employers not to contact their current places of employment.

When potential employers call to schedule interviews, applicants are sometimes unavailable. Therefore, it is crucial for applicants to record professional voicemail messages on appropriate telephones. Mobile numbers are generally appropriate contact points for potential employers.

In Practice

Jerome is looking for employment as a medical assistant. He has submitted his resume at several offices and has been waiting for telephone calls requesting interviews. When those calls come, the potential employers hear an unprofessional voicemail greeting left by Jerome and his roommate and decide to leave no message. What should Jerome do to increase his chances of gaining employment?

Preparing for the Interview

Before interviewing, medical assistants should research the offices they will be visiting. Knowledge of the facility suggests interest in the practice and may win special attention from the employer. Assume, for example, an office is known for its success with a certain type of therapy. The applicant who asks about that therapy during the interview shows an interest and will likely stand out in the candidate pool. In addition to research, applicants should think of one or two appropriate questions to ask their prospective employers. Figure 22-7 ◆ identifies some questions to avoid, as well as other interview "don'ts." In general, questions about an office's history or industry trends are among the acceptable. Like research, such questions demonstrate applicants' interest. They also prepare applicants should employers ask for questions when the interviews close, and they give employers the chance to talk about themselves.

Dressing for the Interview

When it comes time for the interview itself, several items are vital, including a working black or blue pen, a notepad, at least two copies of the resume, and copies of reference letters, certifications, and awards. Appropriate dress is also a crucial part of the interview. Clothing should be clean and conservative as well as professional. Men should opt for a jacket and tie; women should wear clothing that fits properly and is cut modestly (Figure 22-8 ◆).

Applicants' personal hygiene, like their clothing, must be impeccable. Hands, nails, and teeth should be clean and groomed, and perfumes and colognes should be nearly imper-

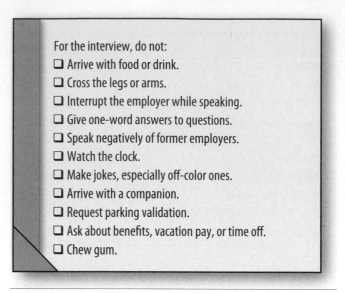

For the interview, do not:
❏ Arrive with food or drink.
❏ Cross the legs or arms.
❏ Interrupt the employer while speaking.
❏ Give one-word answers to questions.
❏ Speak negatively of former employers.
❏ Watch the clock.
❏ Make jokes, especially off-color ones.
❏ Arrive with a companion.
❏ Request parking validation.
❏ Ask about benefits, vacation pay, or time off.
❏ Chew gum.

Figure 22-7 ◆ Interview don'ts.

ceptible. Smokers should try to erase all evidence of smoke on the clothing and the breath as all applicants should be pleasant and odor free. Men and women both should avoid large jewelry, although earrings, necklaces, and wristwatches are appropriate when tasteful. Tattoos, whenever possible, should be covered; visible piercings other than in the ears are generally undesired and should be removed prior to the interview.

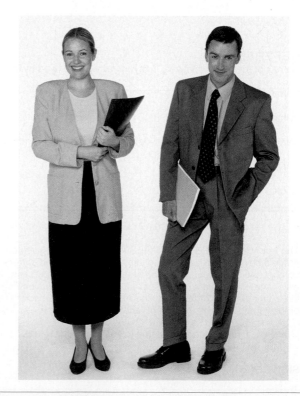

Figure 22-8 ◆ Professional attire is appropriate for the medical office interview.

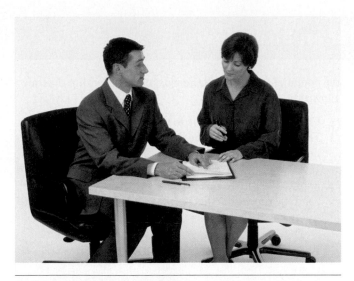

Figure 22-9 ◆ The office manager interviews an applicant.

Presenting the Right Image

Upon initial employer meetings, applicants should stand and shake their interviewers' hands. Eye contact should be direct when speaking; avoidance is viewed as deceptive. During the interview, applicants should strive to convey confidence. They should sit straight and speak in a calm, measured tone. Body language communicates a great deal to prospective employers.

Even when walking, applicants should maintain proper posture and avoid shuffling. When applicants are prone to nerves, they can take notes on notepads to keep hands busy (Figure 22-9 ◆).

Following Up After the Interview

Interview followup increases the likelihood of hiring. Followup both reminds employers of candidates and allows those candidates to ask questions, extend courtesies, and emphasize their interest in employment. The day after the interview is held, the candidate should send a handwritten thank-you note (Figure 22-10 ◆).

Changing Jobs

Unlike 50 years ago, employees today tend to switch jobs every 3 to 5 years. As in all facets of medical assisting, it is important to maintain professional protocol when leaving a job. To leave positions on desired terms, medical assistants should give their employers at least 2 weeks' notice in writing (4 weeks' if a supervisory position). During that period, it should be business as usual. Assistants should remain positive and continue performing their duties to the best of their abilities. They should clearly communicate the status of all projects, and they should also clean their workspace and return any office items. Finally, assistants should ask their employers for letters of recommendation (Figure 22-11 ◆).

September 4, 2009

Dear Dr. Bryant:

Thank you for taking the time to interview with me on Monday. I enjoyed hearing about the advances you have made in the area of foot care for diabetic patients. As I stated during our meeting, I am very interested in working in the administrative area of your clinic and feel my qualifications are perfectly suited to what you are looking for in an administrative medical assistant.

If you would like to discuss the position further, I can be reached at (602) 555-0923. I welcome the opportunity to work with you in your clinic and hope that I will hear from you soon.

Sincerely,

Oksana Simonenko, CMA (AAMA)

Figure 22-10 ◆ Sample interview thank-you note.

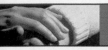

PROCEDURE 22-3 Follow Up After an Interview

Theory and Rationale
Many medical offices interview several applicants for a single opening. To stand out in desired ways, medical assistants must find ways to make potential employers remember and want to hire them.

Materials
- Note card
- Blue or black pen

Competency
(**Conditions**) With the necessary materials, you will be able to (**Task**) follow up after an interview with a thank-you note to the potential employer (**Standards**) correctly within the time allowed by the instructor.

1. Handwrite or type a note to the interviewer.
2. Thank the person for the interview time.
3. List something about the position or office that inspires you to want to work there.
4. Express a desire to meet again.
5. Send the note immediately after the interview.

November 11, 2009

Re: Martin Hawkins, RMA (AMT)

To Whom It May Concern:

I have had the pleasure of working with Martin Hawkins from January 2004 to November 2007 when Martin and his family decided to relocate to Texas.

Martin has demonstrated a tremendous desire to learn, along with a drive to become the best he can be within his chosen profession within the health care field. His ability to work both alone and within groups is unsurpassed, and his attention to detail, especially in the area of patient confidentiality, will serve his future employer well.

I would highly recommend Martin Hawkins, RMA (AMT) for employment in a medical setting. He will make a valued asset to the medical office that recognizes his talents and abilities, and the patients he cares for will be fortunate to have him as their advocate.

Sincerely,

Sharon Tsete, MHA
Clinical Office Manager
Shoreline Family Medicine
(206) 555-9472

Figure 22-11 ◆ Sample recommendation letter.

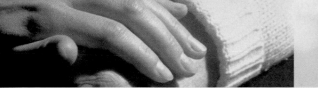

REVIEW

Chapter Summary

- An externship program offers benefits for the medical assistant, the externship site, and the medical assisting program.
- Attractive and effective resumes are critical tools for job seekers, whether those applicants are recently graduated students or established medical assistants.
- When resumes are clear, accurate, and written using action words, they can help medical assisting candidates secure jobs.
- Cover letters, like resumes, support job-searching initiatives by explaining to the potential employer the reasons why the applicant is right for the job.
- Medical assistants can search for job opportunities in varied places, such as newspapers, job fairs, local medical assisting programs, and on the Internet.

- Proper dress and body language are vital while interviewing.
- Interview followup can make the difference between candidates securing the desired position or not. Followup techniques include sending a thank-you note to the potential employer and calling to see if the interviewer has any additional questions of the applicant.
- When medical assistants decide to seek new employment, they should take all steps to leave their employers on good terms. Requesting a recommendation letter upon leaving the office may help secure a future position.

Chapter Review

Multiple Choice

1. During the extern program, the student medical assistant should try to participate in areas devoted to:
   a. administration
   b. clinical procedures
   c. administration and clinical procedures
   d. none of the above

2. Which of the following is an "action" word?
   a. Monitored
   b. Willing
   c. Working
   d. All of the above

3. Which of the following is inappropriate for an interview?
   a. Three-inch pumps
   b. Neck tie
   c. Suit jacket
   d. All of the above

4. When job applicants change phone numbers, they should reflect the change on their resumes by:
   a. crossing through the old number and handwriting the new one
   b. whiting out the old number and handwriting the new one
   c. placing a note over the old number about the change
   d. retyping the number and reprinting the resume

True/False

T F 1. The U.S. Department of Labor predicts that medical assisting will be among the fastest growing professions between the years 2004 and 2014.

T F 2. All externship programs require 240 hours for accreditation.

T F 3. Before witnessing patient procedures, student medical assistants should ask for patients' permission.

T F 4. Before starting externship programs, student medical assistants should sign a HIPAA compliance form stating that they will disclose no patient information.

T F 5. Sloppy and poorly written resumes suggest that work in the medical office will be similarly poor.

T F 6. For medical assistants, scrubs are appropriate interview attire.

T F 7. Resumes should reflect competencies such as fluency in sign language.

T F 8. Attractive resumes gain attention through their appearance.

T F 9. To gain attention, resumes should appear on bright paper, like bright pink or red.

T F 10. It is acceptable to leave portions of employment applications blank.

T F 11. Applicants who follow up with the employer after interviews are more likely to be hired.

Short Answer

1. Why is it important to get permission from professional references?

2. What is the purpose of the cover letter?

3. List several places the medical assistant may seek employment.

4. Why is it important to research offices before interviews?

5. Name several items that should not be taken to an interview.

Research

1. Looking at the jobs advertised for medical assistants in your area, what is the starting wage for a new medical assistant?

2. Search online for information on how to compose a professional resume. What information did you find?

3. Ask one of your instructors to review your resume and give you feedback on how you might improve it.

Externship Application Experience

While the medical assisting student is completing an externship in a family practice office, that assistant notices the physician appears to have made an error in a patient's medication. How should the assistant handle this situation?

Resource Guide

Absolutely Health Care (online community for posting resumes)
http://www.healthjobsusa.com/

Americans with Disabilities Act
http://www.ada.gov/workta.htm

Monster (Internet site for seeking employment)
www.monster.com

MedMedia

http://www.MyMAKit.com

More on this chapter, including interactive resources, can be found on the Student CD-ROM accompanying this textbook and on http://www.MyMAKit.com.

Correlation of Text to the General and Administrative Skills of the CMA (AAMA)

General Skills

Communication

Skill	Chapter
Recognize and respect cultural diversity	3, 4, 5, 6, 7, 8, 20
Adapt communications to individual's understanding	4, 5, 6, 7, 8, 9, 16, 20
Employ professional telephone and interpersonal techniques	7, 16, 21
Recognize and respond effectively to verbal, nonverbal, and written communications	5, 6, 7, 8, 9, 16, 20, 21
Utilize and apply medical terminology appropriately	5, 6, 7, 8, 9, 16, 17, 18, 19
Receive, organize, prioritize, store, and maintain transmittable information utilizing electronic technology	6, 7, 9, 10, 11, 12, 13, 19, 20, 21
Serve as "communication liaison" between the physician and patient	5, 6, 7, 8, 12, 16, 17, 18, 19
Serve as patient advocate professional and health coach in a team approach in health care	5, 6, 7, 8, 9, 16, 17, 18, 19
Identify basics of office emergency preparedness	15, 21

Legal Concepts

Skill	Chapter
Perform within legal (including federal and state statutes, regulations, opinions, and rulings) and ethical boundaries	4, 6, 7, 15, 17, 18, 19, 21
Document patient communication and clinical treatments accurately and appropriately	4, 5, 6, 7, 8, 9, 12, 21
Maintain medical records	4, 6, 7, 10, 11
Follow employer's established policies dealing with the health care contract	3, 4, 6, 7, 9, 13, 14, 16, 17, 18, 19, 21
Comply with established risk management and safety procedures	4, 14, 15, 21
Recognize professional credentialing criteria	3, 4, 21
Identify and respond to issues of confidentiality	3, 4, 5, 6, 7, 8, 9, 10, 11, 16, 19, 20, 21

Instruction

Skill	Chapter
Function as a health care advocate to meet individual's needs	3, 7, 8, 9
Educate individuals in office policies and procedures	5, 7, 8, 9
Educate the patient within the scope of practice and as directed by supervising physician in health maintenance, disease prevention, and compliance with patient's treatment plan	5, 8, 9
Identify community resources for health maintenance and disease prevention to meet individual patient needs	14
Maintain current list of community resources, including those for emergency preparedness and other patient care needs	15
Collaborate with local community resources for emergency preparedness	15
Educate patients in their responsibilities relating to third-party reimbursements	16

Operational Functions

Skill	Chapter
Perform inventory of supplies and equipment	13
Perform routine maintenance of administrative and clinical equipment	13
Apply computer and other electronic equipment techniques to support office operations	6, 7, 8, 10, 11, 12, 16, 17, 18, 9, 20
Perform methods of quality control	13, 20

Administrative Skills

Administrative Procedures

Skill	Chapter
Schedule, coordinate, and monitor appointments	9
Schedule inpatient/outpatient admissions and procedures	9
Apply third-party and managed care policies, procedures, and guidelines	15
Establish, organize, and maintain patient medical record	10, 11
File medical records appropriately	10, 11
Perform procedural and diagnostic coding for reimbursement	17, 18
Perform billing and collection procedures	15
Perform administrative functions, including bookkeeping and financial procedures	6, 7, 8, 9, 12, 13, 7, 18, 19, 20
Prepare submittal ("clean") insurance forms	15

Medical Terminology Word Parts

Medical terms are like individual jigsaw puzzles. Once you divide the terms into their component parts and learn the meaning of the individual parts, you can use that knowledge to understand many other new terms. Four basic component parts are used to create medical terms:

Root	The basic, or core, part that makes up the essential meaning of the term. The root usually, but not always, denotes a body part. Root words usually come from the Greek or Latin languages. For example, *bronch* is a root that means "the air passages in the lungs" or "bronchial tubes." *Cephal* means "head." An extensive list of root words is given on pages 445–447.
Prefix	One or more letters placed before the root to change its meaning. Prefixes usually, but not always, indicate location, time, number, or status. For example, the prefix *bi-* means "two" or "twice." When *bi* is placed before the root *lateral* ("side"), to form *bilateral*, the meaning is "having two sides." An extensive list of prefixes is given on page 443.
Suffix	One or more letters placed after the root to change its meaning. Suffixes usually, but not always, indicate the procedure, condition, disorder, or disease. For example, the suffix *-itis* means "inflammation," that is, damaged tissue that is red and painful. The medical term *bronchitis* means "inflammation of the bronchial tubes." Another example is the suffix *-ectomy*, which means "removal." Hence, *appendectomy* means "removal of the appendix." An extensive list of suffixes is given on pages 447–448.
Combining vowel	A letter used to combine roots with other word parts. The vowel is usually an *o*, but sometimes it is an *a* or *i*. When a combining vowel is added to a root, the result is called a combining form. For example, in the word encephalogram, the root is *cephal* ("head"), the prefix is *en-* ("inside"), and the suffix is *-gram* ("something recorded"). These word parts are joined by the combining vowel *o* to make a word more easy to pronounce. *Cephal/o* is the combining form. An *encephalogram* is an X-ray of the inside of the head.

Analyzing a Medical Term

You can often decipher the meaning of a medical term by breaking it down into its separate parts. Consider the following examples:

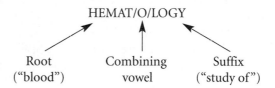

The term *hematology* is divided into three parts. When you analyze a medical term, begin at the end of the word. The ending is called the suffix. Almost all medical terms contain suffixes. The suffix in *hematology* is *-logy,* which means "study of." Now look at the beginning of the word. *Hemat* is the root word, which means "blood." The root word gives the essential meaning of the term.

The third part of this term, which is the letter *o*, has no meaning of its own, but is an important connector between the root (*hemat*) and the suffix (*logy*). It is the combining vowel. The letter *o* is the combining vowel usually found in medical terms.

Putting together the meanings of the suffix and the root, the term *hematology* means "the study of blood."

The combining vowel plus the root is called the combining form. A medical term can have more than one root word; therefore, there can be two combining forms. For example:

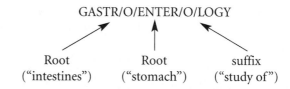

The two combining forms are *gastr/o* and *enter/o*. The entire term (reading from the suffix, back to the beginning of the term, and across) means "the study of the stomach and the intestines."

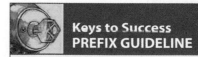
Keys to Success
PREFIX GUIDELINE

A prefix does not require a combining vowel. Do not place a combining vowel between a prefix and a root word.

Keys to Success
WORD PART GUIDELINES

1. A single root word with a combining form cannot stand alone. A suffix must be added to complete the term.
2. The rules for the use of combining vowels apply when adding a suffix.
3. When a suffix begins with a consonant, a combining vowel such as O, is placed before the suffix.

Rules for Using Combining Vowels

1. A combining vowel is not used when the suffix begins with a vowel (*a-e-i-o-u*). For example, when *neur/o* (nerve) is joined with the suffix *-itis* (inflammation), the combining vowel is not used because *-itis* begins with a vowel. *Neuritis* (new-RYE-tis) is an inflammation of a nerve or nerves.
2. A combining vowel is used when the suffix begins with a consonant. For example, when *neur/o* (nerve) is joined with the suffix *-plasty* (surgical repair), the combining vowel *o* is used because *-plasty* begins with a consonant. *Neuroplasty* (NEW-roh-plas-tee) is the surgical repair of a nerve.
3. A combining vowel is always used when two or more root words are joined. As an example, when *gastr/o* (stomach) is joined with *enter/o* (small intestine), the combining vowel is used with *gastr/o*. *Gastroenteritis* (gas-troh-en-ter-EYE-tis) is an inflammation of the stomach and small intestine.

Suffixes and Medical Terms Related to Pathology

Pathology is the study of disease and the following suffixes describe specific disease conditions. (A more complete list of suffixes appears on pages 447–448.)

Suffix	Meaning
-algia	pain and suffering
-dynia	pain
-ectomy	surgical removal
-graphy	process of recording a picture or record
-gram	record or picture
-necr/osis	death (tissue death)
-scler/osis	abnormal hardening
-sten/osis	abnormal narrowing
-centesis	surgical puncture to remove fluid for diagnostic purposes or to remove excess fluid
-plasty	surgical repair
-scopy	visual examination with an instrument

The Double RRs Suffixes

The following suffixes are often referred to as the "double RRs,"

* -rrhage and -rrhagia	Bursting form; an abnormal excessive discharge or bleeding. *Note: -rrhage* and *-rhagia* refer to the flow of blood.
* -rrhaphy	To suture or stitch.
* -rrhea	Abnormal flow or discharge; refers to the abnormal flow of most bodily fluids. *Note:* Although *-rrhea* and *-rrhage* both refer to abnormal flow, they are not used interchangeably.
* -rrhexis	Rupture.

Contrasting and Confusing Prefixes

The following contrasting prefixes can be confusing. Study this list to make sure you know the differences between the contrasting terms. (A more complete list of prefixes appears on page 443.)

Ab- Means "away from." *Abnormal* means not normal or away from normal.

Ad- Means "toward" or "in the direction." *Addiction* means drawn toward or a strong dependence on a drug or substance.

Dys- Means "bad," "difficult," "painful." *Dysfunctional* means an organ or body that is not working properly.

Eu- Means "good," normal, well, or easy. Euthyroid (you-THIGH-roid) means a normally functioning thyroid gland.

Hyper- Means "excessive" or "increased." *Hypertension* (high-per-TEN-shun) is higher than normal blood pressure.

Hypo- Means "deficient" or "decreased." *Hypotension* (high-poh-TEN-shun) is lower than normal blood pressure.

Inter- Means "between" or "among." *Interstitial* (in-ter-STISH-al) means between, but not within, the parts of a tissue.

Intra- Means "within" "into." *Intramuscular* (in-trah-MUS-kyou-lar) means within the muscle.

Sub- Means "under," "less," or "below." *Subcostal* (sub-KOS-tal) means below a rib or ribs.

Supra- Means "above." *Supracostal* (sue-prah-KOS-tal) means above or outside the ribs.

Singular and Plural Endings

Many medical terms have Greek or Latin origins. As a result of these different origins, the rules for changing a singular word into a plural form are unusual. Additionally, English endings have been adopted for some commonly used terms.

Keys to Success
USING A MEDICAL DICTIONARY

Learning to use a medical dictionary is an important part of mastering the correct use of medical terms. Some dictionaries use categories such as "Diseases and Syndromes" to group disorders with these terms in the titles. For example:

- Venereal disease would be found under "disease, venereal."
- Fetal alcohol syndrome would be found under "syndrome, fetal alcohol."

When you come across a term and cannot find it listed by the first word, the next step is to look under the appropriate category.

Guidelines to Unusual Plural Forms

Guideline	Singular	Plural
1. If the term ends in an *a*, the plural is usually formed by adding an *e*.	bursa vertebra	bursae vertebrae
2. If the term ends in *ex* or *ix*, the plural is usually formed by changing the *ex* or *ix* to *ices*.	appendix index	appendices indices
3. If the term ends in *is*, the plural is usually formed by changing the *is* to *es*.	diagnosis metastasis	diagnoses metastases
4. If the term ends in *itis*, the plural is usually formed by changing the *is* to *ides*.	arthritis meningitis	arthritides meningitides
5. If the term ends in *nx*, the plural is usually formed by changes the *x* to *ges*.	phalanx meninx	phalanges meninges
6. If the term ends in *on*, the plural is usually formed by changing the *on* to *a*.	criterion ganglion	criteria ganglia
7. If the term ends in *um*, the plural is usually formed by changing the um to *a*.	diverticulum ovum	diverticula ova
8. If the term ends in *us*, the plural is usually formed by changing the *us* to *i*.	alveolus malleolus	alveoli malleoli

Basic Medical Terms

The following subsections discuss basic medical terms that are used to describe diseases and disease conditions, major body systems, and body direction.

Keys to Success
ACCURACY IN SPELLING

Accuracy in spelling medical terms is extremely important! Changing just one or two letters can completely change the meaning of the word—and this difference could literally be a matter of life or death for the patient.

Terms Used to Describe Diseases and Disease Conditions

The basic medical terms used to describe diseases and disease conditions are listed here.

- A *sign* is evidence of disease, such as fever, that can be observed by the patient and others. A sign is objective because it can be evaluated or measured by others.
- A *symptom,* such as pain or a headache, can only be experienced or defined by the patient. A symptom is subjective because it can be evaluated or measured only by the patient.
- A *syndrome* is a set of signs and symptoms that occur together as part of a specific disease process.
- *Diagnosis* is the identification of disease. To diagnose is the process of reaching a diagnosis.
- A *differential diagnosis* attempts to determine which of several diseases may be producing the symptoms.
- A *prognosis* is a forecast or prediction of the probable course and outcome of a disorder.
- An *acute* disease or symptom has a rapid onset, a severe course, and relatively short duration.
- A *chronic* symptom or disease has a long duration. Although chronic symptoms or diseases may be controlled, they are rarely cured.
- A *remission* is the partial or complete disappearance of the symptoms of a disease without having achieved a cure. A remission is usually temporary.
- Some diseases are named for the condition described. For example, *chronic fatigue syndrome* (CFS) is a persistent overwhelming fatigue that does not resolve with bed rest.
- An *eponym* is a disease, structure, operation, or procedure that is named for the person who discovered or described it first. For example, Alzheimer's disease is named for Alois Alzheimer, a German neurologist who lived from 1864 to 1915.
- An *acronym* is a word formed from the initial letter or letters of the major parts of a compound term. For example, the acronym AMA stands for American Medical Association.

Terms Used to Describe Major Body Systems

The following is a list of the major body systems and some common related combining forms used with each.

Major Structures and Body System	Related Roots with Combining Forms
Skeletal system	bones (oste/o)
	joints (arthr/o)
	cartilage (chondr/o)
Muscular system	muscles (my/o)
	ligaments (syndesm/o)
	tendons (ten/o, tend/o, tendin/o)
Cardiovascular system	heart (card/o, cardi/o)
	arteries (arteri/o)
	veins (phleb/o, ven/o)
	blood (hem/o, hemat/o)
Lymphatic and immune systems	lymph, lymph vessels, and lymph nodes (lymph/o), (lymphangi/o)
	tonsils (tonsill/o)
	spleen (splen/o)
	thymus (thym/o)
Respiratory system	nose (nas/o, rhin/o)
	pharynx (pharyng/o)
	trachea (trache/o)
	larynx (laryng/o)
	lungs (pneum/o, pneumon/o)
Digestive system	mouth (or/o)
	esophagus (esophag/o)
	stomach (gastr/o)
	small intestines (enter/o)
	large intestines (col/o)
	liver (hepat/o)
	pancreas (pancreat/o)
Urinary system	kidneys (nephr/o, ren/o)
	ureters (ureter/o)
	urinary bladder (cyst/o, visic/o)
	urethra (urethr/o)
Integumentary system	glands (aden/o)
	skin (cutane/o, dermat/o, derm/o)
	sebaceous glands (seb/o)
	sweat glands (hidraden/o)
Nervous system	nerves (neur/o)
	brain (encephal/o)
	spinal cord (myel/o)
	eyes (ocul/o, ophthalm/o)
	ears (acoust/o, ot/o)
Endocrine system	adrenals (adren/o)
	pancreas (pancreat/o)
	pituitary (pituit/o)
	thyroid (thyr/o, thyroid/o)
	parathyroids (parathyroid/o)
	thymus (thym/o)
Reproductive system	*Male:*
	testicles (orch/o, orchid/o)
	Female:
	ovaries (oophor/o, ovari/o)
	uterus (hyster/o, metr/o, metri/o, uter/o)

Terms Used to Describe Body Direction

Certain terms are used to describe the location of body parts relative to the trunk or other parts of the anatomy. See Figure B-1 ◆.

Ventral (VEN-tral) refers to the front or belly side of the body or organ (*ventr* means "belly side" of the body and *al* means "pertaining to").

Dorsal (DOR-sal) refers to the back of the body or organ (*dors* means "back of body" and *al* means "pertaining to").

Anterior (an-TEER-ee-or) means situated in the front. It also means on the forward part of an organ (*anter* means "front" or "before" and *ior* means "pertaining to"). For example, the stomach is located anterior to (in front of) the pancreas. *Anterior* is also used in reference to the ventral surface of the body.

Posterior (pos-TEER-ee-or) means situated in the back. It also means on the back portion of an organ (*poster* means "back" or "after" and *ior* means "pertaining to"). For example, the pancreas is located posterior to (behind) the stomach. Posterior is also used in reference to the dorsal surface of the body.

Superior means uppermost, above, or toward the head. For example, the lungs are superior to (above) the diaphragm.

Inferior means lowermost, below, or toward the feet. For example, the stomach is located inferior to (below) the diaphragm.

Cephalic (seh-FAL-ick) means toward the head (*cephal* means "head" and *ic* means "pertaining to").

Caudal (KAW-dal) means toward the lower part of the body (*caud* means "tail" or "lower part" of the body and *al* means "pertaining to").

Proximal (PROCK-sih-mal) means situated nearest the midline or beginning of a body structure. For example, the proximal end of the humerus (the bone of the upper arm) forms part of the shoulder. Or, it may be easier for you to think of it as "closer to the origin of the body part or the point of attachment of a limb to the body trunk."

Distal (DIS-tal) means situated farthest from the midline or beginning of a body structure. For example, the distal end of the humerus forms part of the elbow.

Medial means the direction toward or nearer the midline. For example, the medial ligament of the knee is near the inner surface of the leg.

Lateral means the direction toward or nearer the side and away from the midline. For example, the lateral ligament of the knee is near the side of the leg.

Bilateral means relating to, or having, two sides.

Planes of the Body

Medical professionals often refer to sections of the body in terms of anatomical planes (flat surfaces). These planes are imaginary lines—vertical or horizontal—drawn through an upright body. The following terms are used to describe a specific body part (see Figure B-2 ◆):

- Coronal plane (frontal plane): A vertical plane running from side to side; divides the body or any of its parts into anterior and posterior portions.

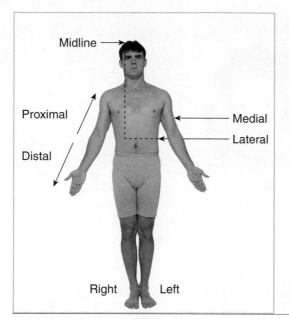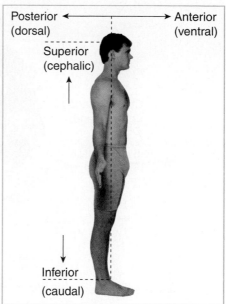

Figure B-1 ◆ Directional anatomical terms.

- Sagittal plane (median plane): A vertical plane running from front to back; divides the body or any of its parts into right and left sides.
- Axial plane (transverse plane): A horizontal plane; divides the body or any of its parts into upper and lower parts.

Prefixes, Root Words, and Suffixes

The most common medical prefixes, root words, and suffixes are listed here. Knowing these common prefixes, roots, and suffixes will help you decipher medical terms.

Prefixes

a	without or absence of
ab	from; away from
ad	to; toward
an	without or absence of
ante	before
anti	against
bi	two
bin	two
brady	slow
con	together
contra	against
de	from; down from; lack of
dia	through; complete; between; apart
dis	to undo; free from
dys	difficult; labored; painful; abnormal
ec	out
ecto	outside
endo	within
epi	on; upon; over
eso	inward
eu	normal; good
ex	outside; outward
exo	outside; outward
extra	outside of; beyond
hemi	half
hyper	above; excessive
hypo	below; incomplete; deficient
in	in; into; not
infra	under; below
inter	between
intra	within
mal	bad
meso	middle
meta	after; beyond; change
micro	small
multi	many
neo	new
nulli	none
pan	all; total
para	outside; beyond; around
per	through
peri	surrounding (outer)
poly	many; much
post	after
pre	before; in front of
pro	before
quadri	four
re	back
retro	back; behind
semi	half
sub	under; below
super	over; above
supra	above; beyond; on top
sym	together; joined
syn	together; joined
tachy	fast; rapid
tetra	four
trans	through; across; beyond
tri	three
ultra	beyond; excess
uni	one

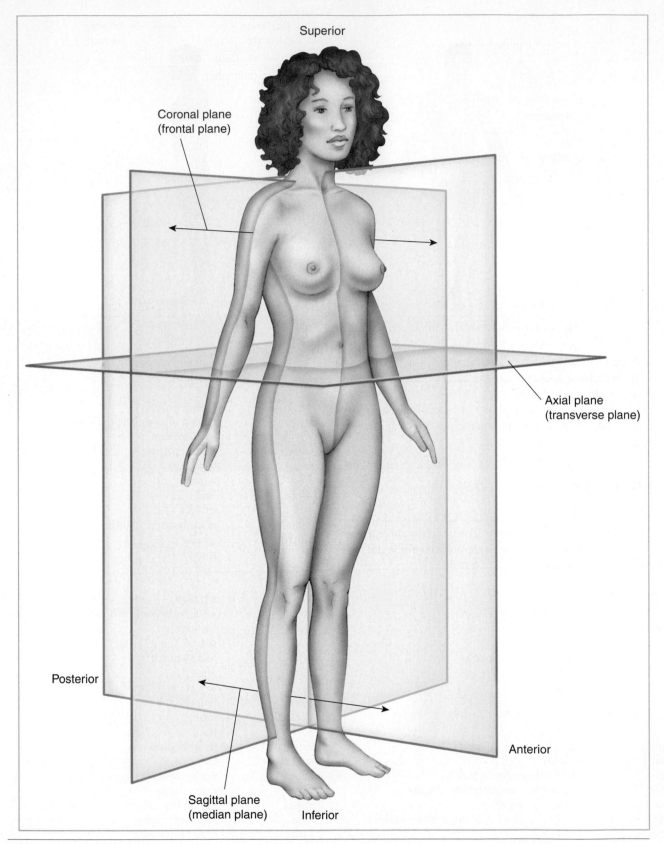

Figure B-2 ◆ Anatomical planes.

Root Words

abdomin	abdomen		erythr	red
aden	gland		esophag	esophagus
adren	adrenal gland		esthesi	sensation; feeling; sensitivity
adrenal	adrenal gland		eti	cause (of disease)
aer	air; oxygen; gas		exocrin	secrete out of
alveol	alveolus		faci	face
angi	(blood) vessel; (lymph) vessel		fasci	fascia; fibrous band
ankyl	crooked; stiff; bent		fract	break; broken
appendic	appendix		galact	milk
arteri, arter	artery		gastr	stomach
arteriol	arteriole (small artery)		ger	old age; aged
arthr	joint		geront	old age; aged
ather	yellowish; fatty plaque		gingiv	gums
aur	ear		glauc	gray
aut	self		gloss	tongue
bil	bile		gluc	sweetness; sugar
bio	life		glyc	sugar; glucose
blephar	eyelid		glycos	sugar; glucose
bronch	airway; bronchus		gnos	knowledge; a knowing
bronchiol	bronchiole		gonad	gonad; sex glands
burs	bursa		gyn	woman
carcin	cancer		gynec	woman
cardi	heart		gyr	turning; folding
caud	tail; toward lower part of the body		hem	blood
cephal	head		hemat	blood
cerebell	cerebellum		hepat	liver
cerebr	cerebrum; brain		hidr	sweat
cervic	neck; cervix		hist	tissue
cheil	lip		hom	same
chiro	hand		home	sameness; unchanging
cholangi	bile duct		hydr	water
chole	gall; bile		hyster	uterus
chondr	cartilage		ile	ileum
coccyg	coccyx; tailbone		ili	ilium
col	colon; large intestine		immun	immune
conjunctiv	conjunctiva		irid	iris
corne	cornea		kerat	horny tissue; hard
coron	heart; crown of the head		kin	movement
cost	rib		kinesi	movement; motion
crani	cranium; skull		labi	lips
cutane	skin		lacrim	tear duct; tear
cyan	blue		lact	milk
cyst	bladder; sac		lapar	abdomen
cyt, cyte	cell		laryng	larynx
dacry	tears; tear duct		later	side
dactyl	fingers or toes		lei	smooth
dent	tooth		leuk	white
derm	skin		lingu	tongue
dermat	skin		lip	fat
dipl	two; double		lith	stone; calculus
diverticul	diverticulum		lob	lobe
dors	back (of the body)		lymph	lymph
duoden	duodenum		macr	abnormal largeness
ectop	located away from usual place		mamm	breast
edema	swelling		mast	breast
electr	electricity; electrical activity		meat	opening or passageway
encephal	brain		melan	black
endocrin	endocrine		men	menstruation
enter	intestines (usually small intestine)		mening	meninges
epiglott	epiglottis		ment	mind
epitheli	epithelium		mes, meso	middle

metr	uterus	py	pus
mon	one	pyel	renal pelvis
morbid	disease; sickness	pylor	pylorus
muc	mucus	pyr	fever; heat
my, myos	muscle	quadr	four
myc	fungus	rect	rectum
myel	bone marrow; spinal cord	ren	kidney
myelon	bone marrow	retin	retina
myring	eardrum	rhin	nose
narc	stupor; numbness	sacr	sacrum fallopian (uterine)
nas	nose	salping	tube
nat	birth	sanit	soundness; health
necr	death (cells; body)	sarc	flesh; connective tissue
nephr	kidney	scler	sclera; white of eye; hard
neur	nerve	scoli	crooked; curved
noct	night	seb	sebum; oil
nyct	night	seps	infection
nyctal	night	sept	infection; partition; septum
ocul	eye	sial	saliva
onc	tumor	sinus	inus
onych	nail	somat	body
oophor	ovary	somn	sleep
ophthalm	eye	son	sound
or	mouth	sopor	sleep
orth	straight	sperm	sperm, spermatazoa; seed
oste	bone	spermat	sperm, spermatazoa; seed
ot	ear	spher	round; sphere; ball
ox	oxygen	sphygm	pulse
palpat	touch; feel; stroke	spin	spine; backbone to
pancreat	pancreas	spir	breathe
par, part	bear; give birth to; labor	splen	spleen
parathyroid	parathyroid	spondyl	vertebra; spinal or vertebral column
path	disease; suffering	staphyl	grapelike clusters
pector	chest; muscle	stern	(breastbone)
ped	child; foot	steth	chest (muscles)
pelv	pelvis; pelvic bone	stoma	mouth; opening
pen	penis	stomat	mouth; opening
perine	perineum	strab	squint; squint-eyed
peritone	peritoneum	synovi	synovia; synovial membrane
petr	stone; portion of temporal bone	system	system
phac, phak	lens of the eye	ten, tend	tendon
phag	eat; swallow	tendin	tendon
phalang	finger or toe bone	test	testis; testicle
pharyng	pharynx, throat	therm	heat
phas	speech	thorac	thorax; chest
phleb	vein	thromb	clot
phot	light	thym	thymus gland; soul
phren	mind	thyr	thyroid gland
physi	nature	thyroid	thyroid gland
pleur	pleura	tom	cut; section
pneum	lung; air	ton	tension; pressure
pneumat	lung; air	tone	to stretch
pneumon	lung; air	tonsill	tonsils
pod	foot	top	place; position; location
poli	gray matter	tox, toxic	poison; poisonous
polyp	polyp; small growth	trach, trache	trachea; windpipe
poster	back (of body)	trachel	neck; necklike
prim	first	trich	hair
proct	rectum	tubercul	little knot; swelling
pseud	fake; false	tympan	eardrum; middle ear
psych	mind	ulcer	sore; ulcer
pulmon	lung	ungu	nail

ur	urine; urinary tract
ureter	ureter
urethr	urethra
uria	urination; urine
urin	urine or urinary organs
uter	uterus
uvul	uvula; little grape
vagin	vagina
valv	valve
valvul	valve
vas	vessel; duct
vascul	blood vessel; little vessel
ven	vein
versicul	seminal vesicles; blister
vertebr	vertebra; backbone
vesic	urinary bladder
vir	poison; virus
viril	masculine; manly
vis	seeing; sight
visc	sticky
viscer	viscera; internal organs sternum
viscos	sticky
vit	life
xanth	yellow
xen	strange; foreign
xer	dry
zygot	joined together

Additional Rootwords

caus	burning sensation; capable of burning
cusp	point; cusp
flexion	bending
genital	pertaining to birth
lumb	lumbar; loin region
mediastin	mediastinum
tens, tensi	pressure, force, stretching

Suffixes

Suffixes Meaning "Pertaining to"

ac
al, ine
ar, ior
ary, ory
eal, ous
ial
ic
ical, tic

Suffixes Meaning "Abnormal Conditions"

ago	abnormal condition, disease
esis	abnormal condition, disease
ia	abnormal condition, disease
iasis	abnormal condition, disease
ion	condition
ism	condition, state of abnormal condition
osis	disease

Common Suffixes Used in Medical Terminology

algia	pain, suffering
asthenia	weakness
cele	hernia, protrusion
centesis	surgical puncture to remove fluid
cidal	killing
clasia	break
clasis	break
clast	break
clysis	irrigating; washing
coccus	berry shaped (a form of bacterium)
crine	separate; secrete
crit	to separate
cyte	cell
desis	fusion; to bind; tie together
drome	run; running
ductor	to lead or pull
dynia	pain
ectasis	stretching out; dilation; expansion
ectomy	excision or surgical removal
ectopia	displacement
emesis	vomiting
emia	blood; blood condition
gen	producing, forming
genesis	producing; forming
genic	producing, forming
gnosis	a knowing
gram	record; X-ray
graph	instrument used to record
graphy	process of recording; X-ray filming
ictal	seizure; attack
ism	state of
itis	inflammation
lepsy	seizure
logist	specialist
logy	study of
lysis	destruction; reduce; separation
malacia	softening
mania	madness; insane desire
megaly	enlargement
meter	instrument used to measure
metry	measurement
morph	form; shape
oid, ode	resembling
oma	tumor; mass
opia	vision (condition)
opsy	to view
oxia	oxygen
paresis	slight paralysis
pathy	disease
penia	abnormal reduction in number; lack of
peps, pepsia	digestion
pexy	surgical fixation; suspension
phagia	eating; swallowing
philia	love
phily	love
phobia	abnormal fear of or adversion to specific objects or things
phonia	sound or voice
phoria	feeling
physis	growth

plasia	formation; development; a growth	scopy	visual exam with an instrument
plasm	growth; formation; substance	sepsis	infection
plasty	plastic or surgical repair	sis	state of
plegia	paralysis; stroke	spasm	sudden involuntary muscle contraction
pnea	breathing	stalsis	contraction; constriction
porosis	lessening in density; porous condition	stasis	control; stop; standing still
praxia	in front of; before	stat	to stop
ptosis	drooping; sagging; prolapse	stenosis	narrowing; constriction
ptysis	spitting	stomy	new artificial opening
rrhage	bursting forth, an abnormal excessive discharge or bleeding	therapy	treatment
		tome	instrument used to cut
rrhagia	bursting forth, an abnormal excessive discharge or bleeding	tomy	cutting into; surgical incision
		tripsy	crushing
rrhaphy	to suture or stitch	trophy	nourishment
rrhea	abnormal flow or discharge	ule	little
rrhexis	rupture	uria	urine; urination
schisis	split; fissure		
sclerosis	hardening		
scope	instrument used for visual exam		
scopic	visual exam		

Source: Adapted from Vines, Deborah, Braceland, Ann, Rollins, Elizabeth, and Miller, Susan. *Comprehensive Health Insurance: Billing, Coding, and Reimbursement.* © 2008. Pearson Education. Upper Saddle River, NJ.

Registered Medical Assistant (RMA) Medical Assisting Task List

MEDICAL ASSISTING TASK LIST

The various tasks that medical assistants perform include, but are not necessarily limited to, those on the following list. The tasks presented in this inventory are considered by American Medical Technologists to be representative of the medical assisting job role. This document should be considered dynamic, to reflect the medical assistant's evolving role with respect to contemporary health care. Therefore, tasks may be added, removed, or modified on an on-going basis.

Medical Assistants that meet AMT's qualifications and pass a certification examination are **certified** as a Registered Medical Assistant (RMA).

I. GENERAL MEDICAL ASSISTING KNOWLEDGE

A.   Anatomy and Physiology
1. Body systems
2. Disorders and diseases of the body

B.   Medical Terminology
1. Word parts
2. Medical terms
3. Common abbreviations and symbols
4. Spelling

C.   Medical Law
1. Medical law
2. Licensure, certification, and registration

D.   Medical Ethics
1. Principles of medical ethics
2. Ethical conduct
3. Professional development

E.   Human Relations
1. Patient relations
2. Interpersonal skills
3. Cultural diversity

F.   Patient Education
1. Identify and apply proper communication methods in patient instruction
2. Develop, assemble, and maintain patient resource materials

II. ADMINISTRATIVE MEDICAL ASSISTING

A.   Insurance
1. Medical insurance terminology
2. Various insurance plans
3. Claim forms
4. Electronic insurance claims
5. ICD-9/CPT Coding applications
6. HIPAA mandated coding systems
7. Financial applications of medical insurance

B.   Financial Bookkeeping
1. Medical finance terminology
2. Patient billing procedures
3. Collection procedures
4. Fundamental medical office accounting procedures
5. Office banking procedures
6. Employee payroll
7. Financial calculations and accounting procedures

C.   Medical Secretarial – Receptionist
1. Medical terminology associated with receptionist duties
2. General reception of patients and visitors
3. Appointment scheduling systems
4. Oral and written communications
5. Medical records management
6. Charting guidelines and regulations
7. Protect, store and retain medical records according to HIPAA regulations
8. Release of protected health information adhering to HIPAA regulations
9. Transcription of dictation
10. Supplies and equipment management
11. Medical office computer applications
12. Compliance with OSHA guidelines and regulations of office safety

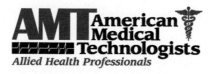

AMT American Medical Technologists
Allied Health Professionals

8/05

III.   CLINICAL MEDICAL ASSISTING

A.   Asepsis
1.   Medical terminology
2.   State/Federal universal blood borne pathogen/body fluid precautions
3.   Medical/Surgical asepsis procedure

B.   Sterilization
1.   Medical terminology associated with sterilization
2.   Sanitization, disinfection, and sterilization procedures
3.   Record keeping procedures

C.   Instruments
1.   Specialty instruments and parts
2.   Usage of common instruments
3.   Care and handling of disposable and re-usable instruments.

D.   Vital Signs / Mensurations
1.   Blood pressure, pulse, respiration measurements
2.   Height, weight, circumference measurements
3.   Various temperature measurements
4.   Recognize normal and abnormal measurement results

E.   Physical Examinations
1.   Patient history information
2.   Proper charting procedures
3.   Patient positions for examinations
4.   Methods of examinations
5.   Specialty examinations
6.   Visual acuity / Ishihara (color blindness) measurements
7.   Allergy testing procedures
8.   Normal / abnormal results

F.   Clinical Pharmacology
1.   Medical terminology associated with pharmacology
2.   Commonly used drugs and their categories
3.   Various routes of medication administration
4.   Parenteral administration of medications (Subcutaneous, Intramuscular, Intradermal, Z-Tract)
5.   Classes or drug schedules and legal prescriptions requirements for each
6.   Drug Enforcement Agency regulations for ordering, dispensing, storage, and documentation of medication use
7.   Drug Reference books (PDR, Pharmacopeia, Facts and Comparisons, Nurses Handbook)

G.   Minor Surgery
1.   Surgical supplies and instruments
2.   Asepsis in surgical procedures
3.   Surgical tray preparation and sterile field respect
4.   Prevention of pathogen transmission
5.   Patient surgical preparation procedures
6.   Assisting physician with minor surgery including set-up
7.   Dressing and bandaging techniques
8.   Suture and staple removal
9.   Biohazard waste disposal procedures
10.   Instruct patient in pre- and post-surgical care

H.   Therapeutic Modalities
1.   Various standard therapeutic modalities
2.   Alternative/complementary therapies
3.   Instruct patient in assistive devices, body mechanics and home care

I.   Laboratory Procedures
1.   Medical laboratory terminology
2.   OSHA safety guidelines
3.   Quality control and assessment regulations
4.   Operate and maintain laboratory equipment
5.   CLIA waived laboratory testing procedures
6.   Capillary, dermal and venipuncture procedures
7.   Office specimen collection such as: Urine, throat, vaginal, wound cultures – stool, sputum, etc
8.   Specimen handling and preparation
9.   Laboratory recording according to state and federal guidelines
10.   Adhere to the M A Scope of Practice in the laboratory

J.   Electrocardiography
1.   Standard, 12 Lead ECG Testing
2.   Mounting techniques for permanent record
3.   Rhythm strip ECG monitoring on Lead II

K.   First Aid
1.   Emergencies and first aid procedures
2.   Emergency crash cart supplies
3.   Legal responsibilities as a first responder

American Medical Technologists
10700 W. Higgins Road
Rosemont, Illinois 60018
Phone: (847) 823-5169 – Fax: (847) 823-0458
Website: www.amt1.com

How to Become a Successful Student

What Kind of Learner Are You?

In order to become a successful student, it is important to evaluate the type of learner you are. Following are the characteristics of the visual, auditory, and tactile learner.

The visual learner

- Tries to envision the word when spelling it out.
- Dislikes listening for long periods of time.
- Becomes distracted by movement when trying to concentrate.
- May not remember names, but will typically remember faces.
- Prefers face-to-face meetings.
- Prefers to read or hear descriptions when learning new material.
- Likes to look at pictures when learning new material.

The auditory learner

- Tries to sound out the word when spelling it out.
- Enjoys listening rather than talking.
- Becomes distracted by sounds or noises when trying to concentrate.
- Prefers the telephone to face-to-face meetings.
- Prefers verbal instructions.

The tactile learner

- Writes a word out when learning to spell it.
- Uses gestures and expressive movements when talking.
- Becomes distracted by activity when trying to concentrate.
- Prefers to talk while participating in activities.
- Is not necessarily a good reader—prefers stories that are action oriented.
- Tends to figure things out as they go along rather than read directions.

Skill Sets

Once you've realized the type of learner you are, take steps to use the skills you have in learning new material.

The visual learner might try

- Looking at pictures or diagrams when learning new material.
- Studying in a quiet room with no distractions.
- Asking for descriptions or asking instructors to explain how a topic might apply in the real world. For example, "Would you demonstrate that skill to the class?"

The auditory learner might try

- Reading aloud or taping their voice and playing it back to study new material.
- Taping the instructor's lecture and replaying it later to study.
- Studying in a quiet room with no distractions.
- Working with study groups where students discuss the material they've learned.

The tactile learner might try

- Writing material down several times in order to memorize it.
- Studying in a quiet area with no distractions.
- Asking the instructor to give examples of how a topic is addressed. For example, "Would you allow the class to role-play that activity so we can see what it feels like?"
- Practicing activities or skills in order to commit them to memory.

Time Management

One of the greatest difficulties for new students is time management and organization of priorities. For those students who have trouble in this area, the following steps may help:

- Set aside blocks of time for studying.
- Take periodic breaks when studying—get up and move around, get a drink, close your eyes for a few moments.

- Prioritize your assignments. Many students find it helpful to write down their assignments and place numbers next to each to indicate the order in which they need to be done.

- Study or read while doing other activities. Students can study or read while exercising, or at the gym.

- Review study material just prior to class on test day.

- Create "to do" lists.

- Use a daily/weekly/monthly calendar. Write down dates of upcoming tests or project due dates then back track to add in dates when certain stages of the project should be completed. For example, if a paper is due four weeks from today, add a note to the calendar for one week from today that the outline should be completed. Two weeks from today that the rough draft should be completed, and so on.

- Look for study partners for each class. Link up with study partners who are "good" students, not those who are not as dedicated as you are to learning the material. Spend time together each week going over the material from the class and studying or preparing for tests or projects.

Students should always be able to consult the course instructor for clarification of subject matter, or for verification of course progress. Students must keep aware of their progress in any given class and take an active part in assuring their own success.

Preparing for the CMA and RMA Certification Exams

The AMT Examination

The certification received after passing the AMT examination is Registered Medical Assistant (RMA). This exam consists of 200 to 210 multiple-choice questions. Those questions consist of approximately 43 percent general, 22 percent administrative, and 35 percent clinical topics. The AMT classifies general questions as those pertaining to anatomy and physiology, medical terminology, medical law and ethics, human relations, and patient education. Administrative questions are those pertaining to insurance, financial bookkeeping, and medical reception. Clinical questions are those pertaining to asepsis, sterilization, instruments, vital signs, physical examinations, clinical pharmacology, minor surgery, therapeutic modalities, laboratory procedures, electrocardiography, and first aid. The AMT weighs questions according to the difficulty of the question. The AMT test format consists of either a test booklet with answers written in pencil or on a computer. You have 2 hours to take the computer exam and 3 hours to take the written exam.

Eligibility Requirements

In order to be eligible for the RMA examination, applicants must meet the following requirements:

- Be of good moral character and at least 18 years of age

- Be a graduate of an accredited high school or acceptable equivalent

- Meet one of the following criteria:
  - Be a graduate of a medical assisting program that is accredited by the ABHES or the CAAHEP, or
  - Be a graduate of a medical assisting program that is accredited by a Regional Accrediting Commission or by a national accrediting organization approved by the U.S. Department of Education. The program must include a minimum of 720 hours of training in medical assisting skills, including a clinical externship.
  - Have been employed in the profession of medical assisting for a minimum of 5 years, with no more than 2 years of that time spent as an instructor in a medical assisting program.

- Applicants who have passed a generalist medical assisting certification examination offered by a medical assisting certification association that is approved by the AMT

Board of Directors, and have been working as a medical assistant for 5 years, and who meet the training and experience requirements of the AMT may be considered for the RMA certification without further examination.

Application Process

Applications for the RMA examination may be downloaded from the AMT Web site at http://www.amt1.com/site/epage/15334_315.htm. The application must be filled out and mailed to the AMT at:

American Medical Technologists
10700 West Higgins Road, Suite 150
Rosemont, IL 60018

The application may also be filled out and submitted online at the same Web site. Whether filled out online or downloaded and mailed to the AMT, the applicant must submit all applicable signatures and notarized documents in order to have the application processed. These documents are to be submitted to the AMT along with the payment for the examination. The application fee is currently $90.00.

The AAMA Examination

The certification received after passing the AAMA examination is Certified Medical Assistant (CMA). This exam consists of 300 multiple-choice questions divided into three sections—general, administrative, and clinical. General questions include: anatomy and physiology, medical terminology, medical law and ethics, pyschology, and communication. Administrative questions include: data entry, equipment, computer concepts, opening and delivering mail, medical records management, appointment scheduling, finding community resources, managing the physician's professional schedule, office management, office policies and procedures, and medical practice finances. Clinical questions include: principles of asepsis, assisting the physician, preparing patients, maintaining the treatment area, interviewing the patient, collecting and processing specimens, diagnostic testing, preparing and administering medications, handling emergencies, and nutrition. All questions are scored equally. As of January 5, 2009, the CMA (AAMA) Certification Examination began to be offered via computer-based testing. Candidates are able to select locations and flexible testing times at conveniently located computer-based testing centers throughout the United States.

Eligibility Requirements

In order to be eligible to sit for the AAMA examination, the applicant must have graduated from an accredited medical assisting program. The program must have been accredited by the Commission on Accreditation of Allied Health Education Programs (CAAHEP) or the Accrediting Bureau of Health Educations Schools (ABHES).

Grounds for Denial of Eligibility

The AAMA lists the following reasons for denial of sitting for the examination:

- Obtaining or attempting to obtain certification or recertification of the CMA credential through fraud or deception

- Knowingly assisting someone else in obtaining or attempting to obtain certification or recertification of the CMA credential through fraud or deception

- Making a misstatement of material fact or failure to make a statement of material fact in application for certification or recertification

- Falsifying information required for admission to the CMA Examination, impersonating another examinee, or falsifying education or credentials

- Copying answers, permitting another to copy answers, or providing or receiving unauthorized advice about examination content during the CMA Examination

- Unauthorized possession or distribution of examination materials, including copying and reproducing examination questions and problems

Generally, individuals who have been found guilty of a felony, or pleaded guilty to a felony, are not eligible to take the CMA exam. The Certifying Board may grant a waiver based upon certain circumstances. In order to apply for this waiver, an applicant must submit the following information to the Certifying Board:

- The age at which the crime was committed

- The circumstances surrounding the crime

- The nature of the crime committed

- The length of time since the conviction

- The individual's criminal history since the conviction

- The individual's current employment references

- The individual's character references

- Other evidence demonstrating the ability of the individual to perform the professional responsibilities competently, and evidence that the individual does not pose a threat to the health or safety of patients

Application Process

The exam fee for the computer-based test is $125 for CAAHEP and ABHES graduating students, recent CAAHEP and ABHES graduates, and AAMA members. The exam fee is $250 for non-recent CAAHEP and ABHES graduates and nonmembers. Exam fees are nonrefundable.

After taking the computer-based exam, preliminary pass/fail results will be provided Official scores will be mailed directly to candidates within five to six weeks.

Recertification

As of 2005, all newly certified and recertifying CMAs will hold their certification through the last day of their birth month in the sixth calendar year following their last certification/recertification. Recertification may be achieved either by sitting for the CMA Examination again or through accumulation of continuing education units (CEUs). If the applicant is recertifying through accumulation of continuing education units, the total points needed is 60. Of that total, 15 points must come from topics in the general category, 15 from the administrative category, and 15 from the clinical category. The remaining 15 points may be accumulated from any of the three categories. In addition, at least 20 of the 60 points must be accumulated from AAMA-approved continuing education units.

When accumulating CEUs, the medical assistant is responsible for keeping documentation of the CEUs earned. This documentation includes:

- The date the CEU was obtained

- The sponsor of the CEU (the group or organization issuing the CEU credits)

- The name of the program attended

- The amount and type of CEU obtained (general, administrative, clinical)

- The number of CEU credits received from each event

How to Prepare for the Examination

Just as when studying for any exam, it is important to observe certain techniques in order to achieve the maximum amount from your study time. The following are suggested study tactics:

- Find a quiet place to study.

- Inform those around you that you are not to be disturbed during study time.

- Avoid any possible disruptions, such as having a television or radio on. Turn off the ringer on your telephone.

- Use flashcards to memorize details if this method works for you.

- Use rhymes to memorize details if this method works for you.

- Research medical assisting exam review classes in your area.

- Join or form a study group.

- Purchase a pretest book and use it to take the practice exams. After scoring these practice exams, you will have a better idea of the area(s) you need to focus on for further study.

On the Day of the Exam

- Both of the exams consist of multiple-choice questions. In order to do well on these types of tests, it is important to read thoroughly the question and each answer before making your choice.

- Eliminate the answers you know are wrong. When you have eliminated the wrong answers, consider the answers remaining. Though more than one of them may be correct, remember that one of them is more appropriate than the other.

- Keep an eye on the clock. Considering the number of questions you have to answer, be sure you do not spend more than 45 seconds on any one question. If a question takes longer than that for you to answer, leave it and move on. If you have time after finishing the rest of the questions, come back to consider the ones you skipped.

- Be careful with "all of the above" or "none of the above" answers. If any one of the answers does *not* apply, "all of the above" cannot be the correct choice. Likewise, if even one of the answers *does* apply, "none of the above" cannot be the correct choice.

- Be careful when you see the words, "always," "never," "all," or "none." If you can think of even one exception to the word used, that answer is not correct.

- If you cannot choose between two or more answers, it is in your best interest to guess at the answer. Both the AMT and AAMA take away points for answers left blank.

Translation of English–Spanish Phrases

Would you prefer a morning or an afternoon appointment?
¿Usted prefiere una cita en la manana o' en la tarde?

Are you covered by medical insurance?
¿Tiene aseguranza medica?

Do you need directions to the office?
¿Necesita direccion de nuestra oficina?

Is your visit due to an accident?
¿Es su visita relacionado por un accidente?

What is your home telephone number?
¿Qua les el numero de telefono de su casa?

What is your work telephone number?
¿Qua les el numero de telefono de su trabajo?

Your co-payment for today is $_____.

Su co-pago de este dia es $_____.

Please take a seat, the medical assistant will take you back in just a moment.
Por favor tome asiento, el asistente medico va a tender en un momento.

Can you bring someone with you who speaks English?
¿Puede traer a alguien con usted que pueda abler ingles?

The doctor is running behind schedule, there will be a 20 minute wait.
El doctor esta atrasado, va a ver una espera de viente minutos.

Children may not be left unattended in the reception room.
No dese solos a los ninos en el cuarto de espera.

I need to take a photocopy of your driver's license.
Necesito tomar una fotocopia de su licensia.

Has someone referred you to our office?
¿Quien le recomendo nuestra clinica?

Which doctor did you want to see?
¿Que doctor quiere ver?

Is there a day of the week you would prefer for your appointment?
¿Que dia de la semana prefiere usted su cita?

Please bring your insurance information with you when you come in for your appointment.
Por favor traiga la informacion de su asguranza cuando venga a sue cita.

Please take this slip to the laboratory.
Por favor lleve esta hoja al laboratorio.

This form is our HIPAA privacy agreement.
Este formulario de HIPPA es nuestro aquerdo de privacidad.

I see that you are upset. Let me show you to a private room where we can talk.
Entiendo que esta molesto pasemos a un cuarto privado parea dialogar.

This pamphlet contains written information about your condition.
Este panfieto contiene informacio escrita sobre su condicion.

How long have you had problems with this?
¿Desde cuando tiene este tipo do problemas?

What is your name?
¿Como se llama usted?

Do you speak English?
¿Habla usted ingles?

Can you read English?
¿Sabe usted leer en ingles?

Thank you
Gracias

You are welcome.
De nada

Please
Por favor

It is nice to meet you.
Es un placer conocerle.

Common Medical Abbreviations

AAO	alert, awake, and oriented		COPD	chronic obstructive pulmonary disease
A&O	alert & oriented		CP	cerebral palsy
ABD	abdomen		CPAP	continuous positive airway pressure
ABG	arterial blood gas		CPR	cardiopulmonary resuscitation
abs	absent		CT	computerized tomography
AC	before eating		CVA	cerebrovascular accident
ACLS	advanced cardiac life support		CXR	chest X-ray
ADH	anti-diuretic hormone		DC	discontinue or discharge
adm	admission		DNR	do not resuscitate
ADR	adverse drug reaction		DOA	dead on arrival
ad lib	as much as needed		DTR	deep tendon reflexes
AFP	alpha-fetoprotein		DVT	deep venous thrombosis
amb	ambulatory		DX	diagnosis
amt	amount		ECG	electrocardiogram
ant	anterior		EMG	electromyogram
ante	before		ENT	ears, nose, and throat
AOB	alcohol on breath		FBS	fasting blood sugar
AP	anteroposterior		FTT	failure to thrive
ASAP	as soon as possible		FU	followup
BCP	birth control pills		Fx	fracture
BE	barium enema		GI	gastrointestinal
bid	twice a day		GSW	gunshot wound
BM	bowel movement		GTT	glucose tolerance test
BMR	basal metabolic rate		HA	Headache
BP	blood pressure		HBP	high blood pressure
BPH	benign prostatic hypertrophy		HCG	human chorionic gonadotropin
BPM	beats per minute		HCT	hematocrit
BS	bowel or breath sounds		HDL	high density lipoprotein
BX	biopsy		HEENT	head, eyes, ears, nose, throat
c	with		Hgb	hemoglobin
CA	cancer		HIV	human immunodeficiency virus
Ca	calcium		HO	history of
CAD	coronary artery disease		H&P	history and physical examination
CAT	computerized axial tomography		HR	heart rate
CBC	complete blood count		HS	at bedtime
CC	chief complaint		HSV	herpes simplex virus
CHF	congestive heart failure		HTN	hypertension
CNS	central nervous system		Hx	history
C/O	complaining of		I&D	incision and drainage

ICU	intensive care unit	qd	every day
ID	infectious disease	qh	every hour
IG	immunoglobulin	qid	four times a day
IM	intramuscular	qod	every other day
INF	intravenous nutritional fluid	R	right
IV	Intravenous	RA	rheumatoid arthritis
L	left	RBC	red blood cell
LLL	left lower lobe	R/O	rule out
LMP	last menstrual period	ROM	range of motion
LOC	loss of consciousness or level of consciousness	ROS	review of systems
LPN	licensed practical nurse	RTC	return to clinic
MAO	monoamine oxidase	s	without
MBT	maternal blood type	SOAP	subjective, objective, assessment, plan
MI	myocardial infarction or mitral insufficiency	SOB	shortness of breath
		SQ	subcutaneous
mL	milliliter	STAT	immediately
MMR	measles, mumps, rubella	Sx	symptoms
MRI	magnetic resonance imaging	T&C	type and cross
MRSA	methicillin resistant staph aureus	TB	tuberculosis
MS	multiple sclerosis	tid	three times a day
MVA	motor vehicle accident	TIG	tetanus immune globulin
NG	nasogastric	TMJ	temporo mandibular joint
NKA	no known allergies	TNTC	too numerous to count
NKDA	no known drug allergies	TO	telephone order
NMR	nuclear magnetic resonance	TPN	total parenteral nutrition
NPO	nothing by mouth	TSH	thyroid stimulating hormone
NSAID	nonsteroidal anti-inflammatory drugs	TT	thrombin time
NSR	normal sinus rhythm	Tx	treatment
OB	obstetrics	UA	urinalysis
OPV	oral polio vaccine	UAO	upper airway obstruction
OR	operating room	UBD	universal blood donor
PA	posteroanterior	URI	upper respiratory infection
PC	after eating	US	ultrasound
PDR	*Physician's Desk Reference*	UTI	urinary tract infection
PE	physical exam	VO	verbal order
PKU	phenylketonuria	WBC	white blood cell
PMH	previous medical history	WD	well developed
PO	by mouth	WF	white female
PR	by rectum	WM	white male
PRN	as needed	WNL	within normal limits
PT	prothrombin time, or physical therapy	WO	written order
Pt	patient	yo	years old
PTT	partial thromboplastin time	YOB	year of birth
PUD	peptic ulcer disease	yr	year
q	every (e.g. q6h = every 6 hours)	ytd	year to date

Answers to Chapter Case Studies/ Critical Thinking Questions

Chapter 1

Dr. Kenyon will be giving a presentation on the history of medicine to a local community group. She has asked her medical assistant to prepare some background materials for this event. Because Dr. Kenyon is a surgeon, she wants her medical assistant to find information about early medical practices, including how patients were anesthetized and operated on in early days.

CTQ 1-1: What are the historical roots of modern medicine?

Answer: Modern medicine can trace its roots back to the time of the caveman. Early practitioners used snakes, and all parts of plants and flowers to treat patients. Many treatments were painful and some were fatal. Most people believed disease and illness was caused by demons or gods.

CTQ 1-2: Why was Hippocrates called "The Father of Medicine"?

Answer: Hippocrates helped shift medical care from a religious and superstitious practice to a scientific one by basing his practice of medicine on the belief that illness was the result of a physical condition.

CTQ 1-3: Why did chloroform replace ether in anesthesia use?

Answer: Because ether had many side effects, **chloroform** replaced it as an anesthetic agent in 1853.

CTQ 1-4: Why were Dr. Semmelweiss's colleagues skeptical of hand washing's benefits?

Answer: Dr. Semmelweiss's colleagues did not understand that the condition of childbed fever was being caused by germs being transferred by the physician from one patient to another.

CTQ 1-5: How can research from the Human Genome Project improve the delivery of contemporary health care?

Answer: Scientists hope to use the information discovered in the Human Genome Project to learn how diseases work from the molecular level and thereby find cures for many diseases.

CTQ 1-6: Why has the number of women attending medical school in the United States increased so dramatically since 1970?

Answer: The role of women in health care has continued to grow as women have moved into more and more professional positions. The traditional role of women staying home to raise their children has changed on a cultural level, with women moving into fields once dominated by men.

Chapter 2

Karla Wilkins and the medical assistant were friends in high school. By the time the two unexpectedly meet at the local grocery store, they have not been in touch for several months. The medical assistant tells Karla about becoming certified in the field and includes such details as course load and topics. Looking confused, Karla responds, "If medical assistants don't *have* to be certified, why waste the time going to school? Why not just find a job and learn on the job?"

CTQ 2-1: Referring to the case study at the beginning of this chapter, what evidence supports the argument that medical assistants should have a standardized base of knowledge?

Answer: With dramatic changes in health care over the past decade, including shorter hospital stays and managed care, physicians must rely on allied health personnel like medical assistants to help care for patients. With technology advancing and patient safety increasingly a focal point, many physicians today insist on hiring medical assistants who have been formally trained in accredited medical assisting programs.

CTQ 2-2: Why do medical assistants who have completed accredited programs have more health care knowledge than those lacking formal training?

Answer: Medical assistants who completed an accredited program have taken anywhere from 6 months to 2 years to complete their training. This ensures that graduates will have a knowledge base as a foundation for caring for patients.

CTQ 2-3: How do certification discounts on physicians' medical malpractice insurance policies impact job opportunities for medical assistants?

Answer: These discounts encourage physicians to hire certified or registered medical assistants. This places the medical assistant with certification in a better place in the health care market.

CTQ 2-4: How does an externship support the educational goals of an accredited medical-assisting program?

Answer: Externships involve working as a medical assistant under a physician's supervision. Externships can run anywhere from 60 to 240 hours, but many medical-assisting programs require externships of more than 240 hours. While externships are unpaid, students earn credits toward their medical assisting certificates. The externship is an opportunity for the medical assistant to practice his or her newly learned skills in a safe, supervised environment.

Chapter 3

William Johanson is a patient of Dr. Chan's. Because the office medical assistant is responsible for arranging specialist referrals for patients, Dr. Chan has asked the medical assistant to arrange for Mr. Johanson to see a podiatrist and an ophthalmologist as part of his diabetes care plan. Mr. Johanson is unsure what those specialists do.

CTQ 3-1: Referring to the case study at the beginning of the chapter, why is the process of building trust with Mr. Johansen an important part of patient advocacy? In what way can the medical assistant in the case study gain Mr. Johansen's trust?

Answer: While patient care is part of medical assisting, the medical assistant's main responsibility is to be the patient's advocate. Because medical assistants will likely spend more time with patients than the physicians, medical assistants must develop a rapport with patients. Patients must be able to trust medical assistants, because those patients are more likely to share their personal information with assistants they trust. Patients may feel uncomfortable sharing their personal information with physicians, especially physicians they do not trust.

Medical assistants can earn their patient's trust by listening to the patient and acting in a position as an advocate for the patient.

CTQ 3-2: Imagine Mr. Johanson asks the medical assistant about his referrals in a public area of the office. How can the medical assistant best answer Mr. Johanson's questions while maintaining the patient's privacy?

Answer: The medical assistant should move the patient to a private area of the office, out of the hearing range of other patients, before going over the questions the patient has about her referrals.

CTQ 3-3: Imagine Dr. Chan is referring Mr. Johanson to a podiatrist the medical assistant dislikes. How might the medical assistant disguise his feelings in front of Mr. Johanson?

Answer: The medical assistant must be sure to keep his facial expressions and body language neutral so that the patient does not suspect the medical assistant does not like the podiatrist in question.

CTQ 3-4: Referring to the case study at the beginning of the chapter, imagine the medical assistant is leaving the office at the end of her shift when Dr. Chan asks her to schedule the referral for Mr. Johanson. How should the medical assistant handle this situation?

Answer: The medical assistant should handle the referrals for the physician and patient before leaving the office. In the event the medical assistant is not able to stay late to handle the referrals, he or she should find another medical assistant who is available to handle this task before leaving the office.

CTQ 3-5: Medical assistants are often asked to refer patients to such specialists as podiatrists and ophthalmologists. What type of information could the medical assistant keep on hand to help answer patient questions?

Answer: The medical assistant could keep brochures from the specialists on hand to give to the patients. If no brochure is available, the medical assistant could find material on the Internet about the specialties and, after gaining the physician's approval, give copies of that information to the patients.

Chapter 4

Victoria Mason is a medical assistant in Dr. Kozlowski's office. Victoria takes a telephone call from a man named Bart. He tells Victoria that one of his employees is a patient of Dr. Kozlowski's and asks her to tell him when his employee was last in the office and what treatment she received.

CTQ 4-1: How does the case study outlined at the beginning of this chapter illustrate one of the torts in Table 4-2? Please specify the tort.

Answer: The case study illustrates the tort of invasion of privacy. The medical assistant cannot release any information about a patient to another individual without the patient's consent or a court order.

CTQ 4-2: Referring to the case study at the beginning of the chapter, assume that Victoria revealed information about the patient's care to the patient's employer. What is the potential impact on the patient?

Answer: The employer might use the information gained about the patient's care to fire her or to deny her advancement to a better position.

CTQ 4-3: In the case study at the beginning of the chapter, the patient's employer obtained a subpoena for her medical information. How would the medical assistant determine which information to release? What is the proper procedure?

Answer: The medical assistant would want to verify the subpoena has been duly signed. The medical assistant would then seek to determine exactly what information the subpoena covers—the dates of service or condition that are specifically being requested.

CTQ 4-4: Assume that the patient was fired after the medical office gave her employer her private health information without her permission. How should she go about filing a complaint with HIPAA?

Answer: Victoria would need to ask the medical office for a complaint form and file the complaint with the office.

Chapter 5

Katerina Bolshoy is a Russian patient who speaks broken English. The medical assistant, who does not speak Katerina's language, must schedule several appointments for Katerina, as well as explain insurance coverage to her.

CTQ 5-1: How can the medical assistant enhance communication with non-native English speakers like Katerina?

Answer: The medical assistant should be careful to use proper English, without using slang terms. The medical assistant might also try writing things down for the patient; often the patient will better understand English they see written rather than hearing it spoken.

CTQ 5-2: What is the value of written communication for patients like Katerina, who speak English as a second language? What characteristics would make that written communication most effective?

Answer: Often the patient who is not a native English speaker will better understand the written

word over the spoken word. A patient may have someone at home who understands English better and the written communication could be used to help the patient relay to family members the information given by the office. Any written communication should be clear and concise.

CTQ 5-3: How does the reflecting conversation technique help ensure that medical assistants understand the concerns of patients like Katerina? What sort of questions would support this technique?

Answer: Using the reflecting conversation technique, the medical assistant is able to repeat information back to the patient, thereby ensuring that the patient's information was correctly understood. Questions that would support this technique would be, "Mrs. Dow, you said that for 2 weeks you have been having pain in your right shoulder and arm and that the pain has been running down to your right hand. Is that right?"

Chapter 6

Dr. Calvin Jones brings the medical assistant a business card from the medical equipment salesperson he just had lunch with and asks the assistant to type a letter to the salesperson. In the letter, the physician would like to thank the salesperson for showing him a new electrocardiogram (EKG) machine and indicate that while he is uninterested in purchasing the machine now, the salesperson should call after the first of the year to assess the physician's willingness to change that stance.

CTQ 6-1: Referring to the case study at the beginning of this chapter, how can the medical assistant help ensure that the typed letter contains no errors?

Answer: Using spellcheck software and proofreading documents help ensure that a typed letter contains no errors.

CTQ 6-2: What are the possible ramifications to Dr. Jones if the medical assistant does not use accurate grammar, spelling, and punctuation?

Answer: Incorrectly typed letters can result in misunderstanding, misdiagnosis, or even malpractice lawsuits in certain circumstances.

CTQ 6-3: Which courtesy title is appropriate for a letter to a sales representative, and why?

Answer: A letter to a sales representative should use the courtesy title "Mr." or "Ms." These titles are professional and indicate a professional relationship between the sales representative and the medical office.

Chapter 7

Martha Hagen, one of the medical office's established patients, calls to notify the office that she is having chest pains. Martha is not sure if she should make an appointment to come into the office or if she should to go the emergency room.

CTQ 7-1: While Martha Hagen is on the phone with her possibly life-threatening condition, how should the medical assistant handle the other calls that are holding?

Answer: The medical assistant should alert a coworker to handle the other callers.

CTQ 7-2: If the medical office mentioned in the case study lacks a triage notebook, how should the medical assistant go about creating one?

Answer: The medical office should hold a staff meeting to discuss the need for the notebook, the conditions that should be listed in the notebook, and the questions to be asked of the patients along with steps for the medical assistant to follow while on each type of telephone call.

Chapter 8

When Marilyn Peterson enters the medical office for a new patient appointment, the medical assistant greets her and gives her paperwork to complete. In response, Marilyn frowns and says, "I don't want to fill all of that out. I'm only here to see the doctor about a sore throat. I don't have time for paperwork."

CTQ 8-1: How can the medical assistant demonstrate caring and concern to Marilyn?

Answer: The medical assistant should explain to Marilyn the correlation between filling out the paperwork and receiving appropriate care and diagnosis from the physician. If the patient is unwilling to fill out the paperwork, the medical assistant should take the patient to a private location and ask the questions of the patient, then write down the given answers.

CTQ 8-2: Thinking back to the case study at the beginning of the chapter, how can the medical assistant argue to the physician or office manager that sending new patient history forms before patients' first visits will in fact benefit the office?

Answer: The medical assistant could point out to the physician or office manager that sending the information to the patient will save time for the patient. Also, if the patient is running late when he/she comes in, having the paperwork already filled out will save the office time.

CTQ 8-3: How should the medical assistant respond to Marilyn? What is appropriate for facial expression and tone of voice?

Answer: The medical assistant should explain to Marilyn the importance of having a correct history of the patient. The medical assistant's facial expression and tone of voice should relay concern and compassion rather than impatience.

Chapter 9

When Glenn Jenson calls the office to set up an appointment, he says he has never been in to see the physician before. When the medical assistant asks him why he must see the physician, he responds, "I'd rather not go into that with you. I'll tell the doctor when I see her."

CTQ 9-1: If Glenn fails to state his reason for requesting a physician visit, how can the medical assistant determine the time to allot for the appointment?

Answer: Without knowing the reason for the visit, the medical assistant would not know how much time to schedule the patient for.

CTQ 9-2: How should the medical assistant respond if Glenn refuses to disclose his insurance information?

Answer: In this event, the medical assistant would need to notify the patient of the amount of time he or she was setting aside, clarifying that if the patient's condition or complaint needed more time than that set aside that the patient would need to reschedule for a second visit.

CTQ 9-3: Assume Glenn will be taking the bus to the office. What steps can the medical assistant take to ensure Glenn obtains correct route information?

Answer: The medical assistant should have a list of bus routes available at the front desk in order to give that information to patients.

Chapter 10

When Melissa begins working for Dr. Miranda Kingsley, Caroline, one of the physician's longtime medical assistants, is charged with training her. One day, as Caroline pulls charts for patients scheduled for that afternoon, she points out a note on the outside of Robert Olson's chart that reads, "Problem." Caroline explains that the note alerts the medical assistants and the physician to patients who are "hard to work with." She says these patients complain, are late to their appointments, or are just generally unpleasant.

CTQ 10-1: Recall the case study at the beginning of this chapter. How would writing "Problem" on the patient's chart work against the physician's office?

Answer: If the patient noticed the word on his chart and asks about it, the medical assistant would be forced to either lie to the patient or to tell the truth—which would likely result in an angry patient.

CTQ 10-2: What are the potential implications of abbreviations for "problem patients"? How does this approach compare to full notes on patient charts, as described in the chapter-opening case study?

Answer: Writing abbreviations on the patients chart is no better than writing out the entire term. If the patient asks about the abbreviation, the medical assistant would either have to lie to the patient or tell the truth, causing the patient to be either hurt or angry.

CTQ 10-3: Imagine that the medical office has decided to discontinue notes like "Problem" on patient charts. How should the office go about removing such notes from patient files?

Answer: Since using correction fluid or any other method to obliterate portions of the medical record may cause the office to be looked upon with suspicion in the event of a legal case, the only way to remove the notes is to draw a single line through the note as with any other error in the medical chart, and date and sign the correction.

Chapter 11

Walter Reardon is an 80-year-old patient in Dr. Rand's office. Dr. Rand has recently converted his patient files from paper medical records to electronic medical records. David is Dr. Rand's medical assistant. David escorts Mr. Reardon to the examination room and then begins to perform his initial assessment using the electronic medical record he accesses from the computer in the examination room. When he notices this, Mr. Reardon becomes upset saying he doesn't trust computers and doesn't want his private medical information "out there for everyone to see."

CTQ 11-1: Recall the case study at the beginning of this chapter. What can you tell Mr. Reardon about the safety of his private patient information as it is contained within the electronic health record? How can you reassure him that his information isn't "out there"?

Answer: The medical assistant should tell Mr. Reardon that his information is well protected as is all information within the medical office computer system. The medical assistant should let Mr. Reardon know that the medical office will not release any information about patients unless the patient directs them to do so, or unless the office receives a court order to release the information.

CTQ 11-2: Recall the case study at the beginning of this chapter. What might you say to Mr. Reardon to convince him the change from paper to electronic medical records is in his best interests?

Answer: The medical assistant should outline the benefits of having medical records electronically instead of on paper. These benefits include the higher level of accuracy in typed entries as opposed to hand-written entries; the ability of more than one staff member to access the patient's file at the same time—which translates into faster insurance processing, and quicker turnaround time for patient inquiries.

CTQ 11-3: Referring to the case study at the beginning of the chapter, what sort of health maintenance reminders do you think a patient such as Mr. Reardon might benefit from receiving?

Answer: A patient such as Mr. Reardon might benefit from receiving reminders about yearly physical exams, regular colonoscopy exams, and yearly flu shots.

CTQ 11-4: Recall the case study at the beginning of this chapter. Do you think you could convince Mr. Reardon that having access to his medical records online might be helpful to him?

Answer: The medical assistant could explain to Mr. Reardon that he might enjoy being able to look at his medical records from home or to be able to allow his family or other physicians to access the medical records. Also, Mr. Reardon might enjoy having the ability to access his medical records while he is traveling away from home, especially in the event of a medical emergency while he is out of town.

Chapter 12

Dr. Crates has asked the medical assistant to research options for adding a new computer terminal to the office. The physician wants to ensure that the chosen system can run all the latest software in addition to the practice management software and electronic health record software used in the office.

CTQ 12-1: What must the medical assistant know about the medical office's computer needs? How does office need dictate computer choice?

Answer: The medical assistant should know the requirements of any software programs run by the office in addition to the planned budget for the computer system.

CTQ 12-2: What factors would justifiably influence the medical office to fund a flat-screen monitor?

Answer: If the computer monitor was going to be located in a location that is tight on space, a flat-screen monitor might be the appropriate choice.

CTQ 12-3: What type of information can the medical assistant gather to give the physician an accurate idea of printer costs?

Answer: The medical assistant should gather information on the cost of the printer and the cost and availability of the supplies.

Chapter 13

During a medical office's weekly staff meeting, several staff members voice their frustration over frequently running out of clerical supplies before new supplies are received. As the person in charge of inventory and supply ordering in the administrative office, the office manager asks the medical assistant to devise a system to address the situation.

CTQ 13-1: How does rotating the person in charge of inventory each week benefit the medical office's inventory process?

Answer: By rotating the person in charge of the inventory-taking process, the medical office will have a fresh set of eyes looking at the inventory each week. Also, if only one person takes care of inventorying supplies, the office may well run short of items when that one person takes a vacation or is out sick.

Chapter 14

Monte Taylor recently passed the medical assisting certification exam and has just obtained his first job as a registered medical assistant. Dr. Wilma Radcliff, an internist who shares her office space with several other physicians, has hired Monte. On Monte's first day, he asks the office manager if there is a manual that outlines office procedures. The office manager tells Monte that office staff have never taken the time to compose a procedures manual. She asks Monte if he would be willing to take on such a task.

CTQ 14-1: What type of policies and procedures should Monte start identifying for his office?

Answer: Monte should make a list of items that should be included in the book. These might include personnel policies regarding benefits as well as instructions on how certain tasks are handled within the office.

CTQ 14-2: If Monte's office lacks a mission statement, how should he go about explaining its importance to the physician?

Answer: Monte should explain to the physician that a mission statement is helpful in giving all members of the staff a common vision for the clinic.

CTQ 14-3: How should Monte determine which policies should appear in his office's policy manual?

Answer: Monte should make a list of commonly performed tasks in the office, such as an opening and closing routine that should be included in the policy manual.

Chapter 15

Mark Whitford is a 70-year-old patient in Dr. Hardy's office. As Mark walks toward the reception desk, he stumbles, loses his balance, and falls. Mark strikes his head on a cabinet, loses consciousness, and sustains a gash on his forehead that is bleeding profusely.

CTQ 15-1: How could the medical office have helped prevent Mark Whitford's injury?

Answer: The medical office could make sure there are no objects that a patient would hit his head upon in the office. The receptionist could have come out from behind the desk to assist the patient as soon as he or she notices the patient was unsteady.

CTQ 15-2: Imagine that when Mark Whitford falls, the reception room is full of other patients waiting to see their physicians. How should the medical assistant handle this situation?

Answer: The medical assistant's first duty is to the injured patient. After attending to the patient and alerting the necessary clinical staff, the medical assistant should go about calming those patients in the reception area and cleaning up any mess from the incident.

CTQ 15-3: When patients lose consciousness after hitting their heads, what should medical assistants do?

Answer:
1. If the patient collapses with no warning, do not move the patient. The patient may have sustained neck or back injury.
2. Notify the physician.
3. Loosen any tight clothing, and cover the patient with a blanket for warmth.
4. If the physician directs, use a footstool to support the patient's legs in a raised position.
5. If the physician directs, call for emergency services.

6. Once the emergency passes, document all activities in the patient's medical record.

CTQ 15-4: How should the medical assistant try to control the patient's bleeding?

Answer: For bleeding patients, the medical assistant should don appropriate protective equipment and then apply several layers of sterile dressing material directly to any wounds. Direct pressure should stop or slow bleeding until emergency personnel arrive.

CTQ 15-5: How would a medical assistant recognize the signs of shock in Mark Whitford?

Answer: The most common signs of shock include pale, gray, or bluish skin; moist, cool skin; dilated pupils; a weak, rapid pulse; shallow, rapid respirations; and extreme thirst.

Chapter 16

Martin Zamora is a patient at Woodway Health Care. Martin has recently gotten married and his new wife has health coverage through her employer. Martin says he believes his wife's coverage is better than the one he has through his own employer, and he wants her policy billed for his care, instead of his own.

CTQ 16-1: How should the medical assistant explain to Martin that his wife will need to add him to her policy if she has not yet done so?

Answer: The medical assistant should explain that it is not typically automatic for a new spouse to be added onto an insurance policy. The medical assistant should encourage Martin to have his wife contact her human resources department to find out the necessary steps to add him to her policy.

CTQ 16-2: Is it advisable to call the insurance carrier of Martin's wife to check on benefits? Why or why not?

Answer: The medical assistant should be able to determine the insurance coverage if he or she calls Martin's wife's insurance carrier.

CTQ 16-3: Assume the medical assistant determined that Martin's wife's insurance plan was not one of the physician's preferred plans. What should the medical assistant say to Martin?

Answer: The medical assistant should explain the nonpreferred status of the physician to Martin in addition to explaining how that status affects his coverage in that office.

CTQ 16-4: Using the birthday rule as a guide, what types of questions should the medical assistant ask Martin?

Answer: The medical assistant would need to determine Martin's spouse's date of birth. This in-formation would only be needed if there were children between Martin and his spouse, for whom the medical assistant would need to bill the insurance company.

Chapter 17

Recently hired in the billing area of Dr. Johnson's medical office, Mary is asked to assign a diagnostic code to a patient's visit and bill for the charges. Unfortunately, Mary has a difficult time deciphering Dr. Johnson's handwriting. After deciding she cannot read the writing in the patient's chart, she says, "Well, it looks like the visit has something to do with the patient's ear, so I'll just code the visit as an earache."

CTQ 17-1: When Mary guesses at the patient's diagnostic code in the chapter-opening case study, what is the potential harm?

Answer: Mary may be giving the patient a harmful diagnosis, which may cause the patient to lose insurance coverage or be denied insurance one day. Using the wrong diagnosis may also result in the claim being denied, delayed, or underpaid.

CTQ 17-2: When Mary cannot decipher the physician's handwriting, what should she do?

Answer: Mary should go to the physician and ask him or her to translate the notes.

Chapter 18

At Monday morning's staff meeting, Dr. Anderson mentions she is unhappy with the amount she is being reimbursed for her Medicare patients' office visits. To boost reimbursement, Dr. Anderson asks her medical assistant, Lydia, to use higher codes for those patients.

CTQ 18-1: What should Lydia tell Dr. Anderson about the relationship between appropriate codes and medical chart documentation?

Answer: Lydia should explain to Dr. Anderson that all codes used should be properly reflected in the patient's chart notes. Since insurance companies may request copies of their insured's chart notes at any time, improper coding may result in an audit of the practice.

CTQ 18-2: Assuming Lydia complied with Dr. Anderson's request to bill Medicare for higher codes, what might Medicare do, and why?

Answer: Medicare may request copies of patients' chart notes and conduct a lengthy audit of Dr. Anderson's practice. If Medicare's audit results in a finding of fraud, Dr. Anderson may lose her ability to treat Medicare patients, pay a fine, or be charged with a criminal offense.

CTQ 18-3: How would Lydia describe upcoding to Dr. Anderson?

Answer: Upcoding is the act of assigning a higher value code to a procedure with the intent to charge more money than the proper code would earn. Upcoding is illegal and unethical.

Chapter 19

Millie Alonso owes $550 for services her young son received, but she has made no payments for 2 months. As a result, her account now appears as past due. The medical assistant must call Millie to determine when she will send payment, either in full or by installment.

CTQ 19-1: Would Millie be more or less likely to have a balance due if someone in the medical office had discussed a payment plan when services were rendered? Why?

Answer: Millie would be less likely to have a balance due in the office if someone had discussed a payment plan before or at the time services were rendered. If Millie had a financial concern about payment, it could have been raised at that time.

CTQ 19-2: Should medical offices have policies to offer discounts to patients like Millie when those patients agree to pay their full bills via credit card during collection calls? Why?

Answer: Medical offices should have policies in place to offer discounts to patients who pay their bill in full. This practice allows the office to save the future costs of collecting on this account by discounting the bill and having it paid in full now.

CTQ 19-3: Imagine that Millie agrees to pay $100 on her credit card now and $100 per month for the next 4 months. What is the best means the medical assistant has for tracking this agreement?

Answer: The medical assistant should get a written agreement from the patient that outlines the payments agreed to. The medical assistant should then enter this information into a calendar system of some sort in order to follow up on the appropriate days to be certain Millie has sent her payment as agreed.

Chapter 20

Francie, who works as the medical office's receptionist, recently married a man with three children. Francie asks the medical assistant, who is in charge of payroll, to help her change her tax deductions so that fewer taxes are taken from her paycheck.

CTQ 20-1: What should the medical assistant do with Francie's employee file now that she has provided new information?

Answer: The medical assistant must update Francie's employee file with the new information so that Francie's tax deductions will be correct.

CTQ 20-2: What form must Francie complete for her employee file to ensure withholding allowances are processed properly?

Answer: Francie must fill out a new W-4 form.

CTQ 20-3: Because the medical assistant, and not an outside agency, handles the medical office's payroll, what can the assistant tell Francie about the time it will take to change her payroll deductions?

Answer: The medical office should have a policy that outlines the length of time it will take for payroll changes to go into effect. Typically, these changes will go into effect no less than 1 week and no more than 2 weeks from the time the employee fills out the change in paperwork.

Chapter 21

Juanita Ryan is the office manager at Valley View Medical Clinic, which has three physicians, one of whom arrives late every morning and returns late after lunch. Juanita has spoken with the physician, Dr. Whittier, several times. Patients are angry and frustrated by their long waits.

CTQ 21-1: As the office manager, how should Juanita address Dr. Whittier's tardiness issue?

Answer: Juanita should speak to Dr. Whittier in a private location and explain how the patients are reacting to the extended wait times.

CTQ 21-2: How could Juanita use a staff meeting to address the issue of Dr. Whittier's tardiness?

Answer: Juanita could bring up the issue at a staff meeting and ask staff members for their input on how to best handle the issue.

CTQ 21-3: Imagine that the chronically late physician, Dr. Whittier, fails to attend the staff meeting at which the issue is addressed. How should Juanita inform him of the staff meeting's discussion?

Answer: Juanita should give Dr. Whittier a copy of the staff meeting minutes, which should outline the discussion and any possible solutions.

CTQ 21-4: How could Juanita communicate to the chronically tardy physician the potential impact of his actions on patient care?

Answer: Juanita could explain to the physician that angry patients will sometimes file malpractice lawsuits. In addition, angry patients may discuss the physician in a negative manner in the community, with their family and friends. This could cause a decrease in the number of patients who see this physician.

Chapter 22

Karim Yousef, a medical assisting graduate seeking employment in health care, lacks personal transportation. Because Karim must rely on public transportation, he has arrived late to a few interviews.

CTQ 22-1: Should Karim note his lack of personal transportation on his resume? Why or why not?

Answer: Karim should not point out his lack of transportation on his resume. This information could be used against Karim and may cost him a chance to interview for the job.

CTQ 22-2: Karim was fired from his last two jobs due to chronic tardiness. Should he mention those terminations in his cover letter? Why or why not?

Answer: Karim should not mention his terminations in his cover letter. If this information comes up in an interview, Karim will have the opportunity to address the topic face to face with the potential employer.

CTQ 22-3: If Karim lacks personal transportation, how should he seek employment?

Answer: Karim should look for employment in a clinic or facility that is within walking distance of his home or is located in a place he can easily access with public transportation.

Answers to In-Practice Scenarios

Chapter 2

In coming years, the scope of medical assisting will expand to meet the needs of an aging population and to fill a continued nursing shortage. As it does, new graduates will acquire new skills. How will current medical assistants keep their skills up to date? What resources can assistants use to further their training?

Current medical assistants will be able to keep their skills up to date by attending their local, county, and state association events. Through these agencies the medical assistant can keep up to date on possible continuing education opportunities to learn any needed new skills.

Chapter 3

A new patient in town, Isaiah Rodriguez, arrives at the office needing a physician. According to Isaiah, his last physician had an unpleasant receptionist. Isaiah tells the medical assistant, "If I didn't like my doctor so much, I would have found another one." He adds that the person who answered his call for this appointment seemed like she was in a hurry. How should the medical assistant handle this situation? What can the medical assistant say to Isaiah? Should the medical assistant bring the situation to the doctor's attention? Why or why not?

The medical assistant should let Isaiah know that he will not experience similar events in this office and that the staff is dedicated to patient satisfaction. The medical assistant should bring this information to the physician's attention, just as she should bring any comments such as these to the physician's attention.

Chapter 4

Jan has been working as an administrative medical assistant for Dr. Borse for 7 years. Dr. Borse frequently asks Jan to add charges to a patient account for services he did not perform.

Jan is paid well and feels she is harming no patients by complying with the doctor's requests. Dr. Borse says he only submits the false claims to make up for the money he loses by treating Medicare and Medicaid patients. One day, Dr. Borse is arrested for insurance fraud. He eventually serves 2 years in prison and loses his license to practice medicine. Jan has a very hard time getting a new job. Dr. Borse's story has been in all the local papers, and employers do not want to work with unethical staff. How could Jan have changed the course of events? What advice would have helped Jan while she was working with Dr. Borse?

Jan could have refused to add the fraudulent charges to the patient bills. She could have told Dr. Borse that it was illegal and unethical and that she would not participate. Jan likely now knows that the money she made working for Dr. Borse was not worth the shunning she is now experiencing in her community from employers who are reluctant to hire someone who knowingly worked for a physician who committed insurance fraud.

Chapter 5

Mark Minton is completing paperwork in the reception area. Two of the medical assistant's coworkers, who are standing behind the assistant at the front desk, begin a conversation about last night's episode of their favorite television show. Their conversation is loud enough to be heard in the reception area. What should the medical assistant do?

The medical assistant should remind the coworkers that their conversation can be overheard by patients. This conversation is inappropriate and should not continue in front of the patient.

Chapter 6

Dr. Mohammad asks Joanne Brennan, his new administrative medical assistant, to type a letter to a patient while he dictates. During dictation, Dr. Mohammad uses words unfamiliar to Joanne, so she asks, "Can I guess how to spell some words? The patient probably won't notice."

What is the proper response to Joanne? What is the proper course of action if Joanne continues to guess at word spellings? Why is this issue important?

Joanne must spell the words correctly. A misspelling can result in incorrect information being sent to the patient, which may result in a misunderstanding that could have a catastrophic consequence.

Chapter 7

Established patient Josie Welton often arrives early for her appointments. While she waits in the reception area, Josie uses the patient phone to make a call during which she details her health care problems and other personal information. The other patients in the reception area overhear the entire conversation. How should the medical assistant address this situation?

The medical assistant should ask Josie if she would like to be moved to a private location to use the telephone. If Josie declines and continues her conversation, the medical assistant should alert the clinical staff to take Josie to a treatment room as soon as possible.

Since Josie is the one talking about her own health care issues, there is no violation of HIPAA privacy laws in this scenario. However, it is inappropriate to have a patient discuss these issues, especially in the detail Josie appears to be using, in front of other patients. Some patients may have a queasy stomach, or become frightened by Josie's description of her symptoms.

Chapter 8

The small physician's office where Jenny works as a front-desk medical assistant is on the first floor of a building where cars are parked outside the door. When Marion Wilson arrives for her appointment, she approaches the front desk and tells Jenny that she is going to leave her 2-year-old son sleeping in his car seat because Jenny can see the car from her desk. How should Jenny respond to Marion? What are some appropriate suggestions?

Jenny needs to let Marion know that it is not safe to leave a child in the car and that she will not be able to watch him while Marion is in the office. Under no circumstances should Jenny agree to allow Marion to leave the child in the car unattended.

Chapter 9

Dr. Brosnan performed a vasectomy on William Grissom and asked him, as he asks all patients who have undergone this procedure, to have a followup evaluation and laboratory work to determine the procedure's effectiveness. Mr. Grissom, however, failed to show for his followup appointment. Three months later, Dr. Brosnan received a notice that Mr. Grissom had filed a malpractice suit. According to the notice, Mr. Grissom is alleging that Dr. Brosnan was negligent because Mr. Grissom's wife is newly pregnant. How could Dr. Brosnan's office have protected itself against this situation?

Dr. Brosnan's office should have clearly documented the missed appointment by Mr. Grissom. The office should also have sent a certified letter to Mr. Grissom alerting him to the importance of the return visit. Documentation that the letter was signed for should have been placed within Mr. Grissom's file. With this information, Mr. Grissom would have a hard time proving that Dr. Brosnan was negligent in not determining whether the vasectomy procedure was a success.

Chapter 10

Dylan McElvaney, RMA, has taken a telephone call from Lynn Kinney, a patient in the office. Lynn states she is very unhappy with the office because she has been waiting for three days for her laboratory results to be conveyed to her. She says she won't be coming back to the office and will be calling to have copies of her medical file sent to another facility. What should Dylan say to Lynn? How should Dylan chart this telephone call in Lynn's medical record?

Dylan should attempt to calm Lynn down and should apologize for the tardiness of the return of her laboratory results. Dylan should offer to transfer Lynn's telephone call to the clinical nurse to hear her results right away, or to the physician, if he or she is available. If Lynn is unwilling to budge from her resolve to change physicians, Dylan should record the following in the patient's chart:

"(Date of the call) Patient called stating she has been waiting for three days for her laboratory results. Patient is unhappy over the unexpected wait time. Offered to transfer patient to the clinical nurse (or physician) and patient declined. Patient states she will be requesting transfer of her medical records to a new physician. Dylan McElvaney, RMA"

Chapter 11

Dr. Jonas runs a private practice and makes rounds in two local hospitals. He uses one type of electronic medical records software in his private office and two other packages in the two hospitals. Not only must Dr. Jonas learn three software systems, he may at times be unable to move patient information between those systems due to incompatibility. What might Dr. Jonas do to address these issues?

Dr. Jonas could contact the software vendors for all three programs to find out if there is a bridging program he could use that would allow him to translate documents from one system to another. In lieu of that, Dr. Jonas could purchase software that matches one of the two hospitals he rounds within.

Chapter 12

Dr. Victor is giving a presentation on a new procedure she is performing for scar-tissue removal. Dr. Victor has asked Jamie, her medical assistant, to use the Internet to find information on other, similar procedures for comparison. How should Jamie begin, and where? What key words would be appropriate for the search engine?

In order to perform this search, Jamie should go to reputable professional medical Web sites online. Dr. Victor is likely subscribed to one or more of these sites and Jamie should visit them all to perform a search for any information pertaining to procedures for scar tissue removal. After locating the information, Jamie should compose a list of the findings and present that list to Dr. Victor, along with information on the Web site where the information was found.

Jamie should begin by visiting only reputable medical information Web sites or search engines. She should be certain to use the key words provided by Dr. Victor and should keep the name of each Web site available to refer to should Dr. Victor have further questions.

Chapter 13

Before the medical assistant was hired, the medical office lacked a system for ordering supplies. Members of the health care team simply ordered supplies as they felt necessary. As a result, the office now has cupboards full of supplies that will expire in a month. As a new employee, the medical assistant is charged with devising a system for tracking office inventory. Where should the assistant start? What steps will help ensure that all supplies are counted correctly?

First a policy should be put into place that spells out who will take inventory, how often inventory will be performed, and who is responsible for the ordering of all supplies. The office needs an inventory supply log to track inventory, and a regular system of tracking the supplies being used in the office in order to keep an adequate supply on hand at all times.

Chapter 14

Anka is a registered medical assistant working for Dr. Mock. While Anka is finishing a blood draw on a patient, she accidentally sticks herself with the contaminated needle. How will Anka know what to do now that this injury has happened?

Anka should report the needle stick injury to her supervisor. She should then consult the policy manual to determine the exact steps she should take for documenting her injury, and the need for any testing or vaccinations she may require.

Chapter 15

When Courtney Molino enters the medical office for her physical exam, she says she feels unwell after choosing the stairs over the elevator. In fact, she says she is having chest pain and extreme dizziness. What should the medical assistant do?

The medical assistant should immediately escort Courtney to an examination room and alert the physician and clinical staff of the possible emergency. The medical assistant should stay with Courtney until other clinical staff take over and should remain available should emergency services need to be contacted.

Chapter 16

Georgia Collins calls the medical office to schedule an appointment as a new patient. When the medical assistant asks her about her insurance coverage, she says she is unsure of her insurance company's name and cannot locate her insurance card. How should the medical assistant respond? Is insurance information needed before patients seek care? Why? If Georgia becomes angry, how should the medical assistant react?

Since Georgia cannot locate her insurance card while on the phone, the medical assistant should politely let her know that her coverage may vary greatly depending upon the type of health insurance she has. It is important to let her know that with some managed care plans she may not be covered for ser-

vices in the office; it is impossible to be able to tell her for sure unless it is known which insurance plan she has.

If she still cannot locate the insurance card, confirm her appointment and ask her to call you back if she finds the card prior to her visit. Politely let her know that if she is with a managed care plan that your office is not contracted with, she may be responsible for the entire fee for the visit.

Chapter 17

Sharon is the administrative medical assistant who completes billing work in the office. One day when she pulls a patient file, Sharon notices that the fee slip the physician completed indicates that he drained a cyst on the patient's wrist. When Sharon reviews the chart notes to assign a diagnosis code, she finds that the physician has written nothing in the chart about the cyst or the procedure. In situations like these, Sharon usually just "jots something" in the chart. What might be wrong with this scenario?

Anything charted in the medical chart should be charted *only* by the person who performed the service. Since Sharon did not perform or witness the procedure performed on this patient, it would be fraud for her to "jot something" in the medical record in order to make it match what the fee slip says. Instead, Sharon should give the file to the physician and ask him or her to complete the charting for that day.

Chapter 18

During the 5 years Audrey has worked for Dr. Suarez, the physician has often asked her to bill for services he did not perform. Audrey has never objected, in part because she feels patients are unharmed by the practice. She also believes she is blameless, because she receives no additional money from the process.

One day Audrey arrives at work to find that Dr. Suarez has been arrested. Later, the physician is convicted and sentenced to 2 years in jail. The office closes, and Audrey loses her job. Audrey begins a job search but finds that her association with Dr. Suarez is a negative. In fact, several potential employers have turned her away as a result. One of those employers said, "I'm sorry, but we just can't trust someone who worked for a doctor involved in insurance fraud." How could Audrey have avoided this situation?

Audrey could have avoided this situation by doing one of two things—either explain to Dr. Suarez that what he is doing is insurance fraud and she refuses to be a part of it, or to quit her job. Audrey didn't realize that the actions of the physician she worked for would follow her, and are now keeping her from getting a new job.

Chapter 19

Dr. Bowman wants to raise his prices for certain services. He tells his medical assistant he fails to understand why insurance companies do not pay him more simply because he has begun charging more. What can the medical assistant say about fee schedule determination?

Dr. Bowman doesn't understand how fee schedules are made. The medical assistant will need to explain to him how the RBRVS and RVU numbers are assigned by Medicare and how those assigned numbers are standard. He can raise his fees, but until Medicare raises the RSRVS and RVU, he will not receive a higher allowed fee for his services.

Chapter 20

Wendy Lu, a registered medical assistant who works for Dr. Patch, is responsible for balancing the office's petty cash fund. When Wendy tries to balance the fund today, however, she notices the account is $40 short. What should she do to find the error?

Wendy should recount the funds for the day and if she continues to find them $40 short she should review the receipts written and posted to determine if the error is a posting error. Sometimes asking a coworker to check the work can reveal an error as well.

Chapter 21

Carrie is an administrative medical assistant working the medical office's reception desk. Mrs. Carnes enters the office and begins loudly complaining about a bill she has received.

She demands that Carrie explain why the bill is so high. During the exchange, several other patients in the reception room watch Carrie for her reaction. What should Carrie do to defuse this scene?

Carrie should attempt to move Mrs. Carnes out of the reception area and into a private area as soon as possible. Carrie should remain calm and soothing to Mrs. Carnes and she should let her know that she will take care of the problem as quickly as possible. If the office manager is available, Carrie should take Mrs. Carnes to the office manager's office and should explain the problem to the office manager before leaving Mrs. Carnes there.

Chapter 22

Jerome is looking for employment as a medical assistant. He has submitted his resume at several offices and has been waiting for telephone calls requesting interviews. When those calls come, the potential employers hear the voicemail greeting Jerome shares with his roommate: "Hi. This is Jerome and Terrence. We're either not home, or we're too hung over to answer the phone right now. Leave a message." When the potential employers hear this message, they decide to leave no messages. What should Jerome do to increase his chances of gaining employment?

Jerome should change his voicemail message to one that is professional, or he should use his mobile telephone number on his resume so that calls will not be received on his home voicemail.

Introduction to Medisoft Advanced (version 12) and Medisoft Simulation

Medisoft Advanced is a medical practice management software program that offers choices of actions through a series of menus. Commands are issued by clicking an option on the menu bar or by clicking a shortcut button on the toolbar. All data, whether a patient's address or a charge for a procedure, is entered into Medisoft through menus on the menu bar or through the buttons on the toolbar. Selecting an option from the menus or toolbar brings up a dialog box. The TAB key is used to move between text boxes within a dialog box.

The menu bar lists the names of the menus in Medisoft: File, Edit, Activities, Lists, Reports, Tools, Window, Services, and Help. Beneath each menu name is a pull-down menu of one or more options.

Menu Bar Titles

The purpose of each menu is briefly described as follows:

File Menu The File menu is used to enter information about the medical office practice when first setting up Medisoft. It is also used to back up data, maintain files, and set up program options.

Edit Menu The Edit menu contains the basic commands needed to move, change, or delete information. These commands are Undo, Cut, Copy, Paste, and Delete.

Activities Menu Most medical office data collected on a day-to-day basis is entered through options on the Activities menu. This menu is used to enter information about patients' office visits, including diagnoses and procedures performed. Transactions, including charges, payments, and adjustments, are also entered via the Activities menu.

Lists Menu Information on new patients, such as name, address, and employer, is entered through the Lists menu. The Lists menu also provides access to lists of codes, insurance carriers, and providers.

Reports Menu The Reports menu is used to print reports about patients' accounts and other reports about the practice.

Tools Menu The calculator is accessed through the Tools menu. Other options on the Tools menu can be used to view the contents of a file as well as a profile of the computer system.

Window Menu Using the Window menu, it is possible to switch back and forth between several open windows.

Services Menu This menu contains links for electronic transmission of insurance claims, electronic prescriptions, and electronic eligibility verification.

Help Menu The Help menu is used to access Medisoft's Help feature.

Basic Medisoft Actions

In this section we discuss some of the basic tasks that all medical office specialists should be able to perform with the Medisoft software.

Saving Data

Information entered into Medisoft is saved by clicking the Save button that appears in most dialog boxes (those in which data is input).

Deleting Data

The majority of Medisoft dialog boxes have buttons for the purpose of deleting data.

Exiting Medisoft

Medisoft is exited by clicking Exit on the File menu or by clicking the Exit button on the toolbar.

Entering Patient Information into Medisoft

Patient information is entered in the Patient/Guarantor dialog box, accessed by clicking Patient/Guarantors and Cases on the **Lists** menu. The Patient List dialog box displays a list of established patients. Information on a new patient is entered by clicking the *New Patient* button at the bottom of the dialog box. The Patient/Guarantor dialog box contains four tabs: the **Name, Address** tab, **Other Information** tab, **Payment Plan** tab, and **Custom** tab (Figure J-1 ◆).

Name, Address Tab

This tab is completed with information provided by a new patient on the practice's patient information form. Most of the information is demographic: name, address, phone numbers, birth date, gender, and Social Security number. Phone numbers must be entered without parentheses or hyphens. The birth date is entered using the eight-digit MMDDCCYY format. The nine-digit Social Security number should be entered *with*

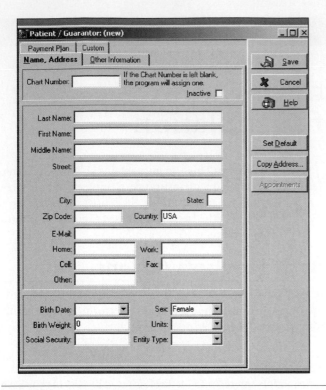

Figure J-1 ◆ The Name, Address tab in the Patient/Guarantor window (dialog box).

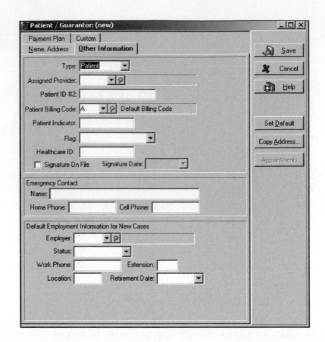

Figure J-2 ◆ The Other Information tab in the Patient/Guarantor window.

hyphens. Some of the boxes, such as the cell phone number and fax number boxes, are optional.

Chart Number: The chart number is a unique number that identifies each patient. The most common method of assigning a number is to use the first three letters of the last name, the first two letters of the first name, and the digit 0, which represents head of household. If the last name has less than five letters, use more letters of the first name and even of the middle name if necessary. It is not necessary to enter a chart number when entering a new patient. If you choose not to enter one, Medisoft will assign one for you. It is important to note that once the Chart Number is set it cannot be changed. To correct an incorrect chart number, the patient and case information would have to be deleted then re-created with the correct Chart Number.

Other Information Tab

The Other Information tab (Figure J-2 ◆) contains facts about a patient's employment and other miscellaneous information. The major fields in the Other Information tab are:

Type: The Type drop-down list designates whether, for billing purposes, an individual is a patient or a guarantor. A guarantor is someone who is responsible for insurance and payment.

Assigned Provider: The code for the specific doctor who provides care to this patient is selected.

Signature on File: A check mark in the Signature on File check box means that the patient's signature is on file for the purpose of submitting insurance claims.

Signature Date: The date keyed in the Signature Date box is the date the patient signed the release of information form.

Emergency Contact: The name the patient/guarantor has written on the patient information form as an emergency contact is keyed in here, along with any phone numbers provided.

Employer: The name of the patient's employer is selected from the drop-down list of employers stored in the database.

Payment Plan Tab

The Payment Plan tab (Figure J-3 ◆) contains data regarding a patient who has signed a financial agreement to pay the facility the balance on the account over a specific period of time.

Custom Tab

The Custom tab is designed by the particular facility to contain information important to that facility. In the tutorial data for Medisoft, the Custom tab contains height, weight, and cigarette smoking data.

Cases

Information about a patient's insurance coverage, billing account, diagnosis, and condition are stored in cases. When a patient comes for treatment, a case is created. Cases are set up to contain the transactions that relate to a particular condition. For example, all treatments and procedures for bronchial asthma would be stored in a case called "Bronchial Asthma." Services performed and charges for those services are entered in the system linked to the bronchial asthma case.

In Medisoft cases are created, edited, and deleted from within the **Patient List** dialog box. When the Case radio button

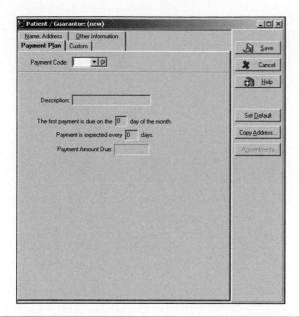

Figure J-3 ◆ The Payment Plan tab in the Patient/Guarantor window.

in the Patient List dialog box is clicked, the following buttons appear at the bottom of the Patient List dialog box: Edit Case, New Case, Delete Case, Copy Case, and Close. These buttons perform their respective functions on cases. For example, to create a new case, the New Case button is clicked. Data recorded in the Case dialog box is stored by clicking the Save button on the right side of the Case dialog box.

Entering Case Information

Information on a patient is entered in 11 different tabs within the Case dialog box: Personal, Account, Diagnosis, Policy 1, Policy 2, Policy 3, Condition, Miscellaneous, Medicaid and Tricare, Comment, and EDI. A 12th tab, Custom One, allows the facility to create and design its own Custom tabs as well.

Personal Tab

The Personal tab (Figure J-4 ◆) contains basic information about a patient and his or her employment. The most important boxes that must be completed in the Personal tab are as follows:

> **Case Number:** The case number is a unique sequential number *assigned by Medisoft*.
> **Description:** Information entered in the Description box indicates a patient's complaint, or reason for seeing the physician.
> **Guarantor:** The Guarantor box lists the name of the person responsible for paying the bill.

Account Tab

The Account tab includes information on a patient's assigned provider, referring provider, referral source, as well as other information that may be used in some medical practices but not

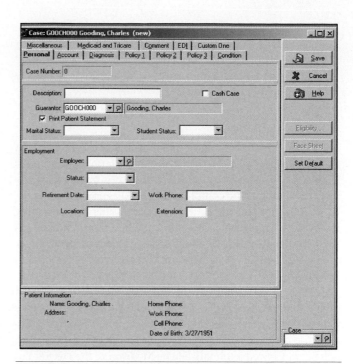

Figure J-4 ◆ Case window, Personal tab.

others (Figure J-5 ◆). The most important boxes that must be completed in the Account tab are as follows:

> **Assigned Provider:** The Assigned Provider box is automatically filled in with the code number and name of the assigned provider listed in the Patient/Guarantor dialog box.
> **Referring Provider:** If the patient was referred to the facility by another provider, choose the referring provider's name from the drop-down list.
> **Facility:** Choose the correct facility name from the drop-down box for the place the services were rendered.

Figure J-5 ◆ Case window, Account tab.

Authorization Number: For patients whose insurance carrier requires a referral/authorization number for services, the number issued should be entered here along with the number of visits authorized and the referral expiration date.

Diagnosis Tab

The Diagnosis tab contains a patient's diagnosis, information about allergies, and electronic medical claim (EMC) notes (Figure J-6 ◆). The Allergies and Notes box is the most important box that must be completed in the Diagnosis tab:

Allergies and Notes: If the patient is allergic to anything it should be entered here. This information is taken from the patient information form. Notes regarding payment arrangements, a forgotten copayment, or anything else are entered in this area as well.

You will not complete the Default Diagnosis 1 through 4 boxes. When you are setting up the case, you will not know the patient's diagnosis. After you have posted the charge transaction, the diagnosis code entered into the charge information will be transferred automatically by Medisoft to the Default Diagnosis boxes in this tab.

Policy 1, 2, and 3 Tabs

The Policy tabs are where information about a patient's insurance carrier and coverage is recorded (Figure J-7 ◆). If a patient has more than one insurance policy, the Policy 2 and 3 tabs are used. The following boxes are the most important ones to be completed in the Policy tabs:

Insurance 1: The Insurance 1 box lists the patient's insurance carrier name, which is chosen from the drop-down list.

Policy Holder 1: This box shows the name of the insured person, which is chosen from the drop-down list. (This may or may not be the patient.) The guarantor

Figure J-6 ◆ Case window, Diagnosis tab.

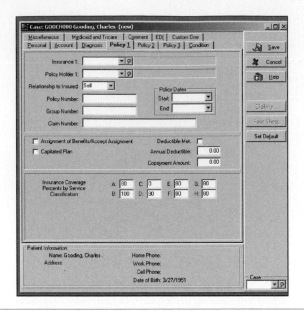

Figure J-7 ◆ Case window, Policy 1 tab.

must be entered in to the Patient List so that he or she can be chosen from the drop-down list here.

Relationship to Insured: This box indicates the patient's relationship to the individual listed in the Policy Holder 1 box.

Policy Number: The patient's insurance policy or ID number is entered in the Policy Number box.

Group Number: If there is a group number for a patient's policy, it is entered in the Group Number box.

Assignment of Benefits/Accept Assignment: Check this box if the patient has assigned insurance benefits to the provider.

Insurance Coverage Percents by Service Classification: The percentage of fees that an insurance carrier covers is entered in the Insurance Coverage Percents . . . box. The default entry in this box is 80. The default can be changed by highlighting the default entry and keying the correct percentage over the default. Some insurance policies pay different percentages of charges based on the type of service rendered. For example, a carrier may pay 100% for well-man or well-woman exams and 50% for lab charges.

Condition Tab

The Condition tab stores data about a patient's illness, accident, disability, and hospitalization. This information is used by insurance carriers to process claims (Figure J-8 ◆).

The top portion of the Condition tab is completed with the date of the illness, injury, or last menstrual period (if the patient is pregnant). Make the appropriate choice from the Illness Indicator drop-down list. If treatment rendered was for an emergency condition, check the box next to Emergency. If the case is for treatment of an accident, select the correct type from the Accident drop-down list. If the "accident" was just a

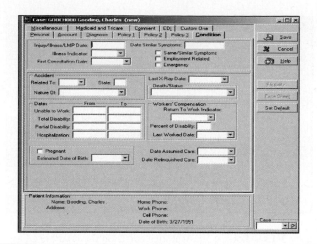

Figure J-8 ◆ Case window, Condition tab.

fall at home, it is not considered a true accident. If the Accident box is marked, the insurance carrier may delay processing of the claim to research whether another insurance carrier should be the primary payer. If the case/treatment is workers' compensation related, the boxes for Unable to Work, Total Disability, Partial Disability, and Hospitalization may be completed. The Return To Work Indicator, Percent of Disability, and Last Worked Date all relate to workers' compensation cases.

Miscellaneous Tab

The Miscellaneous tab records a variety of miscellaneous information about the patient and his or her treatment, including outside lab work, prior authorization numbers, and other information (Figure J-9 ◆). For the authorization number to print out on the CMS-1500 form, it must be entered in the Miscellaneous tab.

Medicaid and Tricare Tab

For patients covered by Medicaid or TRICARE, the Medicaid and Tricare tab is used to enter additional information about the government program (Figure J-10 ◆).

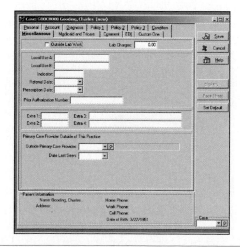

Figure J-9 ◆ Case window, Miscellaneous tab.

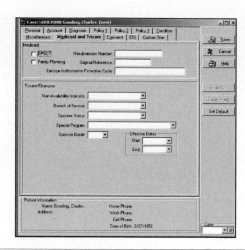

Figure J-10 ◆ Case window, Medicaid and Tricare tab.

Comment Tab

Any comments or notes pertinent to this patient's case may be entered into the Comment tab (Figure J-11 ◆).

EDI Tab

Information necessary for the processing or transmission of electronic data interchange (EDI) data is entered in the EDI tab (Figure J-12 ◆).

Adding the Insurance Carriers

If, when you are in the patient's Case window and entering the insurance carrier name, you notice the insurance carrier you are looking for is *not* in the drop-down list, you must go to the **Insurance Carrier List** to add it (Figure J-13 ◆). This can be accessed via a shortcut button or the Lists menu.

Click on the **New** button to add a new carrier name and address.

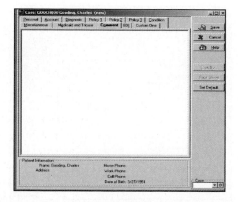

Figure J-11 ◆ Case window, Comment tab.

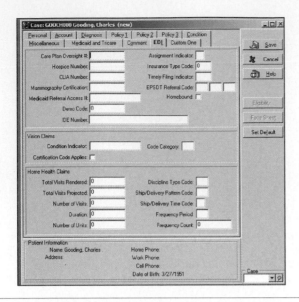

Figure J-12 ◆ Case Window, EDI tab.

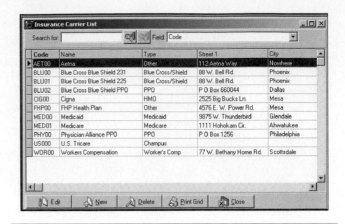

Figure J-13 ◆ Adding an insurance carrier in the Insurance Carrier window.

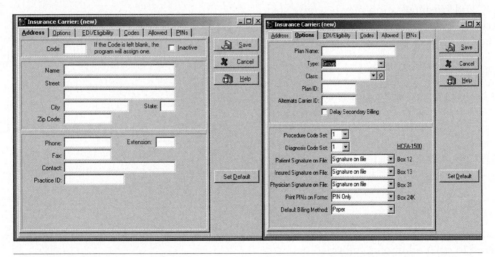

Figure J-14 ◆ New Insurance Carrier window, Address tab (left) and Options tab (right).

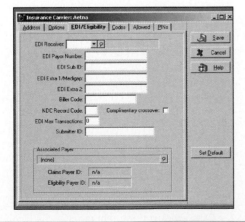

Figure J-15 ◆ Insurance Carrier window, EDI/Eligibility tab.

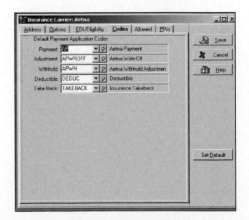

Figure J-16 ◆ Insurance Carrier window, Codes tab.

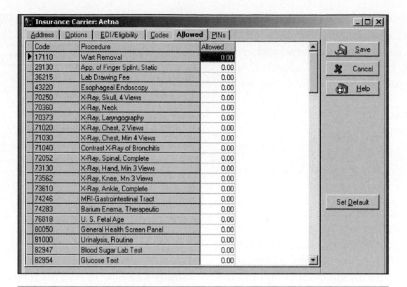

Figure J-17 ◆ Insurance Carrier window, Allowed tab.

In the **Address** tab of the new Insurance Carrier window, enter the insurance carrier's name, address, telephone number, fax number, and contact name if you have one (Figure J-14 ◆).

The **Options** tab in the new Insurance Carrier window is vitally important because it is here that you choose the insurance plan type and indicate whether or not "Signature On File" (SOF) should appear on the claim form. SOF indicates that you have the patient's authorization to release this information and that the patient has assigned benefits directly to the provider (Figure J-14). (So the payment for the claim will be sent directly to your provider and not the patient.) "Signature on File" should *always* appear on the claim forms you submit.

The **EDI/Eligibility** tab is used to enter important EDI information for that insurance carrier (Figure J-15 ◆).

The Codes tab is for entering default transactions codes (Figure J-16 ◆).

The Allowed tab may be used to enter the contractual allowed amount per procedure code for that particular insurance carrier (Figure J-17 ◆).

The **PINs** tab in the Insurance Carrier List is also very important (Figure J-18 ◆). You must first Save your new carrier, then go back in and Edit it to add the provider PINs. PINs are specific to each carrier. Be sure to enter the correct insurance carrier PIN for each participating provider. The appropriate qualifier should also be entered so that it prints on the CMS-1500 claim form.

Entering Employers

When entering patient and case information, it will be necessary to add the patient's or guarantor's employer name/address into Medisoft. This is accomplished in the **Address List,** which is accessed from the taskbar using the Address List shortcut button (Figure J-19 ◆).

The Address List contains not only employer addresses, but also referral sources (other than physicians), facility addresses, and attorney addresses (Figure J-20 ◆).

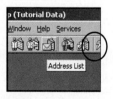

Figure J-19 ◆ Address List shortcut button on the taskbar.

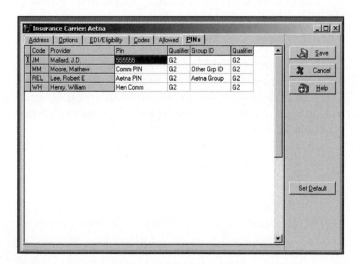

Figure J-18 ◆ Insurance Carrier window, PINs tab.

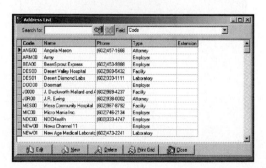

Figure J-20 ◆ Address List window.

Click on the **New** button to begin (Figure J-21 ◆). Add the employer name, address and telephone number.

If you are entering an employer (and not a referral source, etc.), in the Type field, be sure Employer is shown (Figure J-22 ◆). Click Save when you have finished entering the information.

You can now select the Employer name from the drop-down list in the Patient List or Case windows.

Reviewing a Completed Superbill

The completed superbill is the primary source of information a medical office specialist needs to record procedure charges. The completed superbill includes the following information: the provider's name, patient's name and chart/account number, date the services were performed, diagnosis, charge amounts, amount of payment received at the time of service, and the next appointment time needed.

After a physician completes a patient exam, he or she will place a check mark (or an X or circle) on the superbill next to the procedures performed. As you may recall, the superbill includes only the most common procedures provided by the medical office. If the physician performs a procedure not listed on the superbill, he or she writes the procedure in the "Other Procedures" area or in a blank space on the form.

Insurance carriers will not pay for treatment without a diagnosis code. The *diagnosis* is the physician's opinion of the patient's condition based on the examination. Therefore, the physician must record this information on the superbill so that it may be included as part of the procedure charge. If a procedure code or diagnosis is not marked on the superbill, you will need to ask the physician to mark it. Never demand that the physician do so and never accuse the physician of forgetting to mark the superbill. Always use respect and tact when addressing members of your medical practice.

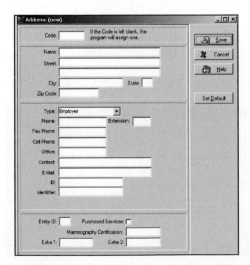

Figure J-21 ◆ New Address window.

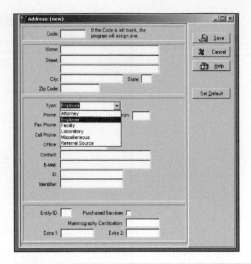

Figure J-22 ◆ In the Type field of the new Address window, be sure to choose "Employer" when entering a new employer.

Entering a Procedure Charge

After you review a patient's superbill, you are ready to enter the transaction into Medisoft to record the procedure charge and diagnosis code. You will process all transactions (charges, payments, and adjustments) in the **Transaction Entry** window. To access this window, you can use the **Activities** menu and click on Enter Transactions, click the **Transaction Entry** shortcut buttonor click the **Accounting** menu on the **Medisoft** side bar and choose Enter Transactions.

After you have opened the Transaction Entry window, *the first thing you must do is choose the correct patient's chart number and case number to post a charge to.*

Step 1: Choose a patient chart number and case number (Figure J-23 ◆).

Step 2: After the correct patient and case have been chosen, click on the **New** button in the *middle* of the screen (to access the top of the screen) (Figure J-24 ◆).

Medisoft will add today's date by default to the screen. If the date of service is not today's date, type the correct date in the Date field.

Click your mouse inside the **Procedure** field next to the date. A drop-down menu will be shown. You may either search for the correct procedure code marked on the superbill or type it in.

Once you have entered the CPT® code, press Enter or Tab to be taken to the Units field. Most of the time you will not need to change the default units entry.

Press Tab or Enter to move to the **Amount** field. Medisoft has already entered a dollar amount associated with that CPT code. If this amount is incorrect, key in the correct amount.

Press Tab or Enter again to be taken to the **DIAG1** field. Type in the primary diagnosis code or use the drop-down menu

CPT is a registered trademark of the American Medical Association.

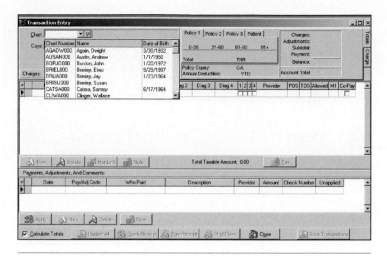

Figure J-23 ◆ Begin working in the Transaction Entry window by choosing a patient chart number and case number.

to search for the correct diagnosis. You may enter up to four diagnosis codes per charge transaction.

Tab over to the **Provider** field to make sure the correct provider is being credited with seeing this patient.

The **POS** (place of service) and **TOS** (type of service) fields will automatically be filled in based on the information in the CPT code database.

The **Allowed** amount field is also completed by default per information in the CPT code and insurance database.

The **M1** field is used to enter a two-character CPT modifier if one is marked on the patient superbill.

Complete all of these steps again to enter another procedure charge.

When you have finished entering charges, click on the **Save Transactions** button at the lower right of the screen or the **Update All** button near the lower left side of the window. When the Update All button is used to save transactions, the Medisoft program checks all fields for missing or invalid information and will display a message if information is needed or invalid.

Posting a Payment

When the patient (or his or her insurance carrier) makes a payment on the patient's account, you must enter this into the accounting software. Payments are posted in the **Transaction Entry** window (Figure J-25 ◆). Remember, you cannot enter a transaction without first choosing a patient chart number and case number. It is important to make sure you have chosen the correct case—especially when posting payments from insurance carriers.

After opening the Transaction Entry window and choosing the appropriate chart and case number, click on the **New** button toward the *bottom* of the window within the Payments, Adjustments, And Comments section.

Medisoft will start a new entry by adding today's date.

Click in the **Pay/Adj Code** field and choose the method of payment (personal check, cash, Aetna payment, etc.).

Tab over to the **Who Paid** field and choose the party that is making the payment.

Enter a description if necessary.

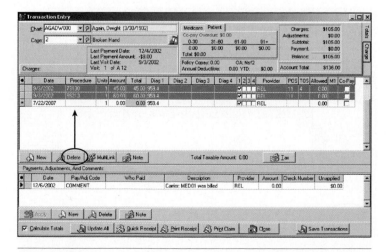

Figure J-24 ◆ After choosing the correct patient and case, choose the New button from the middle of the screen.

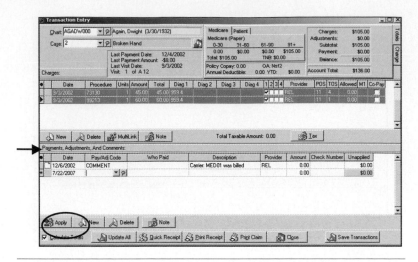

Figure J-25 ◆ Posting payments in the Transaction Entry window.

Make sure the correct provider is shown in the **Provider** field.

Enter the amount of the payment in the **Amount** field. Enter a check number if appropriate in the next field.

Next, *you must apply the payment to the correct charge(s)*. To do this, click on the **Apply** button at the bottom left-hand side of the window, to the left of the New button (Figure J-26 ◆).

A new window will open on top of your Transaction Entry window. This is the **Apply Payment to Charges** window. It is here that you can apply the payment to a specific charge or charges. This is called *line item posting*.

It is most important to post the payment to the correct date of service and the correct procedure code. One payment can be divided among many charges if it is "broken down" that way on the EOB/ERA or the patient has many separate charges and is paying for all of them.

When you have applied the payment to the correct charge(s), click the **Close** button at the bottom of the Apply Payment to Chargeswindow.

Your **Unapplied** column in the Payment, Adjustment, And Comments section of the Transaction Entry window should read $0.00 if you applied the entire payment. (A patient's account may have an unapplied balance if he or she is prepaying on surgery, for example.) You must now save the payment transaction.

Click on the **Update All** or **Save Transactions** button at the bottom of the window.

Posting an Adjustment

Entering an adjustment into a patient's account is similar to entering a payment and is also performed in the **Transaction Entry** window. To begin, you must first choose the patient chart number and case number.

Click on the **New** button towards the *bottom* of the window.

Medisoft will start a new transaction by entering today's date by default.

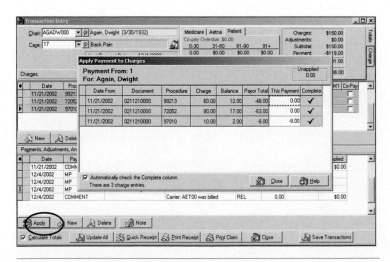

Figure J-26 ◆ Applying a payment to the correct charges.

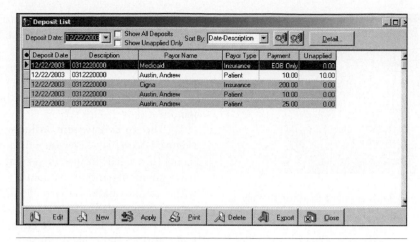

Figure J-27 ◆ Deposit List window (Enter Deposits and Apply Payments).

In the **Pay/Adj Code** field, select the correct type of adjustment (insurance write-off, charge reversal, courtesy discount, etc.).

Tab over to the **Description** entry field and type a note about why the adjustment is needed.

Tab over to the **Provider** field and choose the correct provider, then tab over to the **Amount** field.

If you are *subtracting* an amount from the patient's account, you will need to enter a *minus (–)* sign before typing the amount. If you are adding an amount to a patient's account, you do not need to enter a plus sign before the amount.

Note: Medisoft will assume all adjustments are positive unless you type in a minus (–) sign before the amount.

When you have entered the amount, click on the **Apply** button at the bottom left of the Transaction Entry window.

When you are applying the adjustment, make sure to choose the correct date(s) of service and CPT code(s). *You must enter a minus sign before the amount in the Apply Adjustment to Charges window.*If you do not, Medisoft will *add* the amount to the patient's account.

When you have entered all of the adjustments, click on the **Close** button to take you back to the Transaction Entry window.

To save all of your hard work, be sure to click on **Update All** or **Save Transactions.**

Using the Enter Deposits and Apply Payments Window

It is easiest to post payments that patients make at the time of service in the Transaction Entry window. However, if you receive a large insurance check that covers claims for many different patients, it is easier to post this in the **Enter Deposits and Apply Payments** window. This window can be accessed by clicking the **Enter Deposits and Apply Payments** shortcut button, opening the **Activities** menu and choosing Apply Deposits/Payments, or by clicking on the **Accounting** shortcut button on the **Medisoft** side bar and choosing Enter Deposits/Payments. A Deposit List window will open (Figure J-27 ◆) that contains the following fields:

Deposit Date: The current date is automatically entered. It can be changed by typing a different date in the field.

Show All Deposits: This check box displays all payments entered regardless of date.

Show Unapplied Only: If this box is checked, only the payments that have not been fully applied to charges are shown.

Sort By: This is a drop-down list that allows you to sort deposits by amount, patient chart number, and payer.

Locate and Locate Next: These shortcut buttons allow you to search for a particular deposit.

Detail: This button is used to view a specific deposit in more detail. Highlight the deposit in the window and then click the Detail button.

To enter a new deposit, click on the **New** button at the bottom of the Deposit List window. After the New Deposit window opens (Figure J-28 ◆), you must choose a **Payor Type** (patient, insurance carrier, capitation).

Choose the **Payment Method** (check, cash, credit card, electronic) and Enter or Tab over to the **Check Number** field to enter the check number.

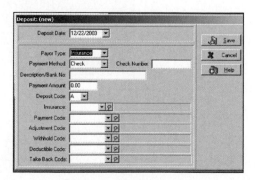

Figure J-28 ◆ New Deposit window.

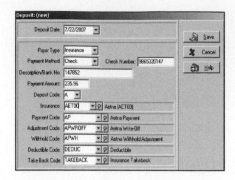

Figure J-29 ◆ The various code fields are filled in automatically when the insurance carrier is selected from the Insurance drop-down box.

The **Description/Bank No.** field is used to enter an (optional) description of the check.

Enter the dollar amount of the payment in the **Payment Amount** field.

The **Deposit Code** drop-down menu is used by some practices to sort deposits according to practice-defined categories.

Select the insurance carrier making payment from the drop-down menu in the **Insurance** field.

After you have selected the carrier, the other **Code** fields are automatically completed (Figure J-29 ◆).

When finished, click **Save.**

After entering the check information, the next step is to apply the payment.

Click the **Apply** button at the bottom of the Deposit List window.

The **Apply Payment/Adjustments to Charges** window (Figure J-30 ◆) is where you will apply payments and adjustments (if needed) to specific patient accounts. You are able to enter payments and adjustments as well as deductibles and withhold information at virtually the same time.

When you have finished entering payment information on one patient, click the **Save Payments/Adjustments** button at the bottom right side of the window.

If you have the **Print Statements Now** box at the bottom of the window checked, after clicking Save, Medisoft will ask what type of statement you would like to print.

If you have another patient to apply payments to, follow the same steps as before.

The **Unapplied Amount** indicator in the top right-hand corner of the window will allow you to keep track of how much you have posted and how much you still have to post (Figure J-31 ◆).

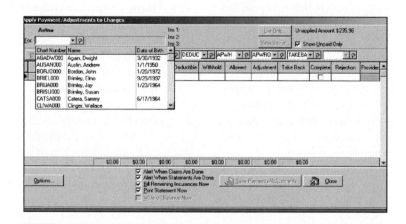

Figure J-30 ◆ The Apply Payments/Adjustments to Charges window.

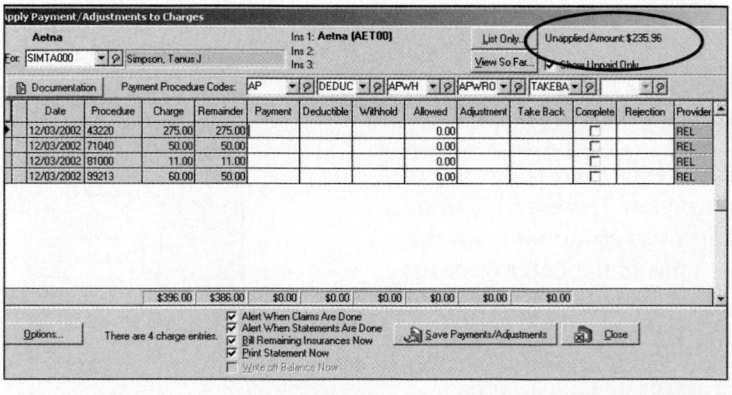

Figure J-31 ◆ The Unapplied Amount indicate tells you how much of a deposit remains to be posted.

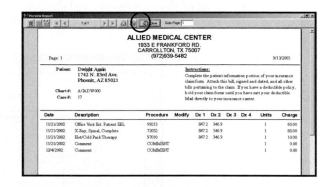

Figure J-32 ◆ Quick Receipt button.

Walkout Receipts

Throughout the simulation at the end of this appendix, you will be responsible for printing a walkout receipt for each patient who has seen the provider. This task is performed in the Transaction Entry window.

After you have posted the patient's charges and/or payments, click the **Quick Receipt** button at the bottom of the window to print a receipt for today's visit only (Figure J-32 ◆). A **Print Report Where?** window will open. After choosing to print to the printer, the receipt will automatically print.

If the patient would like a more comprehensive receipt (one that includes previous visits), click the **Print Receipt** button instead.

When the **Open Report** window opens, choose Walkout Receipt (All Transactions), then click the OK button (Figure J-33 ◆). A **Print Report Where?** window opens after you have clicked OK (Figure J-34 ◆).

After selecting where to print the report, a **Data Selection Questions** window opens. Choose the date ranges for your receipt and click the OK button.

If you choose to preview the report on the screen, you will see a screen similar to that shown in Figure J-35 ◆. To print from the preview screen, click the picture of the printer across the top of the screen. To close the preview screen, click the Close button.

Printing Reports in Medisoft

Let's take a moment to discuss the different reports available in Medisoft.

Patient Day Sheet Report

The Patient Day Sheet report can be accessed in either of two ways: by clicking on the **Reports** menu or by clicking the **Daily Reports** menu on the **Medisoft** side bar.

For the simulation that follows, you will be instructed to stop entering transactions and "batch out." You will need to compile and run the Patient Day Sheet report. This report, as stated earlier in the text, shows all transactions posted in the database for the day. For our purposes, we will use "today's" date.

After clicking on **Patient Day Sheet** in the Reports menu (Figure J-36 ◆), a **Print Report Where?** window will open. After choosing where to print the report (our example printed it to

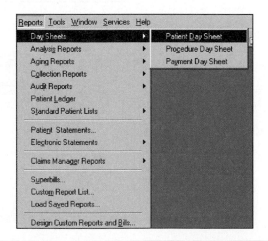

Figure J-35 ◆ Sample walkout receipt.

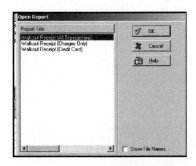

Figure J-33 ◆ Open Report window.

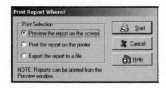

Figure J-34 ◆ Print Report Where? window.

Figure J-36 ◆ Selecting the Patient Day Sheet report from the Reports drop-down menu.

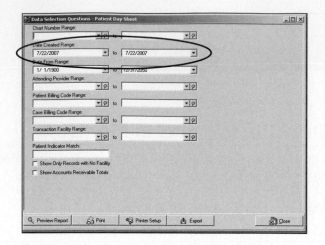

Figure J-37 ◆ Data Selection Questions for Patient Day Sheet Reports.

the screen), another window/dialog box will open: **Data Selection Questions: Patient Day Sheet** (Figure J-37 ◆).

Click in the **Date Created Range** field and choose **today's date** for both the From and To boxes, then click the OK button.

Using the arrows at the top of the screen, go to the last page of the report for your totals. Your totals here should match your totals from all the superbills/EOBs you posted throughout the day (Figure J-38 ◆).

Creating and Printing Insurance Claims

During the simulation that follows, you will be responsible for printing paper CMS-1500 claim forms at the end of each day for the patients' accounts you posted charges to. This task is accomplished in the **Claim Management** window.

The Claim Management window can be accessed by clicking the **Claim Management** shortcut button, clicking the **Accounting** button on the **Medisoft** side bar, or by opening the **Activities** menu and clicking Claim Management.

After opening the Claim Management window, the first thing to do is create the insurance claims you want to send. To do this you click the **Create Claims** button at the bottom of the window (Figure J-39 ◆).

The majority of medical practices print claims several times a week. You will notice, again, that you can sort your claim report many different ways: by transaction dates, chart numbers, primary insurance carrier—you can even create claims for one particular provider name. For the simulation you will be using today's date in the **Transaction Dates** field (Figure J-40 ◆). After entering the dates, click the **Create** button on the right side of the window.

As you create a claim, the Claim Management window will be automatically updated. It will show the claims you've just created as "Ready to Send" in the Status 1 column of the Claim Management window (Figure J-41 ◆).

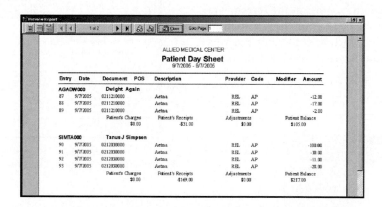

Figure J-38 ◆ Sample Patient Day Sheet report.

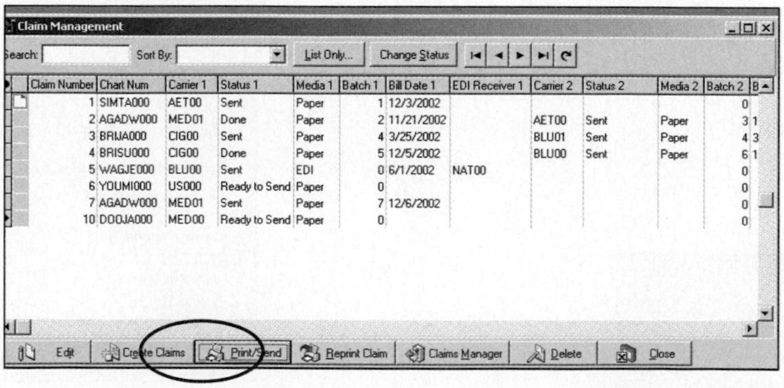

Figure J-39 ◆ To process new insurance claims, click the Create Claims button in the Claim Management window.

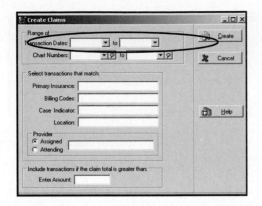

Figure J-40 ◆ The Transaction Dates field in the Create Claims window.

The next step is to look over your claims *before* you print them to make sure they are "clean" claims (meaning no information is missing and all information is correct).

To do this, click on the **Print/Send** button at the *bottom* of the Claim Management window (Figure J-42 ◆).

A Print/Send Claims window will open asking you to choose how you wish to send the claims, either on paper or electronically. For our simulation, you will choose the Paper method for claims. Click the OK button on the right side of the window (Figure J-43 ◆).

An Open Report window will open next (Figure J-44 ◆). If you are printing Medicare claims, you will need to choose the CMS-1500 (Primary) Medicare Centuryreport option. If you are printing claims for any other carrier, choose the CMS-1500 (Primary)report option. It is important to choose the

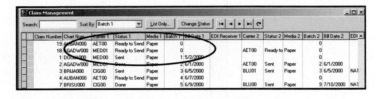

Figure J-41 ◆ The Status 1 column indicates which newly created claims are ready to send to insurance carriers.

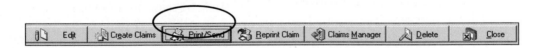

Figure J-42 ◆ Print/Send button at the bottom of the Claim Management window.

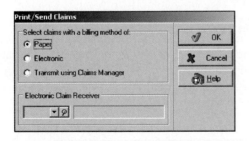

Figure J-43 ◆ Print/Send Claims window.

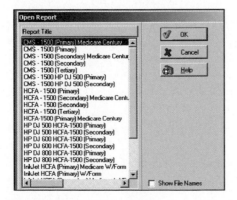

Figure J-44 ◆ Open Report window.

correct report type for claims. Medicare prefers a minimum of information on claims, so be sure to choose the correct report/claim format when submitting claims to Medicare. After choosing the report style, click the OK button.

When the **Print Report Where?** window opens, choose to **Preview the report on the screen** and click Start (Figure J-45 ◆). You will look over the claims on the screen to be sure they are clean before printing.

A Data Selection Questions dialog box will open for you to choose which claims you want to preview. Use today's date in the **Date Created Range** fields. You can "filter" those claims you would like to review. Filtering is selecting certain criteria. For example, you may choose to only review claims for a particular insurance carrier (e.g. Medicaid). In order to do that,

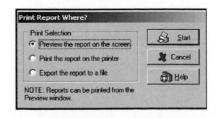

Figure J-45 ◆ Preview the report on the screen.

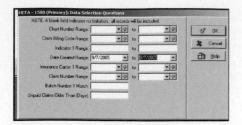

Figure J-46 ◆ Data Selection Questions dialog box.

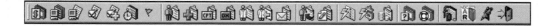

Figure J-47 ◆ Sample CMS-1500 Primary claim printed to screen. Note that the locator boxes do not show on screen.

you would select the name of the insurance carrier from the drop down menu from the Insurance Carrier 1 Range boxes. This would filter out all the other insurance carrier claims and only show you the claims for the carrier you chose from the drop down menu. You can filter claims by Chart Number Range, Claim Billing Code Range or Claim Number Range. After choosing your filters, click OK (Figure J-46 ◆). If you want to see all claims created, complete only the Date Created Range boxes.

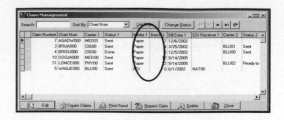

Figure J-48 ◆ Medisoft will update your Claim Management window to indicate that the claims have been sent.

The claims will be shown on the screen in the format you chose. Note that the CMS-1500 locator boxes will not actually show on the screen because they are instead printed on the blank claim form originals that you will insert into your printer when you're ready to print claims. However, you may want to refer to a blank printed claim form while checking your claims on screen to see if any information is missing (Figure J-47 ◆).

Once you have checked all of your claims and corrected any mistakes if necessary, you are ready to print your claims on CMS-1500 forms that you have loaded into your printer's paper tray.

After you have printed your claims, Medisoft will update your Claim Management window (Status 1 column) to show that the claims have been sent (on paper or electronically) (Figure J-48 ◆).

Table J-1 shows the relationship between the form locators on the CMS-1500 claim form and the dialog boxes in Medisoft. If, when looking over the claim forms before printing, you notice data missing on the claim, consult this table to discern where to enter it in Medisoft.

Medisoft Shortcut Buttons

The Shortcut Button toolbar is a quick way to navigate to the most commonly used windows/areas within Medisoft. As a helpful reminder, each button is labeled here with a brief description of what the window is used for.

TABLE J-1 PATIENT/GUARANTOR AND PROVIDER INFORMATION AND THE CMS-1500 FORM

PATIENT/GUARANTOR INFORMATION AND THE CMS-1500 FORM

CMS Form Locator	Medisoft		
	DIALOG BOX	TAB (in Dialog Box)	FIELD (in Dialog Box)
1	Insurance Carrier	Options	Type
1a	Case	Policy	Policy Number
2	Patient/Guarantor	Name, Address	Last Name, First Name, Middle Initial
3	Patient/Guarantor	Name, Address	Birth Date, Sex
4	Case	Policy	Policy Holder
5	Patient/Guarantor	Name, Address	Street, City, State, Zip Code, Phones
6	Case	Policy	Relationship to Insured
7	Patient/Guarantor	Name, Address	Street, City, State, ZIP Code, Phones
8	Case	Personal	Marital Status
8	Patient/Guarantor	Other Information	Employment Status
9	Patient/Guarantor	Name, Address	Last Name, First Name, Middle Initial
9a	Case	Policy	Policy Number
9b	Patient/Guarantor	Name, Address	Birth Date, Sex
9c	Patient/Guarantor	Other Information	Employer
9d	Insurance Carrier	Options	Plan Name
10a	Case	Condition	Employment Related
10b	Case	Condition	Accident Related To
10c	Case	Condition	Accident Related To
10d	Case	Miscellaneous	Local Use A, Local Use B
11	Case	Policy	Policy Number
11a	Patient/Guarant or	Name, Address	Birth Date, Sex
11b	Patient/Guarantor	Other Information	Employer
11c	Insurance Carrier	Options	Plan Name
11d	Case	Policy 2	Insurance 2
12	Patient/Guarantor	Other Information	Signature on File
13	Patient/Guarantor	Other Information	Signature on File

PROVIDER INFORMATION AND THE CMS-1500 FORM

CMS Form Locator	Medisoft		
	DIALOG BOX	TAB (in Dialog Box)	FIELD (in Dialog Box)
14	Case	Condition	Injury/Illness/LMP Date
15	Case	Condition	Same/Similar Symptoms and First Consultation Date
16	Case	Condition	Dates Unable to Work
17	Referring Provider	Address	First Name, Middle Initial, Last Name
17a	Referring Provider	NPI, Qualifiers, PINs, and IDs	Varies with carrier
17b			
18	Case	Condition	Hospitalization
19	Case	Miscellaneous	Local Use A, Local Use B
20	Case	Miscellaneous	Outside Lab Work and Lab Charges
21	Case	Diagnosis	Default Diagnosis 1–4
22	Case	Medicaid	Resubmission Number and Original Reference
23	Case	Miscellaneous	Prior Authorization Number
24A	Transaction Entry	Charge	Dates
24B	Procedure Code	General	Place of Service
24C	Emergency	Condition	Emergency check box
24D	Transaction Entry	Charge	Procedure and Modifiers
24E	Transaction Entry	Charge	Default Diagnosis 1–4
24F	Transaction Entry	Charge	Amount
24G	Transaction Entry	Charge	Units
24H	Case Provider List/Insurance	Medicaid	EPSDT
24I	Carrier List	PINS	PINs/National Identifier
24J			
25	Provider	PINs and IDs	SSN/Federal Tax ID
26	Patient/Guarantor	Name, Address or Other Information	Chart Number or Patient ID #2
27	Case	Policy	Accept Assignment or Transaction Default
28	Transaction Entry	Charge	Amount
29	Transaction Entry	Payment	Amount
30	Transaction Entry		Case Balance
31	Provider	Address	Signature on File
32	Case	Account	Facility
33	Provider	PINs and IDs	Last Name, Middle Initial, First Name, Street, City, State, Zip Code, Phone

Transaction Entry—Use this window to post charges, payments, and adjustments in patient accounts.

 Claim Management—Use this window to create, print, and send insurance claims.

 Statement Management—Use this window to print and send statements.

 Collection List—Use this window to check on open accounts that require collection follow-up and add tickler notes.

 Add Collection List Items—Use this window to add multiple collection items at once to the Collection List based on specific criteria chosen from the screen.

 Appointment Book—Use this window to set appointments for the practice's providers.

 View Eligibility Verification Results—This feature allows the facility to check a patient's insurance coverage online. It is a fee-based service for which the facility must enroll.

 Patient/Case (Guarantor) List—Use this window to add or edit patient, guarantor, or case information.

 Insurance Carrier List—Use this window to add or edit insurance carriers in the Medisoft database.

 Procedure Code List—Use this window to edit or add procedure, payment, or adjustment codes in the Medisoft database.

 Diagnosis Code List—Use this window to add or edit diagnostic codes in the Medisoft database.

 Provider List—Use this window to add or edit practice providers in the Medisoft database.

 Referring Provider List—Use this window to add or edit names of physicians that refer patients to the practice.

 Address List—Use this window to add or edit patient/guarantor, employer, attorney, or facility names to the Medisoft database.

 Patient Recall List—Use this window to enter appointment recall information.

 Custom Report List—Use this window to view every report choice in Medisoft database.

 Quick Ledger—Use this window to quickly view any patient's full financial ledger.

 Quick Balance—Use this window to view any patient's financial balance.

 Enter Deposits and Apply Payments—Use this window as an alternative way to enter patient/guarantor or insurance payments to patients' accounts.

 Show/Hide Hints

 Medisoft Help Menu

 Edit Patient Notes in Final Draft—If notes were entered anywhere in the system, they may be edited here.

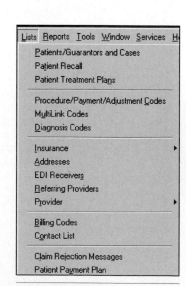 **Launch Advanced Reporting**—Advanced Reporting provides users with enhanced reporting and data viewing capabilities including ad hoc reporting and a set of standard reports that may be customized by users with the report writer.

 LAUNCH Work Administrator—The Work Administrator program lets the staff streamline the work process. Use this feature to organize tasks for users and user groups.

 Exit Medisoft Program

Medisoft Menus

Each Medisoft menu is shown here as a navigation reminder. Each menu was explained on page 475.

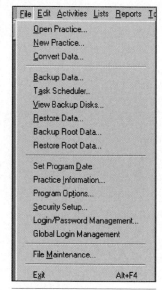

File menu.

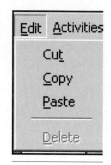

Edit menu.

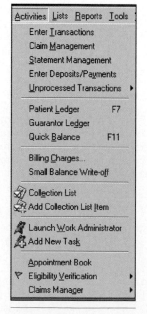

Activities menu.

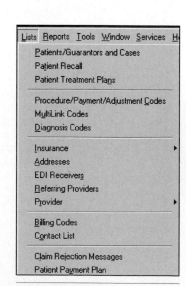

Lists menu.

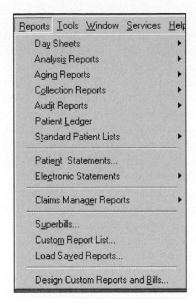

Reports menu.

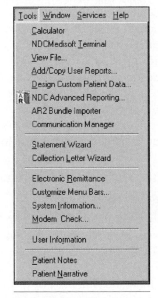

Tools menu.

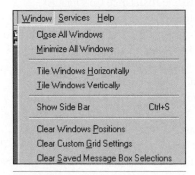

Window menu.

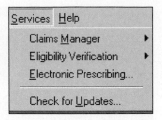

Services menu.

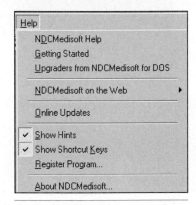

Help menu.

Medisoft Side Bar Shortcut Menus

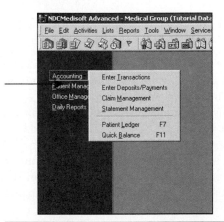

Accounting menu

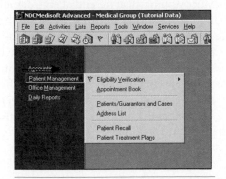

Patient Management menu.

......

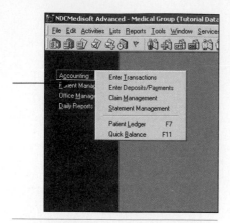

Office Management menu.

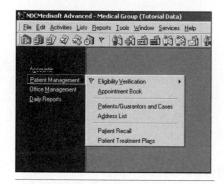

Daily Reports menu.

Simulation Instructions

Please use the patient information forms, encounter forms, and Explanation of Benefits forms located at the end of this appendix to complete this simulation exercise.

For this simulation, you are the medical business office specialist for your medical practice. It is your job to enter all patient demographic information, post charges, payments, and adjustments. **It is necessary to enter the ICD-9 and CPT codes and charges exactly as they appear on the superbills.** This may require you to enter them into the Medisoft database (as a new code) as well as the specific patient's account.

You are responsible for printing a walkout receipt for each patient's account to which you post charges. It is your responsibility to balance your batch at the end of each day and to print insurance claim forms for the patients with insurance.

Some patients may need to come back to the office for follow-up appointments. This will be noted at the bottom of the superbill. If a return appointment is needed, you will need to schedule the appointment for the patient (in Office Hours).

Before class ends each day, you may be instructed to stop posting transactions and "batch out." Access the **Reports** menu and run the **Patient Day Sheet** report for today's date. After

CPT is a registered trademark of the American Medical Association.

printing your report, you will use it to make sure you "balance." To do this, you must separately add up all the charges, payments and adjustments from all the superbills (or EOBs) you posted during the day. Your charges should add up to the amount on the **Total Charges** line on the Patient Day Sheet report. Your payments should equal the negative amount on the **Total Receipts** line of the report, and your adjustments should match the **Total Adjustments** line. If the amounts you totaled from your superbills/EOBs do not match the report totals, you will need to go over the report patient by patient as you look at each patient superbill/EOB to find the discrepancy.

After you have balanced your totals, your instructor may require you to batch your superbills/EOBs and correct Patient Day Sheet report together and turn them in before you leave each day. If this is the case, it means you will have to remove or copy the superbills/EOBs you posted from your textbook. The Patient Day Sheet report is to be placed on top of your superbills/EOBs, followed by your walkout receipts, and stapled together.

Once your batch is complete, it is time to create insurance claims for the patients for whom you entered transaction information. Medisoft allows you to view your insurance claims on screen prior to printing them or sending them electronically. You must look over the claims on the computer screen to make sure there are no errors. If you find any errors, close the claims window and go back to the specific patient's account in the computer and correct it. The claim will automatically be updated with the corrected information. Check your electronic claim batch again to make sure all claims are correct. When you are sure there are no errors, print the claims.

Paper clip your CMS-1500 forms to the bottom of your batch material and turn it in to your instructor.

Tips for Entering Information into Medisoft Advanced

1. First, look over the patient information form. Check the Address List to see if the employer name is already listed in Medisoft. If it is not, add the employer to the Address List.
2. Check the Insurance Carrier List to see if the patient's primary and secondary insurance carrier is already listed in Medisoft. Remember the insurance carrier address must be **exactly the same** as what is written on the patient information form. If the carrier is not listed, add the carrier(s) to the Insurance Carrier List.
3. Check to see if the patient has a Referring Physician (or PCP) listed on the patient information form. If one is listed, check the Referring Provider List to see if the physician is already listed in Medisoft. If the provider is not listed, add the provider.
4. Add the patient to the Patient/Guarantor List if the patient is new. If the patient is not the guarantor, add the guarantor to the Patient/Guarantor List.
5. Make a new Case for the patient. Entering the employer, insurance carrier, and referring provider **prior** to making a patient case allows you to have all the data already

entered when you come to the drop down menus (in the case and the patient/guarantor list) for employer, insurance carrier, etc. This saves the hassle of closing the patient case, opening the Address Book (or Insurance Carrier List, etc.), adding the data, saving and closing the window and then opening the patient case again.

Before beginning the simulation, you will need to enter your physician's information into the Medisoft database. Open the **Provider List** (accessed either by shortcut button or Lists menu) and click **New.**

Enter the following information in the *Address* folder in the window:

Your Name
1933 E. Frankford Rd. #110
office telephone: 972-555-5482
home phone: 214-555-8888
Carrollton, TX 12345
cell phone: 469-555-3657
fax: 972-555-5416
Medicare Participating, Signature on File
License no.: B1740
Specialty: General Practice

In the *Default PINs* folder enter: 75-1234567 for Federal Tax ID Indicator

Medicare PIN: B94765
Medicaid: K89J2
UPIN: B94765
NPI: 1234569860

Be sure to save any data entered. All of the patients you enter during the simulation will be seeing you.

There are two more things to do before you begin. Open the File menu in Medisoft and click on Practice Information. Click in the Practice name box. Enter your name as Your Name Medical Clinic.

Click the Save button on the right side of the window.

Go the Address List and enter a new Facility. The facility will be Your Name Medical Clinic, with the address on Frankford Road that you entered for the Practice Name. Click Save and exit the Address List.

You are ready to begin the simulation.

Allied Medical Center
REGISTRATION FORM
(Please Print)

Today's date: _____   PCP: _____

PATIENT INFORMATION

Patient's last name: DUPONT	First: MARGARET	Middle: B	☐ Mr. ☒ Mrs.	☐ Miss ☐ Ms.	Marital status (circle one) Single / (Mar) / Div / Sep / Wid

Is this your legal name? ☒ Yes ☐ No	If not, what is your legal name?	(Former name):	Birth date: 09/21/1946	Age:	Sex: ☐ M ☒ F

Street address: 12 BRIAR LANE	Social Security no.: 717-87-0054	Home phone no.: (214) 555-9871

P.O. box:	City: DALLAS	State: TX	ZIP Code: 12345

Occupation: MANAGER	Employer: SHARON'S BRIDAL SHOPPE	Employer phone no.: (214) 555-8878

Chose clinic because/Referred to clinic by (please check one box): ☐ Dr.   ☒ Insurance Plan   ☐ Hospital

☐ Family   ☐ Friend   ☐ Close to home/work   ☐ Yellow Pages   Other

Other family members seen here: LISA DUPONT	**REASON FOR THIS VISIT:** Persistent cough

INSURANCE INFORMATION

(Please give your insurance card to the receptionist.)

Person responsible for bill: SELF	Birth date: / /	Address (if different):	Home phone no.: ( )

Is this person a patient here? ☒ Yes ☐ No

Occupation:	Employer:	Employer address:	Employer phone no.: ( )

Is this patient covered by insurance? ☒ Yes ☐ No

Please indicate primary insurance:	PHYSICIAN ALLIANCE PPO	Claims Mailing Address:	P O BOX 1256	Philadelphia, PA	12345
		PHONE: 800-555-5522			

Subscriber's name: SELF	Subscriber's S.S. no.:	Birth date: / /	☐ M ☐ F	Group no.: A435	Policy no.: 621382	Co-payment: $10.00

Patient's relationship to subscriber: ☒ Self ☐ Spouse ☐ Child ☐ Other

Name of secondary insurance (if applicable): BLUE CROSS BLUE SHIELD TX PPO	Subscriber's name and DOB: FRANK DUPONT 07/21/1941	☒ M ☐ F	Group no.: 126	Policy no.: BHR716830061

Patient's relationship to subscriber: ☐ Self ☒ Spouse ☐ Child ☐ Other   Claims Mailing Address: P O BOX 660044 DALLAS 12345

IN CASE OF EMERGENCY

Name of local friend or relative (not living at same address): SHARON THELANER	Relationship to patient: SISTER	Home phone no.: (469) 555-3259	Work phone no.: (817) 555-8114

The above information is true to the best of my knowledge. I authorize my insurance benefits to be paid directly to the physician. I understand that I am financially responsible for any balance. I also authorize ALLIED MEDICAL CENTER or insurance company to release any information required to process my claims.

Maggie Dupont

_____   _____
Patient/Guardian signature   Date

ENCOUNTER FORM

Patient Information		Payment Method		Visit Information	
Patient ID number		**Primary**	Physician's Alliance	Visit date	
Patient name	Margaret Dupont	Primary ID number	621382	Visit number	
Address	12 Briar Lane	Primary group number	A435	Rendering physician	
City/State	Dallas, TX 12345	**Secondary**	BCBS TX	Referring physician	
Phone number	214-555-9871	Secondary ID number	BHR716830061	Reason for visit	Cough
Date of birth	09/21/1946	Secondary group no.	126		
Age		Cash/credit card			
		Other billing			

E/M Modifiers	Procedure Modifiers	DIAGNOSIS:
21 — Prolonged E&M Service	22 — Unusual, excessive procedure	
24 — Unrelated E/M service during postop.	50 — Bilateral procedure	ACUTE SINUSITIS 461.9
25 — Significant, separately identifiable E/M	51 — Multiple surgical procedures in same day	
32 — Mandated Service	52 — Reduced/incomplete procedure	
57 — Decision for surgery	55 — Postop. management only	
	59 — Distinct multiple procedures	

CATEGORY	CODE	MOD	FEE	CATEGORY	CODE	MOD	FEE
Office Visit — New Patient				**Wound Care**			
Minimal office visit	99201			Debride partial thickness burn	11040		
20 minutes	99202			Debride full thickness burn	11041		
30 minutes	99203			Debride wound, not a burn	11000		
45 minutes	99204	X	135.00	Unna boot application	29580		
60 minutes	99205			Unna boot removal	29700		
Other				Other			
Office Visit — Established				**Supplies**			
Minimal office visit	99211			Ace bandage, 2"	A6448		
10 minutes	99212			Ace bandage, 3"-4"	A6449		
15 minutes	99213			Ace bandage, 6"	A6450		
25 minutes	99214			Cast, fiberglass	A4590		
40 minutes	99215			Coban wrap	A6454		
Other				Foley catheter	A4338		
General Procedures				Immobilizer	L3670		
Anoscopy	46600			Kerlix roll	A6220		
Audiometry	92551			Oxygen mask/cannula	A4620		
Breast aspiration	19000			Sleeve, elbow	E0191		
Cerumen removal	69210			Sling	A4565		
Circumcision	54150			Splint, ready-made	A4570		
DDST	96110			Splint, wrist	S8451		
Flex sigmoidoscopy	45330			Sterile packing	A6407		
Flex sig. w/ biopsy	45331			Surgical tray	A4550		
Foreign body removal—foot	28190			Other			
Nail removal	11730			**OB Care**			
Nail removal/phenol	11750			Routine OB care	59400		
Trigger point injection	20552			Postpartum care only (separate procedure)	59430		
Tympanometry	92567			Ante partum 4–6 visits	59425		
Visual acuity	99173			Ante partum 7 or more visits	59426		
Other				Other			
Other				Other			

Other Visit Information: _____

Lab Work to Order: _____

Referral to: _____

Provider Signature: _____

Next Appointment: _____ RETURN IN A FEW DAYS IF NOT BETTER

Fees:

Total Charges: $ 135.00

Copay Received: $ 10.00

Other Payment: $_____

Total Due: **$125.00**

Allied Medical Center
REGISTRATION FORM
(Please Print)

Today's date: _____ PCP: _____

PATIENT INFORMATION

Patient's last name:	First:	Middle:	☐ Mr. ☐ Mrs.	☐ Miss ☐ Ms.	Marital status (circle one)
SMYTH	SAMANTHA	M			(Single) / Mar / Div / Sep / Wid

Is this your legal name? ☐ Yes ☐ No	If not, what is your legal name?	(Former name):	Birth date: 03/17/1968	Age:	Sex: ☐ M ☒ F

Street address: 9401 Winding Valley	Social Security no.: 455-94-8204	Home phone no.: (972) 555-9871

P.O. box:	City: PLANO	State: TX	ZIP Code: 12345

Occupation: FOOD SERVER	Employer: WENDY'S HAMBURGERS	Employer phone no.: (972) 555-8936

Chose clinic because/Referred to clinic by (please check one box): ☐ Dr. ☐ Insurance Plan ☐ Hospital

☐ Family ☐ Friend ☐ Close to home/work ☐ Yellow Pages Other

Other family members seen here: _____ **REASON FOR THIS VISIT:** Cholesterol check

INSURANCE INFORMATION
(Please give your insurance card to the receptionist.)

Person responsible for bill: SAMANTHA SMYTH	Birth date: 03/17/1968	Address (if different): same	Home phone no.: ( )

Is this person a patient here? ☐ Yes ☐ No

Occupation:	Employer:	Employer address:	Employer phone no.: ( )

Is this patient covered by insurance? ☐ Yes ☐ No

Please indicate primary insurance:	NONE	Claims Mailing Address:	
		PHONE:	

Subscriber's name:	Subscriber's S.S. no.:	Birth date: / /	☐ M ☐ F	Group no.:	Policy no.:	Co-payment: $

Patient's relationship to subscriber: ☐ Self ☐ Spouse ☐ Child ☐ Other

Name of secondary insurance (if applicable):	Subscriber's name and DOB:	☐ M ☐ F	Group no.:	Policy no.:

Patient's relationship to subscriber: ☐ Self ☐ Spouse ☐ Child ☐ Other Claims Mailing Address:

IN CASE OF EMERGENCY

Name of local friend or relative (not living at same address): CARRIE TINKHAM	Relationship to patient: FRIEND	Home phone no.: (972) 555-1502	Work phone no.: (972) 555-0074

The above information is true to the best of my knowledge. I authorize my insurance benefits to be paid directly to the physician. I understand that I am financially responsible for any balance. I also authorize ALLIED MEDICAL CENTER or insurance company to release any information required to process my claims.

Samantha Smyth

Patient/Guardian signature _____ _Date_

ENCOUNTER FORM

Patient Information		Payment Method		Visit Information	
Patient ID number		**Primary**		Visit date	
Patient name	Samantha Smyth	Primary ID number		Visit number	
Address	9401 Winding Valley	Primary group number		Rendering physician	
City/State	Plano, TX 12345	**Secondary**		Referring physician	
Phone number	972-555-9871	Secondary ID number		Reason for visit	Cholesterol Check
Date of birth	03/17/1968	Secondary group no.			
Age		Cash/credit card	CHECK		
		Other billing			

E/M Modifiers	Procedure Modifiers	DIAGNOSIS:
21 — Prolonged E&M Service	22 — Unusual, excessive procedure	Hypercholesteremia 272.00
24 — Unrelated E/M service during postop.	50 — Bilateral procedure	
25 — Significant, separately identifiable E/M	51 — Multiple surgical procedures in same day	
32 — Mandated Service	52 — Reduced/incomplete procedure	
57 — Decision for surgery	55 — Postop. management only	
	59 — Distinct multiple procedures	

CATEGORY	CODE	MOD	FEE	CATEGORY	CODE	MOD	FEE
Office Visit — New Patient				**Wound Care**			
Minimal office visit	99201			Debride partial thickness burn	11040		
20 minutes	99202			Debride full thickness burn	11041		
30 minutes	99203			Debride wound, not a burn	11000		
45 minutes	99204			Unna boot application	29580		
60 minutes	99205			Unna boot removal	29700		
Other				Other			
Office Visit — Established				**Supplies**			
Minimal office visit	99211			Ace bandage, 2"	A6448		
10 minutes	99212	X	35.00	Ace bandage, 3"-4"	A6449		
15 minutes	99213			Ace bandage, 6"	A6450		
25 minutes	99214			Cast, fiberglass	A4590		
40 minutes	99215			Coban wrap	A6454		
Other				Foley catheter	A4338		
General Procedures				Immobilizer	L3670		
Anoscopy	46600			Kerlix roll	A6220		
Audiometry	92551			Oxygen mask/cannula	A4620		
Breast aspiration	19000			Sleeve, elbow	E0191		
Cerumen removal	69210			Sling	A4565		
Circumcision	54150			Splint, ready-made	A4570		
DDST	96110			Splint, wrist	S8451		
Flex sigmoidoscopy	45330			Sterile packing	A6407		
Flex sig. w/ biopsy	45331			Surgical tray	A4550		
Foreign body removal—foot	28190			Other			
Nail removal	11730			OB Care			
Nail removal/phenol	11750			Routine OB care	59400		
Trigger point injection	20552			Postpartum care only (separate procedure)	59430		
Tympanometry	92567			Ante partum 4–6 visits	59425		
Visual acuity	99173			Ante partum 7 or more visits	59426		
Other	82465	X	30.00	Other			
Other				Other			

Other Visit Information: _____

Lab Work to Order: _____

Referral to: _____

Provider Signature: _____

Next Appointment: _____ RETURN IN A FEW DAYS IF NOT BETTER _____

Fees:

Total Charges: $65.00

Copay Received: $_____

Other Payment: $65.00 CK #1235

Total Due: $0

Allied Medical Center 1933 E. Frankford Rd. Carrollton, TX 12345 **972-555-5482**

Allied Medical Center
REGISTRATION FORM
(Please Print)

Today's date:	PCP:

PATIENT INFORMATION

Patient's last name: BAILEY	First: EILEEN	Middle: B	❏ Mr. ❏ Mrs.	❏ Miss ❏ Ms.	Marital status (circle one) Single / Mar / Div / Sep / (Wid)

Is this your legal name? ❏ Yes ❏ No	If not, what is your legal name?	(Former name): EILEEN STANFORD	Birth date: 04/26/1961	Age:	Sex: ❏ M ❏ F

Street address: 2531 BENT TREE COURT	Social Security no.: 555-63-2112	Home phone no.: (972) 555-6058

P.O. box:	City: DALLAS	State: TX	ZIP Code: 12345

Occupation: SUPERVISOR	Employer: DISCOUNT COMPUTER WAREHOUSE	Employer phone no.: (972) 555-6577

Chose clinic because/Referred to clinic by (please check one box):	❏ Dr.	❏ Insurance Plan	❏ Hospital

❏ Family	❏ Friend	❏ Close to home/work	❏ Yellow Pages	Other

Other family members seen here: **REASON FOR THIS VISIT:** Yearly Physical

INSURANCE INFORMATION

(Please give your insurance card to the receptionist.)

Person responsible for bill: EILEEN BAILEY	Birth date: / /	Address (if different): Same	Home phone no.: ( )

Is this person a patient here? ❏ Yes ❏ No

Occupation:	Employer:	Employer address:	Employer phone no.: ( )

Is this patient covered by insurance? ❏ Yes ❏ No

Please indicate primary insurance:	PHYSICIAN'S CHOICE EPO	Claims Mailing Address:	P O BOX 9873	Dover, OH	12345
		PHONE: 800-555-8637			

Subscriber's name: EILEEN BAILEY	Subscriber's S.S. no.: 555-63-2112	Birth date: 04/26/1961	❏ M ❏ F	Group no.: K1047	Policy no.: 13056	Co-payment: $

Patient's relationship to subscriber:	❏ Self	❏ Spouse	❏ Child	❏ Other

Name of secondary insurance (if applicable):	Subscriber's name and DOB:	❏ M ❏ F	Group no.:	Policy no.:

Patient's relationship to subscriber:	❏ Self	❏ Spouse	❏ Child	❏ Other Claims Address:

IN CASE OF EMERGENCY

Name of local friend or relative (not living at same address): MALCOLM JOHNSON	Relationship to patient: FRIEND	Home phone no.: (214) 555-5277	Work phone no.: (214) 555-8788

The above information is true to the best of my knowledge. I authorize my insurance benefits to be paid directly to the physician. I understand that I am financially responsible for any balance. I also authorize ALLIED MEDICAL CENTER or insurance company to release any information required to process my claims.

Eileen Bailey

_____   _____
Patient/Guardian signature   *Date*

ENCOUNTER FORM

Patient Information		Payment Method		Visit Information	
Patient ID number		**Primary**	Physician's Choice EPO	Visit date	
Patient name	Eileen Bailey	Primary ID number	13056	Visit number	
Address	2531 Bent Tree Ct	Primary group number	K1047	Rendering physician	
City/State	Dallas, TX 12345	**Secondary**		Referring physician	
Phone number	972-555-6058	Secondary ID number		Reason for visit	Yearly Physical
Date of birth	04/26/1961	Secondary group no.			
Age		Cash/credit card	CHECK		
		Other billing			

E/M Modifiers	Procedure Modifiers	DIAGNOSIS:
21 — Prolonged E&M Service	22 — Unusual, excessive procedure	Routine Exam V70.0
24 — Unrelated E/M service during postop.	50 — Bilateral procedure	
25 — Significant, separately identifiable E/M	51 — Multiple surgical procedures in same day	
32 — Mandated Service	52 — Reduced/incomplete procedure	
57 — Decision for surgery	55 — Postop. management only	
	59 — Distinct multiple procedures	

CATEGORY	CODE	MOD	FEE	CATEGORY	CODE	MOD	FEE
Office Visit — New Patient				**Wound Care**			
Minimal office visit	99201			Debride partial thickness burn	11040		
20 minutes	99202			Debride full thickness burn	11041		
30 minutes	99203			Debride wound, not a burn	11000		
45 minutes	99204			Unna boot application	29580		
60 minutes	99205	X	160.00	Unna boot removal	29700		
Other				Other			
Office Visit — Established				**Supplies**			
Minimal office visit	99211			Ace bandage, 2"	A6448		
10 minutes	99212			Ace bandage, 3"-4"	A6449		
15 minutes	99213			Ace bandage, 6"	A6450		
25 minutes	99214			Cast, fiberglass	A4590		
40 minutes	99215			Coban wrap	A6454		
Other				Foley catheter	A4338		
General Procedures				Immobilizer	L3670		
Anoscopy	46600			Kerlix roll	A6220		
Audiometry	92551			Oxygen mask/cannula	A4620		
Breast aspiration	19000			Sleeve, elbow	E0191		
Cerumen removal	69210			Sling	A4565		
Circumcision	54150			Splint, ready-made	A4570		
DDST	96110			Splint, wrist	S8451		
Flex sigmoidoscopy	45330			Sterile packing	A6407		
Flex sig. w/ biopsy	45331			Surgical tray	A4550		
Foreign body removal—foot	28190			Other			
Nail removal	11730			OB Care			
Nail removal/phenol	11750			Routine OB care	59400		
Trigger point injection	20552			Postpartum care only (separate procedure)	59430		
Tympanometry	92567			Ante partum 4–6 visits	59425		
Visual acuity	99173			Ante partum 7 or more visits	59426		
Other	82465			Other			
Other				Other			

Other Visit Information: _____

Lab Work to Order: _____

Referral to: _____

Provider Signature: _____

Next Appointment: _____ AS NEEDED _____

Fees:

Total Charges: $160.00

Copay Received: $ 32.00

Other Payment: $_____

Total Due: **$128.00**

Allied Medical Center 1933 E. Frankford Rd. Carrollton, TX 12345 **972-555-5482**

Allied Medical Center
REGISTRATION FORM
(Please Print)

Today's date: _____ PCP: _____

PATIENT INFORMATION

Patient's last name: CATHER	First: JIM	Middle: S	❑ Mr. ❑ Mrs.	❑ Miss ❑ Ms.	Marital status (circle one) Single / (Mar) / Div / Sep / Wid

Is this your legal name? ☒ Yes ❑ No	If not, what is your legal name? JAMES CATHER	(Former name):	Birth date: 10/01/1953	Age:	Sex: ❑ M ❑ F

Street address: 425 LAVENDER STREET	Social Security no.: 188-38-3833	Home phone no.: (972) 555-3394

P.O. box:	City: GARLAND	State: TX	ZIP Code: 12345

Occupation: SALESPERSON	Employer: MERRY MILER VANS	Employer phone no.: (972) 555-3337

Chose clinic because/Referred to clinic by (please check one box):	☒ Dr. LESLIE MCNEICE	❑ Insurance Plan	❑ Hospital

❑ Family	❑ Friend	❑ Close to home/work	❑ Yellow Pages	Other **AUTH # A569874, 30 DAYS, 3 VISITS**

Other family members seen here: _____ **REASON FOR THIS VISIT:** Hyperglycemia check up

INSURANCE INFORMATION
(Please give your insurance card to the receptionist.)

Person responsible for bill: JIM CATHER	Birth date: / /	Address (if different): SAME	Home phone no.: ( )

Is this person a patient here? ❑ Yes ❑ No

Occupation:	Employer:	Employer address:	Employer phone no.: ( )

Is this patient covered by insurance? ❑ Yes ❑ No

Please indicate primary insurance:	PHYSICIAN'S ALLIANCE HMO	Claims Mailing Address:	P O BOX 65	TOLEDO, OH	12345
		PHONE: 800-555-9865			

Subscriber's name: SAME AS PATIENT	Subscriber's S.S. no.: 188-38-3833	Birth date: / /	❑ M ❑ F	Group no.: 145	Policy no.: 188383833	Co-payment: $25.00

Patient's relationship to subscriber: ❑ Self ❑ Spouse ❑ Child ❑ Other

Name of secondary insurance (if applicable):	Subscriber's name and DOB:	❑ M ❑ F	Group no.:	Policy no.:

Patient's relationship to subscriber: ❑ Self ❑ Spouse ❑ Child ❑ Other Claims Address:

IN CASE OF EMERGENCY

Name of local friend or relative (not living at same address): MARILYN CATHER	Relationship to patient: SIBLING	Home phone no.: (214) 555-3329	Work phone no.: (469) 555-8200

The above information is true to the best of my knowledge. I authorize my insurance benefits to be paid directly to the physician. I understand that I am financially responsible for any balance. I also authorize ALLIED MEDICAL CENTER or insurance company to release any information required to process my claims.

Jim Cather

_____ _____
Patient/Guardian signature   Date

ENCOUNTER FORM

Patient Information / Payment Method / Visit Information

Patient Information		Payment Method		Visit Information	
Patient ID number		**Primary**	Physician's Alliance HMO	Visit date	
Patient name	Jim Cather	Primary ID number	188383833	Visit number	
Address	425 Lavender St	Primary group number	145	Rendering physician	
City/State	Garland, TX 12345	**Secondary**		Referring physician	Leslie McNeice
Phone number	972-555-3394	Secondary ID number		Reason for visit	Hyperglycemia CK
Date of birth	10/01/1953	Secondary group no.			
Age		Cash/credit card			
		Other billing			

E/M Modifiers	Procedure Modifiers	DIAGNOSIS:
21 — Prolonged E&M Service	22 — Unusual, excessive procedure	Hyperglycemia 790.6
24 — Unrelated E/M service during postop.	50 — Bilateral procedure	
25 — Significant, separately identifiable E/M	51 — Multiple surgical procedures in same day	
32 — Mandated Service	52 — Reduced/incomplete procedure	
57 — Decision for surgery	55 — Postop. management only	
	59 — Distinct multiple procedures	

CATEGORY	CODE	MOD	FEE	CATEGORY	CODE	MOD	FEE
Office Visit — New Patient				**Wound Care**			
Minimal office visit	99201			Debride partial thickness burn	11040		
20 minutes	99202			Debride full thickness burn	11041		
30 minutes	99203			Debride wound, not a burn	11000		
45 minutes	99204			Unna boot application	29580		
60 minutes	99205			Unna boot removal	29700		
Other				Other			
Office Visit — Established				**Supplies**			
Minimal office visit	99211			Ace bandage, 2"	A6448		
10 minutes	99212			Ace bandage, 3"-4"	A6449		
15 minutes	99213			Ace bandage, 6"	A6450		
25 minutes	99214	X	65.00	Cast, fiberglass	A4590		
40 minutes	99215			Coban wrap	A6454		
Other				Foley catheter	A4338		
General Procedures				Immobilizer	L3670		
Anoscopy	46600			Kerlix roll	A6220		
Audiometry	92551			Oxygen mask/cannula	A4620		
Breast aspiration	19000			Sleeve, elbow	E0191		
Cerumen removal	69210			Sling	A4565		
Circumcision	54150			Splint, ready-made	A4570		
DDST	96110			Splint, wrist	S8451		
Flex sigmoidoscopy	45330			Sterile packing	A6407		
Flex sig. w/ biopsy	45331			Surgical tray	A4550		
Foreign body removal—foot	28190			Other			
Nail removal	11730			OB Care			
Nail removal/phenol	11750			Routine OB care	59400		
Trigger point injection	20552			Postpartum care only (separate procedure)	59430		
Tympanometry	92567			Ante partum 4–6 visits	59425		
Visual acuity	99173			Ante partum 7 or more visits	59426		
Other	93000	X	45.00	Other			
Other	82954	X	12.00	Other			

Other Visit Information: _____

Lab Work to Order: _____
Referral to: _____
Provider Signature: _____
Next Appointment: _____

Fees:
Total Charges: $122.00
Copay Received: $ 25.00
Other Payment: $____
Total Due: **$97.00**

Allied Medical Center 1933 E. Frankford Rd. Carrollton, TX 12345 **972-555-5482**

Allied Medical Center
REGISTRATION FORM
(Please Print)

Today's date:	PCP:

PATIENT INFORMATION

Patient's last name: BAE	First: YONG	Middle: JOON	☒ Mr. ☐ Mrs.	☐ Miss ☐ Ms.	Marital status (circle one) Single / (Mar) / Div / Sep / Wid

Is this your legal name? ☒ Yes ☐ No	If not, what is your legal name?	(Former name):	Birth date: 02/23/1972	Age:	Sex: ☒ M ☐ F

Street address: 4549 EXPLORER DRIVE #110	Social Security no.: 661-39-2520	Home phone no.: (469) 555-0719

P.O. box:	City: FRISCO	State: TX	ZIP Code: 12345

Occupation: SUPERVISOR	Employer: SUGARLAND DAIRY FARM	Employer phone no.: (903) 555-8663

Chose clinic because/Referred to clinic by (please check one box): ☒ Dr. MALCOLM MAZOW	☐ Insurance Plan	☐ Hospital

☐ Family	☐ Friend	☐ Close to home/work	☐ Yellow Pages	☐ Other REFERRAL # FOR TODAY–1644401

Other family members seen here: **REASON FOR THIS VISIT:** Shoulder Pain

INSURANCE INFORMATION
(Please give your insurance card to the receptionist.)

Person responsible for bill: PATIENT	Birth date: / /	Address (if different): SAME	Home phone no.: ( )

Is this person a patient here?   ☒ Yes   ☐ No

Occupation:	Employer:	Employer address:	Employer phone no.: ( )

Is this patient covered by insurance?   ☒ Yes   ☐ No

Please indicate primary insurance:	METLIFE HMO	Claims Mailing Address:	P O BOX 6983	NEWARK, DE	12345
		PHONE: 800-555-6897			

Subscriber's name: SELF	Subscriber's S.S. no.: 661-39-2520	Birth date: / /	☐ M ☐ F	Group no.: 62440	Policy no.: 661392520-01	Co-payment: $10.00

Patient's relationship to subscriber:	☒ Self	☐ Spouse	☐ Child	☐ Other

Name of secondary insurance (if applicable):	Subscriber's name and DOB:	☐ M ☐ F	Group no.:	Policy no.:

Patient's relationship to subscriber: ☐ Self	☐ Spouse	☐ Child	☐ Other Claims Address:

IN CASE OF EMERGENCY

Name of local friend or relative (not living at same address): YUJIN JEONG	Relationship to patient: MOTHER	Home phone no.: (214) 650-9801	Work phone no.: ( )

The above information is true to the best of my knowledge. I authorize my insurance benefits to be paid directly to the physician. I understand that I am financially responsible for any balance. I also authorize ALLIED MEDICAL CENTER or insurance company to release any information required to process my claims.

Yong Joon Bae

Patient/Guardian signature	Date

ENCOUNTER FORM

Patient Information		Payment Method		Visit Information	
Patient ID number		**Primary**	MetLife HMO	Visit date	
Patient name	Yong Joon Bae	Primary ID number	661392520-01	Visit number	
Address	4549 Explorer Dr	Primary group number	62440	Rendering physician	
City/State	Frisco, TX 12345	**Secondary**		Referring physician	Malcolm Mazow
Phone number	469-555-0719	Secondary ID number		Reason for visit	Shoulder Pain
Date of birth	02/23/1972	Secondary group no.		Auth # for today: 1644401	
Age		Cash/credit card			
		Other billing			

E/M Modifiers	Procedure Modifiers	DIAGNOSIS:
21 — Prolonged E&M Service	22 — Unusual, excessive procedure	Bursitis, Shoulder 726.10
24 — Unrelated E/M service during postop.	50 — Bilateral procedure	
25 — Significant, separately identifiable E/M	51 — Multiple surgical procedures in same day	
32 — Mandated Service	52 — Reduced/incomplete procedure	
57 — Decision for surgery	55 — Postop. management only	
	59 — Distinct multiple procedures	

CATEGORY	CODE	MOD	FEE	CATEGORY	CODE	MOD	FEE
Office Visit — New Patient				**Wound Care**			
Minimal office visit	99201			Debride partial thickness burn	11040		
20 minutes	99202			Debride full thickness burn	11041		
30 minutes	99203			Debride wound, not a burn	11000		
45 minutes	99204			Unna boot application	29580		
60 minutes	99205			Unna boot removal	29700		
Other				Other			
Office Visit — Established				**Supplies**			
Minimal office visit	99211			Ace bandage, 2"	A6448		
10 minutes	99212			Ace bandage, 3"-4"	A6449		
15 minutes	99213	X	45.00	Ace bandage, 6"	A6450		
25 minutes	99214			Cast, fiberglass	A4590		
40 minutes	99215			Coban wrap	A6454		
Other				Foley catheter	A4338		
General Procedures				Immobilizer	L3670		
Anoscopy	46600			Kerlix roll	A6220		
Audiometry	92551			Oxygen mask/cannula	A4620		
Breast aspiration	19000			Sleeve, elbow	E0191		
Cerumen removal	69210			Sling	A4565		
Circumcision	54150			Splint, ready-made	A4570		
DDST	96110			Splint, wrist	S8451		
Flex sigmoidoscopy	45330			Sterile packing	A6407		
Flex sig. w/ biopsy	45331			Surgical tray	A4550		
Foreign body removal—foot	28190			Other			
Nail removal	11730			OB Care			
Nail removal/phenol	11750			Routine OB care	59400		
Trigger point injection	20552			Postpartum care only (separate procedure)	59430		
Tympanometry	92567			Ante partum 4–6 visits	59425		
Visual acuity	99173			Ante partum 7 or more visits	59426		
Other				Other			
Other				Other			

Other Visit Information: _____ **Fees:**
Lab Work to Order: _____ Total Charges: $45.00
Referral to: _____ Copay Received: $10.00
Provider Signature: _____ Other Payment: $_____
Next Appointment: _____ **Total Due: $35.00**

Allied Medical Center 1933 E. Frankford Rd. Carrollton, TX 12345 **972-555-5482**

Source: Adapted from Vines, Deborah, Braceland, Ann, Rollins, Elizabeth, and Miller, Susan. *Comprehensive Health Insurance: Billing, Coding, and Reimbursement.* © 2008. Pearson Education. Upper Saddle River, NJ.

abstract—the process of locating data in multiple source documents and accurately transferring it to a form.

abuse—improper behavior and billing practices that result in financial gain but are not fraudulent.

accept assignment—physician agrees to accept the amount approved by the insurance company as payment in full for a given service.

accounts receivables—the amount of money that is owed to the medical practice.

accredited—the process of becoming accredited with an overseeing agency. Accredited programs must provide education along the guidelines of the agency that offers the accreditation. In medical assisting, being accredited allows a program to bestow a certificate in medical assisting to the graduate.

Accrediting Bureau of Health Education School—accrediting agency offering medical assistant education programs the ability to offer a certified medical assisting certificate.

active patient files—normally refers to patient files for patients who currently have appointments to be seen, or who have been in to see the physician recently.

acupuncture—a procedure adapted from Chinese medicine in which needles are inserted into various areas of the body for therapeutic purposes.

ADA form—the standard billing form from the American Dental Association for use in billing for dental services.

add-on code—a CPT code designated by the plus sign (+) that cannot be used alone; must be used together with another CPT code.

addendum—something that has been added on to a patient's medical record after the date of the visit.

administrative—pertaining to office functions (e.g., computer operation, medical records management, coding and billing).

administrative duties—medical assisting duties such as computer applications, medical records management, coding and billing, and medical law and ethics.

administrative law—laws that are passed by governmental agencies.

advance beneficiary notice—a form patients sign agreeing to pay for covered Medicare services that may be denied due to medical necessity or frequency.

advance directives—documents outlining a patient's wishes regarding health care in the event the patient is unable to speak for themselves.

adverse outcome—a treatment outcome that is different (worse) than what was expected.

adverse reaction—unexpected or dangerous reaction to a drug.

advocate—standing up for the rights of another.

agenda—a schedule or list of items to be addressed during a meeting.

aging report—a report showing how much money is owed to the medical practice and how long those accounts have been outstanding.

allowed amount—the dollar amount for a service that an insurance company considers acceptable and uses to determine benefit payments; also called *approved amount*.

alphabetical index—alphabetical listing of CPT codes by procedure name, condition, eponym, and acronym.

ambulatory care centers—health care clinics where patients are seen for short visits.

American Association of Medical Assistants (AAMA)—national professional association for medical assistants.

American Medical Technologists (AMT)—professional association for individuals who work as medical technologists.

American Red Cross—humanitarian organization that provides emergency assistance, including disaster relief, inside the United States.

Americans with Disabilities Act—federal law that outlines how patients or employees with disabilities must be treated or accommodated.

anatomy—the study of the structure and organization of living organisms.

ancillary coverage—insurance coverage for services provided by other than a physician or hospital, such as dental, vision, or chiropractic care.

and—interpreted as *either/and/or* in a diagnostic code description.

anesthesia—method of numbing an area for surgery, or method of rendering an individual unconscious for surgery.

annotation—the process of reading a document and highlighting pertinent information for someone else.

antisepsis—the practice of using antiseptic to prevent growth and reproduction of bacteria and viruses.

antiseptic—substance that prevents growth and reproduction of bacteria and viruses.

appeal—a process that varies from one insurance plan to the next. The process of asking for a review of a denied service or claim, in an attempt to see the insurance company's denial reversed or overturned.

approved amount—see *allowed amount*.

assault—the threat of touching or doing harm to another without their consent.

assessing—determining what your patient needs to learn and what you will need to have on hand to teach them.

assignment of benefits—request made by a patient to allow the insurance carrier to pay the health care professional directly rather than issuing monies to the patient.

associate degree—degree awarded by community colleges after a course of study of approximately 2 years.

assumption of risk—a defense to medical malpractice; the physician must prove the patient was fully informed as to the risks involved in the procedure.

astrology—the practice of studying the planets and stars in an attempt to understand how things work on earth.

attitude—a state of mind, a way of carrying oneself.

audit—a review process that verifies that every detail of a CPT code is clearly documented in the medical record.

auditors—persons who work for an agency, such as the IRS, who perform the task of reviewing a person's or company's bank or tax records.

automatic dialer—a telephone feature allowing the user to program commonly called numbers into their system; also called a speed dialer.

automatic routing unit—telephone equipment that allows callers to self-select their call destinations via an automated, electronic prompt system.

autopsy—examination of a corpse in order to determine the cause of death.

balance billing—billing a patient for the dollar difference between the provider's charge and the insurance approved amount; usually not permitted for participating providers.

bar code scanners—devices used to scan or view a bar code, which then enters the information into a computer.

battery—the act of touching or abusing another person without their consent.

battery backup systems—a battery system that protects the computer in the event of a power surge or power outage.

beneficiary—person who is eligible to receive benefits/services under an insurance policy.

bilateral—refers to something that is occurring on both sides of the body.

bioethics—issues surrounding life and death situations in health care, such as cloning, artificial insemination, or abortion.

biofeedback—using monitoring devices to gain some voluntary control over that function.

birthday rule—a rule used by insurance companies when processing claims for minors who are covered under both parents' insurance plans. The parent with the birthday earlier in the year is the primary carrier, and the parent with the later birthday is the secondary carrier under this rule.

body (of letter)—main portion of a business letter.

body language—the way in which our nonverbal actions tell others how we feel.

brochure—a printed document containing information about a topic within the medical office.

buffer time—an appointment scheduling method of leaving certain times of day open to accommodate things like patients who call for same-day appointments or physicians who need to catch up on charting.

bundling—combining multiple services under a single all-inclusive CPT code and one charge.

caduceus—emblem of the medical profession.

call forwarding—telephone feature allowing the user to forward incoming calls to a different number.

capitation plans—health care plans where the provider is paid a set fee per month per member patient. When the patient comes in for a visit, there may be an additional co-payment collected. Other than the possible copayment, no other payment comes from the insurance company or the patient when the patient comes in for care.

caretaker—person or entity responsible for determining when and if a patient needs specific types of health care; also called gatekeeper or primary care provider (PCP).

carve outs—services that are reimbursed in addition to the base rate for the patient.

catastrophic—expensive health care for large, usually unforeseen events such as accidents, treatment for terminal illnesses, or long-term illness.

categorically needy—Medicaid-eligible patients who qualify for cash assistance as well as medical services.

category—a three-digit code in ICD-9-CM tabular list.

category I codes—CPT codes numbered 00100 to 99999 representing widely used services and procedures approved by the FDA.

category II codes—supplemental tracking codes that can be used for performance measurement; four numbers followed by the letter F, such as 1002F.

category III codes—temporary codes for data collection and tracking the use of emerging technology, services, and procedures; four numbers followed by the letter T, such as 0162T.

Centers for Medicare and Medicaid Services—federal agency responsible for monitoring laws and regulations surrounding Medicare and Medicaid services.

central processing unit (CPU)—the computer's ability to process information.

certificate of coverage—a letter from the insurance company that provides proof of type and timeframe of coverage when a patient terminates a health insurance policy.

certified letter—a letter sent via the postal service sent certified is one that must be signed for by the recipient.

Certified Medical Assistant (CMA)—a graduate of an accredited medical assisting program who has passed the AAMA certification examination.

chapter—one of 17 major sections of ICD-9-CM Volume I tabular list, organized by body system and etiology.

charge slip—also called an encounter form or a routing slip. These forms vary from one office to the next and usually contain the procedural and diagnostic codes commonly used in that clinic. A charge slip is generated on each patient coming in for care each day; these are a record of the charges and diagnoses for that patient for that date of service. Usually completed by the health care provider who performed the service.

charitable contributions—donations, including cash, that are given to charitable organizations.

checklist—a preprinted reminder list of activities or steps to take to perform a task.

chemical waste—waste drugs, cleaning solutions, and germicides.

chief complaint—statement in the patient's own words of the reason for seeking medical care.

chiropractic—health care profession that focuses on correcting misalignments of the spine.

chloroform—early method of general anesthesia.

circular E—yearly booklet published by the IRS that outlines the proper federal tax deductions to be taken from an individual's wages, depending upon marital status and number of exemptions.

civil law—laws that relate between two or more citizens.

clean claim—insurance claim form (either electronic or on paper) that contains no errors nor omissions.

clinical duties—medical assisting duties such as drawing blood samples, taking vital signs, and assisting with surgery.

close-ended question—question that can be answered with yes or no.

closed patient files—normally refers to patient files for patients who will not be returning to the clinic.

closing—ending portion of a business letter.

cluster scheduling—a scheduling method allowing patients with similar appointments to be clustered around the same time of day.

coinsurance—percentage of the medical charges the patient will be responsible for according to their insurance plan contract.

collection agency—company that will pursue overdue accounts for a fee.

combination code—a single code that describes two or more conditions that frequently occur together.

commercial insurance—see *private insurance*.

commercial law—laws that relate to businesses or companies.

Commission of Accreditation of Allied Health Education Programs (CAAHEP)—accrediting agency offering medical assistant education programs the ability to offer a certified medical assisting certificate.

common descriptor—the portion of a standalone code before the semicolon that is shared with the indented codes that follow.

common law—laws that stem from the English legal system.

community college—educational institution that provides 2-year undergraduate education, offering certificates, diplomas, and Associate's Degrees.

community property laws—laws that cause one spouse to be financially responsible for the debts of the other.

comparative negligence—defense to medical malpractice where the physician proves the patient was partly responsible for their own injury.

competency—list of skills that accredited programs must teach students.

complementary and alternative medicine—referred to as CAM, natural remedies and methods that do not use medications or surgeries to care for or cure disease and illness.

computed tomography—CT scan; two-dimensional X-rays.

computer peripherals—devices that connect to the computer to add some function or use.

computer viruses—programs written for the purpose of disrupting a computer's functions.

conference call—telephone feature allowing three or more persons in different locations to participate in a call.

confidentiality—state of keeping what one person says from being heard by anyone else.

conscience clauses—clauses that allow persons who work in health care to refuse to work in situations with which they have a religious objection.

Consolidated Omnibus Budget Reconciliation Act (COBRA)—Allows workers to continue their health insurance coverage (at their own expense) after being fired, laid off, or having quit.

constitutional law—laws based on the U.S. Constitution.

consultation—visit between the patient and the health care provider where a discussion, but not an examination, takes place.

consumer-directed healthcare—health insurance plans that place the patient in charge of how their health care dollars are spent.

contact information—patient's address and phone numbers.

continuing education—educational program designed to further knowledge in a particular area.

contract—agreement, either verbal or in writing, between two parties.

contract law—laws pertaining to contracts.

contributory factor—three secondary criteria, in addition to the key components, that may influence the selection of an E&M code; include presenting problem, counseling/coordination of care, and physicians' face-to-face time with patients and families.

contributory negligence—defense to medical malpractice where the physician proves that the injury wouldn't have happened if not for the actions of the patient.

conventions—ICD-9-CM coding rules, abbreviations, symbols, or formatting intended to ensure consistency in coding.

conversion factor—a constant dollar value multiplied by the relative value unit to determine the price of individual services.

coordination of benefits—the process of determining which insurance policy should be billed first, second, or third when a patient is covered by multiple policies.

coordination of care—a contributory factor in E&M coding that describes physician's work in arranging care with other providers.

copayment—set dollar fee per visit or service the patient will be responsible for according to their insurance plan contract.

counseling—a contributory factor in E&M coding that describes physician's discussion with patients and family members regarding diagnosis, treatment options, instructions, and follow-up.

courtesy—polite behavior.

cover letter—letter to accompany the resume when sent to an employer.

covered—services potentially eligible for reimbursement.

CPR mouth barrier—disposable barrier device used to prevent infection.

CPT codes—*Current Procedural Terminology*; a book that is updated every year, contains all nondental procedure codes approved by the Centers for Medicare and Medicaid Services.

CPT-4 book—procedural coding book used in all health care settings in the United States.

crash cart—wheeled cart that contains emergency medical equipment.

credibility—quality of believing a person is and does what they say they will do.

criminal law—laws dealing with crimes.

cross-referencing—method of tracking and finding patient files for those patients who may have more than one last name.

damages—the amount of money a patient is awarded for the damages they have sustained.

day sheet—used with a manual pegboard system.

debit—an addition to an account, usually performed in order to remove a credit balance.

décor—the way an office is decorated.

deductible—amount of money the patient must pay out of pocket for health care services before health insurance benefits begin to pay.

deductions—number of withholding allowances an individual wishes to have withheld from their wages.

defamation of character—to say negative things about another person that causes that person some form of harm.

defibrillator—device that delivers an electric shock to a patient.

delegate—to assign projects to others.

denied—a claim processed by an insurer and determined not eligible for payment.

dependability—the quality of following through with what is expected of you.

dependent—a family member or other individual who qualifies for coverage on the insured's policy; also called *beneficiary*. See also *insured; policyholder*.

Dietary Supplement and Education Act—federal act enacted in 1990 directing how nutritional supplements are to be labeled.

dietary supplements—vitamins, herbs, or minerals administered in a variety of ways to alleviate symptoms or to maintain health in a natural, noninvasive manner.

direct telephone lines—telephone numbers that reach a person directly, rather than routing the calls through an operator or receptionist.

disability insurance—insurance that covers lost wages and certain other benefits due to a disability that prevents the individual from working.

disability policies—policies that cover an individual's lost income in the event of a temporary or long-term disability.

discovery rule—legal term pertaining to medical malpractice cases; this is the period of time within which a patient has to file a medical malpractice lawsuit from the day the injury was discovered, rather than the date of the injury itself.

discriminating—acting against a person's interest solely because of a perceived difference, such as race, gender, or economic status.

documenting—process of writing in the patient's chart.

double booking—scheduling more than one patient for the same appointment time.

downcode—to assign a code for a lower level of service than was actually performed; done by some insurance companies to save money; done by some physicians to avoid fraud or abuse charges.

drug samples—small samples of drugs given to physicians by pharmaceutical companies to be dispensed to patients.

dual fee schedule—a facility or health care provider having two fees for the same service.

duress—act of coercing someone into an act.

e-billing—health insurance claims that are sent electronically.

E codes—diagnosis codes used to indicate the external cause of an illness or poisoning.

elective procedure—procedure that will benefit the patient but does not need to be scheduled immediately.

electronic mail—e-mail; electronically sending a message from one person to another using computers.

electronic medical records—medical records that are kept electronically, on a computer.

electronic sign-in sheet—device attached to a computer allowing a person to sign their name so it appears in the computer.

electronic signature—electronic version of a person's signature to be used in electronic medical records.

eligibility—the process to determine if a patient is qualified to receive coverage/paid benefits according the insurance policy guidelines.

empathy—ability to identify with and understand another person's feelings.

employee handbook—also called a policy manual; list of policies regarding employment within the office.

encounter form—also called a charge slip or a routing slip. These forms vary from one office to the next and usually contain the procedural and diagnostic codes commonly used in that clinic. A charge slip is generated on each patient coming in for care each day; these are a record of the charges and diagnoses for that patient for that date of service. Usually completed by the health care provider who performed the service.

end-stage renal disease—total or nearly complete failure of the kidneys.

endorsement stamp—rubber stamp that contains the banking information for the receiving agency.

ergonomic—designed for proper posture of the body while using the equipment.

escort—to accompany someone.

established patient—patient who has seen the same provider, or another provider of the same specialty in the same practice, within the past three years.

ether—early method of general anesthesia.

etiology—cause of a disease or illness.

evaluation—process of verifying a patient's progress.

Evaluation and Management (E&M)—CPT codes used for billing physician services to evaluate and manage patient care, such as office visits.

evidence-based medicine—theory of medicine that states health care methods should be scientifically proven to work.

examination—a key component of E&M coding that describes the complexity of the physical assessment of the patient.

examples—asking the patient to give an example of how they are feeling.

exclusions—procedures or services that are not covered under a particular insurance plan.

exclusive provider organization—a managed care contract with a smaller network of providers under which the employer agrees to not use any other networks in return for favorable pricing.

expert witnesses—witness in a lawsuit who is considered an expert in their given field.

expiration dates—the date something expires; the date it should not be used past.

explanation of benefits—a statement that accompanies payment from the insurance company which summarizes how the payment for each billed service was calculated and gives reasons for any items not paid.

expressed consent—agreement, either verbally or in writing.

expressed contract—agreement to a contract, either verbally or in writing.

external hard drives—devices that attach to a computer system to allow extra hard drive capacity.

externship program—the final phase of the medical assisting education in an accredited program; consists of hands-on work in a medical office for a specified number of hours.

face-to-face time—a contributory factor in E&M coding that measures the amount of time the provider spent in the presence of the patient and/or family, as opposed to time spent documenting the visit or arranging referrals.

Fair Debt Collection Act—laws outlining how debts may be legally collected.

Fair Labor Standards Act—passed by Congress passed in 1938; addressed several issues relating to workers, including setting a federal minimum wage.

faith healer—Practitioners who use prayer, rather than medicine, to heal their patients.

Federal Insurance Contributions Act (FICA)—addresses Social Security withholding taxes.

federal minimum wage—dollar amount, set by Congress, that is the minimum amount an employer may pay an employee per hour in wages.

Federal Unemployment Tax Act (FUTA)—addresses federal unemployment tax withholdings.

fee schedule—The list of approved fees insurance carriers agree to pay to participating providers who agree to contract with the carrier. Also refers to the standard set of fees the provider charges to all insurers.

fee-for-service—term used to identify the process of insurance companies paying providers a fee for each individual service provided to a covered patient.

feedback—relating to another person what you think you heard them say.

financial information—information about a patient consisting of their health insurance identification numbers and policy numbers.

first listed—the diagnosis that is chiefly responsible for the outpatient services provided; formerly called *primary diagnosis*.

fixed appointment scheduling—a scheduling system of giving every patient a specific appointment time.

flash drives—small, external computer storage devices; also called thumb drives.

flexible spending account—account set up by employers. Employees are allowed to place pretax earnings into these accounts and then submit receipts to the employer for allowed medical expenses; also called *health care reimbursement account*.

flexibility—willingness to change direction or plans when needed or requested.

flow charts—graphs that are used in the patient's medical record to track things such as weight gain or growth of a newborn.

font—typestyle used within a word processing program.

forgiven—with regard to collections, to forgive an account is to stop attempting to collect from the debtor.

form locators—the boxes to be completed on the CMS-1500 claim form.

formulary—tiered list of drugs covered by a particular insurance company. Normally, generic or less expensive drugs are covered at a higher rate (with a smaller copay, if any), whereas name brand or more expensive drugs are covered at a lower rate (with a higher copay). Each insurance company constructs their own formulary list. Some insurance plans will *only* covered preferred (lower cost) drugs.

fossil—ancient mineralized remains of plants, animals, or other organisms.

Four Ds of negligence—refers to malpractice; patients must prove duty, dereliction of duty, direct cause, and damages.

fraud—to intentionally bill for services that were never given, including billing for a service that has a higher reimbursement than the service provided.

front desk—place in a medical office where the receptionist welcomes the patients as they enter.

garnished—to have monies withheld from a person's wages due to a court order.

generic drugs—lower cost, non-name brand prescription drugs that duplicate their brand name counterparts in active ingredient and effect.

generic message—telephone answering messages that are not specific to any individual office.

geographic adjustment factor (GAF)—a numeric multiplier used by Medicare to adjust fees for the varying costs of practicing medicine in different areas of the country.

Geographical Practice Cost Index (GPCI)—Medicare system of adjusting fees based on the country in which the health care provider practices.

Good Samaritan Act—laws that protect a person when they perform life-saving care to a stranger outside the medical setting.

gross pay—amount of money a person earns before any taxes or deductions are taken out.

group health insurance—a commercial insurance policy with rates based on a group of people, usually offered by an employer.

guidelines—specific instructions at the beginning of each section of the CPT manual that define terms and describe specific information about how to use codes in that section.

hands-free telephone device—headsets or headphones that contain both a speaker and a microphone, worn by an individual who is using a telephone and does not wish to hold the receiver.

hardship agreement—agreement a patient signs to indicate an inability to pay full health care costs due to financial hardship.

hazard—something that is dangerous, or possibly dangerous.

HCFA 1500 form—former name for the CMS-1500 claim form.

Health Care Financing Administration—former name for the Centers for Medicare and Medicaid Services.

health care reimbursement account—see *flexible spending account.*

health care savings account—similar to a flexible spending account. Employees are allowed to place pretax earnings into an account set up by their employer. They then submit receipts to the employer for covered medical expenses. This type of account can normally roll over from one year to the next if the employee does not use all of the funds and can often be taken with the employee from one job to another.

Healthcare Common Procedure Coding System (HCPCS)—contains coding for all procedures and services.

Health Insurance Portability and Accountability Act (HIPAA)—legislation that addresses patient privacy.

health maintenance organization—a group of physicians or medical center that provides comprehensive service to members under a capitated payment plan; members' care is covered only when using these designated providers.

health savings account—tax-free savings accounts used for medical expenses in conjunction with a high-deductible health plan.

health-related calculators—programs that allow the user to determine information about health-related conditions, such as target body weight.

HIPAA compliant—in line with laws regarding patient confidentiality.

Hippocrates—"Father of Medicine"; Greek physician who began moving the practice of medicine to a scientific nature.

Hippocratic oath—oath of ethics thought to be written by Hippocrates. Still recited at medical school graduations.

history—a key component of E&M coding that describes the background, onset, and progression of the patient's current condition.

hold feature—telephone feature allowing the user to place callers on hold, allowing the user to take other telephone calls.

holistic—natural, nonmedical treatment.

hospice—facility or service provided for patients who are given a diagnosis of a terminal illness, with 6 months or less to live. Services may be provided in the hospice facility, in the hospital, skilled nursing facility, or the patient's home. Care is normally palliative (comfort-based) in nature.

hospital services—patient care provided by a licensed acute care hospital.

hourly—amount of money to be paid to an employee per hour worked.

Human Genome Project—project designed to map out the human genes.

hypnosis—artificially induced altered state of consciousness, usually accompanied by an increased receptiveness to suggestion.

identification numbers—numbers given by the insurance carrier that identify the insured. These numbers have taken the place of using the insured's Social Security number.

immunity—unable to be held accountable for one's actions.

implementation—putting a plan into place.

implied contract—to agree to a contract by one's actions, without speaking or writing.

inactive patient files—normally refers to patient files for patients who have not been in to see the physician for an extended period of time.

indecipherable—unreadable.

indemnity—see *fee-for-service.*

indented code—a CPT code whose description is indented 3 spaces under another (standalone) code and whose definition includes the portion before the semicolon (;) in the standalone code; done to save space in the CPT manual.

individual insurance—a commercial insurance policy with rates based on individual health criteria.

individual practice association—HMOs that are the most decentralized and involve contracting with individual physicians to create a healthcare delivery system.

infectious waste—any garbage exposed to bodily fluids or any laboratory cultures or blood products.

informed consent—when a physician goes over the risks associated with a procedure with a patient, including the risks of nontreatment and the accepted alternatives to treatment.

initiative—taking it upon oneself to begin a task, without being asked by someone else to do it.

inpatient—a person who is formally admitted to the hospital for a minimum of 24 hours.

instructional notes—directions in the tabular index, which appear in parentheses before or after a code entry, to point the user to alternative codes for closely related procedures or to codes than must or must not be used together.

insured—term used to identify the person who holds or owns an insurance policy. See *policyholder*.

intentional tort—to purposefully hurt or harm another.

interdisciplinary—multiple health care specialties.

interest—to charge a percentage fee each month on overdue account balances.

Internal Revenue Service—federal agency responsible for collecting federal taxes due from individuals and companies.

international law—laws pertaining to two or more countries.

Internet search engines—Web sites that search the Internet for information based on words entered by an individual.

interview—a meeting, usually face-to-face, between an employer and an applicant.

invasion of privacy—to give out information about another person without permission.

inventory—supplies that are on hand; counting the supplies that are in the office.

job application—a paper to fill out when applying for a job; contains questions about the applicant.

Joint Commission for the Accreditation of Healthcare Organizations (JCAHO)—this organization is mandatory for hospitals; an accrediting agency that identifies patient care and safety standards.

key component—three primary determining criteria in selecting an E&M code; include history, examination, and medical decision making.

laryngeal nerve—nerve that controls the muscles of the larynx in the throat; controls the ability for making vocal sounds.

last number redial—telephone feature allowing the user to push one button to dial the last number dialed from that telephone.

late effect—current condition that is the result or byproduct of a previous, resolved condition.

ledger card—used with manual pegboard systems; each patient has their own ledger card to track services rendered and payments made.

legible—writing that others can read.

letterhead—professional quality stationery containing the name, address, and telephone number of the medical office.

Level I codes—same as CPT.

Level II codes—HCPCS alphanumeric codes created by CMS to bill supplies, drugs, and certain services.

Level III codes—HCPCS alphanumeric codes created by regional Medicare carriers; being phased out under HIPAA.

liability insurance—covers injuries that occur on, in, or because of the insured's property.

licensed—process of registering as a health care professional. Those professionals who are bound by law to be licensed in order to practice.

lifetime maximum benefit—amount of money allowed by an insurance carrier for a covered member's covered expenses over the course of the member's lifetime. Often set at $1 million.

limiting charge—the maximum amount a Medicare non-PAR provider may bill the patient on an unassigned claim; 115% of the non-PAR fee schedule.

litigation—legal action taken against another.

logo—artwork used by the medical office in their letterhead or on other printed materials.

Long—American physician who developed the use of general anesthesia.

long-term disability insurance—insurance that covers lost wages and certain other benefits due to a disability that prevents the individual from working, usually for more than one year.

long-term care facilities—health care facilities designed to care for patients who need care on a long-term basis, and may not be able to be cared for in their home.

loyalty—devotion to another; standing by another even in hard times.

M codes—identify neoplasm type and tumor behavior; used by tumor registries.

magnetic resonance imaging—method of using powerful magnets to provide two-dimensional images of the inside of objects.

magnetic therapy—therapy with magnets.

main term—words by which conditions and diseases are alphabetized in ICD-9-CM Volume II; may be name of condition, eponym, acronym, or synonym, but not an anatomical site; may also be words by which procedures and services are alphabetized in the CPT index; may be a procedure, service, anatomic site, condition, synonym, eponym, or abbreviation.

maintained—to keep something in good working order.

malfeasance—performing an incorrect treatment.

malpractice insurance policy—liability insurance that covers injuries patients receive due to acts or omissions by health care providers.

malpractice premium—amount of money an insurance carrier charges a health care provider in exchange for a malpractice insurance policy.

malware—computer programs written with the purpose of destroying computers or their programs.

managed care—a system of healthcare delivery focused on reducing costs by transferring risk to the provider and may limit the type and frequency of care members may receive.

manifestation—outward or associated condition resulting from an underlying disease.

massage—using the hands to relax the muscles of the body.

matrix—process of blocking out times in the appointment schedule when the provider is unavailable or out of the office.

Medicaid—a joint federal and state program that helps with medical costs for some people with low incomes and limited resources.

medical decision making (MDM)—a key component of E&M coding that describes the complexity of establishing a diagnosis and/or selecting a management option.

medical information—information about a patient's medical care and history.

medical management software—software the medical office uses to perform day-to-day functions.

medical necessity—criteria establishing when a service is appropriate.

medical record—legal document consisting of medical information obtained from the patient via consultations, examinations, and tests.

medical research program—program where research is conducted to determine the effectiveness or harm of certain medications or medical treatments.

medical savings account—tax-free savings account for small employers and self-employed; used for medical expenses in conjunction with a high-deductible health plan.

medically needy—Medicaid-eligible patients who are eligible for medical services, but not cash assistance.

Medicare—federal program covering medical expenses for the elderly, those with end-stage renal disease, and those with a long-term disability. Part A covers hospitalization; Part B covers medical, laboratory, and equipment expenses; and Part D covers prescription drugs.

Medicare managed care plan—managed care plan for Medicare recipients. Less costly than Medicare Part B benefits, and with more restrictions.

meditation—deep concentration on a matter.

member—the person who owns the insurance policy.

memo—interoffice note.

mentor—the preceptor; person who supervises the extern within the health care facility during the program.

merit—with regard to malpractice, when a case has substance or is more likely to be found in the patient's favor.

misfeasance—performing a procedure incorrectly.

mission statement—a written statement that describes the office's reason for existence.

modified wave scheduling—scheduling system where two or three patients are scheduled at the beginning of each hour, followed by single patient appointments every 10 to 20 minutes for the rest of that hour.

modifier—two-digit alphanumeric codes appended to CPT or Level II codes to further describe circumstances.

modifying term—descriptive words in the alphabetic index that appear indented under the main term to further describe the service or procedure.

morbidity—the cause of illness or injury.

mortality—the cause of death.

multidisciplinary—many disciplines; multiple specialties.

multiple coding—a diagnosis that requires more than one ICD-9-CM code to completely describe it; often indicated by a second code in slanted brackets.

narrative—type of medical charting where the health care provider writes a narrative version of contact with the patient.

national commercial insurance carrier—insurance plans available from a variety of companies nationwide. These can be purchased by groups or individuals. Benefits will vary greatly.

national conversion factor—number released by Medicare each year that determines fee schedules for all health care services.

national standard—providing a standard that is used throughout the United States.

naturopath—type of therapy that uses natural remedies to treat illness.

negligence—term to describe medical malpractice.

negotiated fee schedule—a common reimbursement method in managed care whereby the MCO develops a list of fees for providers that they agree to accept in the participating provider contract. Fees may be determined based on a percentage of the provider's usual fee or arrived at through negotiation.

neoplasm—the medical term for an abnormal growth of new tissue; often referred to as a tumor.

net pay—amount of an individual's paycheck after all deductions and taxes are taken out.

new patient—patient who has not seen the same provider, or another provider of the same specialty in the same practice, for more than three years.

new patient checklist—preprinted list of information needed from a new patient when they call to schedule an appointment.

no carbon required (NCR)—paper that, when written on, makes an exact copy beneath it, without the need for carbon paper.

noncompliance—when a patient refuses to follow the physician's instructions.

noncovered—services not eligible for reimbursement under any circumstance.

nonessential modifiers—words in parentheses after a main term in the ICD-9-CM; they clarify the main term, but need not be present in the medical record.

nonfeasance—delaying treatment or failing to perform a treatment.

nonparticipating provider—health care provider who has not contracted with a particular health insurance carrier.

nontherapeutic research—research programs that do not create any benefit for the patients in the study; these studies are designed to test if the drug or treatment is harmful to the healthy participant/patient.

nontoxic—not harmful to the body.

not elsewhere classified (NES)—diagnosis code that cannot be found elsewhere in the coding book.

not otherwise specified (NOS)—a general code used when details are not available in the medical record.

notice—with regard to legal cases, notice means notice of an impending lawsuit filed.

nurse practitioner—registered nurse who has completed advanced education and training in the management of common medical illnesses.

obliterate—to make the original entry completely unreadable.

observation status—a designated type of care in which a patient is hospitalized for monitoring, but not formally admitted.

office brochure—pamphlet outlining the staff and services offered within a clinic.

Office of the Insurance Commissioner—each state has its own Insurance Commissioner. This office oversees all aspects of insurance within the state, including health insurance.

office policy—an agreed-upon policy used within the office so all similar situations are handled in the same way.

omission—to leave something out.

Omnibus Budget Reconciliation Act—passed by Congress in 1993; created a formula by which all health care service fees are calculated.

open-ended question—a question that requires more than a simple yes or no answer.

open hours—scheduling method that allows patients to come in at their leisure, without a set appointment time.

opening the office—the steps to take to be sure the office is opened properly at the beginning of the day.

organizational chart—breakdown of the chain of command in a business.

OSHA—Occupational Safety and Health Administration; a federal agency responsible for oversight of safety in the workplace.

outliers—exceptional circumstances that cost far more or less than the average.

outpatient—patient who has been not formally admitted to a facility, such as for office visits, emergency department, and observation status.

outsourced—sending work outside of the office to a separate company.

overhead—amount of money it costs to sustain a business (rent, salaries, utilities, etc.).

overtime—wages paid to an individual beyond a regular 40-hour work week; usually paid at 1.5 times the normal hourly wage of that individual.

pacemaker—implantable device used to regulate the heartbeat.

packing slip—list of the supplies that were ordered and included in a shipment.

parent code—see *standalone code*.

participating provider—health care provider who has contracted with a particular health insurance carrier.

past timely filing limits—the time beyond which an insurance claim will be accepted by an insurance carrier. Usually set at one year from the date of service, though some plans will not accept claims beyond 90 days from the date of service.

pasteurization—method of heating liquids in order to kill bacteria.

patient billing statements—statements sent to patients, usually monthly, indicating the amount of money they owe to the clinic or provider for health care services.

patient status—classification of patients as new or established.

Patients' Bill of Rights—laws pertaining to patients' rights regarding their health care.

payor number—unique identifying number assigned to each insurance carrier for the purpose of directing electronic claims.

payroll—process of calculating wages and deductions; calculating the amount to be paid to employees for work performed.

payroll taxes—monies withheld from employees' wages for federal income taxes, Social Security, and Medicare.

pegboard accounting system—manual system of bookkeeping.

penicillin—antibiotic drug useful in killing some forms of bacteria.

per case—*per case* payment method used for hospitals. Under this method, the hospital receives a pre-established amount per patient for the entire stay, based on the patient's diagnosis, regardless of how long they are in or what services are provided.

per diem—*per day* payment method whereby the facility is paid a flat amount per day the patient remains, regardless of what services are provided.

personal digital assistants (PDAs)—small, portable devices used to keep and transmit information.

personal information—information about a patient's personal habits or social activities.

personal space—unseen "bubble" around each of us that outlines the parameter we are not comfortable with others entering.

personnel file—file to be kept on all employees in a company; includes original applications, federal withholding requests, dates and copies of evaluations.

personnel manual—also called an employee handbook, a list of policies relating to employment in an individual office.

pharmaceuticals—drugs, medicines, chemical compounds.

physical status modifier—two-digit alphanumeric codes (P1 to P6) appended to anesthesia codes which indicate the health status of the patient at the beginning of the procedure.

physician services—patient care provided by a licensed physician.

physician's assistant—nonphysician clinician licensed to practice medicine under a physician's supervision.

Physician's Desk Reference (**PDR**)—published every year, containing up-to-date information on all drugs available for legal sale in the United States.

physiology—study of the mechanical, physical, and biochemical functions of living organisms.

planning—researching the actions or steps needed to implement something.

point of service—an insurance offering in which a patient has access to multiple plans, such as an HMO, PPO, and indemnity, and may choose to use any of them for any given service.

policy—statement of guidelines, or rules, on a given topic in the office.

policy and procedure manuals—manuals kept in the office, outlining the ways staff should handle/perform certain activities.

policy number—number given by insurance carriers that identify a group of insureds.

policyholder—same as the member or the insured; term used to identify the person who holds or owns an insurance policy.

portability—being able to take an insurance policy from one employer to another.

postage meter—electronic machine capable of printing postage in the office.

posting—adding charges or payments to a patient's account.

postoperative—period of time after an operative procedure.

postoperative period—the number of days following a procedure during which follow-up visits are bundled with the primary procedure and are not billed separately.

preapprovals—process of calling a patient's insurance carrier prior to a service in order to obtain preapproval or authorization for the service to be performed.

preauthorization—approval for treatment or service obtained from an insurance company before the care is provided.

precedence—to decide a legal case in court, which then relates to all cases that come after it.

preceptor—mentor; person who supervises the extern within the health care facility during the program.

precertification—see *preauthorization*.

pre-existing condition—condition for which a patient received treatment in a certain period prior to beginning coverage with a new insurance plan. Rules vary from one insurance plan to another.

preferred—services or providers covered at a higher (less cost to the patient) fee.

preferred provider organization—organization that contracts with independent providers to perform services for members at discounted rates.

preferred providers—physician who has signed a contract to accept the conditions outlined by a managed care health plan.

premium—dollar amount paid to the insurance company to have coverage in force; usually paid monthly; employers may pay part or all of the premium as an employee benefit.

presenting problem—a contributory factor in E&M coding that consists of a disease, condition, illness, injury, symptom, sign, finding complaint, or other reason for the encounter, as stated by the patient.

primary care provider—term used to define the physician, usually a general or family practice doctor, who oversees all care needed or desired by their patient. The primary care provider is referred to as the PCP and many managed care plans require the PCP be the one to determine when the patient needs care or services, such as a referral to a specialist.

primary diagnosis—see *first-listed*.

primary insurance—insurance plan that pays first for a covered patient's services.

principal diagnosis—the reason determined, after study, to be responsible for an inpatient stay.

private insurance—insurance not provided by the government but by an independent not-for-profit or for-profit company; also called *commercial insurance*.

problem-oriented medical record charting—type of medical record charting that focuses on the patient's health care problems and addresses those problems at each visit.

procedural coding—coding for services and procedures in health care.

procedure—list of steps describing how to perform a given task or project.

procedures—services such as surgery or therapy performed on a patient by a health care provider.

professional appointments—appointments the doctor makes with other health care providers, associates, or colleagues.

professional courtesy—to give a patient a discount, or free service, due to the fact that they are a health care professional.

professional distance—keeping a professional relationship with patients.

progress notes—notes in the patient's medical chart outlining their progress or complaints.

proofreader's marks—list of marks commonly used when proofreading documents.

proofreading—the process of reading and reviewing a document for possible errors.

public health—the overall health of a community.

public law—laws pertaining to citizens.

purge—to remove closed or inactive patient medical records from the medical office.

qualified—diagnosis statement accompanied by terms such as possible, probable, suspected, rule out (R/O), or working diagnosis, indicating the physician has not determined the root cause.

quality improvement programs—programs designed to improve the quality of a service, such as patient care.

quarterly payroll reports—reports of amount of taxes withheld from employees' wages to be filed quarterly (four times per year).

radioactive waste—any waste contaminated with radioactive material.

radiocarbon dating—procedure that uses the measure of carbon in a substance to determine its age.

radium—radioactive chemical element.

rapport—mutual trust and affection for one another.

reasonable and necessary skill and care—care a reasonable person would render to a patient; the skills a health care provider is expected to have.

reception area—waiting area for patients in the medical office.

receptionist—medical staff member who greets patients, answers the telephone, and directs the office flow.

recertification—process of renewing a certificate.

reference initials—in a professional letter, these are the initials of the author of the letter followed by the initials of the person who typed the letter (AJF/cmm).

referral—one health care provider sending a patient to another provider. Usually required for coverage with a specialist in managed care plans.

reflecting—repeating to the patient what you believe they are saying to you.

registered medical assistant (RMA)—credential given a medical assistant who has passed the RMA certification examination.

regulatory laws—laws regarding government regulations.

reimbursement—payment sent to the health care provider for services rendered.

rejected—a claim that is returned to the provider without processing due to a technical error.

relative value unit (RVU)—unit of measure assigned to medical services based on the resources required to provide it; includes work, practice expense, and liability insurance.

remotely—to access something, such as a computer system, while away from the office.

res judicata—Latin for the thing has been decided.

resource-based relative value scale—the methodology Medicare uses to establish physician fees, based on the relative value unit, the geographic adjustment factor, and the conversion factor.

respect—to hold another in a place of high esteem.

respite care—temporary care provided by an outside party to relieve the usual caregiver.

respondeat superior—Latin for let the master answer.

resume—professional document outlining the educational and job experience of an applicant for a job.

retirement plan—benefit provided by an employer whereby money (either from the employer only or from both the employer and the employee) can be put aside for the employee's eventual retirement.

risk management—identifying possible risks that may cause injury to a patient or employee in a health care setting.

role delineation chart—list created by the AAMA which identifies all clinical, administrative, and general procedures medical assistants are trained for.

route—to direct telephone calls to a particular extension.

rubber stamp signature—rubber stamp image of a person's signature to be used when obtaining the actual signature is not possible.

salaried—employee who is paid a set amount for a period of time regardless of the hours worked.

salutation—greeting that begins a professional letter (Dear _____).

scanners—similar to a copier; capable of taking an exact image of a photo or document and placing it into the computer.

scope of practice—the range of skills a particular health care professional is expected to have and operate within.

secondary diagnoses—conditions, diseases, or reasons for seeking care in addition to the first-listed diagnosis; they may or may not be related to the first-listed diagnosis.

secondary insurance—insurance plan that pays second for a covered patient's services.

section—an organizational division of a chapter that groups together multiple categories; also is one of six major divisions of the CPT manual: evaluation and management; anesthesia; surgery; radiology; pathology and laboratory; medicine.

security envelope—envelope that cannot be seen through.

segregation—to keep two parties apart due to differences, such as race or gender.

self-insurance—type of insurance where rather than purchasing a commercial insurance policy, an employer sets aside a large reserve fund to directly reimburse employees for medical expenses.

semicolon (;)—a punctuation mark in a standalone code; the part of the definition before the semicolon is used by the indented codes that follow.

sentinel event—an event in the health care setting where someone was injured, or could have been injured.

sequelae—an abnormal condition resulting from a previous injury, condition, or disease.

served—with regard to legal cases, being served is to be given notice of an impending lawsuit filed.

service animal—animal that has been trained to assist a person with a handicap.

settled—when an offer of money is extended and accepted in order to drop a legal lawsuit.

sexual harassment—unwanted sexual attention or comments in the workplace.

shaman—religious or spiritual figure.

shingling—process of attaching small pieces of paper to standard-size sheets of paper so the small items are easy to locate in patients' charts.

sign—a physical sign of a condition that can observed or measured by a physician.

sign-in sheet—place where patients sign their name upon entry to the office; may be on paper or electronic.

skilled nursing facility—a licensed facility which primarily provides inpatient, skilled nursing care to patients who require medical, nursing, or rehabilitative services but does not provide the level of care or treatment available in a hospital.

slack time—appointment scheduling method of leaving certain times of day open to accommodate things like patients who call for same-day appointments or physicians who need to catch up on charting.

sliding fee scale—a provider's fee schedule that charges varying fees for a service based on a patient's financial ability to pay.

small claims court—the place to file claims against a debtor who owes a small amount of money; the amount of money varies from one state to another.

SOAP note charting—type of charting that takes into account the patient's subjective and objective findings, the provider's assessment of the patient's condition, and the prescribed plan of action for treatment.

social information—information about a patient's social habits such as tobacco, drug, or alcohol use.

Social Security Act—passed by Congress in 1935 as a means to provide financial security to workers and their families; a process where money is taken from an employee's wages in order to give it back to them after retirement.

solid waste—paper, cans, cups and other garbage from non-clinical areas.

speaker telephone—allows the user to place the caller on a speaker, which permits anyone in the room with the user to hear and be heard by the caller.

special instructions—directions within each section describing specific rules and definitions for use of codes within a particular category or subcategory.

specialist—health care provider who specializes in a particular area, such as a cardiologist (heart) or dermatologist (skin).

speed dial—telephone feature allowing the user to program commonly called numbers into their system; also called an automatic dialer.

spell check—software that comes with most word processing programs enabling the user to verify the correct spelling of many words.

staff model HMO—employs salaried physicians who treat members in facilities owned and operated by the HMO.

standalone code—a CPT code that contains a full description and is not dependent on another code for complete meaning.

standard of care—legal term to describe the type of care a reasonable health care provider is expected to provide under the same situation.

standard precautions—infection control techniques.

standardized—uniform practice.

statute of limitations—time within which a patient has to file a lawsuit after an injury has occurred.

stem cells—cells that are capable of forming into any other cell type.

stereotyping—holding an opinion of another person based solely on something about their group status, such as race, gender, or economic status.

stop loss—the maximum amount the patient must pay out-of-pocket for copayments and coinsurance.

subcategory—a four-digit code in the ICD-9-CM tabular list.

subclassification—a five-digit code in the ICD-9-CM tabular list.

subject line—in a professional letter, this is the subject of the letter.

subpoena—court order demanding someone's appearance in court, or for copies of the medical record to be sent to a third party.

subscriber—same as the member or the insured; a term used to identify the person who holds or owns an insurance policy.

subsection—subdivisions within a CPT section of the tabular index.

subterm—indented two spaces under the boldfaced main term in the ICD-9-CM and further describes the condition in terms of etiology, co-existing conditions, anatomic site, episode, or similar descriptor.

superbill—also called an encounter form or a routing slip. These forms vary from one office to the next and usually contain the procedural and diagnostic codes commonly used in that clinic. A charge slip is generated on each patient coming in for care each day; these are a record of the charges and diagnoses for that patient for that date of service. Usually completed by the health care provider who performed the service.

supporting documentation—copies sent to an insurance company at its request (and with the patient's permission) in order to determine the medical necessity of a requested procedure. Usually consists of medical chart notes, lab reports, operative reports, or pathology reports.

surgical package—refers to all services that are covered under one surgical code.

suspected condition—condition the physician suspects the patient may have.

sympathy—feeling pity for another person.

symptom—indication of a condition reported by the patient that the physician cannot observe or measure.

synonyms—words of equivalent meaning.

tabular index—the numerical listing of all CPT codes, accompanied by guidelines and notes.

tabular list—Volume I of ICD-9-CM, which lists all diagnostic codes in numerical order.

take home pay—the amount of an individual's paycheck after all deductions and taxes are taken out.

tax audits—a function of the IRS where an individual or company's records are reviewed to verify that taxes were paid correctly.

technical educational programs—programs designed to teach skills to students without the need for higher education. Also called vocational programs.

ten-key calculator—calculator, usually electronic, that has the keys from 1 to 0 laid out similar to a telephone key pad.

thesaurus—resource for locating alternate words that have similar meanings.

third-party administrator—a company that processes paperwork for claims for a self-insured employer.

thumb drives—also called flash drives; small-sized external storage devices.

tickler file—reminder method for keeping track of events needing attention in the future.

time clock—piece of equipment where an employee uses a card to have arrival and departure from work times stamped for the purposes of payroll.

tort law—laws that relate to one party injuring another.

tort of outrage—to intentionally inflict emotional upset on another.

tracing claims—process of calling an insurance company when an insurance claim has not been paid in a timely manner.

traditional laws—also known as common law.

training manual—a book that details the type of training needed to use a certain piece of equipment and the date and signature indicating when an individual employee was trained.

transcribe—to listen to a spoken word (usually via tape recording) and type it into a printed document.

transcription machines—machine that allows the user to listen to a tape while typing the words into a printed document.

transdisciplinary duties—general medical assisting duties, such as acting in a professional manner, treating patients with respect, and protecting patient privacy.

transplant—method of removing an organ from a donor and implanting it into a recipient.

traveler's checks—checks that are more secure for use during travel.

treatment regimen—prescribed or recommended plan of treatment made by the health care provider.

triage notebook—notebook kept near the administrative medical assistant responsible for answering incoming telephone calls. The notebook contains questions and steps to follow in the event a caller has a potentially life-threatening condition. The purpose of the notebook is to allow the administrative medical assistant to determine if the patient needs to be seen in the office or referred to emergency medical services.

triaging—process of sorting patients into a priority order based upon their needs.

TRICARE—health insurance administered by the U.S Department of Defense for active duty military personnel, retired service personnel, and their eligible dependents. Formerly known as Civilian Health and Medical Program (CHAMPUS).

ultrasound—method of using sound waves to portray 3-D images.

unbundling—billing multiple services with separate CPT codes and separate charges that should be combined under a single CPT code and one charge.

uncertain—see *qualified*.

uncollectible—account that the clinic does not believe will ever be paid.

undue influence—to persuade someone to do something they do not want to do.

unemployment insurance—insurance that allows employees to be paid unemployment benefits in the event they should lose their job.

unintentional tort—to harm another person accidentally.

upcode—to code and bill for a higher level of service than was actually provided.

urgent care clinics—facilities, such as emergency rooms, that care for patients who have urgent care needs.

user manual—document that describes how something (e.g., equipment) is used.

usual, customary, and reasonable (UCR) fee—a fee determined by third-party payers to reimburse providers based on the provider's normal fee, the range of fees charged by providers of the same specialty in the same geographic area, and other factors to determine appropriate fees in unusual situations.

V codes—used to classify the reason for the visit, other than the disease or illness.

verify—take steps to confirm something, such as a patient's health care coverage.

vocational programs—educational programs designed to teach skills to students without the need for higher education. Also called technical educational programs.

W-2 form—federal form that is given the each employee by January 31st for wages paid in the previous year; this form is sent in by each employee with their federal tax return.

W-4 form—federal form filled out by all employees to indicate their marital status and the number of exemptions they wish to claim for the purpose of federal tax withholding.

wages—amount of money paid to an employee for work performed.

waiting period—period of time after a new health insurance plan begins during which certain services are not covered. Varies from one health plan and policy to another.

waiver—see *advance beneficiary notice*.

warranty—period within which a piece of equipment will be repaired without cost to the buyer.

wave scheduling—scheduling system where patients are scheduled only during the first half of each hour.

with—interpreted as *both, together with* in a diagnostic code description.

withholding allowances—the number of exemptions, such as children, an employee wishes to claim on federal tax forms.

worker's compensation—insurance coverage for job-related illness or injury provided by law by employers for employees. Covers medical expenses, lost wages, and job retraining for injuries received by employees while on the job.

write off—to remove a balance from a patient account.

yoga—a natural therapy that consists of a series of exercises designed to promote control over the body and mind.

References

Books and Manuals

Fisher, Leonard Everett (1980). *The Hospitals*. New York: Holiday House.

Harris, Philip R., and Robert T. Moran (1977). *Managing Cultural Differences*. Houston, TX: Gulf Publishing Co.

Holland, Alex (2000). *Voices of Qi: An Introductory Guide to Traditional Chinese Medicine*. Northwest Institute of Acupuncture and Oriental Medicine. New York: North Atlantic Books.

Maciocia, Giovanni (2005). *The Foundations of Chinese Medicine: A Comprehensive Text for Acupuncturists and Herbalists*. London: Churchill Livingstone.

Porter, R. (1999). *The Greatest Benefit to Mankind: A Medical History of Humanity from Antiquity to the Present*. New York: W.W. Norton and Company.

Vallejo-Manzur, F., et al. (2003). "The resuscitation greats. Andreas Vesalius: The concept of an artificial airway." *Resuscitation* 56:3–7. Tamaulipas, Mexico: Autonomous University of Tamaulipas.

Wells, Susan, PhD (2001). *Out of the Dead House: Nineteenth-Century Women Physicians and the Writing of Medicine*. Madison, WI: University of Wisconsin Press.

Internet-Based References

www.alz.org: Alzheimer's Association

www.alsa.org: The ALS Association

www.amrad.org: Amateur Radio Research and Development Corporation Telecommunications for the Deaf

www.aapc.com: American Academy of Professional Coders

www.aama-ntl.org: American Association of Medical Assistants

www.aamt.org: American Association of Medical Transcription

www.diabetes.org: American Diabetes Association

www.ahima.org: American Health Information Management Association

www.americanheart.org: American Heart Association

www.aha.org/aha_app/index.jsp: American Hospital Association

www.lungusa.org: American Lung Association

www.amt1.com: American Medical Technologists

www.apdaparkinson.org: American Parkinson Disease Association

www.cdc.gov/: Centers for Disease Control and Prevention

www.cms.hhs.gov/: Centers for Medicare and Medicaid Services

www.cebm.net/: Centre for Evidence-Based Medicine

www.cfhi.org: Child Family Health International

www.epicsystems.com: Epic

www.ftc.gov: Federal Trade Commission

www.hpso.com: Health Care Providers Service Organization

http://www.hhs.gov/ocr/hipaa/: Health Insurance Portability and Accountability Act

www.americanhospice.org: Hospice

www.ornl.gov/sci/techresources/Human_Genome/home.shtml: Human Genome Project

www.ingenix.com/: Ingenix

http://www.iom.edu: The Institute of Medicine

www.jointcommission.org/SentinelEvents/: Joint Commission

www.medrecinst.com/: Medical Records Institute

http://nccam.nih.gov/: National Center for Complementary and Alternative Medicine

www.payroll-taxes.com: Payroll-Taxes.com

www.pbs.org/healthcarecrisis/history.htm: PBS's Health Care Crisis: Health Care Timeline

www.powermed.com/: PowerMed

www.citizen.org: Public Citizen

www.shrinershq.org/Hospitals/_Hospitals_for_Children/: Shriner's Hospital for Children

www.skillpath.com: SkillPath Seminars

www.sorryworks.net/: Sorry Works

www.tricare.org/: U.S. Department of Defense Military Health System

www.hhs.gov/ocr/hipaa/: U.S. Department of Health and Human Services

www.usdoj.gov/: U.S. Department of Justice

www.dol.gov: U.S. Department of Labor

www.bls.gov/: U.S. Department of Labor Bureau of Labor Statistics

www.dot.gov: U.S. Department of Transportation (USDOT)

www.nlm.nih.gov/medlineplus: U.S. National Library of Medicine

www.who.org: World Health Organization

Numbers in italics refer to figures; those followed by t refer to tables.